The
Medical &
Health Sciences
Word Book

THIRD EDITION

Compiled by Ann Roe-Hafer

Houghton Mifflin Company

BOSTON   NEW YORK

Library of Congress Cataloging-in-Publication Data

The Medical & health sciences word book/compiled by Ann Roe-Hafer — 3rd ed.
    p.   cm.
1. Medicine — Terminology. 2. Medical sciences — Terminology.
I. Roe-Hafer, Ann II. Title: Medical and health sciences word book.
[DNLM: 1. Nomenclature.   W 15 R699m]
R123.M38, 1992
610'.14 — dc20
DNLM/DLC
for Library of Congress   92-1535
                                                           CIP

ISBN   0-395-60664-0

PRINTED IN THE UNITED STATES

BP 10 9 8 7 6 5 4 3 2

Contents

Executive Editor   Robert B. Costello

Editor for the Third Edition   Ann-Marie Imbornoni

Consultants

How to Use This Book

The Medical & Health Sciences Word Book, Third Edition, has been revised in order to continue providing the most accurate information on the spelling of the terms currently being used in medicine, nursing, and other health sciences. You will find, listed in alphabetical order, over 64,000 such terms that have been divided into syllables and given stress marks to indicate pronunciation according to the same morphological and phonetic criteria applied in *The American Heritage Dictionary, Third Edition.*

The sources of technical terms in *The Medical & Health Sciences Word Book, Third Edition,* were many: the latest and most comprehensive medical dictionaries and technical and professional journals, the *Index Medicus,* and additional items supplied by citation readers and medical and nursing consultants. This ensures that the vocabulary selected for inclusion in the list is as comprehensive and up-to-date as possible.

Words in common usage have been omitted unless they have technical senses; obsolete terms have been eliminated. Proper nouns have been entered only when they form part of a phrase or other compound in the scientific lexicon. Additional words that may be formed with such suffixes as *-ly* and *-ment* have as a general rule been omitted from the list unless the suffixed form is distinct in meaning from the base form.

The Medical & Health Sciences Word Book, Third Edition, has a number of useful features, including a list of abbreviations; a list of trade names of drugs; a table of elements; a table of Latin and Greek terms used in prescriptions; a list of medical signs and symbols; a table of weights and measures; tables for converting apothecary weights and measures into the metric system; and a table of thermometric equivalents. Also included is a chart of the plurals of Latin and Greek nouns and a special table of sound-spelling correspondences to aid in locating words whose pronunciation is known but whose spelling may present difficulties.

The following guide to the book will enable you to make the maximum use of its special features.

ORDER OF ENTRIES

The entries are listed in strict alphabetical order. Therefore, open compounds and phrases of two or more words are alphabetized as if the letters formed one word:

> Ab'be-Est'lan·der operation
> Ab'be lip flap
> Ab'be-Zeiss' cell

Series of multiword phrases sharing a common first element are listed under the key word in the following style:

cal'ci•no'sis
—cu'tis cir'cum•scrip'ta
—cutis u'ni•ver•sa'lis

In such a series the dash functions as a ditto mark, indicating that the key word (in this case *calcinosis*) is repeated in each subsequent phrase: *calcinosis cutis circumscripta* and *calcinosis cutis universalis.*

DIVISION OF WORDS

The Medical & Health Sciences Word Book, Third Edition, shows how words may be divided correctly into syllables. With the exception of a few foreign words, and in particular foreign proper names, all words have been syllabicated according to English phonetic criteria. Divisions are shown by means of a centered dot, a stress mark, or a hyphen:

ab•dom'i•nal   mel'a•no•cyte'   a•ba'si•a-a•sta'si•a

All standard syllable divisions are shown, even where end-of-line division is not normally recommended. Therefore, although a word may with justification be broken at the end of a line of type wherever a syllable division is indicated, hyphenation restrictions such as those presented in style manuals should be followed wherever adherence to standard printing practice is desired. The following two rules are typical:

1. A syllable consisting of a single letter should not be separated from the rest of the word. Thus, at the end of a line *a•ba'sic* should be divided *aba-sic,* not *a-basic.*

2. A hyphenated word should be divided only at the hyphen.

STRESS

This book indicates which syllables are stressed when a word is pronounced. Two different marks are used. The first, a boldface stress, indicates the syllable that receives the primary stress in the word:

fol'li•cle   mal'a•dy

Normally only one syllable in a word receives primary stress. However, certain compound words may have more than one primary stress:

Fried′rich-Bau′er operation   third′-de·gree′ burn

The second mark, a lighter stress, indicates syllables that are pronounced with less stress than those marked with a primary stress but with stronger stress than unmarked syllables:

ab′em·bry·on′ic   de′cu·ba′tion

INFLECTED FORMS

Inflected forms are given for every entry word exhibiting any irregularity or stress or spelling changes in the inflected forms. These forms include the singulars of nouns (labeled *sing.,* where the plural is the main-entry form) and the plurals of nouns (labeled *pl.*) whenever they are not formed simply by adding -*s* or -*es* to the base form. Other forms given are the third person singular past tense and the past participle and the present participle of verbs whenever they are not formed simply by adding -*ed* or -*ing* to the base form. Such forms have been shortened to save space unless a shift in stress pattern or pronunciation necessitates showing the full form.

ac′e·tab′u·lum *pl.* -lums *or* -la   a·buse′, a·bused′, a·bus′ing
da′ta *sing.* -tum   bite, bit, bit′ten *or* bit, bit′ing
pal·mar′is *pl.* -mar′es′   freeze, froze, fro′zen, freez′ing

In these examples you will notice that verbs may have either two or three inflected forms. If only two forms are shown, the first is both the past tense and the past participle (e.g., *abused*), and the second is the present participle (e.g., *abusing*). If three forms are shown, the first is the past tense (e.g., *froze*), the second is the past participle (e.g., *frozen*) and the third is the present participle (e.g., *freezing*).

Alternate inflected forms are also shown, as the alternate plurals -*lums* and -*la* for *acetabulum* and the alternate past participles *bitten* and *bit* for *bite*.

VARIANTS

A variant is a form of a word that is spelled or pronounced differently from the main form of that word. Variants are included whenever they are in common use in the technical vocabulary. With the exceptions specified below, they are entered separately, even if the main form and the variant are directly adjacent in the alphabetical listing. Inflected forms are given when necessary.

ce·sar′e·an   *also* caesarean
cae·sar′e·an   *var. of* cesarean

a·moe′bu·la *pl.* -las *or* -lae′, *also* amebula
a·me′bu·la *pl.* -las *or* lae′, *var. of* amoebula
em·bed′, -bed′ded, -bed′ding, *also* imbed
im·bed′, -bed′ded, -bed′ding, *var. of* embed

In the case of long lists of spelling variants beginning with a very produc-
tive prefix or combining form (e.g., *haem-, haema-, haemat-, haemato-,* and
haemo-), variants have not been entered separately, but notes are provided to
direct the user to the entries beginning with the main form of the prefix or
combining form:

haem-. See words spelled *hem-.*

Similarly, compound words consisting of a variant spelling of a word
plus another element have not been entered. Thus while both *meter* and *metre*
are included, the entries for such words as *decameter* and *kilometer* do not
show the variants *decametre* and *kilometre.*

WORDS LIKELY TO BE CONFUSED

In *The Medical & Health Sciences Word Book, Third Edition,* short identifying
definitions, or glosses, and cross-references are given for pairs or sets of
words that are likely to be confused. Such words fall into two categories:

1. Homophones, or words that are pronounced precisely the same but are
spelled differently.

il′e·ac′ *(pertaining to the ileum)*
♦ *iliac*

il′i·ac′ *(pertaining to the ilium)*
♦ *ileac*

2. Words that are likely to be confused because they are similar in spelling or pronunciation.

ab·sorb′ *(to take in)*
♦ *adsorb*

ad·sorb′ *(to hold on a surface)*
♦ *absorb*

The glosses provided are not to be regarded as full definitions. They
merely serve to point out possible sources of confusion. A dictionary should
be consulted for more detailed and precise definitions.

PREFIXATION

Many terms beginning with such prefixes as *anti-* (e.g., *antifungal*),
counter- (e.g., *countertransference*), and the like have been included in this
book, but it is impossible to enter all such words. However, the guiding prin-

ciple in hyphenation is that hyphens should be used only when necessary for clarity, that is, as a means of avoiding ambiguity.

1. Always use a hyphen between a prefix and a word beginning with a capital letter (e.g., *anti-Semite*).

2. Use a hyphen when not doing so would create an awkward combination of letters, particularly of vowels (e.g., *contra-angles, pre-exitation, pseudo-oedema*).

3. Use a hyphen after a prefix when the unhyphenated form and the hyphenated form differ in meaning (e.g., *coop* and *co-op*).

The following is a list of the most commonly used prefixes.

ante-	inter-	post-	super-
anti-	intra-	pre-	trans-
bi-	micro-	pro-	tri-
co-	mid-	pseudo-	ultra-
contra-	non-	re-	un-
counter-	out-	semi-	
de-	over-	sub-	

Compounds with these prefixes are usually formed according to rules 1, 2, and 3 mentioned previously. Compounds with the prefixes *all-* and *self-* are always formed with a hyphen.

LATIN AND GREEK PLURALS

Nouns in Latin and Greek are classified according to gender and declension, both of which determine the proper endings in the plural. Therefore, the formation of the plurals of Latin and Greek nouns in the medical vocabulary cannot be reduced to a set of simple rules. However, it is almost always acceptable to pluralize these forms just as English nouns are pluralized. In fact, in most cases the English and foreign plurals exist side by side and are used with about the same frequency.

The chart below provides a typical—but not exhaustive—list of plural endings for Latin and Greek words; while it can be used for guidance, it should be borne in mind that there are exceptions to the rules.

Singular	Plural	
-a	-ae	abscissa, abscissae
-ax	-aces	thorax, thoraces

Singular	Plural	
-en	-ina	flumen, flumina
-er	-era	tuber, tubera
-ex	-ices	apex, apices
-is	-es	analysis, analyses
	-ides	cnemis, cnemides
-ix	-ices	appendix, appendices
-oma	-omata	adenoma, adenomata
-on	-a	phenomenon, phenomena
-os	-i	omphalos, omphali
-u	-ua	cornu, cornua
-um	-a	serum, sera
-ur	-ora	femur, femora
-us	-udes	incus, incudes
	-era	genus, genera
	-i	alveolus, alveoli
	-ora	corpus, corpora
-x	-ces	calx, calces
	-ges	meninx, meninges

A

a'bac·te'ri·al
A'ba·die' sign
ab·ap'i·cal
a'bap·tis'ton'
a·bar'og·no'sis *pl.* -ses'
ab·ar'tic'u·lar
ab·ar'tic'u·la'tion
a·ba'si·a
—trep'i·dans'
a·ba'si·a-a·sta'si·a
a·ba'sic
a·bate', a·bat'ed, a·bat'ing
a·bate'ment
a·bat'ic
ab·ax'i·al
Ab'be-Est'lan·der opera-
tion
Ab'be lip flap
Ab'be-Zeiss' cell
Ab'bott
—method
Ab'bott-Lu'cas approach
Ab'der·hal'den-
Kauf'mann-Lig'nac
syndrome
Ab'der·hal'den reaction
ab'do·men *pl.* -mens *or*
ab·dom'i·na
ab·dom'i·nal
ab·dom'i·no·an·te'ri·or
ab·dom'i·no·car'di·ac'
ab·dom'i·no·cen·te'sis
pl. -ses'
ab·dom'i·no·hys'ter·ec'-
to·my
ab·dom'i·no·hys'ter·
ot'o·my
ab·dom'i·no·jug'u·lar
ab·dom'i·no·pel'vic
ab·dom'i·no·per'i·ne'al
ab·dom'i·no·plas'ty
ab·dom'i·no·pos·te'ri·or
ab·dom'i·nos·co·py
ab·dom'i·no·scro'tal
ab·dom'i·no·tho·rac'ic
ab·dom'i·nous
ab·dom'i·no·u'ter·ot'o·my
ab·dom'i·no·vag'i·nal
ab·dom'i·no·ves'i·cal
ab·duce'

ab·du'cens *pl.* ab'du·cen'tes'
ab·du'cent
ab·duct'
ab·duc'tion
ab·duc'tor *(a muscle that draws
a part away from the axis of the
body or an extremity)*
♦*adductor*
ab'em·bry·on'ic
ab'en·ter'ic
Ab'er·crom'bie degenera-
tion
Ab'er·ne'thy sarcoma
ab·er'ran·cy
ab·er'rant
ab·er'rant·ly
ab'er·ra'tion
a·bet', a·bet'ted, a·bet'ting
a·be'ta·lip'o·pro'tein·e'mi·a
a·bey'ance
ab'i·ence
ab'i·et'ic
A bile
a'bi·o·gen'e·sis *pl.* -ses'
a'bi·o·ge·net'ic
a'bi·og'e·nous
a'bi·on'er·gy
a'bi·o'sis *pl.* -ses'
a'bi·ot'ic
a'bi·o·troph'ic
a'bi·ot'ro·phy
ab·ir'ri·tant
ab·ir'ri·tate', -tat'ed, -tat'ing
ab·ir'ri·ta'tion
ab'lac·ta'tion
a'blas·te'mic
a·blas'tin
ab·late', -lat'ed, -lat'ing
ab·la'ti·o pla·cen'tae'
ab·la'tion
ab·la'tive
a'ble·phar'i·a
a·bleph'a·ron'
a·blep'si·a
ab'lu·ent
ab·lu'tion
ab·mor'tal
ab·ner'val
ab·neu'ral
ab·nor'mal
ab'nor·mal'i·ty
ABO blood group

ab'o·ma·si'tis
ab'o·ma'sum *pl.* -sa
ab·o'rad'
ab·o'ral
a·bort'
a·bort'er
a·bor'ti·cide'
a·bor'tient
a·bor'ti·fa'cient
a·bor'tin
a·bor'tion
a·bor'tion·ist
a·bor'tive
a·bor'tus *pl.* -tus·es
a·bra'chi·a
a·bra'chi·o·ce·pha'li·a
a·bra'chi·o·ceph'a·lus
a·bra'chi·us
a·brad'ant
a·brade', a·brad'ed,
a·brad'ing
a·brad'er
A'brams test
a·bra'si·o cor'ne·ae'
a·bra'sion
a·bra'sive
a·bra'sor
ab're·act'
ab're·ac'tion
Ab'ri·kos'ov tumor *var. of*
Abrikossoff
Ab'ri·kos'soff tumor *also*
Abrikosov
a·bro'si·a
a·brup'tion
ab·rup'ti·o' pla·cen'tae'
a'brus
ab'scess'
ab·sces'sus
—flat'u·o'sus
—per de·cu'bi·tum
ab·scis'sa *pl.* -sas *or* -sae'
ab·scis'sion
ab·scon'si·o'
ab·sco'pal
ab'sence
ab·sen'te' fe'bre'
ab·sen'ti·a ep'i·lep'ti·ca
ab'sinthe
ab'sin'thism
ab·sin'thi·um
ab·sin·thol'

ab'so·lute'
ab·sorb' (*to take in*)
   ♦adsorb
ab·sorb'a·ble
ab·sorb'ance
ab·sor'be·fa'cient
ab·sorb'en·cy
ab·sorb'ent
ab·sorb'er
ab·sorp'ti·om'e·ter
ab·sorp'ti·om'e·try
ab·sorp'tion
ab·sorp'tive
ab'sorp·tiv'i·ty
ab·ster'gent
ab'sti·nence
ab'stract
ab·strac'tion
ab·trop'fung
a·bu'li·a
a·bu'lic
a·bu'lo·ma'ni·a
a·buse', a·bused', a·bus'ing
a·but', a·but'ted, a·but'ting
a·but'ment
a·ca'cia
a'cal·ci·co'sis
a'cal·cu'li·a
a'cal·cu·lous
a·camp'si·a
a·can'tha
a·can'tha·moe·bi'a·sis *pl.*
  -ses'
a·can'thes·the'si·a
a·can'thi·on'
a·can'tho·am'e·lo·blas·
  to'ma *pl.* -mas *or* -ma·ta
A·can'tho·ceph'a·la
a·can'tho·ceph'a·li'a·sis
  pl. -ses'
A·can'tho·chei'lo·ne'ma
  —per'stans'
a·can'tho·chei'lo·ne·mi'-
  a·sis *pl.* -ses'
a·can'tho·cyte'
a·can'tho·cy·to'sis *pl.* -ses'
a·can'thoid'
a·can'tho·ker'a·to·der'mi·a
a·can'tho·ker'a·to'ma
  pl. -mas *or* -ma·ta
ac'an·thol'y·sis *pl.* -ses'
  —bul·lo'sa
a·can'tho·lyt'ic

ac'an·tho'ma *pl.* -mas *or*
  -ma·ta
  —ad'e·noi'des'
  —cys'ti·cum
ac'an·tho'ma·tous
a·can'tho·pel'vis
a·can'tho·pel'yx
a·can'thor·rhex'is
ac'an·tho'sis *pl.* -ses'
  —ni'gri·cans'
ac'an·thot'ic
a·cap'ni·a
a·cap'ni·al
a·cap'nic
a·cap'su·lar
a·car'bi·a
a·car'di·a
a·car'di·ac'
a'car·di·a'cus
  —a·ceph'a·lus
  —a·mor'phus
  —an'ceps'
a·car'di·o·he'mi·a
a·car'di·o·ner'vi·a
a·car'di·us
a·car'i·an
ac'a·ri'a·sis *pl.* -ses'
a·car'i·cid'al
a·car'i·cide'
ac'a·rid
A·car'i·dae'
a·car'i·dan
a·car'i·di·a'sis *pl.* -ses'
Ac'a·ri'na
ac'a·ri·no'sis *pl.* -ses'
ac'a·ro·der'ma·ti'tis
  —ur'ti·car'i·oi'des'
ac'a·roid'
ac'a·rol'o·gist
ac'a·rol'o·gy
ac'a·ro·pho'bi·a
ac'a·ro·tox'ic
ac'a·rus *pl.* -ri'
Ac'a·rus
  —fol·lic'u·lo'rum
  —sca·bi·e'i'
a·car'y·ote'
a·cat'a·la'si·a
a·cat'a·lep'si·a
a·cat'a·lep'sy
a·cat'a·lep'tic
a·cat'a·ma·the'si·a
a·cat'a·pha'si·a

ac'a·ta·sta'si·a
ac'a·ta·stat'ic
ac'a·thex'i·a
ac'a·thex'is
ac'a·this'i·a *var. of* akathisia
a·cau'dal
a·cau'date'
ac·cel'er·ant
ac·cel'er·ate', -at'ed, -at'ing
ac·cel'er·a'tion
ac·cel'er·a'tor
ac·cel'er·in
ac·cel'er·om'e·ter
ac·cen'tu·a'tion
ac·cen'tu·a'tor
ac·cep'tor
ac·ces'sion
ac·ces·so'ri·us
  —ad flex'o'rem dig'i·to'rum
    pro·fun'dum
ac·ces'so'ry
ac'ci·dent
ac'ci·den'tal
ac'ci·dent-prone'
ac·cip'i·ter
ac'cli·mate', -mat'ed,
  -mat'ing
ac·cli'ma'tion
ac·cli'ma·ti·za'tion
ac·cli'ma·tize', -tized',
  -tiz'ing
ac·cliv'i·ty
ac·com'mo·date', -dat'ed,
  -dat'ing
ac·com'mo·da'tion
ac·com'mo·da'tive
ac·couche·ment'
  —for·cé'
ac·cou·cheur'
ac·cou·cheuse'
ac·cre·men·ti'tion
ac·crete', -cret'ed, -cret'ing
ac·cre'ti·o'
ac·cre'tion
Ac'cu-Chek' system
ac·cu'mu·la'tion
ac·cu'mu·la'tor
ac'e·bu'to·lol'
a·cec'li·dine'
ac'e·dap'sone'
a·cel'lu·lar
a·ce'lo·mate'
a·ce'lous

a·ce′nes·the′si·a
a·ce′no·cou·ma·rol′
a·cen′tric
a′ce·pha′li·a
a′ce·phal′ic
a·ceph′a·lism
a·ceph′a·lo·bra′chi·a
a·ceph′a·lo·bra′chi·us
a·ceph′a·lo·car′di·a
a·ceph′a·lo·car′di·us
a·ceph′a·lo·chi′ri·a
a·ceph′a·lo·chi′rus
a·ceph′a·lo·cyst′
a·ceph′a·lo·gas′ter
a·ceph′a·lo·gas·te′ri·a
a·ceph′a·lo·po′di·a
a·ceph′a·lo·po′di·us
a·ceph′a·lor·rha′chi·a
a·ceph′a·lo·sto′mi·a
a·ceph′a·los′to·mus
a·ceph′a·lo·tho·ra·ci·a
a·ceph′a·lo·tho′rax′
a·ceph′a·lous
a·ceph′a·lus
—a·car′di·us
—a·tho′rus
—di·bra′chi·us
—di′pus
—mon′o·bra′chi·us
—mon′o·pus′
—pseu′do·a·cor′mus
—sym′pus
—tho′rus
a·ceph′a·ly
ac′er·ate′
a·cer′bi·ty
ac′er·in
a·cer′vu·line′
a·cer′vu·lus
a·ces′cence
a·ces′cent
a·ces′o·dyne′
ac′e·tab′u·lar
ac′e·tab′u·lec′to·my
ac′e·tab′u·lo·plas′ty
ac′e·tab′u·lum *pl.* -lums *or*
  -la
ac′e·tal′
ac′et·al′de·hyde′
a·cet′a·mide′
a·cet′a·min′o·phen
ac′et·an′i·lid
ac′et·ar′sone′

ac′e·tan′nin
ac′e·tate′
ac′et·a·zol′a·mide′
ac′et·di·mer·sul·fon′a·
  mide′
Ac′e·test′
a·ce′tic
a·ce′ti·fi·ca′tion
a·ce′ti·fy′, -fied′, -fy′ing
ac′e·tim′e·ter
ac′e·tin
ac′e·to·a·ce′tic
ac′e·to·a·ce′tyl-CoA
A·ce′to·bac′ter
ac′e·to·hex′a·mide′
a·cet′o·in
ac′e·to·ki′nase
ac′e·tol′
ac′e·tol′y·sis *pl.* -ses′
ac′e·to·me·naph′thone′
ac′e·to·mor′phine′
ac′e·tone′
ac′e·to·ne′mi·a
ac′e·to·ne′mic
ac′e·to·ni′trile
ac′e·to·nu′ri·a
ac′e·to·phen′a·zine′
ac′e·to·phe·net′i·din
a·ce′to·sal′
ac′e·to·sul′fone′
ac′e·tous
ac′et·phe′no·li′sa·tin
ac′e·tract′
ac′e·tri·zo′ate′
ac′e·tri·zo′ic
a·ce′tum *pl.* -ta
a·cet′u·rate′
ac′e·tu′ric
ac′e·tyl·a·ce′tic
ac′e·tyl·a·den′y·late′
ac′e·tyl·am′i·no·ben′zine′
ac′e·tyl·am′i·no·fluor′ene′
ac′e·tyl·an′i·line
a·cet′y·lase′
a·cet′y·la′tion
a·cet′y·la′tor
ac′e·tyl-be′ta-
  meth′yl·cho′line′
ac′e·tyl·car·bro′mal
ac′e·tyl·cho′line′
ac′e·tyl·cho′lin·es′ter·ase′
ac′e·tyl-CoA
ac′e·tyl·co·en′zyme′ A

ac′e·tyl·cys′te·ine′
ac′e·tyl·dig′i·tox′in
a·cet′y·lene′
ac′e·tyl·hex′os·a·min′i·
  dase′
a·cet′y·lide′
a·ce′tyl·sa·lic′y·late′
a·ce′tyl·sal′i·cyl′ic
ac′e·tyl·stro·phan′thi·din
ac′e·tyl·sul′fa·di′a·zine′
ac′e·tyl·sul′fa·gua′ni·dine′
ac′e·tyl·sul′fa·thi′a·zole′
ac′e·tyl·sul′fon′a·mide′
ac′e·tyl·trans′fer·ase′
ach′a·la′si·a
A·chard′-Cas·taigne′
—method
—test
A·chard′-Thiers′
  syndrome
ache, ached, ach′ing
a·chei′li·a
a·chei′lous
a·chei′lus
a·chei′ri·a *also* achiria
a·chei′ro·po′di·a
a·chei′rus *also* achirus
A·chil′les
—bursa
—jerk
—reflex
—tendon
a·chil′lo·bur·si′tis
a·chil′lo·dyn′i·a
ach′il·lor′rha·phy
a·chil′lo·te·not′o·my
ach′il·lot′o·my
a·chi′ri·a *var. of* acheiria
a·chi′rus *var. of* acheirus
a′chlor·hy′dri·a
a′chlor·hy′dric
a·chlor·op′si·a
a·chlu′o·pho′bi·a
a·cho′li·a
a·chol′ic
a′cho·lu′ri·a
a′cho·lu′ric
a·chon′dro·gen′e·sis
a·chon′dro·pla′si·a
a·chon′dro·plas′tic
a′chor′
a·chor′dal
A·cho′ri·on′

A'chor-Smith' syndrome
a·chre'o·cy·the'mi·a
a·chres'tic
a·chro'a·cyte'
a·chro'a·cy·to'sis *pl.* -ses'
a·chroi'o·cy·the'mi·a
a·chro'ma
a·chro'ma·cyte'
ach'ro·ma·si·a
ach'ro·mat'
ach'ro·mat'ic
a·chro'ma·tin
a·chro'ma·tin'ic
a·chro'ma·tism
a'chro·mat'o·cyte'
a·chro'ma·tol'y·sis *pl.* -ses'
a'chro·mat'o·phil
a·chro'ma·to·phil'i·a
a·chro'ma·top'si·a
a·chro'ma·to'sis *pl.* -ses'
a·chro'ma·tous
a·chro'ma·tu'ri·a
a·chro'mi·a
  —cu'tis
  —par'a·sit'i·ca
a·chro'mic
a·chro'mo·cyte'
a·chro'mo·der'ma
a·chro'mo·phil
a·chro'mo·trich'i·a
a·chro'o·am'y·loid'
a·chro'o·cy·to'sis *pl.* -ses'
a·chro'o·dex'trin
A'chu·cár'ro stain
ach'y
a·chy'la·ne'mi·a
a·chy'li·a
  —gas'tri·ca
  —pan'cre·at'i·ca
a·chy'lic
a·chy'lous
a·chy'mi·a
a·cic'u·lar
ac'id
ac'id·am'i·nu'ri·a
ac'i·de'mi·a
ac'id-fast'
a·cid'ic
a·cid'i·fi'a·ble
a·cid'i·fi·ca'tion
a·cid'i·fi'er
a·cid'i·fy', -fied', -fy'ing
ac'i·dim'e·ter

ac'i·dim'e·try
ac'id·ism
a·cid'i·ty
a·cid'o·cyte'
ac'i·do·cy'to·pe'ni·a
ac'i·do·cy·to'sis *pl.* -ses'
ac'i·do·gen'ic
a·cid'o·phil'
ac'i·do·phil'i·a
ac'i·do·phil'ic
ac'i·doph'i·lism
ac'i·doph'i·lous
ac'i·do'sis *pl.* -ses'
ac'i·dos'te·o·phyte'
ac'i·dot'ic
ac'id-re·sis'tant
a·cid'u·lant
a·cid'u·late', -lat'ed, -lat'ing
a·cid'u·lous
ac'i·du'ri·a
ac'i·du'ric
ac'id·yl
a·cid'y·lat'ed
ac'i·nar
ac'i·ne'si·a
Ac'i·net'o·bac'ter lwof'fi
a·cin'ic
a·cin'i·form'
ac'i·ni'tis
ac'i·nose'
ac'i·no·tu'bu·lar
ac'i·nous
a-c interval
ac'i·nus *pl.* -ni'
a·clac'i·no·my'cin
a·clad'i·o'sis *pl.* -ses'
a'cla·ru'bi·cin
ac'la·sis *pl.* -ses'
a·clas'tic
a·cleis'to·car'di·a
a·clu'sion
ac'me
ac'mes·the'si·a
ac'mic
ac'ne
  —ag'mi·na'ta
  —al'bi·da
  —ar'ti·fi'ci·a'lis
  —a·troph'i·ca
  —ca·chec'ti·co'rum
  —co·ag'mi·na'ta
  —con·glo'ba·ta
  —cys'ti·ca

  —de·cal'vans'
  —in'du·ra'ta
  —ker·a'to·sa
  —me·chan'i·ca
  —med'i·ca·men·to'sa
  —mil'i·ar'is
  —ne·crot'i·ca
  —ne'o·na·to'rum
  —pan'cre·at'i·ca
  —pap'u·lo'sa
  —pus'tu·lo'sa
  —ro·sa'ce·a
  —scrof'u·lo·so'rum
  —tar'si'
  —trop'i·ca
  —ur'ti·ca'ta
  —var'i·o'li·for'mis
  —vul'gar·is
ac'ne·form' *var. of* acneiform
ac'ne·gen
ac'ne·gen'ic
ac·ne'i·form' *also* acneform
ac·ne'mi·a
ac·ni'tis
ac'o·can'ther·in
a·coe'li·a
ac'o·kan'ther·a
ac'o·la'si·a
ac'o·las'tic
a·co'lous
a·con'a·tive
ac'o·nine'
a·con'i·tase'
ac'o·nit'ic
a·con'i·tin
a·con'i·tine'
a·con'u·re'sis
a'cop·ro'sis *pl.* -ses'
a·cop'rous
a'cor'
ac'o·re'a *(absence of the pupil)*
  ♦acoria
a·co'ri·a *(absence of the feeling of satiety), also* akoria
  ♦acorea
a·cor'mus
A·cos'ta disease
a·cou'es·the'si·a *also* acuesthesia
a·cou'me·ter
ac'ou·met'ric
a·cou'o·pho'ni·a
a·cous'ma *pl.* -mas *or* -ma·ta

a·cous'ma·tag·no'sis
a·cous'ma·tam·ne'si·a
a·cous'tic
a·cous'ti·cal
a·cous'ti·co·fa'cial
a·cous'ti·co·mo'tor
a·cous'ti·co·pal'pe·bral
a·cous'ti·co·pho'bi·a
a·cous'tics
a·cous'ti·gram'
ac·quired'
ac'qui·si'tion
ac'ral
a·cra'ni·a
a·cra'ni·al
a·cra'ni·us
a·cra'si·a *(intemperance)*
  ♦acratia
a·cra'ti·a *(impotence)*
  ♦acrasia
a·crat'u·re'sis
Ac'ree-Ro'sen·heim' test
Ac'rel ganglion
ac're·mo'ni·o'sis *pl.* -ses'
ac'rid
ac'ri·dine'
ac'ri·fla'vine'
ac'ri·mo'ny
ac'ri·sor'cin
a·crit'i·cal
ac'ri·to·chro'ma·cy
ac'ro·ag·no'sis
ac'ro·an'es·the'si·a
ac'ro·ar·thri'tis
ac'ro·a·tax'i·a
ac'ro·blast'
ac'ro·brach'y·ceph'a·ly
ac'ro·bys·ti'tis
ac'ro·cen'tric
ac'ro·ce·pha'li·a
ac'ro·ce·phal'ic
ac'ro·ceph'a·lo·pol'y·syn·dac'ty·ly
ac'ro·ceph'a·lo·syn·dac'tyl'i·a
ac'ro·ceph'a·lo·syn·dac'-ty·lism
ac'ro·ceph'a·lo·syn·dac'-ty·ly
ac'ro·ceph'a·ly
ac'ro·chor·do'ma *pl.* -mas *or* -ma·ta
ac'ro·chor'don'

ac'ro·ci·ne'si·a
ac'ro·ci·ne'sis
ac'ro·con·trac'ture
ac'ro·cy'a·no'sis *pl.* -ses'
ac'ro·cy'a·not'ic
ac'ro·der·ma·ti'tis
  —chron'i·ca a·troph'i·cans'
  —con·tin'u·a
  —en'ter·o·path'i·ca
  —hi'e·ma'lis
  —pus·tu·lo'sa per'stans'
ac'ro·der·ma·to'sis *pl.* -ses'
ac'ro·dol'i·cho·me'li·a
ac'ro·dyn'i·a
ac'ro·es·the'si·a
ac'ro·ge'ri·a
ac'rog·no'sis
ac'ro·hy'per·hi·dro'sis
ac'ro·hy'po·ther'mi·a
ac'ro·hy'po·ther'my
ac'ro·ker'a·to'sis *pl.* -ses'
  —ver·ru'ci·for'mis
ac'ro·ki·ne'si·a
ac'ro·ki·ne'sis
a·cro'le·in
ac'ro·mac'ri·a
ac'ro·mas·ti'tis
ac'ro·me·ga'li·a
ac'ro·me·gal'ic
ac'ro·meg'a·loid'
ac'ro·meg'a·loid·ism
ac'ro·meg'a·ly
ac'ro·me·lal'gi·a
ac'ro·mere'
ac'ro·met'a·gen'e·sis
  pl. -ses'
a·cro'mi·al
a·cro'mi·a'le os sec'on·dar'i·um
ac'ro·mic'ri·a
a·cro'mi·o·cla·vic'u·lar
a·cro'mi·o·cor'a·coid'
a·cro'mi·o·hu'mer·al
a·cro'mi·on'
a·cro'mi·o·nec'to·my
a·cro'mi·o·plas'ty
a·cro'mi·o·scap'u·lar
a·cro'mi·o·tho·rac'ic
a·crom'pha·lus
ac'ro·my'o·to'ni·a
ac'ro·my·ot'o·nus
ac'ro·nar·cot'ic
ac'ro·neu·rop'a·thy

ac'ro·neu·ro'sis *pl.* -ses'
ac'ro·nine'
a·cron'y·chous
ac'ro·nyx'
ac'ro·os·te·ol'y·sis
ac'ro·pach'y
ac'ro·pach'y·der'ma
ac'ro·pa·ral'y·sis *pl.* -ses'
ac'ro·par'es·the'si·a
ac'ro·pa·thol'o·gy
a·crop'a·thy
a·crop'e·tal
ac'ro·pho'bi·a
ac'ro·pig'men·ta'tion
ac'ro·pig'men·ta'ti·o'
  re·tic'u·lar'is
ac'ro·pos·thi'tis
ac'ro·pur'pu·ra
ac'ro·scle·ro·der'ma
ac'ro·scle·ro'sis *pl.* -ses'
ac'ro·so'mal
ac'ro·some'
ac'ro·sphe'no·syn·dac·tyl'i·a
ac'ros·te·al'gi·a
ac'ro·te'ri·a
ac'ro·ter'ic
a·crot'ic
ac'ro·tism
ac'ro·tro'pho·neu·ro'sis
ac'ryl·al'de·hyde'
a·cryl'ate'
a·cryl'ic
ac'ry·lo·ni'trile'
ac'tin
ac·tin'ic
ac·tin'i·form'
ac'ti·nism
ac·tin'i·um
ac·ti·no·bac'il·lo'sis *pl.* -ses'
Ac·ti·no·ba·cil'lus
  —lig'ni·er·es'i·i'
  —mal'le·i'
ac'ti·no·chem'is·try
ac'ti·no·der·ma·ti'tis
ac·tin'o·gen
ac'ti·no·gen'e·sis *pl.* -ses'
ac'ti·no·gen'ic
ac'ti·no·gen'ics
ac·tin'o·graph'
ac·tin'o·lite' *var. of* actinolyte
ac·tin'o·lyte' *also* actinolite
ac'ti·nom'e·ter

ac'ti·nom'e·try
ac'ti·no·my·ce'li·al
Ac·ti·no·my'ces'
—bo'vis
—is·ra·e'li·i'
—naes·lun'di·i'
Ac·ti·no·my'ce·ta'ce·ae'
Ac·ti·no·my'ce·ta'les'
ac'ti·no·my'cete'
ac'ti·no·my·ce'tic
ac'ti·no·my·ce'tin
ac'ti·no·my'cin
ac'ti·no·my·co'ma *pl.* -mas
   or -ma·ta
ac'ti·no·my·co'sis *pl.* -ses'
ac'ti·no·my·cot'ic
ac'ti·no·my'co·tin
ac'ti·non'
ac'ti·no·neu·ri'tis
ac'ti·no·phy·to'sis *pl.* -ses'
ac'ti·no·rho'dine'
ac'ti·no·ru'bin
ac'ti·no·spec'to·cin
ac'ti·no·ther'a·py
ac'ti·vase'
ac'ti·vate', -vat'ed, -vat'ing
ac'ti·va'tion
ac'ti·va'tor
ac'tive
ac·tiv'i·ty
ac·tom'e·ter
ac'to·my'o·sin
a·cu·es·the'si·a *var. of*
   acouesthesia
a·cu'i·ty
ac'u·la'li·a
a·cu'le·ate'
a·cu'me·ter
a·cu'mi·nate'
ac'u·pres'sure
ac'u·punc'ture
a'cus
ac'u·sec'tion
ac'u·sec'tor
Ac'u·son' sonography
a·cus'ti·cus
a·cute'
a·cu'ti·cos'tal
ac'u·tor'sion
a·cy'a·no·blep'si·a
a·cy'a·nop'si·a
a·cy'a·not'ic
a·cy'cli·a

a·cy'clic
a·cy'clo·gua'no·sine'
a·cy'clo·vir'
ac'y·e'sis
ac'y·et'ic
ac'yl
ac'y·lase'
ac'yl·a'tion
ac'yl·trans'fer·ase'
a·cys'ti·a
a·cys'ti·ner'vi·a
a·cys'ti·nu'ri·a
a·dac'ry·a
a·dac'tyl
a·dac'tyl'i·a
a·dac'tyl·ism
a·dac'ty·lous *(lacking fingers or
   toes)*
   ♦adactylus
a·dac'ty·lus *(individual with
   congenital absence of fingers or
   toes)*
   ♦adactylous
a·dac'ty·ly
A·dair'-Digh'ton syndrome
ad'a·man'tine'
ad'a·man'ti·no·car'ci·
   no'ma *pl.* -mas *or* -ma·ta
ad'a·man'ti·no'ma *pl.* -mas
   or -ma·ta
ad'a·man'ti·no'ma·toid'
ad'a·man'to·blast'
ad'a·man'to·blas·to'ma
   pl. -mas *or* -ma·ta
ad'a·man'to'ma *pl.* -mas *or*
   -ma·ta
A·dam·kie'wicz
—artery
—reaction
—test
Ad'ams
—clasp
—position
—procedure
Ad'am's ap'ple
ad'ams·ite'
Ad'ams-Stokes' syndrome
Ad'an·so'ni·a
—dig'i·ta'ta
a·dapt'
a·dapt'a·ble
ad'ap·ta'tion
a·dapt'er *also* adaptor

a·dap'tive
ad'ap·tom'e·ter
a·dap'tor *var. of* adapter
ad·ax'i·al
ad'de
ad'de·pha'gi·a
ad'der
ad'dict
ad·dic'tion
ad·dic'tive
Ad'dis
—count
—test
Ad'dis and Shev'ky test
Ad'di·son
—anemia
—disease
—keloid
—point
—syndrome
ad'di·so'ni·an
ad'di·son·ism
ad'di·tive
ad·du'cent
ad·duct'
ad·duc'tion
ad·duc'tor *(a muscle that draws
   a part toward the axis of the
   body or an extremity)*
   ♦abductor
a·del'o·mor'phic
a·del'o·mor'phous
a·del'pho·tax'is
a·del'pho·tax'y
ad'e·nal'gi·a
ad'e·nase'
ad'en·as·the'ni·a
a·den'dric
a'den·drit'ic
ad'e·nec'to·my
ad'en·ec·to'pi·a
a·de'ni·a
a·de'nic
a·den'i·form'
ad'e·nine'
ad'e·ni'tis
ad'e·no·ac'an·tho'ma
   pl. -mas *or* -ma·ta
ad'e·no·am'e·lo·blas·
   to'ma *pl.* -mas *or* -ma·ta
ad'e·no·an'gi·o·sar·co'ma
   pl. -mas *or* -ma·ta
ad'e·no·blast'

ad'e·no·can'croid'
ad'e·no·car'ci·no'ma
  pl. -mas *or* -ma·ta
ad'e·no·cele'
ad'e·no·cel'lu·li'tis
ad'e·no·chon·dro'ma
  pl. -mas *or* -ma·ta
ad'e·no·cyst'
ad'e·no·cys'tic
ad'e·no·cys·to'ma *pl.* -mas *or*
  -ma·ta
  —lym'pho·ma·to'sum
ad'e·no·cys'to·sar·co'ma
  pl. -mas *or* -ma·ta
ad'e·no·cyte'
ad'e·no·dyn'i·a
ad'e·no·ep'i·the'li·o'ma
ad'e·no·fi·bro'ma *pl.* -mas *or*
  -ma·ta
ad'e·no·fi·bro'sis *pl.* -ses'
ad'e·no·gen·e'sis *pl.* -ses'
ad'e·no·gen'ic
ad'e·no·gen'ic
ad'e·nog'e·nous
ad'e·nog'ra·phy
ad'e·no·hy·poph'y·se'al
ad'e·no·hy·poph'y·sec'to·my
ad'e·no·hy·poph'y·sis
  pl. -ses'
ad'e·noid'
ad'e·noi'dal
ad'e·noid·ec'to·my
ad'e·noid·ism
ad'e·noid·i'tis
ad'e·no·lei'o·my'o·fi·
  bro'ma *pl.* -mas *or* -ma·ta
ad'e·no·lei'o·my'o·ma
  pl. -mas *or* -ma·ta
ad'e·no·li·po'ma *pl.* -mas *or*
  -ma·ta
ad'e·no·lip'o·ma·to'sis
  pl. -ses'
ad'e·no·log'a·di'tis
ad'e·no·lym·phi'tis
ad'e·no·lym'pho·cele'
ad'e·no·lym'pho·ma
  pl. -mas *or* -ma·ta
ad'e·no'ma *pl.* -mas *or*
  -ma·ta
  —des'tru·ens
  —ma·lig'num
  —se·ba'ce·um
  —sub·stan'ti·ae' cor'ti·ca'lis
   su'pra·re·na'lis

  —su'do·rip'a·rum
ad'e·no·ma·la'ci·a
ad'e·no'ma·toid'
ad'e·no·ma·to'sis *pl.* -ses'
ad'e·no'ma·tous
ad'e·no·meg'a·ly
ad'e·no·mere'
ad'e·no·my'o·fi·bro'ma
  pl. -mas *or* -ma·ta
ad'e·no·my'o·hy'per·pla'-
  si·a
ad'e·no·my'o'ma *pl.* -mas *or*
  -ma·ta
ad'e·no·my'o·ma·to'sis
  pl. -ses'
ad'e·no·my'o·ma·tous
ad'e·no·my'o·me·tri'tis
ad'e·no·my'o·sal'pin·gi'tis
ad'e·no·my'o·sar·co'ma
  pl. -mas *or* -ma·ta
ad'e·no·my'o·sis *pl.* -ses'
ad'e·no·myx'o·chon'dro·
  sar·co'ma *pl.* -mas *or*
  -ma·ta
ad'e·no·myx·o'ma *pl.* -mas
  or -ma·ta
ad'e·no·myx'o·sar·co'ma
  pl. -mas *or* -ma·ta
ad'e·non'cus
ad'e·no·neu'ral
ad'e·nop'a·thy
ad'e·no·phar'yn·gi'tis
ad'e·no·phleg'mon'
ad'en·oph·thal'mi·a
ad'e·no·sal'pin·gi'tis
ad'e·no·sar·co'ma *pl.* -mas
  or -ma·ta
ad'e·no·sar'co·rhab'do·
  my·o'ma *pl.* -mas *or* -ma·ta
ad'e·no·scle·ro'sis *pl.* -ses'
ad'e·nose'
a·den'o·sine'
  —ar'a·bin'o·side'
  —di·phos'pha·tase'
  —di·phos'phate'
  —mon'o·phos'pha·tase'
  —mon'o·phos'phate'
  —phos'pha·tase'
  —py'ro·phos'phate'
  —tri·phos'pha·tase'
  —tri·phos'phate'
ad'e·no'sis *pl.* -ses'
ad'e·no·tome'

ad'e·not'o·my
ad'e·nous
ad'e·no·vi'rus
ad'e·nyl
  —cy'clase'
a·den'y·late'
ad'e·nyl'ic
ad'e·nyl·py'ro·phos'pha·
  tase'
ad'e·nyl·py'ro·phos'-
  phate'
ad'e·nyl·py'ro·phos·
  phor'ic
a·den'y·lyl
ad'e·pha'gi·a
ad'eps' *pl.* ad'i·pes'
  —an'ser·i'nus
  —ben·zo·i·na'tus
  —la'nae'
  —lanae hy·dro'sus
  —praep'a·ra'tus
  —su·il'lus
ad'e·qua·cy
a·der'mi·a
a·der'mo·gen·e'sis *pl.* -ses'
ad·here', -hered', -her'ing
ad·her'ence
ad·her'ent
ad·he'si·o' *pl.* -he'si·o'nes'
  —in'ter·tha·lam'i·ca
ad·he'sion
ad·he'si·ot'o·my
ad·he'sive
ad·he'sive·ness
a·di'a·bat'ic
a·di'a·ac·tin'ic
a·di'a·do'cho·ki·ne'si·a
a·di'a·do'cho·ki·ne'sis
a·di'a·pho·re'sis
a·di'a·pho·ret'ic
a·di'a·pho'ri·a
a·di'as·to'le
a·di'a·ther'mance
a·di'a·ther'man·cy
a·di'a·ther'mic
a·di'a·the'sic
a·di'a·thet'ic
a·dic'i·ty
A'die
  —pupil
  —syndrome
ad'i·ent
Ad'i·ni'da

ad′i·pec′to·my
ad′i·phen′ine′
a·dip′ic
ad′i·po·cele′
ad′i·po·cel′lu·lar
ad′i·po·cer′a·tous
ad′i·po·cere′
ad′i·po·cyte′
ad′i·po·fi·bro′ma *pl.* -mas *or*
  -ma·ta
ad′i·po·gen′e·sis *pl.* -ses′
ad′i·po·gen′ic
ad′i·pog′e·nous
ad′i·poid′
ad′i·po·ki·ne′sis *pl.* -ses′
ad′i·po·ki·net′ic
ad′i·po·ki′nin
ad′i·po·lyt′ic
ad′i·pol′y·sis
ad′i·po′ma *pl.* -mas *or* -ma·ta
ad′i·po·ne·cro′sis
  —ne′o·na·to′rum
  —sub·cu·ta′ne·a ne′o·na·
    to′rum
ad′i·po·pec′tic
ad′i·po·pex′i·a
ad′i·po·pex′ic
ad′i·po·pex′is
ad′i·po′sa dys·tro′phi·a
  gen′i·ta′lis
ad′i·pose′
ad′i·po′sis *pl.* -ses′
  —cer′e·bra′lis
  —do′lo·ro′sa
  —he·pat′i·ca
  —or·cha′lis
  —tu′be·ro′sa sim′plex′
ad′i·po′si·tas cer′e·bra′lis
ad′i·po·si′tis
ad′i·pos′i·ty
ad′i·po·su′ri·a
a·dip′si·a
a·dip′sy
ad′i·tus *pl.* ad′i·tus *or* -tus·es
  —ad an′trum
  —ad antrum mas·toi′de·um
  —ad aq′uae·duc′tum cer′e·
    bri′
  —glot′ti·dis inferior
  —glottidis superior
  —la·ryn′gis
  —or′bi·tae′
ad′junct′

ad·junc′tive
ad′ju·vant
ad′ju·van·tic′i·ty
ad lib′i·tum
ad·max′il·lar′y
ad·me′di·al
ad·me′di·an
ad′mi·nic′u·lum *pl.* -la
  —lin′e·ae′ al′bae′
ad·min′is·ter
ad·min′is·tra′tion
ad·mix′ture
ad·na′sal
ad nau′se·am
ad·ner′val
ad·neu′ral
ad·nex′a
  —oc′u·li′
  —u′ter·i′
ad·nex′al
ad′nex·i′tis
ad·nex′o·gen′e·sis *pl.* -ses′
ad′o·les′cence
ad′o·les′cent
a·don′in
a·don′i·tol′
ad·o′ral
ad·or′bit·al
a·dre′nal
a·dre′nal·ec′to·mize′
a·dre′nal·ec′to·my
a·dren′a·line′
a·dren′a·li·ne′mi·a
a·dren′a·li·nu′ri·a
a·dre′nal·ism
a·dre′nal·i′tis
a·dren′a·lone′
a·dre′nal·op′a·thy
ad′re·ner′gic
a·dre′nic
a·dre′nin
ad′re·ni′tis
a·dre′no·cep′tor
a·dre′no·chrome′
a·dre′no·cor′ti·cal
a·dre′no·cor′ti·cism
a·dre′no·cor′ti·coid′
a·dre′no·cor′ti·co·mi·
  met′ic
a·dre′no·cor′ti·co·troph′ic
a·dre′no·cor′ti·co·tro′phin
a·dre′no·cor′ti·co·trop′ic
a·dre′no·cor′ti·co·tro′pin

a·dre′no·gen′i·tal
a·dre′no·leu′ko·dys′tro·
  phy
a·dre′no·lyt′ic
a·dre′no·med′ul·lar′y
a·dre′no·meg′a·ly
ad′re·nop′a·thy
a·dre′no·pause′
a·dre′no·re·cep′tor
ad′re·no·ster′one′
a·dre′no·sym′pa·thet′ic
a·dre′no·tox′in
a·dre′no·trope′
a·dre′no·troph′ic
a·dre′no·tro′phin
a·dre′no·trop′ic
a·dre′no·tro′pin
ad′re·not′ro·pism
A′dri·an-Bronk′ law
a·dro′mi·a
Ad′son maneuver
ad·sorb′ (*to hold on a surface*)
  ♦absorb
ad·sor′bate′
ad·sor′bent
ad·sorp′tion
ad·sorp′tive
ad·ster′nal
ad·ter′mi·nal
a·dul′t′
a·dul′ter·ant
a·dul′ter·ate′, -at′ed, -at′ing
a·dul′ter·a′tion
a·dult′hood′
ad·um·bra′tion
ad·vance′
ad·vance′ment
ad·vanc′er
ad′ven·ti′tia
ad′ven·ti′tial
ad′ven·ti′tious
ad·verse′
ad·ver′sive
a′dy·nam′i·a
  —ep′i·sod′i·ca he·red′i·
    tar′i·a
a′dy·nam′ic
a·dy′na·my
A·ë′des′
  —ae·gyp′ti′
ae′lu·rop′sis
ae′quum

aer'ate', -at'ed, -at'ing
aer·a'tion
aer'a'tor
aer·e'mi·a
aer·en'ter·ec·ta'si·a
aer'i·al
aer·if'er·ous
aer'i·form'
aer'o·al'ler·gen
Aer'o·bac'ter
　—aer·og'e·nes'
aer'obe'
aer·o'bi·an
aer·o'bic
aer'o·bi·ol'o·gy
aer'o·bi'o·scope'
aer'o·bi'o·sis pl. -ses'
aer'o·bi·ot'ic
aer'o·cele'
aer'o·col'pos'
aer'o·cys'to·scope'
aer'o·cys·tos'co·py
aer'o·don·tal'gi·a
aer'o·don'ti·a
aer'o·don'tics
aer'o·duc'tor
aer'o·em'bo·lism
aer'o·em'phy·se'ma
aer'o·gel'
aer'o·gen
aer'o·gen'e·sis pl. -ses'
aer'o·gen'ic
aer·og'e·nous (forming gas)
　♦erogenous
aer'o·gram'
aer'o·i'on·i·za'tion
aer'o·i'on·o·ther'a·py
aer'o·med'i·cine
aer·om'e·ter
aer'o·neu·ro'sis pl. -ses'
aer'o·o·ti'tis
aer·op'a·thy
aer'o·pause'
aer'o·per'i·to·ne'um
aer'o·per'i·to'ni·a
aer'o·pha'gi·a
aer'oph'a·gy
aer'o·phil'
aer'o·phil'ic
aer'o·pho'bi·a
aer'o·phore'
aer'o·phyte'
aer'o·pi·e'so·ther'a·py

aer'o·plank'ton
aer'o·ple·thys'mo·graph'
aer'o·pleu'ra
aer'o·scope'
aer·os'co·py
aer'o·si'a·loph'a·gy
aer'o·si'nus·i'tis
aer·o'sis pl. -ses'
aer'o·sol'
aer'o·sol'i·za'tion
aer'o·tax'is
aer'o·ther'a·peu'tics
aer'o·ther'a·py
aer'o·ti'tis
aer'o·to·nom'e·ter
aer'o·to·nom'e·try
aer'o·trop'ic
aer·ot'ro·pism
aer'o·tym'pa·nal
aer'o·u·re'thro·scope'
aer'o·u·re'thros'co·py
a·feb'rile
a·fe'tal also afoetal
af'fect'
af·fec'tion
af·fec'tive
af·fec·tiv'i·ty
af·fec'to·mo'tor
af'fer·ent (directed toward a
　central organ)
　♦efferent
af·fin'i·ty
af'fir·ma'tion
af·fix'
af'flu·ence
af'flu·ent (copious; flowing
　freely)
　♦effluent
af'flux'
af·flux'ion
af·fric'a·tive
af·fu'sion
a'fi·brin'o·gen·e'mi·a
af'la·tox'in
a·foe'tal var. of afetal
af'ter·birth'
af'ter·brain'
af'ter·care'
af'ter·cur'rent
af'ter·damp'
af'ter·dis'charge
af'ter·ef·fect'
af'ter·hear'ing

af'ter·im'age
af'ter·im·pres'sion
af'ter·load'
af'ter·move'ment
af'ter·nys·tag'mus
af'ter·pains'
af'ter·per·cep'tion
af'ter·po·ten'tial
af'ter·pres'sure
af'ter·sen·sa'tion
af'ter·sound'
af'ter·taste'
af'ter·touch'
af'ter·treat'ment
af'ter·vi'sion
a·func'tion·al
a'ga·lac'ti·a
　—con·ta'gi·o'sa
a'ga·lac'tous
ag'a·lor·rhe'a also
　agalorrhoea
ag'a·lor·rhoe'a var. of
　agalorrhea
a·gam'ete'
a'ga·met'ic
a·gam'ic
a·gam'ma·glob'u·lin·e'-
　mi·a
a·gam'ma·glob'u·lin·e'mic
a·gam'o·cy·tog'o·ny
Ag'a·mo·fi·lar'i·a
a·gam'o·gen'e·sis
a·gam'o·ge·net'ic
ag'a·mog'o·ny
Ag'a·mo·mer'mis cu'li·cis
ag'a·mont
a·gam'o·sper'my
a·gam'o·spore'
ag'a·mous
a·gan'gli·on'ic
a·gan'gli·o·no'sis
a'gar'
a·gar'ic
a·gar'i·cin
A·gar'i·cus
ag'a·rose'
a·gas'tri·a
a·gas'tric
a'gas·tro·neu'ri·a
A·ga've
　—a·mer'i·ca'na
age, aged, ag'ing
âge de re·tour'

a'gen·cy
a'ge·ne'si·a
a·gen'e·sis *pl.* -ses'
a·ge·net'ic
a·ge·ni·o·ce·pha'li·a
a·ge·ni·o·ceph'a·lus
a·ge·ni·o·ceph'a·ly
a·gen'i·tal·ism
a·gen'o·so'mi·a
a'gent
ag·er·a'si·a
a·geu'si·a
a·geu'sic
a·geu'sti·a
ag'ger
—na'si'
ag·glom'er·ate
ag·glom'er·a'tion
ag·glu'tin·a·ble
ag·glu'ti·nate', -nat'ed, -nat'ing
ag·glu'ti·na'tion
ag·glu'ti·na'tive
ag·glu'ti·nin
ag'glu·tin'o·gen
ag·glu'ti·no·gen'ic
ag·glu'ti·noid'
ag·glu'ti·no·phil'ic
ag·glu'ti·no·phore'
ag·glu'ti·no·scope'
ag'gre·gate
ag'gre·ga'tion
ag'gre·gen
ag·gres'sin
ag·gres'sion
ag·gres'sive
ag'i·tate', -tat'ed, -tat'ing
ag'i·ta'tion
ag'i·to·graph'i·a
ag'i·to·la'li·a
ag'i·to·pha'si·a
Ag·kis'tro·don'
—con·tor'trix
—pis·civ'o·rus
a·glan'du·lar
a·glau·cop'si·a
a·glo·mer'u·lar
a·glos'si·a
a·glos'so·sto'mi·a
a·glu'cone'
a'glu·ti'tion
a·gly·ce'mi·a
a·gly·ce'mic
a·gly'cone'

a·gly'co·su'ri·a
a·gly'co·su'ric
ag'ma·tine'
ag'mi·nat'ed
ag'nail
ag·na'thi·a
ag·na·tho·ce·pha'li·a
ag·na·tho·ceph'a·lus
ag·na·tho·ceph'a·ly
ag·na'thous
ag·na'thus
ag·na·thy
ag·ne'a *also* agnoea
ag·noe'a *var. of* agnea
ag'no·gen'ic
ag·no'si·a
ag·nos'tic
ag'om·phi'a·sis
a·gom'phi·ous
a·go'nad'al
a·go'nad·ism
ag'o·nal
ag'o·nist
ag'o·ny
ag'o·ra·pho'bi·a
a·gou'ti *or* a·gou'ty
a·graffe'
a·gram'ma·pha'si·a
a·gram'ma·tism
a·gran'u·lar
a·gran'u·lo·cyte'
a·gran'u·lo·cy·the'mi·a
a·gran'u·lo·cyt'ic
a·gran'u·lo·cy'to·pe'ni·a
a·gran'u·lo·cy·to'sis
   pl. -ses'
a·gran'u·lo·plas'tic
a·gran'u·lo'sis *pl.* -ses'
a·graph'es·the'si·a
a·graph'i·a
a·graph'ic
ag'ri·mo'ny
ag'ri·us
Ag'ro·bac·te'ri·um
   —tu'me·fa'ciens
ag'ro·ma'ni·a
ag'ryp·net'ic
a·gryp'ni·a
a·gryp'ni·an'al·ge'si·a
a·gryp'node'
ag'ryp·not'ic
a'gua·miel'
a'gue

a·gy'ri·a
a·gy'ric
A·hu·ma'da-Del Cas·til'lo
   syndrome
a·hyp'ni·a
a'hyp·no'sis
aich'mo·pho'bi·a
AIDS (acquired immune
   deficiency syndrome)
ai'ler·on'
ail'ing
ail'ment
ai·lu'ro·phil'i·a
ai·lu'ro·pho'bi·a
ain'hum
air'-con'trast
air'-flu'id
air'sick'
air'sick'ness
air'way'
a·kan'thes·the'si·a
a·kar'y·o·cyte'
a·kar'y·ote'
ak·a·this'i·a *also* acathisia
a·ker'a·to'sis *pl.* -ses'
Ak'er·feldt test
Ak'er·lund deformity
A'kin bunionectomy
a'ki·ne'si·a
   —al'ger·a
   —am·nes'ti·ca
   —i'ri·dis
a'ki·ne'sic
a'ki·ne'sis *pl.* -ses'
a·kin'es·the'si·a
a'ki·net'ic
a·ko'ri·a *var. of* acoria
A'ku·rey'ri disease
a'la *pl.* a'lae'
   —au'ris
   —cer'e·bel'li'
   —ci·ne're·a
   —cris'tae' gal'li'
   —eth'moi·da'lis
   —il'i·i'
   —lat'er·a
   —lob'u·li' cen·tra'lis
   —mag'na
   —magna os'sis sphe'noi·
      da'lis
   —major ossis sphenoidalis
   —minor ossis sphenoidalis
   —na'si'

—os'sis il'i•i'
—ossis il'i•um
—par'va os'sis sphe'noi•
 da'lis
—tem'po•ra'lis
—vo'mer•is
al'a•bam'ne'
a'lac•ta'si•a
Al'a•jou'a•nine' syndrome
a•la'li•a
al'a•nine'
—a•mi'no•trans'fer•ase'
Al'an•son amputation
al'a•nyl
al'a•nyl•gly'cine'
a'lar
a•la•ryn'ge•al
a•las'trim
a'late'
a'la-tra'gus
a•la'tus
al'ba
Al'bar•ran'
—gland
—test
al•bas'pi•din
al•be'do
Al'bee-Del•bet' operation
Al'bers-Schön'berg'
—disease
—marble bones
Al'bert
—disease
—stain
Al'bert
—disease
—position
al•bes'cent
al'bi•cans'
al'bi•du'ri•a
al'bi•dus
al'bi•nism
al'bi•nis'mus
—cir'cum•scrip'tus
—to•ta'lis
—u'ni•ver•sa'lis
al•bi'no pl. -nos
al'bi•noid'ism
al'bi•not'ic
al'bi•nu'ri•a
al'bo•ci•ne're•ous
Al'bright'-Mc•Cune'-
 Stern'berg' syndrome

Al'bright' syndrome
al'bu•gin'e•a
—oc'u•li'
—o•var'i•i'
—pe'nis
—tes'tis
al'bu•gin'e•ot'o•my
al'bu•gin'e•ous
al•bu'gi•ni'tis
al•bu'go
al•bu'men (a nutritive
 substance)
♦albumin
al•bu'min (a water-soluble
 protein)
♦albumen
al•bu'mi•nate'
al•bu'mi•na•tu'ri•a
al•bu'min•e'mi•a
al•bu'min-glob'u•lin
al•bu'mi•nif'er•ous
al•bu'mi•nim'e•ter
al•bu'mi•nim'e•try
al•bu'mi•no•cy'to•log'ic
al•bu'mi•noid'
al•bu'mi•nol'y•sin
al•bu'mi•nol'y•sis pl. -ses'
al•bu'mi•nom'e•ter
al•bu'mi•nop'ty•sis
al•bu'mi•no'sis pl. -ses'
al•bu'mi•nous
al•bu'min•u•ret'ic
al•bu'mi•nu'ri•a
al•bu'mi•nu'ric
al•bu'mo•scope'
al'bu•mose'
al•bu'mo•se'mi•a
al•bu'mo•su'ri•a
al•bu'te•rol'
al•bu'to•in
Al'ca•lig'e•nes' fe•ca'lis
al•cap'ton var. of alkapton
al•cap'to•nu'ri•a var. of
 alkaptonuria
Al'ci•an blue
Al'cock' canal
al'co•gel
al'co•hol'
al'co•hol•ase'
al'co•hol•ate'
al'co•hol'ic
al'co•hol•ism
al'co•hol'i•za'tion

al'co•hol•ize', -ized', -iz'ing
al'co•hol•om'e•ter
al'co•hol•o•phil'i•a
al'co•hol•u'ri•a
al'co•hol'y•sis pl. -ses'
al'cu•ro'ni•um
al'de•hyde'
Al'der
—anomaly
—phenomenon
al'do•bi'u•ron'ic
al'do•hex'ose'
al'dol'
al'dol•ase'
al•don'ic
al'do•pen'tose'
Al'dor' test
al'dose'
al'do•side'
al•dos'ter•one'
al•dos'ter•on•ism
al•do•ster'o•no'ma
 pl. -mas or -ma•ta
al'do•ster'o•nu'ri•a
al•dox'ime'
Al'drich syndrome
al'drin
a•lec'i•thal
a•lem'mal
A•lep'po boil
a•let'a•mine'
a'leu•ke'mi•a
a'leu•ke'mic
a•leu'ki•a hem'or•rha'gi•ca
a•leu'ko•cyt'ic
a•leu'ko•cy•to'sis pl. -ses'
al'eu•rone'
A•leu'tian disease
Al'ex•an'der
—disease
—operation
a•lex'i•a
a•lex'ic
a•lex'i•dine'
a•lex'in
a•lex'i•phar'mac'
a•ley'dig•ism
Al'ez•zan•dri'ni syndrome
al'fa•cal'ci•dol'
al'ga pl. -gae' or -gas
al'gal
alg•an'es•the'si•a
al'ge•don'ic

al'ge·fa'cient
al'ge·os'co·py
al'ge'si·a
al'ge'sic
al'ge·sim'e·ter
al'ge·sim'e·try
al'ges·the'si·a
al'ges·the'sis
al'ges'tone'
al'get'ic
al'gi·cide'
al'gid
al'gin
al'gi·nate'
al·gin'ic
al'gi·o·mo'tor
al'gi·o·mus'cu·lar
al·glu'cer·ase'
al'go·ge·ne'si·a
al·go·gen'e·sis *pl.* -ses'
al'go·gen'ic
al'go·lag'ni·a
al·gom'e·ter
al·gom'e·try
al'go·phil'i·a
al'go·pho'bi·a
al'go·psy·cha'li·a
al'gor'
—mor'tis
al'go·rithm
al'go·rith'mic
al'go·spasm
al'go·spas'tic
al'i·ble
Al'ice in Won'der·land' syndrome
a'li·ces'
al'i·cy'clic
al'ien·a'tion
a'li·e·na'to men'tis
al'ien·ism
al'i·form'
a·lign'
a·lign'ment
al'i·ment
al'i·men'ta·ry
al'i·men·ta'tion
al'i·men'to·ther'a·py
al'i·na'sal
al'i·phat'ic
al'i·quot'
al'i·sphe'noid'
a·liz'a·rin

al'ka·di'ene'
al'ka·le'mi·a
al'ka·les'cence
al'ka·les'cent
al'ka·li' *pl.* -lis' *or* -lies'
al'ka·lim'e·ter
al'ka·lim'e·try
al'ka·line'
al'ka·lin'i·ty
al'ka·lin'i·za'tion
al'ka·lin·ize', -ized', -iz'ing
al'ka·li·nu'ri·a
al'ka·li·ther'a·py
al'ka·li·za'tion
al'ka·lize', -lized', -liz'ing
al'ka·loid'
al'ka·loi'dal
al'ka·lom'e·try
al'ka·lo'sis *pl.* -ses'
al'ka·lot'ic
al'ka·mine'
al'kane'
al'ka·nol'
al'ka·nol'a·mine'
al·kap'ton *also* alcapton
al·kap'to·nu'ri·a *also* alcaptonuria
al'ka·ver'vir
al'kene'
alk·ox'ide'
alk·ox'y
alk·ox'yl
al'kyl
al'kyl·am'ine'
al'kyl·ate', -at'ed, -at'ing
al'kyl·a'tion
al·kyl'o·gen
al'la·ches·the'si·a
al·lan'to·cho'ri·on'
al·lan'to·gen'e·sis *pl.* -ses'
al'lan·to'ic
al'lan·to'i·case'
al'lan·toid'
al'lan·toi'de·an
al'lan·toi·do'an·gi·op'a·gous
al·lan'to·in
al·lan·to'in·ase'
al·lan·to·in·u'ri·a
al'lan·to'is *pl.* al'lan·to'i·des'
al·las'so·ther'a·py
al·lax'is
al·lele'

al·le'lic
al·lel·ism
al·le'lo·ca·tal'y·sis *pl.* -ses'
al·le'lo·cat'a·lyt'ic
al·le'lo·morph'
al·le'lo·mor'phic
al·le'lo·mor'phism
al·le'lo·tax'is
al·le'lo·tax'y
Al'len
—test
—treatment
al'lene'
al·len'the·sis *pl.* -ses'
al'ler·gen
al'ler·gen'ic
al·ler'gic
al'ler·gid
al'ler·gist
al·ler·gi·za'tion
al'ler·gize'
al·ler·gol'o·gy
al'ler·go·sis *pl.* -ses'
al'ler·gy
Al'les·che'ri·a
—boy'di·i'
al'les·the'si·a
al'le·thrin
al·le'vi·ate', -at'ed, -at'ing
al·le'vi·a'tion
al·le'vi·a'tive
al·le'vi·a·to'ry
al'li·cin
al'li·ga'tion
Al'ling·ham operation
Al'lis sign
al·lit'er·a'tion
Al'li·um
al'lo·al·bu'min·e'mi·a
al'lo·an'ti·gen
al'lo·bar'bi·tal'
al'lo·chei'ri·a
al'lo·ches·the'si·a
al'lo·che'zi·a
al'lo·chro·ma'si·a
al'lo·ci·ne'si·a
al'lo·cor'tex'
al'lo·dip'loid'
al'lo·dip'loi·dy
al'loe·o'sis *pl.* -ses'
al'lo·e·rot'i·cism
al'lo·er'o·tism
al·log'a·my

al'lo·ge·ne'ic
al'lo·gen'ic
al'lo·graft'
al'lo·im·mune'
al'lo·i'so·leu'cine'
al'lo·ker'a·to·plas'ty
al'lo·ki·ne'sis pl. -ses'
al'lo·la'li·a
al·lom'er·ism
al'lo·met'ron
al·lom'e·try
al'lo·mor'phic
al'lo·mor'phism
al'lo·mor·pho'sis pl. -ses'
al'lo·mor'phous
al'lo·path'
al'lo·path'ic
al·lop'a·thist
al·lop'a·thy
al'lo·phan·am'ide'
al'lo·phan'ic
al'lo·phore'
al'lo·pla'si·a
al'lo·plasm
al'lo·plast'
al'lo·plas'tic
al'lo·plas'ty
al'lo·ploid'
al'lo·ploi'dy
al'lo·pol'y·ploid'
al'lo·pol'y·ploi'dy
al'lo·psy'chic
al'lo·pu'ri·nol'
al'lo·rhyth'mi·a
al'lo·rhyth'mic
all'-or-none' law
al'lose'
al'lo·some'
al'lo·ste'ric
al'lo·sy·nap'sis pl. -ses'
al'lo·syn'de·sis pl. -ses'
al'lo·tet'ra·ploid'
al'lo·therm'
al'lo·trans'plan·ta'tion
al·lot'ri·o·don'ti·a
al·lot'ri·o·geus'ti·a
al'lo·tri'o·lith'
al·lot'ri·oph'a·gy
al·lot'ri·u'ri·a
al'lo·trope'
al'lo·troph'ic (rendered nonnutritious by digestion)
♦allotropic

al'lo·trop'ic (exhibiting allotropy)
♦allotrophic
al·lot'ro·pism
al·lot'ro·py
al'lo·tryl'ic
al'lo·type'
al'lo·typ'ic
al'lox·an'
al·lox'a·zine'
al·lox'ur
al·lox·u·re'mi·a
al·lox·u·re'mic
al·lox·u'ri·a
al·lox·u'ric
al'loy'
al·lu'sion
al'lyl
al'lyl·am'ine
al'lyl·ene'
al'ma·drate'
Al'men reagent
a·lo'chi·a
al'oe
Al'oe
al'oe-em'o·din
al'o·et'ic
al'o·e'tin
a·lo'gi·a
al'o·in
A·lo'ka
 —machine
 —scanner
 —system
al'o·pe'ci·a
 —ad·na'ta
 —ar'e·a'ta
 —cic'a·tri·sa'ta
 —cir'cum·scrip'ta
 —con·gen'i·ta'lis
 —mu·ci·no'sa
 —pre'ma·tu'ra
 —se·ni'lis
 —syph'i·lit'i·ca
 —to·ta'lis
 —u'ni·ver·sa'lis
al'o·pe'cic
A'lou·ette' amputation
Al'pers syndrome
al'pha
 —globulin
 —streptococci
al'pha-ad're·ner'gic

al'pha-a·mi'no·a·dip'ic
al'pha-a·mi'no·ca·pro'ic
al'pha-a·mi'no·glu·tar'ic
al'pha-a·mi'no·hy'dro·cin·nam'ic
al'pha-a·mi'no·i'so·ca·pro'ic
al'pha-a·mi'no·i'so·va·ler'ic
al'pha-a·mi'no·pro'pi·on'ic
al'pha-a·mi'no-3-in'dole·pro'pi·on'ic
al'pha-a·mi'no·va·ler'ic
al'pha·di'one'
al'pha-fe'to·pro'tein
al'pha-hy'poph'a·mine'
al'pha-i'o·dine'
al'pha-lo'be·line'
al'pha·my'col'ic
al'pha·naph'thol'
al'pha·pro'dine'
Al'pha·vi'rus
al'phos'
al·pho'sis pl. -ses'
al'pho·zone'
al'phus
Al'port' syndrome
al·pra'zo·lam
al'pren'o·lol'
al'ser·ox'y·lon'
Al'ström syndrome
al'te·plase'
al'ter·ant
al'ter·a'tion
al'ter e'go
al'ter·nans'
Al'ter·nar'i·a
al'ter·nar'ic
al'ter·na'tion
al'ter·na'tor
al'ter·no·bar'ic
Alt'hau'sen test
al·the'a
al·thi'a·zide'
Alt'mann-Gersh' method
Alt'mann granules
al'tri·gen'der·ism
al'trose'
al'um
a·lu'mi·na
al'u·min'i·um
a·lu'mi·no'sis pl. -ses'

a·lu′mi·num
al′ve·at′ed
al·ve′o·lar
al·ve′o·late′
al′ve·o·lec′to·my
al·ve′o·li′
 —den′ta′les′ man·dib′u·lae′
 —dentales max·il′lae′
 —pul·mo′nis
 —pul·mo′num
al·ve′o·lin′gual
al·ve′o·li′tis
al·ve′o·lo·ba′sal
al·ve′o·lo·bas′i·lar
al·ve′o·lo·cla′si·a
al·ve′o·lo·con·dyl′e·an
al·ve′o·lo·den′tal
al·ve′o·lo·la′bi·al
al·ve′o·lo·lin′gual
al·ve′o·lon′
al·ve′o·lo·na′sal
al·ve′o·lo·plas′ty
al·ve′o·lot′o·my
al·ve′o·lus *pl.* -li′
al·ve′o·sub·na′sal
al′ver·ine′
al′ve·us *pl.* -ve·i′
 —hip′po·cam′pi′
al′vus *pl.* -vi′
a·lym′phi·a
a·lym′pho·cy·to′sis *pl.* -ses′
a·lym′pho·pla′si·a
a·lys′mus
al′y·so′sis
Alz′hei′mer
 —cell
 —disease
 —plaque
 —stain
a′ma
a′maas′
am′a·cri′nal
am′a·crine
a·mal′gam
a·mal′ga·mate′, -mat′ed, -mat′ing
a·mal′ga·ma′tion
a·mal′ga·ma′tor
a·man′din
Am′a·ni′ta
 —mus·car′i·a
 —phal·loi′des′
a·man′ta·dine′

a·ma′ra
am′a·ranth′
am′a·roid′
am·a·roi′dal
am′a·se′sis
a·mas′ti·a
a·mas′ti·gote′
am′a·tho·pho′bi·a
am′a·tive
am′a·to′ry
am·au·ro′sis *pl.* -ses′
 —fu′gax′
 —par·ti·a′lis fu′gax′
am·au·rot′ic
a·max′o·pho′bi·a
a·ma′zi·a
am′be·no′ni·um
am′bi·dex′ter
am′bi·dex·tral′i·ty
am′bi·dex′trism
am′bi·dex′trous
am′bi·ent
am′bi·fix·a′tion
am·big′u·ous
am′bi·lat′er·al
am′bi·le′vous
am′bi·oc′u·lar′i·ty
am′bi·o′pi·a
am′bi·sex′u·al
am′bi·sex′u·al′i·ty
am′bi·sin′is·ter
am′biv′a·lence
am·biv′a·len·cy
am·biv′a·lent
am′bi·ver′sion
am′bi·vert′
am′bly·a·cou′si·a
am′bly·a′phi·a
am′bly·chro·ma′si·a
am′bly·chro·mat′ic
Am′bly·om′ma
am′bly·ope′
am′bly·o′pi·a
 —al′bi·nis′mus
 —ex a·nop′si·a
am′bly·o′pic
am′bly·o·scope′
am′bo·cep′tor
am·bo·mal′le·al
am·bo·my′cin
am′bon′
Am·boy′na button
Am·bro′si·a

am·bro′sin
am′bu·lance
am′bu·lant
am′bu·late′, -lat′ed, -lat′ing
am′bu·la′tion
am·bu′la·to′ry
am·bu′phyl·line′
am′bu·side′
am·bus′tion
am·cin′o·nide′
am·di′no·cil′lin
a·me′ba *pl.* -bas *or* -bae′, *var. of amoeba*
am′e·bi′a·sis *var. of amoebiasis*
a·me′bic *var. of amoebic*
a·me′bi·cid′al *var. of amoebicidal*
a·me′bi·cide′ *var. of amoebicide*
a·me′bi·form′ *var. of amoebiform*
a·me′bo·cyte′ *var. of amoebocyte*
a·me′boid′ *var. of amoeboid*
a·me′bo·ma *var. of amoeboma*
a·me′bu·la *pl.* -las *or* -lae′, *var. of amoebula*
am′e·bu′ri·a *var. of amoebu-ria*
am′ei·o′sis *pl.* -ses′
a·mel′a·not′ic
a·mel′ei·a *(apathy)*
 ♦*amelia*
a·mel′i·a *(congenital absence of the extremities)*
 ♦*ameleia*
a·mel′i·fi·ca′tion
a·me′lio·ra′tion
am′e·lo·blast′
am′e·lo·blas′tic
am′e·lo·blas·to′ma *pl.* -mas *or* -ma·ta
am′e·lo·blas·to·sar·co′ma *pl.* -mas *or* -ma·ta
am′e·lo·gen′e·sis
 —im′per·fec′ta
am′e·lo·gen′in
am′e·lus *pl.* -li′
a·me′ni·a
a·men′or·rhe′a
a·men′or·rhe′al

a·men'or·rhe'ic
a·men'sa·lism
a'ment
am·er'i·ci·um
am'er·ism
am·er·is'tic
a·met'a·bol'ic
a·me·tab'o·lon' *pl.* -la
a·me·tab'o·lous
a·meth'o·caine'
a·me·thop'ter·in
a·me'tri·a
a·me'tro·he'mi·a
am·e'trope'
am·e·tro'pi·a
am·e·trop'ic
a·me'trous
am'fo·nel'ic
am·i·an'thine'
am·i·an'thi·nop'sy
am·i·an'thoid'
am·i·an·tho'sis *pl.* -ses'
am·i·ce'tin
a'mi·cro'bic
a'mi·cron'
a·mic'u·lum *pl.* -lums *or* -la
am'i·dase'
am'ide'
am'i·deph'rine'
am'i·din (*soluble starch*)
  ◆amidine
am'i·dine' (*compound containing the univalent radical -C(NH2:NH)*)
  ◆amidin
am'i·do·ben'zene'
am'i·do·ben'zol'
am'i·do·gen'
am'i·done'
am'i·do·py'rine'
am'i·dox'imes
a·mil'o·ride'
a·mim'i·a
am'i·nac'rine
am'i·nate'
a·mine'
a·mi'no
a·mi'no·a·ce'tic
a·mi'no·ac'i·de'mi·a
a'mi'no·ac'i·dop'a·thy
a·mi'no·ac'i·du'ri·a
a·mi'no·ac'ri·dine'
a·mi'no·a·dip'ic
a·mi'no·ben'zene'
a·mi'no·ben'zo·ate'
a·mi'no·ben·zo'ic
a·mi'no·ca·pro'ic
a·mi'no·eth'ane·sul·fon'ic
a·mi'no·eth'a·nol'
a·mi'no·fo'lic acid
a·mi'no·glu'cose'
a·mi'no·glu·tar'ic
a·mi'no·glu·teth'i·mide'
a·mi'no·gly'co·side'
a·mi'no·hep'tane'
a·mi'no·hex'a·no'ic
a·mi'no·hip'pu·ric
a·mi'no·hy'dro·cin·nam'ic
a·mi'no-hy·drox'y·bu'ta·no'ic
a·mi'no-hy·drox'y·pro'pa·no'ic
a·mi'no-in'dole·pro·pi·on'ic
a·mi'no·i'so·ca·pro'ic
a·mi'no·i'so·va·ler'ic
a·mi'no·lip'id
am'i·nol'y·sis
a·mi'no-mer·cap'to·pro·pa·no'ic
a·mi'no-meth'yl·bu'ta·no'ic
a·mi'no·met'ra·dine'
a·mi'no·met'ra·mide'
a·mi'no·pen'ta·mide'
a·mi'no·phen'a·zone'
am'i·noph'er·ase'
a·mi'no·phyl'line'
a·mi'no·pol'y·pep'ti·dase'
a·mi'no·pro·pi·on'ic
a·mi'nop'ter·in
a·mi'no·pu'rine'
a·mi'no·py'rine'
a·mi'no·sa·lic'y·late'
a·mi'no·sal'i·cyl'ic
a·mi'no·su'ri·a
a·mi'no·tol'u·ene'
a·mi'no·trans'fer·ase'
am'i·no·trate'
a·mi'no·va·ler'ic
am'i·nu'ri·a
a·mi'o·da·rone'
am'i·phen'a·zole'
am'i·quin'sin
am'i·so·met'ra·dine'
am'i·thi'o·zone'
am'i·to'sis *pl.* -ses'
am'i·tot'ic
am'i·trip'ty·line'
am'me'ter
am'mo·ac'i·du'ri·a
am'mo·nate'
am'mo·ne·mi·a
Am'mon horn
am·mo'ni·a
am·mo'ni·ac'
am·mo'ni·a·cal
am·mo'ni·at'ed
am·mo'ni·e'mi·a
am·mo'ni·fi·ca'tion
am·mo'ni·um
am·mo'ni·u'ri·a
am·mo·nol'y·sis *pl.* -ses'
am·ne'si·a
am·ne'si·ac'
am·ne'sic
am·nes'tic
am'ni·o·car'di·ac'
am'ni·o·cen·te'sis *pl.* -ses'
am'ni·o·cho'ri·al
am'ni·o·gen'e·sis
am'ni·og'ra·phy
am'ni·on' *pl.* -ons' *or* -ni·a
am'ni·on'ic
am'ni·o·ni'tis
am'ni·o·rrhe'a
am'ni·or·rhex'is *pl.* -es'
am'ni·os'
am'ni·o·scope'
am'ni·os'co·py
Am'ni·o'ta
am'ni·ote'
am'ni·ot'ic
am'ni·o·ti'tis
am'ni·o·tome'
am'ni·ot'o·my
am'o·bar'bi·tal'
am'o·di'a·quine'
a·moe'ba *pl.* -bas *or* -bae', *also* ameba
A·moe'ba
am'oe·bi'a·sis *pl.* -ses', *also* amebiasis
  —cu'tis
a·moe'bic *also* amebic
a·moe'bi·cid'al *also* amebicidal

a·moe′bi·cide′ *also*
  amebicide
A·moe′bi·dae′
a·moe′bi·form′ *also*
  amebiform
a·moe′bo·cyte′ *also*
  amebocyte
a·moe′ boid′ *also* ameboid
am′oe·bo′ma *also* ameboma
A·moe′bo·tae′ni·a
a·moe′bu·la *pl.* -las *or*
  -lae′, *also* amebula
am′oe·bu′ri·a *also* ameburia
a·mo′la·none′
am′or′
  —in·sa′nus
  —les′bi·cus
  —su′i′
a′morph′
a·mor′phi·a
a·mor′phic
a·mor′phin·ism
a·mor′phism
a·mor′pho·syn′the·sis
a·mor′phous *(formless)*
  ♦amorphus
a·mor′phus *(anideus)*
  ♦amorphous
  —glob′u·lus
A′moss sign
a·mo′ti·o′ ret′i·nae′
a·mox′a·pine′
a·mox′i·cil′lin
am′per·age
am′pere′
am′pere·me′ter
am′phe·chlo′ral
am·phet′a·mine′
am′phi·ar·thro′sis *pl.* -ses′
am′phi·ar·throt′ic
am′phi·as′ter
am·phib′i·a
Am·phib′i·a
am·phib′i·ous
am′phi·blas′tic
am′phi·blas′tu·la *pl.* -las *or*
  -lae′
am′phi·bol′ic
am·phib′o·lous
am′phi·ce′lous
am′phi·cen′tric
am′phi·cra′ni·a
am′phi·cre·at′i·nine′

am′phi·cro′ic
am′phi·cyte′
am′phi·des′mic
am′phi·des′mous
am′phi·gas′tru·la *pl.* -las *or*
  -lae′
am′phi·gen·e′sis *pl.* -ses′
am′phi·ge·net′ic
am′phi·gen′ic
am·phig′e·nous
am·phig′o·ny
am′phi·kar′y·on′
am′phi·mix′is
am′phi·mor′u·la *pl.* -lae′
am′phi·phile′
am′phi·tene′
am′phi·the′a·ter
am′pho·cyte′
am′pho·di·pol′pi·a
am′pho·lyte′
am′pho·phil′
am′pho·phil′ic
am·phoph′i·lous
am·phor′ic
am′pho·ter′ic
am·pho·ter′i·cin B
am·pho′ter·ism
am·phot′er·o·di·plo′pi·a
am′pi·cil′lin
am′pli·fi·ca′tion
am′pli·fi′er
am′pli·fy′, -fied′, -fy′ing
am′pli·tude′
am′pro·tro′pine′
am′pule′
am′pul′la *pl.* -lae′
  —can′a·lic′u·li′ lac′ri·ma′lis
  —duc′tus def′e·ren′tis
  —ductus lac′ri·ma′lis
  —hep′a·to·pan·cre·at′i·ca
  —lac·tif′er·a
  —mem′bra·na′ce·a anterior
  —membranacea lat′er·a′lis
  —membranacea posterior
  —membranacea superior
  —of Va′ter
  —os′se·a anterior
  —ossea lat′er·a′lis
  —ossea posterior
  —ossea superior
  —phren′i·ca
  —rec′ti′
  —tu′bae′ u′ter·i′nae′

am·pul′lae′
  —mem′bra·na′ce·ae′
  —os′se·ae′
am·pul′lar
am·pul·lar′y
am·pul·late′
am·pul′lu·la *pl.* -lae′
am′pu·tate′, -tat′ed, -tat′ing
am′pu·ta′tion
am′pu·tee′
am′py·zine′
am·quin′ate′
am′ri·none′
Am′sler grid
a·muck′
a·mu′si·a
Am′us·sat′ operation
am′y·cho·pho′bi·a
am′y·dri′a·sis *pl.* -ses′
a·my′e·len·ce·pha′li·a
a·my′e·len·ce·phal′ic
a·my′e·len·ceph′a·lus
am′y·e′li·a
am′y·el′ic
a·my′e·li·nat′ed
a·my′e·lin′ic
a·my′e·lon′ic
a·my′e·lus
a·myg′da·la *pl.* -lae′
a·myg′da·lase′
am′yg·dal′ic
a·myg′da·lin
a·myg′da·loid′
a·myg′da·loi·dec′to·my
a·myg′da·lo·lith′
a·myg′da·lot′o·my
am′yl
am′y·la′ceous
am′y·lase′
am′y·lene′
am′y·lin
am′y·lo·bar′bi·tone′
am′y·lo·clast′
am′y·lo·clas′tic
am′y·lo·dex′trin
am′y·lo·dys·pep′si·a
am′y·lo·gen·e′sis *pl.* -ses′
am′y·loid′
am′y·loi·do′is *pl.* -ses′
  —cu′tis
am′y·lol′y·sis *pl.* -ses′
am′y·lo·lyt′ic
am′y·lo·mal′tase′

am'y·lo·pec'tin
am'y·lo·pec'ti·no'sis
   pl. -ses'
am'y·lo·phos·pho'ry·lase'
am'y·lo·plast'
am'y·lop'sin
am'y·lor·rhe'a
am'y·lose'
am'y·lo·su'crase'
am'y·lum
am'y·lu'ri·a
a·my'o·es·the'si·a
a·my'o·pla'si·a
  —con·gen'i·ta
a·my'o·plas'tic
a·my'o·sta'si·a
a·my'o·stat'ic
a·my'os·the'ni·a
a·my'os·then'ic
a·my'o·tax'i·a
a·my'o·tax'ic
a·my'o·tax'y
a·my'o·to'ni·a
  —con·gen'i·ta
a·my'o·tro'phi·a
  —spi·na'lis pro'gres·si'va
a·my'o·troph'ic
am'y·ot'ro·phy
a·myx·i·a
a·myx'or·rhe'a
an'a
a·nab'a·sine'
an'a·bat'ic
an'a·bi·o'sis *pl.* -ses'
an'a·bi·ot'ic
an'a·bol'er·gy
an'a·bol'ic
a·nab'o·lin
a·nab'o·lism
a·nab'o·lite'
an'a·camp'tic
an'a·ce'li·a·del'phous
an'a·cho·re'sis
an'a·cho·ret'ic
an'a·cid'i·ty
a·nac'la·sis (*refraction of light or sound*), *pl.* -ses'
  ♦anaclisis
an'a·clas'tic
a·nac'li·sis (*the act of reclining*), *pl.* -ses'
  ♦anaclasis
an'a·clit'ic

an·ac'me·sis *pl.* -ses'
an'a·crot'ic
a·nac'ro·tism
an'a·cu'si·a
an'a·cu'sis
an'a·de'ni·a
an'a·did'y·mus
an'a·dip'si·a
an·aer'obe'
an·aer'o·bi·ase'
an·aer'o·bic
an·aer·o·bi·o'sis *pl.* -ses'
an·aer·o·bi·ot'ic
an·aer·o·gen'ic
an'a·gen
an'a·gen'e·sis *pl.* -ses'
an'a·ge·net'ic
an'a·ges'tone'
an'a·go'ge
an'a·gog'ic
an'a·kat'a·did'y·mus
an'a·ku'sis
a'nal
an'al·bu'min·e'mi·a
an'a·lep'tic
an'al·ge'si·a
  —al'ger·a
  —do'lo·ro'sa
an'al·ge'sic
an'al·ge'sist
an'al·get'ic
an'al·gize', -gized', -giz'ing
a·nal'i·ty
an'al·ler'gic
an'a·log' *var. of* analogue
a·nal'o·gous
an'a·logue' *also* analog
a·nal'o·gy
a·nal'y·sand'
a·nal'y·sis *pl.* -ses'
an'a·lyst
an'a·lyt'ic *or* an'a·lyt'i·cal
an'a·lyze'
an'a·lyz'er
an·am'ne'sis *pl.* -ses'
an'am·nes'tic
An·am·ni'o·ta
an·am'ni·ot'ic
an'a·mor·pho'sis *pl.* -ses'
an·an'a·phy·lax'is
an·an'a·sta'si·a
an'an·cas'ti·a
an'an·cas'tic

an·an'gi·o·pla'si·a
an·an'gi·o·plas'tic
an'a·pau'sis *pl.* -ses'
an'a·pei·rat'ic
an'a·phase'
an·a·phi·a
an'a·pho·re'sis
an'a·pho·ret'ic
an'a·pho·ri·a
an·aph'ro·dite'
an'a·phy·lac'tic
an'a·phy·lac'tin
an'a·phy·lac'to·gen
an'a·phy·lac'to·gen·e'sis
an'a·phy·lac'to·gen'ic
an'a·phy·lac'toid'
an'a·phyl'a·tox'in
an'a·phy·lax'is *pl.* -es'
an'a·phyl'o·tox'in
an'a·pla'si·a
An·a·plas'ma
an·a·plas·mo'sis *pl.* -ses'
an'a·plas'tic
an'a·plas'ty
an'a·ple·ro'sis *pl.* -ses'
an'a·poph'y·sis *pl.* -ses'
an·ap'tic
an'a·rith'mi·a
an·ar'thri·a
  —cen·tra'lis
  —lit'er·a'lis
an·ar'thric
an'a·sar'ca
an'a·sar'cous
an'a·schis'tic
an·a·stal'sis *pl.* -ses'
an·a·stal'tic
a·nas'ta·sis *pl.* -ses'
an'a·state'
an'a·stat'ic
an'as·tig'mat'ic
a·nas'to·le'
a·nas'to·mose', -mosed', -mos'ing
a·nas'to·mo'sis *pl.* -ses'
  —ar·te'ri·o·ve·no'sa
a·nas'to·mot'ic
an·as'tral
an'a·ther'a·peu'sis *pl.* -ses'
an'a·tom'ic *or* an'a·tom'i·cal
an'a·tom'i·cal·ly
an'a·tom'i·co·path'o·log'ic
an'a·tom'i·co·pa·thol'o·gy

a·nat'o·mist
a·nat'o·mist's snuff'box'
a·nat'o·my
an'a·tox'ic
an'a·tox'in
an'a·tri·crot'ic
an'a·tri'cro·tism
an'a·trip'tic
an'a·troph'ic
an'a·tro'pi·a
an'a·trop'ic
an·au'di·a
an'a·ven'in
an·az'o·tu'ri·a
an'chor
an'chor·age
an'cil·lar'y
an·cip'i·tal
an·cip'i·tous
an'co·nad'
an·co'nal or an·co'ne·al
an·co'ne·us *pl.* -ne·i'
　　—in·ter'nus
an'co·noid'
An'cy·los'to·ma
　　—a·mer'i·ca'num
　　—bra·zil'i·en'se'
　　—ca·ni'num
　　—du'o·de·na'le'
An'cy·lo·sto·mat'i·dae'
an'cy·lo·sto·mi'a·sis
　　pl. -ses'
An'der·nach' ossicles
An'dersch ganglion
An'ders disease
An'der·sen
　　—disease
　　—syndrome
An'der·son-Fab'ry disease
an'dra·nat'o·my
an'drei·o'ma *pl.* -mas *or*
　　-ma·ta
An'dré test
An·dré' Thom'as sign
An'drews operation
an'dri·at'rics
an'dri·a·try
an'dro·blas·to'ma *pl.* -mas
　　or -ma·ta
an'dro·cyte'
an'dro·ga·lac'to·ze'mi·a
an'dro·gam'one'
an'dro·gen

an'dro·gen'e·sis
an'dro·gen'ic
an'dro·ge·nic'i·ty
an·drog'e·nous (*of male*
　　offspring)
　　♦*androgynous*
an'dro·gyne'
an'dro·gy·ne'i·ty
an'dro·gy'nic
an·drog'y·nism
an·drog'y·noid'
an·drog'y·nous
　　(*hermaphroditic*)
　　♦*androgenous*
an·drog'y·nus
an·drog'y·ny
an'droid'
an·drom'e·do·tox'in
an'dro·mer'o·gone
an'dro·me·rog'o·ny
an'dro·mi·met'ic
an'dro·mor'phous
an·drop'a·thy
an'dro·phile'
an'dro·phil'ic
an·droph'i·lous
an'dro·pho'bi·a
an'dro·stane'
an'dro·stene·di'ol'
an'dro·stene·di·one'
an·dros'ter·one'
an·e'cho'ic
an·ec'ta·sis *pl.* -ses'
a·ne'de·ous
an'e·lec'tro·ton'ic
an'e·lec'trot'o·nus
A·nel' method
a·ne'mi·a
　　—pseu'do·leu·ke'mi·ca
　　—pseudoleukemica
　　　in'fan'tum
a·ne'mic
an'e·mom'e·ter
A·nem'o·ne
a·nem'o·nin
an'e·mo·pho'bi·a
an'e·mot'ro·phy
an·en'ce·pha'li·a
an·en'ce·phal'ic
an·en'ceph'a·lous
an·en'ceph'a·lus
an·en'ceph'a·ly
an·en'ter·ous

an'en·zy'mi·a
a·neph'ro·gen'e·sis *pl.* -ses'
an·ep'i·a
an·ep'i·plo'ic
an'er·ga'si·a
an'er·gas'tic
an·er'gic
an·er·gy
an·er·oid'
an'e·ryth'ro·blep'si·a
an'e·ryth'ro·cyte'
an'e·ryth'ro·pla'si·a
an'e·ryth'ro·plas'tic
an'e·ryth'ro·poi·e'sis
an'e·ryth·rop'si·a
a·nes'the·ki·ne'si·a
a·nes'the·ki·ne'sis *pl.* -ses'
an·es·the'si·a
　　—do'lo·ro'sa
a·nes'the·sim'e·ter
an·es·the·si·ol'o·gist
an·es·the·si·ol'o·gy
an·es'thet'ic
a·nes'the·tist
a·nes'the·ti·za'tion
a·nes'the·tize', -tized',
　　-tiz'ing
a·nes'the·tom'e·ter
an·es'trum
an·es'trus
an'e·thole'
a·ne'thum
an'e·to·der'ma
an'eu·ploid'
an'eu·ploi'dy
a·neu'ri·a (*deficiency of nervous*
　　energy)
　　♦*anuria*
a·neu'ric (*pertaining to*
　　aneuria)
　　♦*anuric*
a·neu'ri·lem'mic
an'eu·rin
an'eu·rysm
an'eu·rys'mal
an'eu·rys·mat'ic
an'eu·rys·mec'to·my
an'eu·rys·mo·plas'ty
an'eu·rys·mor'rha·phy
an'eu·rys·mot'o·my
an'eu·rys'mus
an·frac'tu·os'i·ty
an·frac'tu·ous

an·gel′i·ca
An′ger camera
An·ghe·les′cu sign
an′gi·as·the′ni·a
an′gi·ec·ta′si·a
an′gi·ec·ta·sis *pl.* -ses′
an′gi·ec·tat′ic
an′gi·ec·to·my
an′gi·ec·to·pi·a
an′gi·ec·top′ic
an′gi·i′tis
an·gi′na
—ab·dom′i·nis
—cor′dis
—cru′ris
—de·cu′bi·tus
—fol·lic′u·lar′is
—hy′per·cy′a·not′i·ca
—in·ver′sa
—lu′di·vig′i·i′
—no′tha
—pa·rot′i·de′a
—pec′to·ris
—pectoris va′so·mo·to′ri·a
an·gi′nal
an·gi′noid′
an·gi′no·pho′bi·a
an·gi′nose′
an·gi′nous
an′gi·o·a·tax′i·a
an′gi·o·blast′
an′gi·o·blas′tic
an′gi·o·blas·to′ma *pl.* -mas
   or -ma·ta
an′gi·o·car′di·o·gram′
an′gi·o·car′di·o·graph′ic
an′gi·o·car′di·og′ra·phy
an′gi·o·car′di·o·ki·net′ic
an′gi·o·car′di·op′a·thy
an′gi·o·car′di·tis
an′gi·o·cath′e·ter
an′gi·o·cav′ern·ous
an′gi·o·chei′lo·scope′
an′gi·o·cho·li′tis
an′gi·o·chon·dro′ma
   pl. -mas *or* -ma·ta
an′gi·o·crine′
an′gi·o·cyst′
an′gi·o·der′ma·ti′tis
an′gi·o·dys·pla′si·a
an′gi·o·dys·plas′tic
an′gi·o·dys·tro′phi·a
an′gi·o·dys′tro·phy

an′gi·o·ec·ta′si·a
an′gi·o·e·de′ma
an′gi·o·el′e·phan·ti′a·sis
an′gi·o·en′do·the′li·o′ma
   pl. -mas *or* -ma·ta
an′gi·o·fi′bro·blas′tic
an′gi·o·fi′bro·blas·to′ma
   pl. -mas *or* -ma·ta
an′gi·o·fi·bro′ma *pl.* -mas *or*
   -ma·ta
an′gi·o·gen′e·sis *pl.* -ses′
an′gi·o·gen′ic
an′gi·o·gen′in
an′gi·o·gli·o′ma *pl.* -mas *or*
   -ma·ta
an′gi·o·gli·o·ma·to′sis
an′gi·o·gram′
an′gi·o·graph′ic
an′gi·o·graph′i·cal·ly
an′gi·og′ra·phy
an′gi·o·he′mo·phil′i·a
an′gi·o·hy′a·li·no′sis
   pl. -ses′
an′gi·o·hy′per·to′ni·a
   (vasoconstriction)
♦angiohypotonia
an′gi·o·hy′po·to′ni·a
   (vasodilatation)
♦angiohypertonia
an′gi·oid′
an′gi·o·ker′a·to′ma *pl.* -mas
   or -ma·ta
—cor′po·ris dif·fu′sum
—corporis diffusum u′ni·
   ver·sa′le′
—For′dyce
—Mi·bel′li
an′gi·o·ki·net′ic
an′gi·o·leu·ki′tis
an′gi·o·li·po′ma *pl.* -mas *or*
   -ma·ta
an′gi·o·lith′
an′gi·o·lith′ic
an′gi·ol′o·gy
an′gi·o·lu′poid′
—of Brocq and Pau′tri·er
an′gi·ol′y·sis *pl.* -ses′
an′gi·o′ma *pl.* -mas *or* -ma·ta
   —ar·te′ri·a′le′ rac′e·mo′sum
   —in·fec′ti·o′sum
   —se·ni′le′
   —ser′pig·i·no′sum
an′gi·o·ma·la′ci·a

an′gi·o·ma·to′sis *pl.* -ses′
   —ret′i·nae′
an′gi·om′a·tous
an′gi·o·meg′a·ly
an′gi·om′e·ter
an′gi·o·my′o·li·po′ma
   pl. -mas *or* -ma·ta
an′gi·o·my·o′ma *pl.* -mas *or*
   -ma·ta
an′gi·o·my′o·neu·ro′ma
   pl. -mas *or* -ma·ta
an′gi·o·my·op′a·thy
an′gi·o·my′o·sar·co′ma
   pl. -mas *or* -ma·ta
an′gi·o·myx·o′ma *pl.* -mas
   or -ma·ta
an′gi·o·neu·rec′to·my
an′gi·o·neu·ro′ma *pl.* -mas
   or -ma·ta
an′gi·o·neu·ro·my·o′ma
   pl. -mas *or* -ma·ta
an′gi·o·neu·rop′a·thy
an′gi·o·neu·ro′sis *pl.* -ses′
an′gi·o·neu·rot′ic
an′gi·o·neu·rot′o·my
an′gi·o·no′ma
an′gi·o·pa·ral′y·sis *pl.* -ses′
an′gi·o·par′a·lyt′ic
an′gi·o·pa·re′sis *pl.* -ses′
an′gi·o·pa·thol′o·gy
an′gi·op′a·thy
an′gi·o·pha·co·ma·to′sis
   pl. -ses′
   —ret′i·nae′ et cer′e·bel′li′
an′gi·o·plas′ty
an′gi·o·pneu′mo·graph′ic
an′gi·o·pneu·mog′ra·phy
an′gi·o·poi·e′sis *pl.* -ses′
an′gi·o·poi·et′ic
an′gi·o·pres′sure
an′gi·o·re·tic′u·lo·en′do·
   the·li·o′ma *pl.* -mas *or*
   -ma·ta
an′gi·o·re·tic′u·lo′ma
   pl. -mas *or* -ma·ta
an′gi·o·ret′i·nog′ra·phy
an′gi·or′rha·phy
an′gi·or·rhex′is *pl.* -es′
an′gi·o·sar·co′ma *pl.* -mas
   or -ma·ta
an′gi·o·scle·ro′sis *pl.* -ses′
an′gi·o·scle·rot′ic
an′gi·o·scope′

an'gi·o·sco·to'ma
an'gi·o·sco·tom'e·try
an'gi·o'sis *pl.* -ses'
an'gi·o·spasm
an'gi·o·spas'tic
an'gi·o·sperm'
an'gi·o·stat'ic
an'gi·o·stax'is
an'gi·o·ste·no'sis
an'gi·os·te·o'sis
an'gi·os·to·my
an'gi·o·stron'gy·li·a·sis
an'gi·os·tro·phy
an'gi·o·tel·ec·ta'si·a
an'gi·o·te·lec'ta·sis *pl.* -ses'
an'gi·o·tel'ec·tat'ic
an'gi·o·ten'ic
an'gi·o·ten'sin
an'gi·o·ten·si·nase'
an'gi·o·ten·sin·o'gen
an'gi·o·ti'tis
an'gi·o·tome'
an'gi·ot'o·my
an'gi·o·ton'ic
an'gi·o·to'nin
an'gi·o·tribe'
an'gi·o·troph'ic
an·gi'tis
an'gle
  —of Lou'is
  —of Lud'wig
  —of Qua'tre·fages'
  —of Ro·lan'do'
  —of Syl'vi·us
An'gle classification
an'gle-clo'sure
an'gle-re·ces'sion
an'go·phra'si·a
an'gor'
  —an'i·mi'
  —noc'tur'nus
  —oc'u·lar'is
  —pec'to·ris
angst
ang'strom *or* ang'ström
An·guil'lu·la
an'gu·lar
an'gu·late
an'gu·la'tion
an'gu·lus *pl.* -li'
  —a·cro'mi·a'lis
  —cos'tae'
  —du'do·vi'ci

—inferior scap'u·lae'
—in'tra·ster·na'lis
—i'ri·dis
—i'ri·do·cor'ne·a'lis
—lat'er·a'lis scap'u·lae'
—man·dib'u·lae'
—mas·toi'de·us os'sis
  pa·ri'e·ta'lis
—oc·cip'i·ta'lis os'sis
  pa·ri'e·ta'lis
—oc'u·li' lat'er·a'lis
—oculi me'di·a'lis
—o'ris
—pa·ri'e·ta'lis a'lae'
  mag'nae'
—posterior py·ram'i·dis
—pu'bis
—sphe'noi·da'lis os'sis
  pa·ri'e·ta'lis
—ster'ni'
—sub·pu'bi·cus
—superior py·ram'i·dis
—superior pyramidis os'sis
  tem'po·ra'lis
—superior scap'u·lae'
an'ha·lo'nine'
an·haus'tral
an'he·do'ni·a
an·he'ma·to·poi·e'sis
an·he'ma·to'sis
an·he'mo·lyt'ic
an·he'mo·poi·e'sis
an'hi·dro'sis *pl.* -ses'
an'hi·drot'ic
an·his'tic
an·his'tous
an'hy'drase'
an'hy·dra'tion
an'hy·dre'mi·a
an'hy'dride'
an'hy'drite'
an·hy'dro·hy·drox'y·pro·
  ges'ter·one'
an·hy'dro·sug'ar
an·hy'drous
an'hyp·no'sis
a·ni'a·ci·no'sis *pl.* -ses'
an'i·an'thi·nop'sy
an'ic·ter'ic
a·nid'e·us
a·nid'i·an
an'ile'
an'i·ler'i·dine'

an'i·lide'
an'i·line'
a'ni·lin'gus
an'il·ism
a·nil'i·ty
an'i·ma
an'i·mal'cule'
an'i·mal'cu'lum *pl.* -la
an'i·ma mun'di'
an'i·ma'tion
an'i·ma·tism
an'i·mism
an'i·mus *(feeling of hatred)*
  ♦*anomous*
an'i'on
an'i·on'ic
an'i·rid'i·a
an'i·sa·ki'a·sis *pl.* -ses'
an'i·sate'
an'ise
an·is·ei·kom'e·ter
an·is·ei·ko'ni·a
an·is·ei·kon'ic
a·nis'ic
an'i·sin·di'one'
an·i·so·chro·ma'si·a
an·i·so·chro·mat'ic
an·i·so·chro'mi·a
an·i·so·chro'mic
an·i·so·co'ri·a
an·i·so·cy'to'sis *pl.* -ses'
an·i·so·dac'ty·lous
an·i·so·dac'ty·ly
an·i·so·dont'
an·i·sog'a·mous
an·i·sog'a·my
an·i·sog'na·thous
an·i·so·gyn'e·co·mas'ti·a
an·i·so·kar'y·o'sis *pl.* -ses'
an·i·so·lat'ed
an·i·so·mas'ti·a
an·i·so·me'li·a
an·i·so·mer'ic
an·i·so·met'rope'
an·i·so·me·tro'pi·a
an·i·so·me·trop'ic
an·i·so·mor'phic
an·i·so·mor'phous
an·i·so·my'cin
an·i·so·nu·cle·o'sis *pl.* -ses'
an·i·so·pho'ri·a
an·i·so'pi·a
an·i·so·pi·e'sis

an·i·so·poi·kil·o·cy·to'sis
  pl. -ses'
an·i'so·sphyg'mi·a
an·i'so·sthen'ic
an·i'so·ton'ic
an·i'so·trop'ic
an·i·so·tro'pine' meth'yl·
  bro'mide'
an'i'sot'ro·py
a·ni'stre·plase'
an'i·su'ri·a
a·ni·trog'e·nous
A·nitsch'kow' cell
an'kle
an'ky·lo·bleph'a·ron'
an'ky·lo·chei'li·a *also*
  ankylochilia
an'ky·lo·chi'li·a *var. of*
  ankylocheilia
an'ky·lo·col'pos'
an'ky·lo·dac·tyl'i·a
an'ky·lo·dac'ty·ly
an'ky·lo·glos'si·a
an'ky·lose', -losed', -los'ing
an'ky·lo'sis *pl.* -ses'
an'ky·lo·sto·mi'a·sis
  pl. -ses'
an'ky·lo'ti·a
an'ky·lot'ic
an'ky·lot'o·my
an'ky·rin
an'ky·roid'
an'la'ge *pl.* -la'gen *or* -la'ges
An·nam' ulcer
an'neal'
an'nec'tent
  —gy'ri'
an'ne·lid
An·nel'i·da
an'ne·lism
an·nex'a
an·nex·i'tis
an'nu·lar
an'nu·late'
an'nu·lo·cus'pid
an'nu·lo·plas'ty
an'nu·lor·rha·phy
an'nu·lose'
an'nu·lo·spi'ral
an'nu·lot'o·my
an'nu·lus *pl.* -li'
  —ab·dom'i·na'lis
  —cil'i·ar'is

—cru·ra'lis
—fem'o·ris
—fi'bro·car'ti·la·gin'e·us
  mem·bra'nae' tym'pa'ni'
—fi'bro'sus
—fibrosus fi'bro·car'ti·lag'-
  i·nis in'ter·ver'te·bra'lis
—in'gui·na'lis ab·dom'i·
  na'lis
—inguinalis sub'cu·ta'ne·us
—i'ri·dis major
—iridis minor
—mi'grans'
—of Zinn
—o'va'lis
—ten·din'e·us com·mu'nis
—tym'pan'i·cus
—um·bil'i·ca'lis
—u're·thra'lis
an'o·chro·ma'si·a
a·no'ci·as·so'ci·a'tion
a·no'ci·the'si·a
a'no·coc'cyg'e·al
a'no·cu·ta'ne·ous
an·od'al
an'ode'
an'o·der'mous
an·od'ic
an·od'i'nous
an·od'mi·a
an'o·don'ti·a
an'o·dyne'
an'o·dyn'i·a
an'o·et'ic
a'no·gen'i·tal
a·no'ma·lo'pi·a
a·nom'a·lo·scope'
a·nom'a·lous
a·nom'a·ly
an'o·mer
a·no'mi·a
a·nom'ic
an'o·mie
an'o·mous (*without shoulders*)
  ♦animus
an'o·nych'i·a
a'no·op'si·a
a'no·pel'vic
a'no·per'i·ne'al
A·noph'e·les'
  —al'bi·man'us
  —ar'gy·ri·tar'sis
  —cru'ci·ans'

—cul'li·ci·fa'ci·es'
—dar·lin'gi'
—gam'bi·ae'
—hyr·ca'nus
—mac'u·li·pen'nis
—quad'ri·mac'u·la'tus
a·noph'e·li·cide'
a·noph'e·li·fuge'
a·noph'e·line'
A·noph'e·li'ni'
a·noph'e·lism
an'o·pho'ri·a
an'oph·thal'mi·a
an'oph·thal'mic
an'oph·thal'mos'
an·o'pi·a
a'no·plas'ty
An'o·plu'ra
an·op'si·a
an·or'chi·a
an·or'chism
an·or'chous (*without testes*)
  ♦anorchus
an·or'chus (*an individual*
  without testes)
  ♦anorchous
a'no·rec'tal
a'no·rec'tic
a'no·rec'to·co·lon'ic
a'no·rec'to·plas'ty
an'o·rec'tous
a'no·rec'tum
an'o·rex'i·a
  —ner·vo'sa
an'o·rex'i·ant
an'o·rex'ic
an'o·rex'i·gen'ic
an'or·gas'mi·a
an'or·gas'mic
an'or·gas'my
an'or·thog'ra·phy
an'or·tho'pi·a
a'no·scope'
a·nos'co·py
a'no·sig'moid·os'co·py
an·os'mi·a
an·os'mic
a·no'sog·no'si·a
a'no·spi'nal
an·os·te·o·pla'sia
an'os·to'sis *pl.* -ses'
an·o'ti·a
an·o'tro'pi·a

an·o′tus
a′no·vag′i·nal
an·o′va·rism
a′no·ves′i·cal
an·o′vu·lant
an·o′vu·lar
an·o′vu·la′tion
an·o′vu·la·to′ry
an·ox·e′mic
an·ox′i·a
an·ox′ic
An′rep′ effect
an′sa pl. -sae′
—cer′vi·ca′lis
—hy′po·glos′si′
—len·tic′u·lar′is
—len·ti·for′mis
—ner′vi′ hy′po·glos′si′
—of Vieus′sens
—pe·dun′cu·lar′is
—sa·cra′lis
—sub·cla′vi·a
—vit′el·li′na
an′sae′
—ner′vi′ spi·na′lis
—ner·vo′rum spi·na′li·um
an′sate′
an′ser·ine
an′si·form′
ant·ac′id
an·tag′o·nism
an·tag′o·nist
an·tag′o·nis′tic
an·tal′gic
ant·al′ka·line′
ant·aph′ro·dis′i·ac′
ant·ar·thrit′ic
ant·asth·mat′ic
an·taz′o·line′
an·te·bra′chi·al
an·te·bra′chi·um pl. -chi·a
an·te·car′di·um pl. -di·a
an·te·ce′dent
an′te ci′bum
an·te·col′ic
an·te·cu′bi·tal
an·te·cur′va·ture
an′te·feb′rile
an′te·flect′
an′te·flex′ion
an·te·go′ni·al
an′te·grade′
an′te·hy·poph′y·sis pl. -ses′

an′te mor′tem n.
an′te mor′tem adj.
an·te·na′tal
an·ten′na pl. -nae′ or -nas
an′te·par′tal
an′te·par′tum
an′te·po·si′tion
an′te·py·ret′ic
an·te′ri·ad′
an·te′ri·or
an·ter·o·ap′i·cal
an·ter·o·clu′sion
an·ter·o·col′lis
an·ter·o·dor′sal
an·ter·o·ex·ter′nal
an·ter·o·fun′dal
an·ter·o·grade′
an·ter·o·in·fe′ri·or
an·ter·o·in·te′ri·or
an·ter·o·in·ter′nal
an·ter·o·lat′er·al
an·ter·o·lis·the′sis
an·ter·o·me′di·al
an·ter·o·me′di·an
an·ter·o·pa·ri′e·tal
an·ter·o·pi·tu′i·tar′y
an·ter·o·pos·te′ri·or
an·ter·o·sep′tal
an·ter·o·su·pe′ri·or
an·ter·o·trans·verse′
an′te·vert′
an′te·vert′ed
an′te·ver′sion
ant·he′lix
ant′hel·min′tic
an′thel·my′cin
an′the·lone′
an·the′ma pl. -mas or -ma·ta
an′ther
an′tho·cy′a·nin
an′tho·cy′a·ni·nu′ri·a
An′tho·my′ia
An′tho·ny stain
an′thra·ce′mi·a
an′thra·cene′
an′thra·ce·ne·di′one
an′thra·cid′al
an′thra·coid′
an′thra·com′e·ter
an′thra·co·ne·cro′sis
    pl. -ses′
an′thra·co·sil′i·co′sis
    pl. -ses′

an′thra·co′sis pl. -ses′
an′thra·cot′ic
an′thra·cy′cline
an′thra·lin
an′thra·nil′ic
an′thra·nol′
an′thra·qui·none′
an′thra·ro′bin
an′thrax′ pl. -thra·ces′
an′throne′
an′thro·po·cen′tric
an′thro·po·cen′trism
an′thro·po·ge·net′ic
an′thro·pog′e·ny
an′thro·pog′ra·phy
an′thro·poid′
An′thro·poi′de·a
an′thro·po·ki·net′ics
an′thro·pol′o·gy
an′thro·pom′e·ter
an′thro·po·met′ric
an′thro·pom′e·try
an′thro·po·mor′phic
an′thro·po·mor′phism
an′thro·poph′a·gy
an′thro·po·phil′ic
an′thro·po·pho′bi·a
an′thro·po·zo′o·no′sis
    pl. -ses′
an′ti·a·bor′ti·fa′cient
an′ti·a·bor′tion
an′ti·a·bor′tion·ist
an′ti·ad′re·ner′gic
an′ti·ag·glu′ti·nat′ing
an′ti·ag·glu′ti·nin
an′ti·ag·gres′sin
an′ti·al′bu·mate′
an′ti·al·bu′min
an′ti·al·bu′mi·nate′
an′ti·al·ler′gic
an′ti·a·lex′in
an′ti·am′bo·cep′tor
an′ti·a·me′bic var. of
    antiamoebic
an′ti·a·moe′bic also
    antiamebic
an′ti·am′y·lase′
an′ti·an·a′a·phy·lac′tin
an′ti·an·a′a·phy·lax′is
    pl. -lax′es′
an′ti·an′dro·gen
an′ti·a·ne′mic
an′ti·an′gi·nal

an'ti·an'ti·bod'y
an'ti·an'ti·dote'
an'ti·an'ti·tox'in
an'ti·anx·i'e·ty
an'ti·ar'ach·nol'y·sin
an'ti·a·rin
an'ti·a'ris
an'ti·ar·rhyth'mic
an'ti·ar·thrit'ic
an'ti·asth·mat'ic
an'ti·bac·te'ri·al
an'ti·bech'ic
an'ti·bi·o'sis *pl.* -ses'
an'ti·bi·ot'ic
an'ti·blas'tic
an'ti·blen'nor·rhag'ic
an'ti·bod'y
an'ti·brad'y·car'di·a
an'ti·cal'cu·lous
an'ti·car·cin'o·gen
an'ti·car·cin'o·gen'ic
an'ti·car'di·o·lip'in
an'ti·car'i·o·gen'ic
an'ti·car'i·ous
an'ti·cat'a·lyst
an'ti·cat'a·lyz'er
an'ti·ca·thex'is
an'ti·cen'tro·mere'
an'ti·ceph'a·lin
an'ti·chei·rot'o·nus
an'ti·cho·les'ter·e'mic
an'ti·cho'lin·er'gic
an'ti·cho'lin·es'ter·ase'
an'ti·cli'nal
an'ti·co·ag'u·lant
an'ti·co·ag'u·la·tive
an'ti·co·ag'u·lin
an'ti·co'don'
an'ti·co·in'ci·dence
an'ti·col'la·gen·ase'
an'ti·com'ple·ment
an'ti·com'ple·men'ta·ry
an'ti·con·cep'tive
an'ti·con·vul'sant
an'ti·con·vul'sive
an'ti·cus
an'ti·cu'tin
an'ti·cy'to·tox'in
an'ti·de·pres'sant
an'ti·de·pres'sive
an'ti·di'a·bet'ic
an'ti·di·ar·rhe'al
an'ti·di·u·re'sis *pl.* -ses'

an'ti·di·u·ret'ic
an'ti·di·u·ret'in
an'ti·dot'al
an'ti·dote'
an'ti·drom'ic
an'ti·dys·en·ter'ic
an'ti·ec'ze·mat'ic
an'ti·e·dem'a·tous
an'ti·em·bol'ic
an'ti·e·met'ic
an'ti·en'zyme'
an'ti·ep·i'·lep'tic
an'ti·ep·i'·the'li·al
an'ti·es'tro·gen
an'ti·feb'rile
an'ti·fer'ment
an'ti·fer·men'ta·tive
an'ti·fer·til'i·ty
an'ti·fi·bril'la·to'ry
an'ti·fi'brin
an'ti·fi'bri·nol'y·sin
an'ti·fi'bri·no·lyt'ic
an'ti·fi·lar'i·al
an'ti·flat'u·lent
an'ti·flux'
an'ti·fun'gal
an'ti·ga·lac'tic
an'ti·gen
an'ti·gen·e'mi·a
an'ti·gen'ic
an'ti·ge·nic'i·ty
an'ti·glob'u·lin
an'ti·goi'tro·gen'ic
an'ti·go·nad'o·trop'ic
an'ti·gon'or·rhe'ic
an'ti·hal·lu'ci·na·to'ry
an'ti·he'lix
an'ti·he·mol'y·sin
an'ti·he'mo·lyt'ic
an'ti·he'mo·phil'ic
an'ti·hem'or·rhag'ic
an'ti·hem'or·rhoi'dal
an'ti·hi·drot'ic
an'ti·his'ta·mine'
an'ti·his'ta·min'ic
an'ti·hor'mone'
an'ti·hy'a·lu·ron'i·dase'
an'ti·hy·drop'ic
an'ti·hy'per·cho·les'ter·
  ol·e'mic
an'ti·hy'per·gly·ce'mic
an'ti·hy'per·lip'i·de'mic
an'ti·hy'per·ten'sive

an'ti·hyp·not'ic
an'ti-ic·ter'ic
an'ti-im·mune'
an'ti-in·fec'tious
an'ti-in·fec'tive
an'ti-in·flam'ma·to'ry
an'ti-i'so·ly'sin
an'ti·ken'o·tox'in
an'ti·ke'to·gen
an'ti·ke'to·gen'e·sis *pl.* -ses'
an'ti·ke'to·gen'ic
an'ti·ki'nin
an'ti·lac'tase'
an'ti·le·thar'gic
an'ti·leu·ke'mic
an'ti·leu·ko·ci'din
an'ti·leu·ko·cyt'ic
an'ti·lew'is·ite'
an'ti·li'pase'
an'ti·li·pe'mic
an'ti·lip·fan'o·gen
an'ti·lip'o·trop'ic
an'ti·lith'ic
an'ti·lu·et'ic
an'ti·lym'pho·cyt'ic
an'ti·ly'sin
an'ti·ly'sis *pl.* -ses'
an'ti·lyt'ic
an'ti·ma·lar'i·al
an'ti·mel'lin
an'ti·me·nin'go·coc'cic
an'ti·men'or·rhag'ic
an'ti·mere'
an'ti·mes'en·ter'ic
an'ti·me·tab'o·lite'
an'ti·me·tro'pi·a
an'ti·mi·cro'bi·al
an'ti·mi·cro'bic
an'ti·mi'to·chon'dri·al
an'ti·mi·tot'ic
an'ti·mon'gol·oid'
an'ti·mo'nic
an'ti·mo'nid
an'ti·mo'ni·um
an'ti·mo'nous
an'ti·mo'ny
an'ti·mo'nyl
an'ti·morph'
an'ti·mor'phic
an'ti·mo·til'i·ty
an'ti·mu'ta·gen
an'ti·my'cin
an'ti·my·cot'ic

an'ti·my'o·sin
an'ti·nar·cot'ic
an'ti·nau'se·ant
an'ti·ne'o·plas'tic
an'ti·ne·phrit'ic
an'ti·neu·ral'gic
an'ti·neu·rit'ic
an'ti·neu·tro·phil'ic
an·tin'i·ad'
an·tin'i·al
an·tin'i·on'
an'ti·no'ci·cep'tive
an'ti·nod'al
an·tin'o·my
an'ti·nu'cle·ar
an'ti·nu'tri·ent
an'ti·o'don·tal'gic
an'ti·on·cot'ic
an'ti·oph·thal'mic
an'ti·op'so·nin
an'ti·o'vu·la·to'ry
an'ti·ox'i·dant
an'ti·par'a·lyt'ic
an'ti·par'a·sit'ic
an'ti·par'kin·so'ni·an
an'ti·path'ic
an'tip'a·thy
an'ti·pe·dic'u·lot'ic
an'ti·pep'sin
an'ti·pep'tone'
an'ti·pe'ri·od'ic
an'ti·per'i·stal'sis pl. -ses'
an'ti·per'i·stal'tic
an'ti·per'spi·rant
an'ti·phag'o·cyt'ic
an'ti·phlo·gis'tic
an'ti·phone'
an'ti·phthi'ri·ac'
an'ti·plas'min
an'ti·plas'tic
an'ti·pneu'mo·coc'cic
an'tip'o·dal
an'ti·pode' pl. an·tip'o·des'
an'ti·pros'tate'
an'ti·pros'ta·ti'tis
an'ti·pro'te·ase'
an'ti·pro'tein·ase'
an'ti·pro·throm'bin
an'ti·pro'to·zo'al
an'ti·pro'to·zo'an
an'ti·pru·rit'ic
an'ti·pso·ri'at'ic
an'ti·psy·chot'ic

an'ti·py'o·gen'ic
an'ti·py·re'sis
an'ti·py·ret'ic
an'ti·py'rine'
an'ti·rab'ic
an'ti·ra·chit'ic
an'ti·re'flux
an'ti·ren'nin
an'ti·re·tic'u·lar
an'ti·rheu·mat'ic
an'ti·rick·ett'si·al
an'ti·sca·bet'ic
an'ti·schis'to·so'mal
an'ti·scor·bu'tic
an'ti·seb'or·rhe'ic
an'ti·se·cre'to·ry
an'ti·sense'
an'ti·sep'sis pl. -ses'
an'ti·sep'tic
an'ti·sep'ti·cize'
an'ti·se·ro'to·nin
an'ti·se'rum pl. -rums or -ra
an'ti·si·al'a·gogue'
an'ti·si·al'ic
an'ti·sid'er·ic
an'ti·so'cial
an'ti·spas·mod'ic
an'ti·spas'tic
an'ti·spi'ro·che'tic
an'ti·staph'y·lol'y·sin
an'ti·ste·ril'i·ty
an'ti·ster'num
an'ti·strep'to·coc'cic
an'ti·strep'to·dor'nase'
an'ti·strep'to·he·mol'y·sin
an'ti·strep'to·ki'nase'
an'ti·strep·tol'y·sin
an'ti·su'do·ral
an'ti·su·do·rif'ic
an'ti·sym'pa·thet'ic
an'ti·syph'i·lit'ic
an'ti·tach'y·car'di·a
an'ti·tach'y·car'di·al
an'ti·tei·cho'ic
an'ti·te·tan'ic
an'ti·the'nar
an'ti·ther'mic
an'ti·throm'bin
an'ti·throm'bo·plas'tin
an'ti·thy'mo·cyte'
an'ti·thy'roid'
an'ti·tox'ic
an'ti·tox'i·gen

an'ti·tox'in
an'ti·trag'ic
an'ti·tra'gus
an'ti·trich'o·mo'nal
an'ti·tris'mus
an'ti·trope'
an'ti·try·pan'o·so'mal
an'ti·tryp'in
an'ti·tryp'tase'
an'ti·tryp'tic
an'ti·tu·ber'cu·lar
an'ti·tu·ber'cu·lin
an'ti·tu·ber'cu·lot'ic
an'ti·tu·ber'cu·lous
an'ti·tu'mor
an'ti·tus'sive
an'ti·ty'phoid'
an'ti·u're·ase'
an'ti·ven'ene'
an'ti·ve·ne're·al
an'ti·ven'in
an'ti·ven'om
an'ti·vi'ral
an'ti·vi·rot'ic
an'ti·vir'u·lin
an'ti·vi'rus
an'ti·vi'ta·min
an'ti·xen'ic
an'ti·xe'roph·thal'mic
an'ti·xe·rot'ic
an'ti·zy·mot'ic
ant'lo·pho'bi·a
An'ton' syndrome
an'tra·cele' var. of antrocele
an'tral
an·trec'to·my
an·tri'tis
an'tro·at'ti·cot'o·my
an'tro·cele' also antracele
an'tro·na'sal
an'tro·phose'
an'tro·py·lor'ic
an'trorse'
an'tro·scope'
an·tros'co·py
an·tros'to·my
an·trot'o·my
an'tro·tym·pan'ic
an'trum pl. -trums or -tra
—car·di'a·cum
—mas·toi'de·um
—of High'more'
—py·lo'ri·cum

—tym·pan'i·cum
a·nu'cle·ar
a'nu·cle'o·lar
an'u·li'
—fi·bro'si' cor'dis
an'u·lus *pl.* -li'
—con'junc'ti'vae'
—fem'o·ra'lis
—fi·bro·car'ti·la·gin'e·us
mem·bra'nae' tym'pa·ni'
—fi·bro'sus dis·ci' in'ter·
ver'te·bra'lis
—in'gui·na'lis pro·fun'dus
—inguinalis su'per·fi'ci·a'lis
—i'ri·dis major
—iridis minor
—ten·din'e·us com·mu'nis
—tym·pan'i·cus
—um'bil·i·ca'lis
an'u·re'sis *pl.* -ses'
an'u·ret'ic
an·u'ri·a *(failure of urinary function)*
◆aneuria
an·u'ric *(pertaining to anuria)*
◆aneuric
an·u'rous
an'u·ry
a'nus *pl.* a'nus·es *or* a'ni'
—vag'i·na'lis
—ves'i·ca'lis
—vul'vo·vag'i·na'lis
an'vil
anx·i'e·tas'
—pre'se·ni'lus
—tib'i·ar'um
anx'i·o·lyt'ic
a·or'ta *pl.* -tas *or* -tae'
—ab·dom'i·na'lis
—as·cen'dens
—de·scen'dens
—of Val·sal'va
—tho'ra·ca'lis
—tho·rac'i·ca
a·or'tal
a·or'tal'gi·a
a·or'tic
a·or'ti·co·pul'mo·nar'y
a·or'ti·co·pul·mon'ic
a·or'ti·co·re'nal
a·or·ti'tis
a·or'to·ar'te·ri'tis
a·or'to·bi'fem'o·ral

a·or'to·ca·rot'id
a·or'to·ca'val
a·or'to·cor'o·nar'y
a·or'to·du'o·de'nal
a·or'to·en·ter'ic
a·or'to·fem'o·ral
a·or'to·gram'
a·or'to·graph'ic
a'or·tog'ra·phy
a·or'to·he·pat'ic
a·or'to·il'i·ac'
a·or'to·il'i·o·fem'o·ral
a·or'to·path'ic
a·or'top'a·thy
a·or'to·plas'tic
a·or'to·plas'ty
a'or·tor'rha·phy
a·or'to·scle·ro'sis *pl.* -ses'
a·or'to·scle·rot'ic
a·or'to·sig'moid'
a'or·tot'o·my
a·or'to·ve·log'ra·phy
a·or'to·ven·tric'u·lo·plas'ty
a·pal'les·the'si·a
a·pal'lic
a·pan'cre·a
a·pan'cre·at'ic
ap·an'dri·a
ap'an·thro'pi·a
a·par'a·lyt'ic
a'pa·reu'ni·a
ap'ar·thro'sis *pl.* -ses'
a·pas'ti·a
a·pas'tic
ap'a·thet'ic
a·path'ic
ap'a·thism
ap'a·thy
ap'a·tite' *(phosphate)*
◆appetite
ap·at'ro·pine'
ap'a·zone'
ap'ei·do'sis *pl.* -ses'
a·pel'lous
Ap'elt test
a·pe'ri·ent
a·pe'ri·od'ic
a·per'i·os'te·al
a·per'i·stal'sis *pl.* -ses'
a·per'i·tive
Ap'ert
—disease
—syndrome

a·per'tog·na'thi·a
ap'er·tom'e·ter
ap'er·tu'ra *pl.* -rae'
—aq'ue·duc'tus coch'le·ae'
—ex·ter'na aq'ue·duc'tus
ves·tib'u·li'
—externa can'a·lic'u·li'
coch'le·ae'
—inferior can'a·lic'u·li'
tym·pan'i·ci'
—lat'er·a'lis ven·tric'u·li'
quar'ti'
—me'di·a'lis ven·tric'u·li'
quar'ti'
—me'di·a'na ven·tric'u·li'
quar'ti'
—pel'vis inferior
—pelvis superior
—pir'i·for'mis
—si'nus fron·ta'lis
—sinus sphe'noi·da'lis
—superior can'a·lic'u·li'
tym·pan'i·ci'
—tho·ra'cis inferior
—thoracis superior
—tym·pan'i·ca can'a·lic'-
u·li' chor'dae'
—tympanica canaliculi
chordae tym'pa·ni'
ap'er·ture
a'pex' *pl.* a'pex·es *or*
a'pi·ces'
—au·ric'u·lae'
—auriculae Dar'win·i'
—cap'i·tis fib'u·lae'
—ca·pit'u·lae' fib'u·lae'
—car'ti·lag'i·nis ar'y·te·
noi'de·ae'
—co·lum'nae' pos·te·ri·o'ris
—cor'dis
—cor'nus pos·te·ri·o'ris
me·dul'lae' spi·na'lis
—cus'pi·dis
—lin'guae'
—na'si'
—os'sis sa'cri'
—par'tis pe·tro'sae' os'sis
tem'po·ra'lis
—pa·tel'lae'
—pros'ta·tae'
—pul·mo'nis
—py·ram'i·dis os'sis
tem'po·ra'lis

—rad′i·cis den′tis
—su′pra·re·na′lis
(glan′du·lae′ dex′trae′)
—ve·si′cae′ u′ri·nar′i·ae′
a′pex·car′di·o·gram′
a′pex·car′di·og′ra·phy
a′pex·i·fi·ca′tion
a′pex′i·graph′
Ap′gar′ score
a·pha′gi·a
—al·ge′ra
a·pha′gic
a·pha′ki·a
a·pha′ki·al
a·pha′kic
aph′a·lan′gi·a
aph′a·lan·gi·a·sis
a·pha′si·a
a·pha′si·ac′
a·pha′sic
a·pha′si·ol′o·gy
A′phas·mid′i·a
ap′he·li·ot′ro·pism
aph′e·lot′ic
a·phelx′i·a
a·phe′mi·a
a·phe′mic
Aph′i·o·chae′ta
a·pho′ni·a
—par′a·no′i·ca
a·phon′ic
a′phose′
a·phot′ic
a·phra′si·a
a·phra′sic
a·phre′ni·a
aph′ro·dis′i·a
aph′ro·dis′i·ac′
aph′tha pl. -thae′
—ep′i·zo·ot′i·ca
—ser′pens
aph′thae′ trop′i·cae′
aph·thenx′i·a
aph·thoid′
aph·thon′gi·a
aph·tho′sis pl. -ses′
aph′thous
a′phy·lac′tic
a′phy·lax′is
ap′i·cal
ap′i·cal·ly
a′pi·cec′to·my
a′pi·ce·ot′o·my

ap′i·ci′tis
ap′i·co·ec′to·my
ap′i·co·lo′ca·tor
ap′i·col′y·sis pl. -ses′
ap′i·cos′to·my
ap′i·cot′o·my
ap′i·ec′to·my
a′pi·o·ther′a·py
A′pis
—mel·lif′er·a
a′pi·tox′in
A′pi·um
—grav′e·o′lens
a′pla·cen′tal
ap′la·na′si·a
ap′la·nat′ic
a·plan′a·tism
a·pla′si·a
—ax′i·a′lis ex′tra·cor′ti·
ca′lis con·gen′i·ta
a·plas′tic
a·pleu′ri·a
ap′ne·a
—va′gi′
—ve′ra
ap′ne·ic
ap′neu·mat′ic
ap′neu·ma·to′sis
ap′neu·mi·a
ap′neu′sis pl. -ses′
ap·neus′tic
ap′o·at′ro·pine′
ap′o·cam·no′sis
ap′o·ce·no′sis
ap′o·chro·mat′ic
ap′o·co′de·ine
a·poc′o·pe′
ap′o·cop′tic
ap′o·crine
ap′o·cy·nam′a·rin
a·poc′y·nin
a·poc′y·num
ap′o·dal
a·po′di·a
ap′o·dous
ap′o·en′zyme′
ap′o·fer′ri·tin
ap′o·gam′i·a
a·pog′a·my
ap′o·gee
ap′o·kam·no′sis pl. -ses′
a·po′lar
ap′o·lip′o·pro′tein

ap′o·mix′i·a
ap′o·mix′is pl. -mix′es′
ap′o·mor′phine′
ap′o·myt′to′sis pl. -ses′
ap′o·neu·rec′to·my
ap′o·neu·ror′rha·phy
ap′o·neu·ro′sis pl. -ses′
—ep′i·cra′ni·a′lis
—lin′guae′
—mus′cu·li′ bi·cip′i·tis
bra′chi·i′
—pal·mar′is
—plan·tar′is
ap′o·neu·ro·si′tis
ap′o·neu·rot′ic
ap′o·neu·ro·tome′
ap′o·neu·rot′o·my
a·pon′ic
a·poph′y·se′al
a·poph′y·sis pl. -ses′
a·poph′y·si·tis
ap′o·plec′tic
ap′o·plec′ti·form′
ap′o·plex′y
ap′o·qui′nine′
ap′o·re·pres′sor
a·po·ri·a pl. -ri·as or -ri·ae′
ap′or·rhip′sis
ap′o·sid′er·in
ap′o·si′ti·a
ap′o·sit′ic
ap′o·some′
a·pos′ta·sis pl. -ses′
ap′o·stax′is pl. -es
a·pos′thi·a
ap′o·trip′sis pl. -ses′
a′po·zem
a′po·ze′ma
ap′o·zy′mase′
ap·pa·ra′tus pl. ap′pa·
ra′tus
—di′ges·to′ri·us
—lac′ri·ma′lis
—re·spi′ra·to′ri·us
—u′ro·gen′i·ta′lis
ap·pear′ance
ap′pend′age
ap′pend′age cell
ap·pen·dec′to·my
ap·pen·dic′e·al
ap·pen·di·cec′to·my
ap·pen′di·ces′
—ep′i·plo′i·cae′

—ve·sic'u·lo'sae' ep'o·oph'-
o·ri'
ap·pen'di·ci'tis
—o·blit'er·ans
ap·pen'di·co·coele'
ap·pen'di·co·en'ter·os'-
to·my
ap·pen'di·co'lith
ap·pen'di·co'li·thi'a·sis
   pl. -ses'
ap·pen'di·col'y·sis pl. -ses'
ap·pen'di·cop'a·thy
ap·pen'di·cos'to·my
ap'pen·dic'u·lar
ap'pen·dic'u·late
ap·pen'dix pl. -dix·es or
   -di·ces'
   —au·ric'u·lar'is
   —ep'i·di·dym'i·dis
   —fi·bro'sa hep'a·tis
   —tes'tis
   —ven·tric'u·li' la·ryn'gis
   —ver'mi·for'mis
ap·pen'do·li·thi'a·sis
ap'per·ceive'
ap'per·cep'tion
ap'per·cep'tive
ap'per·son'i·fi·ca'tion
ap'pe·stat'
ap'pe·tite' (desire)
   ◆apatite
ap'pla·nate'
ap'pla·na'tion
ap'pla·nom'e·ter
ap·pli'ance
ap'pli·ca'tor
ap'pli·qué'
ap·pose', -posed', -pos'ing
ap·po·si'tion
ap'pre·hen'sion
ap·proach'
ap·prox'i·mal
ap·prox'i·mate', -mat·ed,
   -mat'ing
ap·prox'i·ma'tion
ap·prox'i·ma'tor
ap'ra·clon'i·dine'
a·prac'tic
a·prac'tog·no'si·a
a·prax'i·a
a·prax'ic
a·prin'dine'
ap'ro·bar'bi·tal'

a·proc'ti·a
a·proc'tous
a'pron
ap'ro·sex'i·a
   —na·sa'lis
a'pro·so'pi·a
a·pros'o·pus
a·pro'ti·nin
ap·sel'a·phe'si·a
ap'si·thy'ri·a
Apt test
ap'ty·a'li·a
ap·ty'a·lism
a'pu·do'ma pl. -mas or
   -ma·ta
a·pul'mo·nism
a'pus
a·py'e·tous
a·pyk'no·mor'phous
a·py'rase '
a·py'rene'
a'py·ret'ic
a'py·rex'i·a
a'py·rex'i·al
aq'ua pl. -uae' or -uas
   —re'gi·a
aq'ua·pho'bi·a
aq'ue·duct'
   —of Fal·lo'pi·us
   —of Syl'vi·us
aq'ue·duc'tal
aq'ue·duc'tus
   —cer'e·bri'
   —coch'le·ae'
   —ves·tib'u·li'
a'que·ous
a'quos'i·ty
ar'a·ban
ar'a·bic
a·rab'i·no·syl·cy'to·sine '
ar'a·chid'ic
a·rach'i·don'ate'
a·rach'i·don'ic
ar'a·chis
a·rach'ne·pho'bi·a
a·rach'nid
A·rach'ni·da
a·rach'nid·ism
ar'ach·ni'tis
a·rach'no·dac'ty·ly
a·rach'no·gas'tri·a
a·rach'noid'
ar'ach·noi'dal

ar'ach·noi'de·a
   —en·ceph'a·li'
   —spi·na'lis
ar'ach·noi'de·an
a·rach'noid·ism
a·rach'noid·i'tis
   —os·sif'i·cans'
ar'ach·nol'y·sin
a·rach'no·pho'bi·a
a·rach'no·pho'bic
A'ra·ka'wa test
a·ral'de·hyde'
A·ra'li·a
   —rac'e·mo'sa
a·ral'kyl
A·ran'-Du·chenne'
   —dystrophy
   —syndrome
a·ra'ne·ism
a·ra'ne·ous
ar'a·no'tin
A·ran'ti·us
   —ligament
   —ventricle
a·ra'phi·a
ar'a·ro'ba
Ar'a test
ar'bor
ar·bo're·ous
ar·bo·res'cent
ar'bo·ri·za'tion
ar'bo·rize'
ar'bor·vi'tae'
   —cer'e·bel'i'
ar'bo·vi'rus
ar·bu'ta·mine'
ar'bu·tin
arc
ar'cade'
ar·ca'num pl. -na
ar·ca·tu'ra
arc de cer'cle
arch
ar·cha'ic
ar'che·go'ni·um pl. -ni·a
arch'en·ce·phal'ic
arch'en·ceph'a·lon' pl. -la
arch'en·ter'ic
arch·en'ter·on' pl. -ter·a
ar'che·o·cyte'
ar'che·o·ki·net'ic
ar'che·py'on'
ar'che·type'

ar'chi·blast'
ar'chi·coele'
ar'chi·gas'tru·la *pl.* -las *or*
-lae'
ar'chil
ar'chi·neph'ric
ar'chi·neph'ron'
ar'chi·pal'li·um
ar'chi·stome'
ar'chi·tec·ton'ic
ar'chi·tec·tur·al
ar'chi·tec·ture
ar'cho·plasm
ar'cho·plas'ma
ar'cho·plas'mic
ar·chu'si·a
ar'ci·form'
arc·ta'tion
ar'cu·al
ar'cu·a'li·a
ar'cu·ate'
ar'cu·a'tion
ar'cus *pl.* ar'cus
—al've·o·lar'is man·dib'u·
lae'
—alveolaris max·il'lae'
—anterior at·lan'tis
—a·or'tae'
—car'ti·lag'i·nis cri·coi'-
de·ae'
—cos·ta'lis
—cos·tar'um
—den·ta'lis inferior
—dentalis superior
—glos'so·pal'a·ti'nus
—il'i·o·pec·tin'e·us
—ju've·ni'lis
—lum·bo·cos·ta'lis lat·er·a'-
lis
—lumbocostalis me·di·a'lis
—pal'a·ti'ni'
—pal'a·to·glos'sus
—pal'a·to·pha·ryn'ge·us
—pal·mar'is pro·fun'dus
—palmaris su·per·fi·ci·a'lis
—pal'pe·bra'lis inferior
—palpebralis superior
—pe'dis lon'gi·tu'di·na'lis
—pedis trans·ver'sa·lis
—pha·ryn'go·pal'a·ti'nus
—plan·tar'is
—posterior at·lan'tis
—pu'bis

—se·ni'lis
—senilis len'tis
—su'per·cil'i·ar'is
—tar'se·us inferior
—tarseus superior
—ten·din'e·us
—tendineus fas'ci·ae' pel'-
vis
—tendineus mus'cu·li' lev'-
a·to'ris a'ni'
—tendineus musculi so'le·i'
—ve·no'si' dig'i·ta'lis
—ve·no'sus dor·sa'lis pe'dis
—venosus jug'u·li'
—venosus pal'mar'is pro·
fun'dus
—venosus palmaris su'per·
fi'ci·a'lis
—venosus plan·tar'is
—ver'te·brae'
—vo·lar'is pro·fun'dus
—volaris su'per·fi'ci·a'lis
—volaris ve·no'sus pro·
fun'dus
—volaris venosus su'per·fi'-
ci·a'lis
—zy'go·mat'i·cus
ar'dent pulse
ar'dor
—u·ri'nae
—ven·tric'u·li
ar'e·a *pl.* -as *or* -ae'
—a·cu'sti·ca
—Cel'si'
—cen·tra'lis
—cho·roi'de·a
—coch'le·ae'
—cri·bro'sa me'di·a
—cribrosa pa·pil'lae'
re·na'lis
—cribrosa superior
—em'bry·o·na'lis
—ger'mi·na·ti'va
—in'ter·con·dy·lar'is
anterior tib'i·ae'
—intercondylaris posterior
tibiae
—ner'vi' fa'ci·a'lis
—nu'da
—o·pa'ca
—par'a·ter'mi·na'lis
—par'ol·fac'to'ri·a
(Bro'cae')

—pel·lu'ci·da
—pos·tre'ma
—sub'cal·lo'sa
—vas'cu·lo'sa
—ves·tib'u·lar'is
—vestibularis inferior
—vestibularis superior
—vit'el·li'na
ar'e·ae' gas'tri·cae'
ar'e·a'ta
ar'e·a'tus
a're·flex'i·a
a're·gen'er·a'tion
a're·gen'er·a·tive
a're·gen'er·a·to'ry
ar'e·na'ceous
ar'ene'
ar'e·no·vi'rus group
a·re'o·la *pl.* -lae' *or* -las
—mam'mae'
—pap'il·lar'is
a·re'o·lar
ar·gam'bly·o'pi·a
Ar'gas
—per'si·cus
Ar·gas'i·dae'
ar'gen'taf·fin
ar'gen·taf'fi·no'ma *pl.* -mas
or -ma·ta
ar'gen'tic
ar'gen·tine'
ar'gen'to·phil'ic
ar'gen'tum
ar'gil·la'ceous
ar'gi·nase'
ar'gi·nine'
ar'gi·ni·no·suc·cin'ic
ar'gi·ni·no·suc·cin'ic·ac'i·
du'ri·a
ar'gon'
Ar'gyll' Rob'ert·son
—pupil
—sign
ar·gyr'i·a
ar·gyr'ic
ar·gy'ro·phil'
ar·gy'ro·phil'ic
ar·gy'ro·sis *pl.* -ses'
Ar'i·as-Stel'la cells
a·ri'bo·fla'vin·o'sis *pl.* -ses'
ar'i·cine'
A·ris'to·lo'chi·a
—re·tic'u·la'ta

—ser′pen·tar′i·a
a·rith′mo·ma′ni·a
Ar′i·zo′na bacteria
Ar′kan·sas′ stone
ar′ky·o·chrome′
Arlt trachoma
arm
ar′ma·men·tar′i·um *pl.* -i·a
  or -ums
Ar·man′ni-Eb′stein′
  nephropathy
Ar·me′ni·an disease
arm′pit′
Ar′neth
  —classification
  —count
  —formula
  —index
  —method
ar′ni·ca
Ar′nold
  —convolution
  —nerve
  —neuralgia
Ar′nold-Chi·ar′i
  —malformation
  —syndrome
Ar·noux′ sign
a·ro′ma·tase′
ar′o·mat′ic
a·rous′al
ar′oyl
ar·ray′
ar·rec′tor *pl.* ar′rec·to′res′
ar·rec·to′res′ pi·lo′rum
ar·rest′
ar·rhe′no·blas·to′ma
  pl. -mas *or* -ma·ta
ar·rhe′no·to′ci·a
ar·rhin·en′ce·pha′li·a
ar·rhin′i·a
ar·rhin′ic
ar·rhyth′mi·a
ar·rhyth′mic
ar·rhyth′mo·gen′e·sis
  pl. -ses′
ar·rhyth′mo·gen′ic
ar·rhyth′mo·ki·ne′si·a
ar·rhyth′mo·ki·ne′sis
  pl. -ses′
ar′row·root′
ar′se·nate′
ar′se·nic

ar·sen′i·cal
ar·sen′i·cal·ism
ar′se·nide′
ar′se·nite′
ar·se′niu·ret′ed
ar·se·no·cho′line′
ar′sen·ol′y·sis *pl.* -ses′
ar·se·no·ther′a·py
ar′se·nous
ar′sen·ox′ide′
ar′sine′
ar·sin′ic
ar′si·no·gal′lane′
ar·so′ni·um
ar′son·val′i·za′tion
ars·phen′a·mine′
ars′thi·nol′
ar′ter·al′gi·a
ar′ter·ec′to·my
ar·te′re·nol′
ar·te′ri·a *pl.* -ae′
  —ac′e·tab′u·li′
  —al′ve·o′lar′is inferior
  —alveolaris superior
    posterior
  —an′gu·lar′is
  —a·non′y·ma
  —ap′pen·dic′u·lar′is
  —ar′cu·a′ta pe′dis
  —as·cen′dens il′e·o·col′i·ca
  —au′di·ti′va in·ter′na
  —au′ric′u·lar′is posterior
  —auricularis pro·fun′da
  —ax′il·lar′is
  —bas′il·lar′is
  —bra′chi·a′lis
  —brachialis su′per·fi′ci·a′-
    lis
  —buc′ca′lis
  —buc′ci·na·to′ri·a
  —bul′bi′ pe′nis
  —bulbi u·re′thrae′
  —bulbi ves·tib′u·li′
  —ca·na′lis pter′y·goi′de·i′
  —ca·rot′is com·mu′nis
  —carotis ex·ter′na
  —carotis in·ter′na
  —cau′dae′ pan·cre′a′tis
  —ce·ca′lis anterior
  —cecalis posterior
  —cen·tra′lis ret′i·nae′
  —cer′e·bel′li′ inferior
    anterior

  —cerebelli inferior posterior
  —cerebelli superior
  —cer′e·bri′ anterior
  —cerebri me′di·a
  —cerebri posterior
  —cer·vi·ca′lis as·cen′dens
  —cervicalis pro·fun′da
  —cervicalis su′per·fi′ci·a′lis
  —cho′ri·oi′de·a
  —cho·roi′de·a anterior
  —cir·cum·flex′a fem′o·ris
    lat′er·a′lis
  —circumflexa femoris
    me′di·a′lis
  —circumflexa hu′mer·i′
    anterior
  —circumflexa humeri
    posterior
  —circumflexa il′i·i′
    pro·fun′da
  —circumflexa ilii
    su′per·fi′ci·a′lis
  —circumflexa scap′u·lae′
  —coe·li′a·ca
  —col′i·ca dex′tra
  —colica me′di·a
  —colica si·nis′tra
  —col′lat′er·a′lis me′di·a
  —collateralis ra·di·a′lis
  —collateralis ul·nar′is
    inferior
  —collateralis ulnaris
    superior
  —com′i·tans′ ner′vi′
    is′chi·ad′i·ci′
  —com·mu′ni·cans′ anterior
    cer′e·bri′
  —communicans posterior
    cerebri
  —cor′o·nar′i·a dex′tra
  —coronaria si·nis′tra
  —crem′a·ster′i·ca
  —cys′ti·ca
  —def′e·ren′ti·a′is
  —dor·sa′lis cli·to′ri·dis
  —dorsalis na′si′
  —dorsalis pe′dis
  —dorsalis pe′nis
  —duc′tus def′e·ren′tis
  —ep′i·gas′tri·ca inferior
  —epigastrica su′per·fi′ci·a′-
    lis
  —epigastrica superior

—eth'moi·da'lis anterior
—ethmoidalis posterior
—fa'ci·a'lis
—em'o·ra'lis
—fib'u·lar'is
—fron·ta'lis
—gas'tri·ca dex'tra
—gastrica si·nis'tra
—gas'tro·du'o·de·na'lis
—gas'tro·ep'i·plo'i·ca
  dex'tra
—gastroepiploica si·nis'tra
—gen'u inferior lat'er·a'lis
—genu inferior me'di·a'lis
—genu me'di·a
—ge'nus de·scen'dens
—genus inferior lat'er·a'lis
—genus inferior me'di·a'lis
—genus me'di·a
—genus superior lat'er·a'lis
—genus superior me'di·a'lis
—gen'u superior lat'er·a'lis
—genu superior me'di·a'lis
—genu su'pre'ma
—glu'tae·a inferior
—glutaea superior
—glu'te·a inferior
—glutea superior
—haem'or·rhoi·da'lis
  inferior
—haemorrhoidalis me'di·a
—haemorrhoidalis superior
—he·pat'i·ca
—hepatica com·mu'nis
—hepatica pro'pri·a
—hy'a·loi'de·a
—hy'po·gas'tri·ca
—il'e·o·col'i·ca
—i·li'a·ca com·mu'nis
—iliaca ex·ter'na
—iliaca in·ter'na
—il'i·o·lum·ba'lis
—in·fra·or'bi·ta'lis
—in'ter·cos·ta'lis su·pre'ma
—in'ter·os'se·a anterior
—interossea com·mu'nis
—interossea dor·sa'lis
—interossea posterior
—interossea re·cur'rens
—interossea vo·lar'is
—la·bi·a'lis inferior
—labialis superior
—lab'y·rin'thi'

—lac'ri·ma'lis
—la·ryn'ge·a inferior
—laryngea superior
—li'e·na'lis
—lig'a·men'ti' te·re'tis
  u'ter·i'
—lin·gua'lis
—lo'bi' cau·da'ti'
—lum·ba'lis i'ma
—lu·so'ri·a
—mal'le·o·lar'is anterior
  lat'er·a'lis
—malleolaris anterior
  me'de·a'lis
—malleolaris posterior
  lat'er·a'lis
—malleolaris posterior
  me'di·a'lis
—mam·mar'i·a in'ter'na
—mas'se·ter'i·ca
—max'il·lar'is
—maxillaris ex·ter'na
—maxillaris in·ter'na
—me'di·a'na
—me·nin'ge·a anterior
—meningea me'di·a
—meningea posterior
—men·ta'lis
—mes'en·ter'i·ca inferior
—mesenterica superior
—mus'cu·lo·phren'i·ca
—nu·tri'ci·a fem'or·is
  inferior
—nutricia femoris superior
—nutricia fib'u·lae'
—nutricia hu'mer·i'
—nutricia tib'i·ae'
—ob·tu·ra·to'ri·a
—obturatoria ac'ces·so'ri·a
—oc·cip'i·ta'lis
—oph·thal'mi·ca
—o·var'i·ca
—pal'a·ti'na a·scen'dens
—palatina de·scen'dens
—palatina major
—pan'cre·at'i·ca dor·sa'lis
—pancreatica inferior
—pancreatica mag'na
—pan'cre·at'i·co·du'o·de·na'lis
  inferior
—pancreaticoduodenalis
  superior
—pe'nis

—per'fo·rans' pri'ma
—perforans se·cun'da
—perforans ter'ti·a
—per'i·car'di·a·co·phren'i·ca
—per'i·ne·a'lis
—per'i·ne'i'
—per'o·ne·a
—pha·ryn'ge·a a·scen'dens
—phren'i·ca inferior
—plan·tar'is lat'er·a'lis
—plantaris me'di·a'lis
—pop·lit'e·a
—prin'ceps' pol'li·cis
—pro·fun'da bra'chi·i'
—profunda cli·to'ri·dis
—profunda fem'o·ris
—profunda lin'guae'
—profunda pe'nis
—pu·den'da in·ter'na
—pul'mo·na'lis
—pulmonalis dex'tra
—pulmonalis si·nis'tra
—ra'di·a'lis
—radialis in'di·cis
—rec·ta'lis inferior
—rectalis me'di·a
—rectalis superior
—re·cur'rens ra'di·a'lis
—recurrens tib'i·a'lis
  anterior
—recurrens tibialis posterior
—recurrens ul·nar'is
—re·na'lis
—sa·cra'lis lat'er·a'lis
—sacralis me'di·a
—sacralis me'di·a·na
—scap'u·lar'is de·scen'dens
—scapularis dor·sa'lis
—seg·men'ti' an·te'ri·o'ris
—segmenti anterioris
  in·fe'ri·o'ris
—segmenti anterioris
  su·pe'ri·o'ris
—segmenti in·fe'ri·o'ris
—segmenti lat'er·a'lis
—segmenti me'di·a'lis
—segmenti pos·te'ri·o'ris
—segmenti su·pe'ri·o'ris
—sper'mat'i·ca ex·ter'na
—spermatica in·ter'na
—sphe'no·pal'a·ti'na
—spi'na'lis anterior
—spinalis posterior

—ster'no·clei'do·mas·toi'de·a
—sty'lo·mas·toi'de·a
—sub·cla'vi·a
—sub'cos·ta'lis
—sub·lin·gua'lis
—sub'men·ta'lis
—sub·scap'u·lar'is
—su'pra·or'bi·ta'lis
—su'pra·re·na'lis inferior
—suprarenalis me'di·a
—suprarenalis superior
—su'pra·scap'u·lar'is
—su'pra·troch'le·ar'is
—tar'se·a lat'er·a'lis
—tem'po·ra'lis me'di·a
—temporalis pro·fun'da
 anterior
—temporalis profunda
 posterior
—temporalis su'per·fi'ci·a'lis
—tes·tic'u·lar'is
—tho·ra·ca'lis lat'er·a'lis
—thoracalis su·pre'ma
—tho·rac'i·ca in·ter'na
—thoracica lat'er·a'lis
—thoracica su·pre'ma
—tho·ra·co·a·cro'mi·a'lis
—tho'ra·co·dor·sa'lis
—thy're·oi'de·a i'ma
—thyreoidea inferior
—thyreoidea superior
—thy·roi'de·a i'ma
—thyroidea inferior
—thyroidea superior
—tib'i·a'lis anterior
—tibialis posterior
—trans·ver'sa col'li'
—transversa fa'ci·e'i'
—transversa scap'u·lae'
—tym·pan'i·ca anterior
—tympanica inferior
—tympanica posterior
—tympanica superior
—ul'nar'is
—um·bil'i·ca'lis
—u're·thra'lis
—u'ter·i'na
—vag'i·na'lis
—ver'te·bra'lis
—ves'i·ca'lis inferior
—vesicalis superior
—vo'lar'is in'di·cis ra'di·a'-
 lis

—zy'go·mat'i·co·or'bi·
 ta'lis
ar·te'ri·ae'
—al've·o·lar'es' su·pe'ri·o'-
 res' an·te'ri·o'res'
—ar'ci·for'mes'
—ar'cu·a'tae' re'nis
—bron'chi·a'les'
—cer'e·bri'
—cil'i·ar'es' an·te'ri·o'res'
—ciliares pos·te'ri·o'res'
 brev'es'
—ciliares posteriores lon'-
 gae'
—con·junc'ti·va'les' an·te'-
 ri·o'res'
—conjunctivales pos·te'ri·
 o'res'
—dig'i·ta'les' dor·sa'les
 ma'nus
—digitales dorsales pe'dis
—digitales pal·mar'es'
 com·mu'nes'
—digitales palmares
 pro'pri·ae'
—digitales plan·tar'es'
 com·mu'nes'
—digitales plantares
 pro'pri·ae'
—digitales vo·lar'es'
 com·mu'nes'
—digitales volares
 pro'pri·ae'
—ep'i·scle·ra'les'
—gas'tri·cae' brev'es'
—hel'i·ci'nae' pe'nis
—il'e·ae'
—il'e·i'
—in'ter·cos·ta'les' pos'te·ri·
 o'res' I et II
—intercostales posteriores
 III-XI
—in'ter·lo·bar'es' re'nis
—in'ter·lob·u'lar'es'
 hep'a·tis
—interlobulares re'nis
—in·tes'ti·na'les'
—je·ju·na'les'
—la'bi·a'les' an·te'ri·o'res'
 pu·den'di' mu'li·e'bris
—labiales pos·te'ri·o'res'
 pu·den'di' mu'li·e'bris
—lum·ba'les'

—me'di·as'ti·na'les'
 an·te'ri·o'res'
—met'a·car'pe·ae' dor·sa'-
 les'
—metacarpeae pal·mar'es'
—metacarpeae vo·lar'es'
—met'a·tar'se·ae' dor·sa'-
 les'
—metatarseae plan·tar'es'
—na·sa'les' pos·te'ri·o'res',
 lat'er·a'les', et sep'ti'
—nu·tri'ci·ae' hu'mer·i'
—nutriciae pel'vis re·na'lis
—oe·so'pha'ge·ae'
—pal'a·ti'nae' mi·no'res'
—pal'pe·bra'les' lat'er·a'les'
—palpebrales me'di·a'les'
—pan'cre·at'i·co·du'o·de·na'les'
 in·fe'ri·o'res'
—per'fo'ran'tes'
—phren'i·cae' in·fe'ri·o'res'
—phrenicae su·pe'ri·o'res'
—rec'ur·ren'tes' ul'nar'es'
—re'nis
—ret'ro·du'o·de·na'les'
—sa·cra'les' lat'er·a'les'
—scro·ta'les' an·te'ri·o'res'
—scrotales pos·te'ri·o'res'
—sig·moi'de·ae'
—su'pra·du'o·de·na'les'
 su·pe'ri·o'res'
—su·ra'les'
—tar'se·ae' me'di·a'les'
—tem'po·ra'les' pro·fun'-
 dae'
—thy'mi·cae'
—ves'i·ca'les' in·fe'ri·o'res'
—vesicales su·pe'ri·o'res'
ar·te'ri·al
ar·te'ri·al·i·za'tion
ar·te'ri·a'sis pl. -ses'
ar·te'ri·ec'ta·sis pl. -ses'
ar·te'ri·ec·to·my
ar·te'ri·ec·to'pi·a
ar·te'ri·o·cap'il·lar'y
ar·te'ri·o·fi·bro'sis pl. -ses'
ar·te'ri·o·gram'
ar·te'ri·o·graph'
ar·te'ri·o·graph'ic
ar·te'ri·og'ra·phy
ar·te'ri·o'la pl. -lae'
—mac'u·lar'is inferior
—macularis superior

—me′di·a′lis ret′i·nae′
—na·sa′lis ret′i′nae′ inferior
—nasalis retinae superior
—rec′ta
—tem′po·ra′lis ret′i′nae′
 inferior
—temporalis retinae
 superior
ar·te′ri·o′lae′ rec′tae′ re′nis
ar·te′ri·o′lar
ar·te′ri·ole′
ar·te′ri·o·lith′
ar·te′ri·o·lith′ic
ar·te′ri·o·li′tis
ar·te′ri·o′lo·ne·cro′sis
 pl. -ses′
ar·te′ri·o′lo·ne·crot′ic
ar·te′ri·o′lo·scle·ro′sis
 pl. -ses′
ar·te′ri·o′lo·scle·rot′ic
ar·te′ri·o·ma·la′ci·a
ar·te′ri·o·mes′en·ter′ic
ar·te′ri·o·mo′tor
ar·te′ri·o·my′o·ma·to′sis
 pl. -ses′
ar·te′ri·o·ne·cro′sis *pl.* -ses′
ar·te′ri·op′a·thy
ar·te′ri·o·plas′tic
ar·te′ri·o·plas′ty
ar·te′ri·o·pres′sor
ar·te′ri·o·punc′ture
ar·te′ri·o·re′nal
ar·te′ri·or′rha·phy
ar·te′ri·or·rhex′is
 pl. -rhex′es′
ar·te′ri·o·scle·ro′sis *pl.* -ses′
 —o·blit′er·ans′
ar·te′ri·o·scle·rot′ic
ar·te′ri·o·spasm
ar·te′ri·o·spas′tic
ar·te′ri·o·ste·no′sis *pl.* -ses′
ar·te′ri·os·to′sis *pl.* -ses′
ar·te′ri·o·strep′sis *pl.* -ses′
ar·te′ri·o·sym′pa·thec′-
 to·my
ar·te′ri·o·tome′
ar·te′ri·ot′o·my
ar·te′ri·o·ve′nous
ar·te′ri·o·ver′sion
ar·te·ri′tis
 —de·for′mans′
 —o·blit′er·ans′
ar′ter·y

ar·thral′gi·a
 —hys·ter′i·ca
 —sat′ur·ni′na
ar·thral′gic
ar·threc′to·my
ar·thres·the′i·a
ar′thri·flu′ent
ar·thrit′ic
ar′thri·tide′
ar·thri′tis
 —de·for′mans′
 —fun·go′sa
 —u′re·thrit′i·ca
ar·throc′a·ce
ar′thro·cele′
ar′thro·cen·te′sis *pl.* -ses′
ar′thro·chon·dri′tis
ar′thro·cla′si·a
ar′thro·cla′sis *pl.* -ses′
ar′thro·de′si·a
ar′thro·de′sis *pl.* -ses′
ar·thro′di·a *pl.* -ae′
ar·thro′di·al
ar′thro·dyn′i·a
ar′thro·dyn′ic
ar′thro·dys·pla′si·a
ar′thro·em′py·e′sis *pl.* -ses′
ar′thro·en·dos′co·py
ar′thro·e·rei′sis
ar′thro·fi·bro′sis *pl.* -ses′
ar·throg′e·nous
ar′thro·gram′
ar·throg′ra·phy
ar′thro·gry·po′sis *pl.* -ses′
 —mul′ti·plex′ con·gen′i·ta
ar′thro·ka·tad′y·sis *pl.* -ses′
ar′thro·klei′sis *pl.* -ses′
ar′thro·lith′
ar′thro·li·thi′a·sis *pl.* -ses′
ar·throl′o·gy
ar·throl′y·sis *pl.* -ses′
ar′thro·men·in·gi′tis
ar·throm′e·ter
ar·throm′e·try
ar·thron′cus
ar′thro·neu·ral′gi·a
ar′thro·on′y·cho·dys·
 pla′si·a
ar′thro-oph′thal·mop′a·thy
ar′thro·os′te·o·on′y·cho·
 dys·pla′si·a
ar′thro·path′ic
ar·throp′a·thy

ar′thro·phy′ma
ar′thro·phyte′
ar′thro·plas′tic
ar′thro·plas′ty
ar′thro·pod
Ar·throp′o·da
ar′thro·py·o′sis *pl.* -ses′
ar′thro·rheu′ma·tism
ar′thro·scle·ro′sis *pl.* -ses′
ar′thro·scope′
ar·thros′co·py
ar·thro′sis *pl.* -ses′
ar′thro·spore′
ar·thros′to·my
ar′thro·syn′o·vi′tis
ar′thro·tome′
ar′thro·to·mog′ra·phy
ar·throt′o·my
ar′thro·trop′ic
ar′throus
ar′thro·xe·ro′sis *pl.* -ses′
ar·throx′e·sis *pl.* -ses′
Ar′thur performance scale
Ar′thus phenomenon
ar′ti·cle
ar·tic′u·lar
ar·tic′u·lar′e′
ar·tic′u·lar′is gen′us
ar·tic′u·late′, -lat′ed, -lat′ing
ar·tic′u·la′ti·o′
 pl. -la′ti·o′nes′
 —a·cro′mi·o·cla·vic′u·lar′is
 —at′lan′to·ax′i·a′lis lat·er·
  a′lis
 —atlantoaxialis me′di·a′na
 —at′lan′to·ep′i′stroph′i·ca
 —at′lan′to·oc·cip′i·ta′lis
 —cal·ca′ne·o·cu·boi′de·a
 —cap′i·tis cos′tae′
 —ca·pit′u·li′
 —car′po·met′a·car′pe·a
  pol′li·cis
 —coch′le·ar′is
 —com·pos′i·ta
 —con′dy·lar′is
 —cos′to·trans·ver′sar′i·a
 —co′tyl·i′ca
 —cox′ae′
 —cri′co·ar′y·tae·noi′de·a
 —cri′co·ar′y·te·noi′de·a
 —cri′co·thy′re·oi′de·a
 —cri′co·thy′roi′de·a
 —cu′bi·ti′

—cu'ne·o·na·vic'u·lar'is
—el'lip·soi'de·a
—gen'u
—ge'nus
—hu'mer·i'
—hu'mer·o·ra'di·a'lis
—hu'mer·o·ul·nar'is
—in·cu'do·mal'le·ar'is
—in·cu'do·mal'le·o·lar'is
—in·cu'do·sta·pe'di·a
—man·dib'u·lar'is
—ma'nus
—me'di·o·car'pe·a
—os'sis pi'si·for'mis
—pe'dis
—pla'na
—ra·di·o·car'pe·a
—ra·di·o·ul·nar'is dis·ta'lis
—radioulnaris prox'i·ma'lis
—sac'ro·i·li'a·ca
—sel·lar'is
—sim'plex'
—sphe·roi'de·a
—ster'no·cla·vic'u·lar'is
—sub'ta·lar'is
—ta'li' trans·ver'sa
—ta'lo·cal·ca'ne·a
—ta'lo·cal·ca'ne·o·na·vic'u·lar'is
—ta'lo·cru·ra'lis
—ta'lo·na·vic'u·lar'is
—tar'si' trans·ver'sa
—tem'po·ro·man·dib'u·lar'is
—tib'i·o·fib'u·lar'is
—tro·choi'de·a
ar·tic'u·la'tion
ar·tic'u·la'ti·o'nes'
—ca·pit'u·lo'rum cos·
 tar'um
—car'po·met'a·car'pe·ae'
—cos'to·chon·dra'les'
—cos'to·ver'te·bra'les'
—dig'i·to'rum ma'nus
—digitorum pe'dis
—in'ter·car'pe·ae'
—in'ter·chon·dra'les'
—interchondrales cos·tar'um
—in'ter·met'a·car'pe·ae'
—in'ter·met'a·tar'se·ae'
—in'ter·pha·lan'ge·ae'
 ma'nus
—interphalangeae pe'dis
—in'ter·tar'se·ae'
—ma'nus

—met'a·car'po·pha·lan'ge·ae'
—met'a·tar'so·pha·lan'ge·ae'
—os'sic'u·lo'rum au·di'tus
—pe'dis
—ster'no·cos·ta'les'
—tar'so·met'a·tar'se·ae'
ar·tic'u·la'tor
ar·tic'u·la·to'ry
ar·tic'u·lus *pl.* -li'
ar'ti·fact'
ar'ti·fac·ti'tious
ar'ti·fi'cial
ar'y·ep'i·glot'tic
ar'y·ep'i·glot'ti·cus
ar'yl·ar'so·nate'
ar'yl·cy'clo·hex'yl·am'ine
ar'yl·ene'
ar'yl·sul'fo·trans'fer·ase'
ar'yl·trans'fer·ase'
ar'y·te'no·ep'i·glot'tic
ar'y·te'noid'
ar'y·te'noi·dec'to·my
ar'y·te'noi·di'tis
ar'y·te'noi·do·pex'y
ar'y·vo·cal'is
as'a·fet'i·da
a·sa'phi·a
as'a·rum
as·bes'ti·form
as·bes'tos
as·bes·to'sis *pl.* -ses'
as·ca·ri'a·sis *pl.* -ses'
as·car'i·cide'
as·ca'rid *pl.* -rids *or*
 as·car'i·des'
As·ca·rid'i·a
as·car'i·dole'
As·ca·ris
—e·quo'rum
—lum'bri·coi'des'
—meg'a·lo·ceph'a·la
—mys'tax'
—su'um
As·ca·rops
as·cend'
Asch operation
Asch'heim-Zon'dek
—reaction
—test
Asch'ner phenomenon
Asch'off'
—bodies
—cell

—nodules
Asch'off-Ro'ki·tan'sky
 sinus
Asch'off-Ta·wa'ra node
as·ci'tes' *pl.* as·ci'tes'
—ad'i·po'sus
—chy·lo'sus
—sac·ca'tus
—vag'i·na'lis
—vul·ga'ti·or'
as·cit'ic
as'co·carp'
as'co·go·nid'i·um *pl.* -i·a
As·co'li
—test
—treatment
As'co·my·ce'tes'
as'co·my·ce'tous
a·scor'bate'
a·scor'bic
as'co·spore'
as·cribe', -cribed', -crib'ing
as'cus *pl.* -ci'
A·sel'i glands
as'e·ma'si·a
a·se'mi·a
a·sep'sis *pl.* -ses'
a·sep'tic
a·sex'u·al
Ash'er·man syndrome
Ash'man phenomenon
a'si·a'li·a
a·si·a·lo·gly'co·pro'tein'
a·si·a·lor·rhe'a
A'sian influenza virus
a·si·at'i·co'side'
a·sid·er·o'sis *pl.* -ses'
a·sid·er·ot'ic
As'ken·stedt' method
a·so'cial
a·so'ma
a·so'mous
a·so'ni·a
as·pal'a·so'ma
as·par'a·gin·ase'
as·par'a·gine'
as·par'a·gin·ic
as·par'a·gin·yl
as·par'a·mide'
as·par'tame'
as·par'tase'
as·par'tate' a·mi'no·trans'-
 fer·ase'

as·par'tic
as·par'to·cin
as·par'to·ki·nase'
as·par'tyl
a·spas'tic
a·spe·cif'ic
as·pect'
as·per·gil'lic
as·per·gil'lin
as·per·gil·lo'ma *pl.* -mas *or*
  -ma·ta
as·per·gil'lo·sis *pl.* -ses'
as·per·gil'lo·tox'i·co'sis
  pl. -ses'
As·per·gil'lus
as·per·lin
a·sper·mat'ic
a·sper'ma·tism
a·sper'ma·to·gen·e·sis
a·sper'mi·a
a·sper'mous
as·per'sion
as·phal·ge'si·a
a·spher'ic *or* a·spher'i·cal
as·phyx'i·a
  —liv'i·da
  —ne'o·na·to'rum
  —pal'li·da
as·phyx'i·al
as·phyx'i·ant
as·phyx'i·ate', -at'ed, -at'ing
as·pid'i·um
as·pi·do·sper'ma
as·pi·do·sper'mine'
as·pi·rate', -rat'ed, -rat'ing
as·pi·ra'tion
as·pi·ra'tor
as·pi·rin
As'pis
  —cor·nu'tus
a·sple'ni·a
a·sple'nic
a·spo'ro·gen'ic
as·po·rog'e·nous
a·spo'rous
a·spor'u·late'
As·sam' fever
as'say'
as·sess', -sessed', -sess'ing
as·sess'a·ble
as·sess'ment
as·si·dent
as·sim'i·la·ble

as·sim'i·late'
as·sim'i·la'tion
as·sim'i·la'tive
Ass'mann focus
as·so'ci·a'tion
as·so'ci·a·tive
as'so·nance
a·sta'si·a
a·sta'si·a-a·ba'si·a
a·stat'ic
as'ta·tine'
a·sta·xan'thin
a·ste'a·to'sis *pl.* -ses'
a·stem'i·zole'
as'ter
a·ster'e·o·cog·no·sy
a·ster'e·og·no'sis *pl.* -ses'
as·ter'ic
as·te'ri·on' *pl.* -ri·a
as·ter'ix'is
a·ster'nal
a·ster'ni·a
as'ter·o·coc'cus
as'ter·oid'
as·the'ni·a
  —cru'rum par'es·thet'i·ca
  —pig'men·to'sa
  —u'ni·ver·sa'lis con·gen'-
    i·ta
as·then'ic
as'the·no·bi·o'sis
as'the·no·co'ri·a
as'the·nom'e·ter
as'the·nope'
as'the·no·pho'bi·a
as'the·no'pi·a
as'the·nop'ic
as'the·no·sper'mi·a
as'the·nox'i·a
asth'ma
asth·mat'ic
asth·mat'i·form'
asth·mo·gen'ic
a·stig'ma·graph'
as·tig'mat'ic
a·stig'ma·tism
a·stig'ma·tom'e·ter
as·tig'mat'o·scope'
a·stig'mi·a
a·stig'mic
as'tig·mom'e·ter
as'tig·mom'e·try
a·stig'mo·scope'

as'tig·mos'co·py
a·stom'a·tous
a·sto'mi·a
a·sto'mous
a·strag'a·lar
a·strag'a·lec'to·my
a·strag'a·lo·cal·ca'ne·al
a·strag'a·lo·cru'ral
a·strag'a·lo·scaph'oid'
a·strag'a·lo·tib'i·al
a·strag'a·lus *pl.* -li'
as'tral
a·stric'tion
a·strin'gen·cy
a·strin'gent
as·tro·bi·ol'o·gy
as·tro·blast'
as·tro·blas·to'ma *pl.* -mas *or*
  -ma·ta
as·tro·cyte'
as·tro·cyt'ic
as·tro·cy·to'ma *pl.* -mas *or*
  -ma·ta
  —gi·gan'to·cel'lu·lar'e'
as·tro·cy·to'sis *pl.* -ses'
as·trog'i·a
as·trog'li·o'ma *pl.* -mas *or*
  -ma·ta
as'troid'
as·tro'ma *pl.* -mas *or* -ma·ta
as'tro·sphere'
as·tro·spher'ic
As'trup method
a'syl·la·bi·a
a·sym·bo'li·a
a·sym·met'ric *or*
  a·sym·met'ri·cal
a·sym'me·try
a·sym'phy·tous
a·symp'to·mat'ic
as'ymp·tot'ic
a·syn·ap'sis *pl.* -ses'
a·syn'chro·nism
a·syn'chro·nous
a·syn'chro·ny
a·syn'cli·tism
a·syn'de·sis *pl.* -ses'
a·syn'det'ic
a·syn·ech'i·a
a·syn'er'e·sis
a·syn·er'gi·a
a·syn·er'gic
a·syn'er·gy

a'syn·o'vi·a
a'syn·tax'i·a
a'sys·tem'ic
a·sys'to·le
a'sys·to'li·a
a'sys·tol'ic
a·tac'tic
a·tac'ti·form'
at'a·rac'tic
at'ar·al·ge'si·a
at'a·rax'i·a
at'a·rax'ic
at'a·rax'y
at'a·vism
at'a·vis'tic
a·tax'i·a
—cor'dis
a·tax'i·a·gram'
a·tax'i·a·graph'
a·tax'i·am'e·ter
a·tax'i·a·pha'si·a
a·tax'i·a·tel·an'gi·ec·ta'si·a
a·tax'ic
a·tax'i·o·phe'mi·a
a·tax'i·o·pho'bi·a
a·tax'o·phe'mi·a
a·tax'y
at'e·lec'ta·sis *pl.* -ses'
at'e·lec·tat'ic
at'tel'ei·o'sis *pl.* -ses'
at'tel'ei·ot'ic
at'el·en'ce·pha'li·a
at'el·en·ceph'a·ly
a·tel'e·sis *pl.* -ses'
a·te'li·a
a·te'lic
a·tel'i·o'sis *pl.* -ses'
a·tel'i·ot'ic
at'e·lo·car'di·a
at'e·lo·ceph'a·lous
at'e·lo·chei'li·a
at'e·lo·chei'ri·a
at'e·lo·en'ce·pha'li·a
at'e·lo·glos'si·a
at'e·log·na'thi·a
at'e·lo·ki·ne'si·a
at'e·lo·my·e'li·a
at'e·lo·po'di·a
at'e·lo·pro·so'pi·a
at'e·lo·ra·chid'i·a
at'e·lo·sto'mi·a
a·ten'o·lol'
a·the'li·a

ath'er·ec'to·mize'
ath'er·ec'to·my
a·ther'mic
a·ther'mo·sys·tal'tic
ath'er·o·em'bo·lism
ath'er·o·gen'e·sis *pl.* -ses'
ath'er·o·gen'ic
ath'er·o'ma *pl.* -mas *or* -ma·ta
ath'er·o·ma·to'sis *pl.* -ses'
ath'er·om'a·tous
ath'er·o·ne·cro'sis *pl.* -ses'
ath'er·o·scler'o·gen'ic
ath'er·o·scle·ro'sis *pl.* -ses'
—o·blit'er·ans'
ath'er·o·scle·rot'ic
ath'e·toid'
ath'e·to'sic
ath'e·to'sis *pl.* -ses'
ath'e·tot'ic
a·thi'a·min·o'sis *pl.* -ses'
a·threp'si·a
a·threp'tic
ath'ro·cy·to'sis
a·thy'mi·a
a·thy'mic
a·thy're·a
a·thy're·o'sis *pl.* -ses'
a·thy're·ot'ic
a·thy'roid·ism
a·thy'ro·sis *pl.* -ses'
a·thy'rot'ic
At'kin e·piph'y·se'al
   fracture
at·lan'tad
at·lan'tal
at·lan'to·ax'i·al
at·lan'to·bas'i·lar'is
   in·ter'nus
at·lan'to·did'y·mus
at·lan'to·ep'i·stroph'ic
at·lan'to·mas'toid'
at·lan'to·oc·cip'i·tal
at·lan'to·o·don'toid'
at'las
at'lo·ax'oid'
at·mol'y·sis *pl.* -ses'
at·mom'e·ter
at'mos
a·to'ci·a
at'om
a·tom'ic
at'om·ism

at'om·is'tic
at'om·i·za'tion
at'om·ize', -ized', -iz'ing
at'om·iz'er
a·to'ni·a
a·ton'ic
a'to·nic'i·ty
at'o·ny
at'o·pen
a·top'ic
a·top'og·no'si·a
a·top'og·no'sis
at'o·py
a·tox'ic
ATPase
a·trach'e·lo·ceph'a·lus
a·trach'e·lous
at'ra·cu'ri·um
a·trans'fer·ri·ne'mi·a
a'trau·mat'ic
a·tre'mi·a
a·tre'si·a
—a'ni' vag'i·na'lis
—fol·lic'u·li'
—of i'ter
—vul'vae'
a·tre'sic
a·tret'ic
a·tre'to·ceph'a·lus
a·tre'to·cor'mus
a·tre'to·cys'ti·a
a·tre'to·gas'tri·a
a·tre'to·le'mi·a
a·tre'to·me'tri·a
at're·top'si·a
a·tre'tor·rhin'i·a
a·tre'to·sto'mi·a
a·tre'tu·re'thri·a
a'tri·al
a·trich'i·a
a·tri·cho'sis *pl.* -ses'
a·trich'ous
a'tri·o·fas·cic'u·lar
a'tri·og'ra·phy
a'tri·o-His'
—pathway
—tract
a'tri·o-His'i·an
—bypass tract
—fiber
a'tri·o·meg'a·ly
a'tri·o·sep'to·pex'y
a'tri·o·sep'to·plas'ty

a·tri·ot'o·my
a'tri·o·ven·tric'u·lar
a'tri·o·ven·tric'u·lar'is
  com·mu'nis
a'tri·um *pl.* a'tri·a
  —cor'dis
  —cordis dex'trum
  —cordis si·nis'trum
  —dex'trum
  —me·a'tus me'di·i'
  —of infection
  —si·nis'trum
  —va·gi'nae'
at'ro·lac'ta·mide'
a·tro'phi·a
  —bul'bi'
  —cer'e·bri·se·ni'lis sim'-
    plex'
  —cho·roi'de·ae' et ret'i·nae'
  —cu'tis
  —do'lo·ro'sa
  —mac'u·lo'sa cu'tis
  —mus'cu·lo'rum lip'o·
    mas·to'sa
  —pi·lo'rum pro'pri·a
  —se·nil'is
  —stri·a'ta et' mac'u·lo'sa
  —tes·tic'u·li'
  —un'gui·um
a'troph'ic
at'ro·phied'
at'ro·pho·der'ma
  —of Pa·si'ni and Pi'er·i'ni
  —re·tic'u·la'tum
  —ver·mic'u·lar'is
at'ro·phy
at'ro·pine'
at'ro·pin'i·za'tion
at'ro·scine'
at·tach'ment
at·tack'
at'tar
at·ten'tion
at·ten'u·ant
at·ten'u·ate', -at'ed, -at'ing
at·ten'u·a'tion
at'tic
at'tic·i'tis
at·ti·co·an·trot'o·my
at'ti·co·mas'toid'
at'ti·cot'o·my
at'ti·tude'
at·ti·tu'di·nal

at·tol'lens au'rem
at·to'ni·ty
at·trac'tion
at'tra·hens' au'rem
at·tri'tion
a·typ'i·a
a·typ'i·cal
Aub'-Du Bois' standards
Au'ber'ger blood group
Au'bert phenomenon
Auch'mer·o·my'ia
  —lu·te'o·la
au'dile
au'di·mut'ism
au'di·o' analgesia
au'di·o·ep'i·lep'tic
au'di·o·gen'ic
au'di·o·gram'
au'di·ol'o·gist
au'di·ol'o·gy
au'di·om'e·ter
au'di·om'e·trist
au'di·om'e·try
au'di·o-oc'u·lar
au'di·o·vis'u·al
au'di·phone'
au·di'tion
au'di·tive
au'di·tog·no'sis *pl.* -ses'
au'di·to-oc'u·lo·gy'ric
  reflex
au'di·to·ry
au'di·to·sen'so·ry
Au'en·brug'ger sign
Au'er
  —body
  —rod
Au'er·bach'
  —ganglions
  —plexus
au'gen·blick'
au'ger
aug·ment', -ment'ed,
  -ment'ing
aug'men·ta'tion
aug'men·tor
aug·na'thus
Augs'ber'ger rule
Au·jesz'ky disease
au'ra *pl.* -ras *or* -rae'
  —asth·mat'i·ca
  —cur·so'ri·a
  —hys·ter'i·ca

au'ral *(of the ear)*
  ♦oral
au·ra'no·fin
au·ran·ti'a·sis *pl.* -ses'
  —cu'tis
au·ran'ti·um
au'rate'
au·ri'a·sis *pl.* -ses'
au'ric
au'ri·cle
au·ric'u·la *pl.* -lae'
  —a'tri·i'
  —cor'dis
  —dex'tra
  —si·nis'tra
au·ric'u·lar
au·ric'u·lar'e' *pl.* -lar'i·a
au·ric'u·lar'is *pl.* -lar'es'
au·ric'u·lo·breg·mat'ic
au·ric'u·lo·cra'ni·al
au·ric'u·lo·fron·ta'lis
au·ric'u·lo·pal'pe·bral
au·ric'u·lo·pres'sor
au·ric'u·lo·tem'po·ral
au·ric'u·lo·ven·tric'u·lar
au'ri·form'
au'rin
au'ris *pl.* -res'
  —dex'tra
  —ex·ter'na
  —in·ter'na
  —me'di·a
  —si·nis'tra
au'ri·scope'
au'rist
au'ro·chro'mo·der'ma
  pl. -mas *or* -ma·ta
au'ro·pal'pe·bral
au'ro·ther'a·py
au'ro·thi'o·glu'cose'
au'ro·thi'o·gly'ca·nide'
au'rous
au'rum
aus·cult'
aus·cul'tate', -tat'ed, -tat'ing
aus·cul'ta'tion
aus·cul'ta·to'ry
Aus'tin and Van Slyke
  method
Aus'tin Flint
  —murmur
  —phenomenon
Aus'tra'lia antigen

Aus'tra·lor'bis
au'ta·coid'
aut'ar·ce'sis
au·te'cic
au·te'cious
au·te·me'si·a
au'tism
—pau'vre
au·tis'tic
au'to·ag·glu'ti·na'tion
au'to·ag·glu'ti·nin
au'to·al·ler'gic
au'to·am·pu·ta'tion
au'to·a·nal'y·sis *pl.* -ses'
au'to·an·am·ne'sis *pl.* -ses'
au'to·an'ti·bod'y
au'to·an'ti·gen
au'to·an'ti·tox'in
au'to·au'di·ble
au'to·ca·tal'y·sis *pl.* -ses'
au'to·cat'a·lyst
au'to·cat'a·lyt'ic
au'to·ca·thar'sis *pl.* -ses'
au'to·cho'le·cys'to·du'o·
  de·nos'to·my
au'to·cho'le·cys'to·trans'-
  verse·co·los'to·my
au·toch'tho·nous
au'to·cla'si·a
au·toc'la·sis *pl.* -ses'
au'to·clav'a·ble
au'to·clave'
au'to·crine
au'to·cy·tol'y·sis *pl.* -ses'
au'to·cy'to·tox'in
au'to·di·ges'tion
au'to·dip'loi·dy
au'to·ech'o·la'li·a
au'to·ech'o·prax'i·a
au'to·ec·ze'ma·ti·za'tion
au'to·e·rot'ic
au'to·e·rot'i·cism
au'to·er'o'tism
au'to·fluo·res'cence
au'to·fluo·res'cent
au'to·fluor'o·scope'
au'to·fluo·ros'co·py
au'to·fu'sion
au·tog'a·mous
au·tog'a·my
au'to·gen'e·sis *pl.* -ses'
au'to·ge·net'ic
au'to·gen'ic

au'tog'e·nous
au'tog·no'sis
au'to·graft'
au'to·graph'ism
au'to·he'mag·glu'ti·nin
au'to·hem'ag·glu'ti·na'tion
au'to·he·mol'y·sis *pl.* -ses'
au'to·he·mo·ther'a·py
au'to·hy·drol'y·sis
au'to·hyp·no'sis *pl.* -ses'
au'to·hyp·not'ic
au'to·hyp'no·tism
au'to·im·mune'
au'to·im·mu'ni·ty
au'to·im'mu·ni·za'tion
au'to·in·fec'tion
au'to·in·fu'sion
au'to·in·oc'u·la·ble
au'to·in·oc'u·la'tion
au'to·in·tox'i·cant
au'to·in·tox'i·ca'tion
au'to·i·sol'y·sin
au'to·ker'a·to·plas'ty
au'to·ki·ne'sis
au'to·ki·net'ic
au'to·le'sion
au'to·leu'ko·ag·glu'ti·nin
au'tol'o·gous
au'to·lym'pho·cyte'
au·tol'y·sate'
au·tol'y·sin
au·tol'y·sis
au'to·lyt'ic
au'to·lyze', -lyzed', -lyz'ing
au'to·ma·tic'i·ty
au·tom'a·tism
au'to·mat'o·graph'
au·tom'a·ton *pl.* -tons *or* -ta
au·to·mix'is *pl.* -es
au'tom·ne'si·a
au'to·my'so·pho'bi·a
au'to·ne·phrec'to·my
au'to·no·ma'si·a
au'to·nom'ic
au'to·nom'o·trop'ic
au·ton'o·mous
au·ton'o·my
au'to-oph·thal'mo·scope'
au'to-oph'thal·mos'co·py
au'to-ox'i·da'tion
au'to·path'ic
au'top'a·thy
au'to·pha'gi·a

au'to·pha'gic
au'to·phag'o·some'
au'toph·a'gy
au'to·phil'i·a
au'to·pho'bi·a
au'to·pho'ni·a
au·toph'o·ny
aut'oph·thal'mo·scope'
aut'oph·thal·mos'co·py
au'to·plast'
au'to·plas'tic
au'to·plas'ty
au'to·ploid'
au'to·ploi'dy
au'to·pneu'mo·nec'to·my
au'to·pol'y·mer
au'to·pol'y·mer'i·za'tion
au'to·pol'y·mer·iz'ing
  resin
au'to·pol'y·ploi'dy
au'to·pre·cip'i·tin
au'to·pro·throm'bin
au'to·pro·tol'y·sis *pl.* -ses'
au'top·sy
au'to·psy'che
au'to·psy'chic
au'to·psy·cho'sis *pl.* -ses'
au'to·ra'di·o·gram'
au'to·ra'di·o·graph'
au'to·ra'di·og'ra·phy
au'to·reg'u·la'tion
au'to·re'in·fu'sion
au'to·sen'si·ti·za'tion
au'to·sep'ti·ce'mi·a
au'to·se'rum
au'to·site'
au'to·sit'ic
au'to·so'mal
au'to·some'
au'to·sple·nec'to·my
au'to·sta'pling
au'to·sug·gest'i·bil'i·ty
au'to·sug·ges'tion
au'to·syn·de'sis
au'to·ther'a·py
au·tot'o·my
au'to·top'ag·no'si·a
au'to·tox'ic
au'to·tox'in
au'to·trans·fu'sion
au'to·trans'plant'
au'to·trans'plan·ta'tion
au'to·troph'

au'to·troph'ic
au'to·vac'ci·na'tion
au'to·vac'cine'
au·tox'i·da'tion
aux·an'o·gram'
aux'a·no·graph'ic
aux'a·nog'ra·phy
aux·e'sis *pl.* -ses'
aux·et'ic
aux·il'ia·ry
aux'i·lyt'ic
aux'in
aux'o·chrome'
aux'o·cyte'
aux'o·drome'
aux·om'e·ter
aux'o·ton'ic
aux'o·troph'
aux'o·troph'ic
AV
—nicking
—node
A-V
—patterns
—syndromes
av'a·lanche'
a·val'vu·lar
a·vas'cu·lar
a·vas'cu·lar·i·za'tion
a·vas'cu·lar·ize', -ized',
-iz'ing
A·vel'lis
—paralysis
—syndrome
a·ve'nin
a·ver'sion
a·ver'sive
a'vi·an
av'i·din
A·vi'la
—approach
—technique
a·vir'u·lent
a·vi'ta·min·o'sis *pl.* -ses'
A'vo·ga'dro
—constant
—numbe
a·void'ance
a·void'ant
av'oir·du·pois'
a·vulse'
a·vul'sion
a wave

a'xan·thop'si·a
Ax'en·feld' syndrome
a·xen'ic
a'xe·roph'thol'
ax'i·al
ax'i·a'tion
ax·if'u·gal
ax·il'la *pl.* -lae' *or* -las
ax'il·lar'y
ax·il·lo·bi·fem'o·ral
ax·il·lo·fem'o·ral
ax'i·o·buc'cal
ax'i·o·buc'co·cer'vi·cal
ax'i·o·buc'co·gin'gi·val
ax'i·o·buc'co·lin'gual
ax'i·o·cer'vi·cal
ax'i·o·dis'tal
ax'i·o·dis'to·cer'vi·cal
ax'i·o·dis'to·gin'gi·val
ax'i·o·dis'to·in·ci'sal
ax'i·o·dis'to·oc·clu'sal
ax'i·o·gin'gi·val
ax'i·o·in·ci'sal
ax'i·o·la'bi·al
ax'i·o·la'bi·o·gin'gi·val
ax'i·o·la'bi·o·lin'gual
ax'i·o·lin'gual
ax'i·o·lin'guo·cer'vi·cal
ax'i·o·lin'guo·gin'gi·val
ax'i·o·lin'guo·oc·clu'sal
ax'i·o·me'si·al
ax'i·o·me'si·o·cer'vi·cal
ax'i·o·me'si·o·dis'tal
ax'i·o·me'si·o·gin'gi·val
ax'i·o·me'si·o·in·ci'sal
ax'i·o·oc·clu'sal
ax'i·o·pul'pal
ax·ip'e·tal
ax'is *pl.* ax'es'
—bul'bi' ex·ter'nus
—bulbi in·ter'nus
—len'tis
—oc'u·li' ex·ter'na
—oculi in·ter'na
—op'ti·ca
—op'ti·cus
—pel'vis
—u'ter·i'
ax'le
ax'o·den·drit'ic
ax·og'e·nous *(originating in an axon)*
♦*exogenous*

ax'oid'
ax·oi'de·an
ax'o·lem'ma
ax·ol'y·sis *pl.* -ses'
ax'o·mat'ic
ax·om'e·ter
ax'on'
ax'o·nal
ax'on·a·prax'is
ax'one'
ax'o·ne'ma
ax'o·neme'
ax'o·nom'e·ter
ax'on·ot·me'sis *pl.* -ses'
ax·op'e·tal
ax'o·plasm
ax'o·po'di·um
ax'o·style'
a'ya·huas'co
Ay'a·la
—index
—quotient
—test
A·yer'za
—disease
—syndrome
az'a·cy'clo·nol'
az'a·gua'nine'
az'a·me·tho'ni·um
az'a·per·one'
az·ap'e·tine'
az'a·ri'bine'
az'a·ser'ine'
az·at'a·dine'
az'a·thi'o·prine'
a·zed'a·rach'
az·e'la·ic
a'ze·o·trope'
a'ze·o·trop'ic
az'e·pin'a·mide'
az'e·te'pa
az'ide'
az'i·do·thy'mi·dine'
az'ine'
az·lo·cil'lin
az'o·ben'zene'
az'o·car'mine G
az'o·lit'min
a·zo'o·sper'ma·tism
a·zo'o·sper'mi·a
az'o·pro'tein
az'ote'
az'o·te'mi·a

az'o·tem'ic
a·zot'ic
a·zot'i·fi·ca'tion
Az'o·to·bac'ter
az'o·tom'e·ter
az'o·to·my'cin
az'o·tor·rhe'a
az'o·tu'ri·a
az'o·tu'ric
az·tre'o·nam'
az'ul'
az'u·lene'
az'ure
az'u·res'in
a·zu'ro·phil'
az'u·ro·phil'i·a
az'u·ro·phil'ic
az'y·go·ag'na·thus
a·zy'go·gram'
az'y·gog'ra·phy
az'y·gos' (*unpaired anatomic
structure*)
♦*azygous*
az'y·gous (*unpaired*)
♦*azygos*
a·zy'mi·a
a·zy'mic

B

Baas'trup disease
Bab'bitt metal
Bab'cock'
—operation
—test
Bab'cock-Le'vy test
Ba·bés'-Ernst' bodies
Ba·be'si·a
—bi·gem'i·na
—bo'vis
—ca'nis
—e'qui'
—o'vis
bab'e·si'a·sis *pl.* -ses'
ba·be'si·o'sis *pl.* -ses'
Ba·bés' nodules
Ba·bin'ski
—phenomenon
—platysma sign
—pronation phenomenon
—reflex
—sign
—syndrome

—tonus test
Ba·bin'ski-Froeh'lich
disease
Ba·bin'ski-Na·geotte'
syndrome
Ba·bin'ski-Va·quez'
syndrome
bac'cate'
bac'ci·form'
Ba·cel'li sign
Bach'mann bundle
Bach'man test
Bach'ti·a'row' sign
Bac'il·la'ce·ae'
bac'il·lar
bac'il·lar'y
bac'il·le'mi·a
ba·cil'li·form'
ba·cil'lin
bac'il·lo'sis *pl.* -ses'
bac'il·lu'ri·a
ba·cil'lus *pl.* -li'
—Cal'mette'-Gué·rin'
Ba·cil'lus
—ac'i·doph'i·lus
—aer·og'e·nes' cap'su·la'tus
—aer'try·cke
—ag'ni'
—an'thra·cis
—bi'fi·dus
—bo'vi·sep'ti·cus
—brev'is
—co'li'
—diph·the'ri·ae'
—er'y·sip'e·la'tos-su'is
—fe·ca'lis al'ca·lig'e·nes'
—gas·troph'i·lus
—hof·man'ni·i'
—in'flu·en'zae'
—lac'tis aer·og'e·nes'
—lac'u·na'tus
—lep'rae'
—mal'le·i'
—mes'en·ter'i·cus
—mu·co'sus cap'su·la'tum
—oe·de'ma·tis ma'lig'ni'
—par'a·bot'u·li'nus
—par'a·ty·pho'sus A
—paratyphosus B
—per'frin'gens
—per·tus'sis
—pes'tis
—pol'y·myx'a

—pro·dig'i·o'sus
—pro'te·us
—pu'mi·lus
—sub'ti·lis
—su'i·sep'ti·cus
—tet'a·ni'
—tu·ber'cu·lo'sis
—whit·mo'ri'
—xe·ro'sis
bac'i·tra'cin
back'ache'
back'bleed'ing
back'bone'
back'cross'
back'flow'
back'scat'ter
back'wash'
bac'lo·fen
bac'te·re'mi·a
bac'te·re'mic
bac·te'ri·a *sing.* -ri·um
Bac·te'ri·a'ce·ae'
bac·te'ri·al
bac·te'ri·cid'al
bac·te'ri·cide'
bac·te'ri·ci'din
bac'ter·id
bac'ter·in
bac·te'ri·o·flour·res'cin
bac·te'ri·o·chlo'ro·phyll
bac·te'ri·o·oc'la·sis *pl.* -ses'
bac·te'ri·o·er'y·thrin
bac·te'ri·o·fluo·res'cin
bac·te'ri·o·gen'ic
bac·te'ri·og'e·nous
bac·te'ri·o·he·mol'y·sin
bac·te'ri·oid'
bac·te'ri·o·log'ic *or*
   bac·te'ri·o·log'i·cal
bac·te'ri·ol'o·gist
bac·te'ri·ol'o·gy
bac·te'ri·ol'y·sin
bac·te'ri·ol'y·sis *pl.* -ses'
bac·te'ri·o·lyt'ic
bac·te'ri·o·pex'y
bac·te'ri·o·phage'
bac·te'ri·o·pha'gi·a
bac·te'ri·o·phag'ic
bac·te'ri·o·pro'tein
bac·te'ri·op·son'ic
bac·te'ri·op'so·nin
bac·te'ri·o'sis *pl.* -ses'
bac·te'ri·os'ta·sis *pl.* -ses'

bac·te'ri·o·stat'
bac·te'ri·o·stat'ic
bac·te'ri·o·ther'a·py
bac·te'ri·o·tox·e'mi·a
bac·te'ri·o·tox'ic
bac·te'ri·o·tox'in
bac·te'ri·o·trop'ic
bac·te'ri·ot'ro·pin
Bac·te'ri·um
—a·ce'ti'
—ae·rog'e·nes'
—al'ka·les'cens
—am·big'u·um
—a'vi·sep'ti·cum
—bo'vi·sep'ti·cum
—chol'e·rae'-su'is
—co'li'
—dis'par'
—dys'en·ter'i·ae'
—en'ter·it'i·dis
—flex'ner·i'
—fried·län'der·i'
—fu'si·for'mis
—gin'gi·va'lis
—lac'tis aer·og'e·nes'
—mon'o·cy·tog'e·nes'
—par'a·dys'en·ter'i·ae'
—par'a·ty·pho'sum A
—paratyphosum B
—paratyphosum C
—pneu·mo'ni·ae'
—shi'gae'
—son'ne·i'
—su'i·pes'ti·fer
—su'i·sep'ti·cum
—tu'la·ren'se'
—ty'phi·mu'ri·um
—ty·pho'sum
bac·te'ri·u·ri·a
bac'ter·oid'
Bac'ter·oi·da'ce·ae'
Bac'ter·oi'des'
—cor·ro'dens
—frag'i·lis
—fun'di·li·for'mis
—me·lan'i·no·gen'i·cus
—pneu'mo·sin'tes'
bac'ter·u'ri·a
bac'u·lum
Baer treatment
Bäer'en·sprung disease
Baf'fe anastomosis
baf'fle, -fled, -fling

bag
ba·gasse'
bag'as·so'sis pl. -ses'
bagged
Bagh'dad'
—boil
—spring anemia
Ba·hi'a ulcer
Bail·lar·ger'
—bands
—principle
—sign
Bain'bridge' reflex
Ba'ker cyst
bal'ance, -anced, -anc·ing
ba·lan'ic
Bal·a·ni'tes' ae'gyp·ti'a·ca
bal'a·ni'tis
—xe·rot'i·ca ob·lit'er·ans'
bal'a·no·chlam'y·di'tis
bal'a·no·plas'ty
bal'a·no·pos·thi'tis
bal'a·no·pre·pu'tial
bal'a·nor·rha'gi·a
bal'a·nor·rhe'a
bal'an·tid'i·al
bal'an·ti·di·a·sis pl. -ses'
Bal'an·tid'i·um
—co'li'
bal'an·ti·do'sis pl. -ses'
bal'a·nus
Bal'bi·a'ni rings
bald
bald'ness
Bal·duz'zi sign
Bald'win operation
Bal'dy-Web'ster operation
Bal'four operation
Ba'lint syndrome
Bal'lance
—operation
—sign
Bal·let' sign
Bal'lin·gall disease
bal'lism
bal·lis'mus
bal·lis'tic
bal·lis'to·car'di·o·gram'
bal·lis'to·car'di·o·graph'
bal·lis'to·car'di·og'ra·phy
bal·loon'
bal·loon'ing
Ball operation

bal·lot'a·ble
bal·lotte·ment'
balm
bal'ne·o·ther'a·peu'tics
bal'ne·o·ther'a·py
Ba'lo concentric sclerosis
bal'sam
bal·sam'ic
Bal'ser fat necrosis
Bal'tha·zar Fos'ter murmur
Bam'ber·ger sign
ba'meth'an
bam'i·fyl'line'
Ban'croft' filariasis
ban'crof·to'sis pl. -ses'
band
band'age, -aged, -ag·ing
bands of Pic'co·lo·mi'ni
bane
Bang
—ba·cil'lus
—disease
—method
—test
ba·nis'ter·ine'
Ban'kart operation
Ban'nis·ter disease
Ban'ti
—disease
—syndrome
ban'ting·ism
bap'ti·tox'ine'
bar'ag·no'sis pl. -ses'
Bá'rá·ny
—symptom
—test
bar'ba
—am'a·ril'la
bar'ba·loin'
bar'bei'ro
Bar·be'ri·o test
Bar'ber method
bar'bi·tal'
bar'bi·tu·rate'
bar'bi·tu'ric
bar'bi·tu'rism
bar'bo·tage'
Bar'clay niche
Bar·coo' rot
Bar'dach' test
Bar·de·le'ben operation
Bar'den·heu'er operation
Bar·det'-Biedl' syndrome

Bard'-Pic' syndrome
Bard sign
Bär'en·sprung' disease
bar'es·the'si·a
bar'es·the'si·om'e·ter
Bar'foed
—reagent
—test
bar'i·at'ric
bar'i·a·tri'cian
bar'ic
ba·ril'la
Bar incision
bar'i·to'sis *pl.* -ses'
bar'i·um
bark
Bar'ker operation
Bar'kow ligament
Bar'low
—disease
—syndrome
Barns'dale' bacillus
bar'o·cep'tor
bar'o·don·tal'gi·a
bar'og·no'sis *pl.* -ses'
bar'o·graph'
bar'o·graph'ic
bar'o·ma·crom'e·ter
bar'o·met'ro·graph'
bar'o·phil'ic
bar'o·pho'bi·a
bar'o-o·ti'tis
bar'o·re·cep'tor
bar'o·re'flex'
bar'o·scope'
bar'o·si'nus·i'tis
ba·ros'min
bar'o·stat'
bar'o·tax'is *pl.* -ses
bar'o·ti'tis
—ex·ter'na
—me'di·a
bar'o·trau'ma *pl.* -ma·ta'
Bar·ra'quer
—disease
—operation
Bar·ra'quer-Si'mons
disease
Barr body
Bar·ré'
—sign
—syndrome
Bar·ré'-Guil·lain' syndrome

bar'rel-chest'ed
bar'ren
Barr'-Ep'stein' virus
Bar'rett
—epithelium
—esophagus
—ulcer
bar'ri·er
Bart hemoglobin
Barth hernia
Bar'tho·lin
—cyst
—duct
—gland
bar'tho·lin·i'tis
Bar'ton·el'la
bar'ton·el·le'mi·a
bar'ton·el·lo'sis *pl.* -ses'
Bar'ton operation
Bart'ter syndrome
bar'ye
bar'y·es·the'si·a
bar'y·glos'si·a
bar'y·la'li·a
Bar'y·on'yx
bar'y·pho'ni·a
ba·ry'ta
ba'sad
bas'al
bas'al-cell' carcinoma
bas'al·i·o'ma *pl.* -mas *or*
-ma·ta
ba·sa'lis
bas'al·ly
bas'al·oid'
bas'al·o'ma *pl.* -mas *or*
-ma·ta
base
bas'e·doid'
Ba'se·dow' disease
base'line'
Ba'sel'la
base'ment
ba'se·o'sis *pl.* -ses'
base'plate'
bas-fond'
Bash'am mixture
ba'si·al
ba'si·al·ve'o·lar
ba'si·bran'chi·al
ba'si·breg·mat'ic
ba'sic
ba'si·chro'ma·tin

ba·sic'i·ty
ba'si·cra'ni·al
Ba·sid'i·ob'o·lus
ba·sid'i·o·my·cete'
Ba·sid'i·o·my·ce'tes'
ba·sid'i·o·my·ce'tous
ba·sid'i·o·phore'
ba·sid'i·o·spore'
ba·sid'i·um *pl.* -i·a
ba'si·fa'cial
ba'si·hy'al
ba'si·hy'oid'
bas'i·lad'
bas'i·lar
bas'i·lar'is
—cran'i·i'
ba'si·lat'er·al
ba·sil'ic
ba'si·lem'ma
bas'i·lo'ma *pl.* -mas *or* -ma·ta
bas'i·lo·men'tal
bas'i·lo·pha·ryn'ge·al
bas'i·lo·sub·na'sal
ba'si·na'sal
ba'si·o·al·ve'o·lar
ba'si·o·breg·mat'ic
ba'si·oc·cip'i·tal
ba'si·o·glos'sus
ba'si·on'
ba'si·o·tribe'
ba'si·o·trip'sy
ba·sip'e·tal
ba'si·pha·ryn'ge·al
ba'si·pho'bi·a
ba'si·pre·sphe'noid'
ba'si·rhi'nal
ba'sis *pl.* -ses'
—car'ti·lag'i·nis
ar'y·te·noi'de·ae'
—cer'e·bri'
—coch'le·ae'
—cor'dis
—cra'ni·i' ex·ter'na
—cranii in·ter'na
—glan'du·lae' su'pra·re·
na'lis
—lin'guae'
—man·dib'u·lae'
—mo·di'o·li'
—na'si'
—os'sis met'a·car·pa'lis
—ossis met'a·tar·sa'lis
—ossis sa·cri'

—os'si·um met'a·car·pa'-
li·um
—ossium met'a·tar·sa'li·um
—pa·tel'lae'
—pe·dun'cu·li' cer'e·bri'
—pha·lan'gis dig'i·to'rum
ma'nus
—phalangis digitorum
pe'dis
—pros'ta·tae'
—pul·mo'nis
—py·ram'i·dis re·na'lis
—sta'pe·dis
ba'si·sphe'noid'
ba'si·tem'po·ral
ba'si·ver'te·bral
bas'ket
Ba'sle Nom'i·na
An'a·tom'i·ca
ba'so·cyte'
ba·so·cy'to·pe'ni·a
ba·so·cy·to'sis *pl.* -ses'
ba'so·phil'
ba·so·phil'i·a
ba·so·phil'ic
ba·soph'i·lism
ba·so·phil'o·cyt'ic
ba·soph'i·lous
ba·so·plasm
ba·so·squa'mous
Bas'sen-Korn'zweig'
syndrome
Bas·set' operation
Bas·si'ni
—hernia repair
—operation
bas'so·rin
Bas'ti·an-Bruns' law
Batch'-Spitt'ler-Mc·Fad'-
din knee amputation
bath
bath'mo·trop'ic
bath·mot'ro·pism
bath'o·chrome'
bath'o·chro'mic
bath'o·pho'bi·a
bath'ro·ceph'a·ly
bath'y·car'di·a
bath'y·chrome'
bath'y·chro'mic
bath'y·es·the'si·a
bath'y·hy'per·es·the'si·a
bath'y·hyp'es·the'si·a

bath'y·pne'a
bat'o·pho'bi·a
ba·tra'chi·an
bat'ra·cho·plas'ty
bat'ra·cho·tox'in
Bat'son plexus
bat'ta·rism
bat'ta·ris'mus
Bat'ten disease
Bat'ten-May'ou disease
bat'ter
bat'ter·y
Bat'tey operation
Bat'tle sign
Baude·locque'
—diameter
—line
Bau'er test
Bau'er-Ton'dra-Trus'ler
repair
Bau·mes' sign
Baum'gar'ten syndrome
Ba'u·ru' ulcer
bay'ber'ry
Bayle disease
Baz'ett formula
Ba·zin' disease
Bdel'lo·nys'sus
—ba·co'ti
Bdel'lo·vib'ri·o
beak'er
beam
Be·ance' tu·baire'
vol·un·taire'
Beard disease
bear'ing
beat
Beau
—asystole
—disease
—lines
—syndrome
be·bee'rine'
be·bee'ru'
be·can'thone'
bech'ic
Bech·ter'ew nucleus
Beck
—disease
—gastrostomy
—operation
—paste
—triad

Beck'er
—disease
—nevus
Bé·clard '
—amputation
—hernia
bec'lo·meth'a·sone'
Bec·que·rel' ray
be·dew'ing
Bed'nar aphthae
bed'pan'
bed'side'
Bed·so'ni·a
—psit'ta·ci'
bed'sore'
bed'wet'ter
bed'wet'ting
Beer
—dye test
—law
bees'wax'
beet·u'ri·a
Bee'vor sign
be·hav'ior
be·hav'ior·al
be·hav'ior·ism
be·hav'ior·ist
be·hav'ior·is'tic
Beh'çet syndrome
be·hen'ic
Behr
—disease
—pupil
—sign
Behre test
Bei'gel disease
bej'el
Bé'ké·sy audiometry
Bekh·ter'ev
—arthritis
—deep reflex
—fibers
—nucleus
—reaction
—reflex
—sign
Bekh·ter'ev-Men'del reflex
bel
bel'ae fruc'tus
Bell
—disease
—law
—mania

—muscle
—palsy
—phenomenon
—spasm
bel′la·don′na
bel′la·don′nine′
bell′-crowned′
Bell′-Dal′ly dislocation
belle in·dif·fé·rence′
Belle′vue′ scale
Bel′ling ac′e·to·car′mine
 stain
Bel·li′ni
—duct
—ligament
Bell′-Ma·gen·die′ law
bel′lows
bel′ly
bel′ly·ache′
bel′ly·but′ton
Bel′sey
—operation
—repair
Bel′sey Mark II
 fundoplication
bem′e·gride′
ben·ac′ty·zine′
Ben′a·cus
—gris′cus
ben·a′zo·line′
Bence′-Jones′
—cylinders
—protein
Ben′da test
ben′da·zac′
Ben′der gestalt test
Ben′dien′ test
ben′dro·flu′me·thi′a·zide′
bends
be′ne′
Ben′e·dict
—and Franke method
—and Hitch′cock′ reagent
—and New′ton method
—and Theis method
—method
—solution
—test
—uric acid reagent
Ben′e·dikt syndrome
be·nign′
be·nig′nant
Ben′nett

—angle
—cells
—elevator
—fracture
—movement
Benn′hold′ test
be·nor′ter·one′
ben·ox′i·nate′
ben·per′i·dol′
ben′sa·lan′
ben′ton·ite′
benz·al′de·hyde′
benz′al·dox′ime′
benz′al·ko′ni·um
benz·an′thra·cene′
ben′za·thine′
benz·az′o·line′
ben′zene′
ben·zes′trol′
ben′ze·tho′ni·um
ben·zet′i·mide′
benz·hex′ol′
benz·hy′dra·mine′
ben′zi·dine′
ben′zi·lo′ni·um
ben′zi·mi·da′zole′
ben′zin
benz′in·do·py′rine′
ben′zine′
ben′zo·ate′
ben′zo·caine′
benz·oc′ta·mine′
ben′zo·dep′a
ben′zo·di·az′e·pine′
ben′zo·di·ox′an′
ben′zo·di·ox′ane′
ben·zo′ic
ben·zo′in
ben·zo′i·nat′ed
ben′zol′
ben′zole′
ben·zo′na·tate′
ben′zo·ni′trile
ben′zo·phe·none′
ben′zo·qui′none′
ben′zo·qui′no′ni·um
ben′zo·sul′fi·mide′
ben′zo·yl
ben·zo′yl·ec′go·nine′
ben·zo′yl·gly′cine′
ben·zo′yl·guai′a·col′
ben·zo′yl·meth′yl·ec′go·
 nine′

benz·phet′a·mine′
benz·py′rene′
benz′py·rin′i·um
benz·quin′a·mide′
benz·thi′a·zide′
benz·tro′pine′
ben·zyd′a·mine′
ben′zyl
ben·zyl′ic
ben·zyl′i·dene′
ben′zyl·pen′i·cil′lin
ber·ac′tant
ber′ber·ine′
ber′ber·is
Ber′ga·ra-War′ten·berg′
 sign
Ber′gen·hem operation
Ber′ger
—disease
—intercapsular amputation
—operation
—rhythm
—sign
Bergh test
Berg′mann
—astrocytes
—cords
Berg′meis′ter papilla
Ber·go·nié′-Tri·bon·deau′
 law
ber′i·ber′i
Ber′ke·feld′ filter
ber·ke′li·um
Ber·lin′
—blue
—disease
ber′lock′
ber·loque′
Ber·nard′
—canal
—granular layer
—puncture
—syndrome
Ber·nard′-Hor′ner
 syndrome
Bern′hardt′ paresthesia
Bern′hardt-Roth′
 syndrome
Bern′heim′
—syndrome
—therapy
Ber·noul′li
—effect

—equation
—principle
Bern′reu·ter personality
  inventory
Bern′stein′
—gastroscope
—theory
Ber·tel′ position
Ber′ti·el′la
—mu′cro·na′ta
—stu′de·ri′
Ber·til·lon′ system
be·ryl′li·o′sis *pl.* -ses′
be·ryl′li·um
Ber·ze′li·us test
bes′i·clom′e·ter
Bes·nier′-Boeck′ disease
Bes·nier′-Boeck′-
  Schau′mann′ disease
Bes′sey-Low′ry unit
Best
—carmine stain
—disease
bes′ti·al′i·ty
be′syl·ate′
be′ta
—globulin
Be′ta
be′ta·cism
be′ta-d-al′lo·py′ra·nose′
be′ta-en·dor′phin
be′ta·eu′caine′
be′ta-glu′can
be′ta-he′mo·lyt′ic
be′ta·his′ine′
be′ta-hy·poph′a·mine′
be′ta·ine′
be′ta-ke′to·hy·drox′y·
  bu·tyr′ic
be′ta-lac′tam
be′ta-lac′ta·mase′
be′ta·meth′a·sone′
be′ta·naph′thol′
be′ta·naph′thyl
be′ta·top′ic
be′ta·tron′
be·tax′o·lol′
be′ta·zole′
be·than′e·chol′
be·than′i·dine′
Bet′ten·dorff′ test
bet′u·lin
be·tween′brain′

Betz cell
Bev′an operation
bev′a·tron′
bev′el
be′zoar′
Be′zold′
—abscess
—reflex
—sign
Be·zold′-Brück′e effect
Be′zold′-Jar′isch reflex
Bi′al
—reagent
—test
bi′al·am′i·col′
Bi·an′chi syndrome
bi′ar·tic′u·lar
bi′ar·tic′u·late′
bi′a·stig′ma·tism
bi·a′tri·al
bi′au·ric′u·lar
bi·ax′i·al
bi·bal′lism
bi·bas′al·ly
bi·bas′i·lar
bib′li·o·clast′
bib′li·o·ma′ni·a
bib′li·o·ther′a·py
bib′u·lous
bi·cam′er·al
bi·cap′i·tate′
bi·cap′su·lar
bi·car′bon·ate′
bi·car′di·o·gram′
bi·ca′val
bi·cel′lu·lar
bi·ceph′a·lous
bi′ceps′ *pl.* -ceps′es
bi·chlo′ride′
bi·chro′mate′
bi·cip′i·tal
Bick′er·staff encephalitis
bi·con′cave′
bi·con′dy·lar
bi·con′vex
bi·cor′nu·ate′
bi·cor′nu·ous
bi·cor′ti·cal
bi·cou·dé′
bi·cus′pid
bi′cy′cle
bi·dac′ty·ly
Bid′der

—ganglion
—organ
bi′di·rec′tion·al
bid′u·ous
Bie′brich scarlet
Biedl′-Bar·det′ syndrome
Biel·schow′sky
—disease
—sign
—strabismus
Biel·schow′sky-Jan′sky
  disease
Bi·e′mond syndrome
Bier
—block anesthesia
—method
—spots
Bier′mer
—anemia
—disease
Bier·nack′i sign
Bi·ett′ disease
bi·fas·cic′u·lar
bi′fid *pl.* -fid·us
Bi·fid·o·bac·te′ri·um
bi·fo′cal
bi·fron′tal
bi·fur·cate′, -cat·ed, -cat′ing
bi·fur·ca′ti·o′ *pl.* -ca′ti·o′nes′
bi·fur·ca′tion
Big′e·low method
bi·gem′i·nal
bi·gem′i·ny
bi·go′ni·al
bi·is′chi·al
Bik′e·le sign
bi′labe′
bi·lam′i·nar
bi·lat′er·al
bi·lat′er·al·ism
bi·lay′er
bile
Bil·har′zi·a
bil′har·zi′a·sis *pl.* -ses′
bil′i·ar′y
bil′i·cy′a·nin
bil′i·fi·ca′tion
bil′i·fla′vin
bil′i·fus′cin
bil′i·gen′e·sis
bi·lig′u·late′
bi·lig′u·la′tus
bil′i·hu′min

bil'i·leu'kan'
bi'lin
bil'i·neu'rine'
bil'i·o·in·tes'ti·nal
bil'i·o·pan'cre·at'ic
bil'ious
bil'ious·ness
bil'i·pra'sin
bil'i·pur'pu·rin
bil'i·ra'chi·a
bil'i·ru'bin
bil'i·ru'bin·ate'
bil'i·ru'bin·e·mi·a
bil'i·ru'bin·glo'bin
bil'i·ru'bin'ic
bil'i·ru'bi·nu'ri·a
bil'i·u'ri·a
bil'i·ver'din
Bill'roth'
—anastomosis
—gastroenterostomy
—operation
bi·lo'bar
bi·lo'bate'
bi'lobed'
bi·loc'u·lar
bi·loc'u·late'
bi·mal·le'o·lar
bi·man'u·al
bi·mas'toid'
bi·max'il·lar'y
bi'mo'dal
bi'mo·lec'u·lar
bin'an'gle
bi'na·ry
bi·na'sal
bin·au'ral
bin'au·ric'u·lar
bind, bound, bind'ing
bind'er
Bi·net'
—age
—formula
Bi·net'-Si·mon' intelligence
scale
Bing
—sign
—test
binge, binged, bing'ing
binge'-purge' behavior
Bing'-Neel' syndrome
bin·oc'u·lar
bi·no'mi·al

bin·ot'ic
bin·o'vu·lar
bin·ox'ide'
Bins'wang·er disease
bi·nu'cle·ar
bi·nu'cle·ate'
bi·nu'cle·at'ed
bi'nu·cle·a'tion
bi'nu·cle'o·late'
bi'o·a·cous'tics
bi'o·ac·tiv'i·ty
bi'o·as'say'
bi'o·as'tro·nau'tics
bi'o·au'to·graph'ic
bi'o·au·tog'ra·phy
bi'o·a·vail'a·bil'i·ty
bi'ob·jec'tive
bi'o·cat'a·lyst
bi'oc·cip'i·tal
bi'o·ce·no'sis pl. -ses'
bi'o·chem'i·cal
bi'o·chem'is·try
bi'o·che·mor'phic
bi'o·che·mor·phol'o·gy
bi'o·chrome'
bi'o·cid'al
bi'o·cide'
bi'o·cli·mat'ics
bi'o·cli·ma·tol'o·gy
bi'o·com·pat'i·ble
bi'o·cy'ber·net'ics
bi'o·cy'tin
bi'o·de·grad'a·bil'i·ty
bi'o·de·grad'a·ble
bi'o·deg'ra·da'tion
bi'o·de·tri'tus
bi'o·dis'tri·bu'tion
bi'o·dy·nam'ic
bi'o·dy·nam'ics
bi'o·e·col'o·gy
bi'o·e·lec'tric
bi'o·e·lec·tric'i·ty
bi'o·e·lec·tron'ics
bi'o·en·er·get'ics
bi'o·en·gi·neer'ing
bi'o·en·vi'ron·men'tal
bi'o·e·quiv'a·lence
bi'o·feed'back'
bi'o·fla'vo·noid'
bi'o·gen'e·sis pl. -ses'
bi'o·ge·net'ic
bi'o·gen'ic
bi·og'e·nous

bi·og'e·ny
bi'o·ge'o·chem'is·try
bi'o·haz'ard
bi'o·im·ped'ance
bi'o·in·te·gra'tion
bi'o·ki·net'ic
bi'o·ki·net'ics
bi'o·log'ic or bi'o·log'i·cal
bi·ol'o·gist
bi·ol'o·gy
bi'o·lu'mi·nes'cence
bi'o·lu'mi·nes'cent
bi·ol'y·sis pl. -ses'
bi'o·lyt'ic
bi'o·mag'net·ism
bi'o·mass'
bi'o·ma·te'ri·al
bi'o·math'e·mat'ics
bi'ome'
bi'o·me·chan'ics
bi'o·med'i·cal
bi'o·med'i·cine
bi·om'e·ter
bi'o·me·ter·ol'o·gy
bi'o·me·tri'cian
bi'o·met'rics
bi·om'e·try
bi'o·mi'cro·scope'
bi'o·mi'cro·scop'ic
bi'o·mi·cros'co·py
bi'on'
bi'o·ne·cro'sis pl. -ses'
bi·on'ics
bi'o·nom'ics
bi·on'o·my
bi'o·nu'cle·on'ics
bi'o·pa·thol'o·gy
bi·oph'a·gous
bi·oph'a·gy
bi'o·phore'
bi'o·phor'ic
bi'o·pho·tom'e·ter
bi'o·phys'i·cal
bi'o·phys'ics
bi'o·phys·i·og'ra·phy
bi'o·phys·i·ol'o·gy
bi'o·plasm
bi'o·plas'mic
bi'o·plas'tic
bi'o·pros·the'sis
bi'op·sy
bi'o·psy'chic
bi'o·psy'cho·log'i·cal

bi·o·psy·chol'o·gy
bi·op'ter·in
bi·or'bi·tal
bi·o'rhythm
bi·o'rhyth'mic
bi'os
bi·o·science'
bi·o·sci'en·tif'ic
bi·ose'
bi·o·sen'sor
bi·o·spec·trom'e·try
bi·o·spec·tros'co·py
bi·o·sphere'
bi·o·sta·tis'tics
bi·os'ter·ol'
bi·o·syn'the·sis *pl.* -ses'
bi·o·syn·thet'ic
bi·o'ta
bi·o·tax'is
bi·o·tax'y
Bi·ot' breathing
bi·o·tech'no·log'i·cal
bi·o·tech·nol'o·gy
bi·o·tel'e·met'ric
bi·o·te·lem'e·try
bi·o·te'si·om'e·ter
bi·o·te'si·om'e·try
bi·ot'ic
bi·o'tin
bi·o·tox'i·ca'tion
bi·o·tox'i·col'o·gy
bi·o·tox'in
bi·o·trans'for·ma'tion
bi·o·type'
bi·o·typ'ic
bi·o·ty·pol'o·gy
bi·o'vu·lar
bip'a·ra *pl.* -ras *or* -rae'
bi·pa·ren'tal
bi·pa·ri'e·tal
bip'a·rous
bi·par'tite'
bi·ped'
bi·ped'al
bi·ped'i·cled
bi·pen'nate'
bi·pen'ni·form'
bi·per'i·den
bi·pha'sic
bi·phen'yl
bi·phos'phate'
bi·pla'nar
bi·plane'

bi·po'lar
bi·po·lar'i·ty
bi·po·ten'ti·al'i·ty
bi·ra'mous
birch
bird'-beak' configuration
Bird disease
bi're·frac'tive
bi're·frin'gence
bi're·frin'gent
bir'i·mose'
Birk'haug' test
bi'ro·ta'tion
birth
birth'mark'
bis'a·co'dyl
bis·al'bu'min·e'mi·a
bis·an'trene'
Bisch'off' test
bis'cuit
bi·sect'
bi·sec'tion
bi·sex'u·al
bi·sex'u·al'i·ty
bis·fe'ri·ens
bis·fe'ri·ous
bis'hy·drox'y·cou'ma·rin
bis·il'i·ac'
bis in di'e
Bis'kra button
bis'muth
bis·mu'thi·a
bis'muth·o'sis *pl.* -ses'
bis'muth·o·tar'trate'
bis'muth·yl
bis·o'brin
bis·ox'a·tin
bis'sa
bi'ste·phan'ic
bis'tou·ry
bi·stra'tal
bis'tri·min
bi·sul'fide'
bi·sul'fite'
bi·tar'trate'
bite, bit, bit'ten *or* bit, bit'ing
bi·tem'po·ral
bite'wing'
bi·thi'o·nol'
Bi'tis
   —ga·bon'i·ca
   —la·che'sis
   —na'si·cor'nis

Bi·tot' spots
bi'tro·chan·ter'ic
bit'ter·ling
bit'ters
Bitt'ner milk factor
bi·tu'ber·al
bi·tu'men
bi'tu·mi·no'sis *pl.* -ses'
bi·u'rate'
bi·u'ret'
bi·va'lence
bi·va'len·cy
bi·va'lent
bi·valve'
bi·val'vu·lar
bi·ven'ter
bi·ven'tral
bi·ven·tric'u·lar
bi·zy'go·mat'ic
Biz'zo·ze'ro
   —blood platelet
   —nodules
Bjer'rum
   —scotoma
   —screen
   —sign
Black
   —classification
   —test
Black'fan'-Di'a·mond
   syndrome
black'head'
black'out'
blad'der
blade
blade'break'er
blain
Bla'lock-Han'lon operation
Bla'lock-Taus'sig operation
blanch
bland
Blan'din glands
Bland'-White'-Gar'land
   syndrome
Blan'for'di·a
blast
blas·te'ma *pl.* -mas *or* -ma·ta
blas·te'mic
blas'tin
blas'to·chyle'
blas'to·coele'
blas'to·cyst'
Blas'to·cys'tis hom'i·nis

blas'to·cyte'
blas'to·derm'
blas'to·der'mal
blas'to·der'mic
blas'to·disc'
blas'to·gen'e·sis *pl.* -ses'
blas'to·ge·net'ic
blas'to·gen'ic
blas·tog'e·ny
blas'to·ki·ne'sis *pl.* -ses'
blas'to·ki'nin
blas·tol'y·sis *pl.* -ses'
blas'to·ma *pl.* -mas *or* -ma·ta
blas·tom'a·to·gen'ic
blas·tom'a·tous
blas'to·mere'
Blas'to·my'ces'
 —bra·sil'i·en'sis
 —der'ma·tit'i·dis
blas'to·my·cete'
Blas'to·my·ce'tes'
blas'to·my·ce'tic
blas'to·my'cin
blas'to·my·co'sis *pl.* -ses'
blas'to·neu'ro·pore'
blas'toph·tho'ri·a
blas'toph·thor'ic
blas'to·pore'
blas'to·por'ic
blas'to·sphere'
blas'to·spher'ic
blas'to·spore'
blas'to·spor'ic
blas·tot'o·my
blas'tu·la *pl.* -las *or* -lae'
blas'tu·lar
blas'tu·la'tion
Bla·tel'la
 —ger·man'i·ca
Blaud pill
bleb
bleed, bled, bleed'ing
bleed'er
blem'ish
blen'nad·e·ni'tis
blen'no·gen'ic
blen'noid'
blen'noph·thal'mi·a
blen'nor·rha'gi·a
blen'nor·rhe'a
blen'nor·rhe'al
blen'no·tho'rax'
blen·nu'ri·a

ble'o·my'cin
bleph'ar·ad'e·ni'tis
bleph'a·ral
bleph'a·rec'to·my
bleph'ar·e·de'ma
bleph'a·re·lo'sis *pl.* -ses'
bleph'a·rism
bleph'a·ri'tis
 —an'gu·lar'is
 —cil'i·ar'is
 —gan'grae·no'sa
 —mar'gi·na'lis
 —par'a·sit'i·ca
 —sim'plex'
 —squa·mo'sa
 —ul'ce·ro'sa
bleph'a·ro·ad'e·ni'tis
bleph'a·ro·ad'e·no'ma
 pl. -mas *or* -ma·ta
bleph'a·ro·ath'er·o'ma
 pl. -mas *or* -ma·ta
bleph'a·ro·blen'nor·rhe'a
bleph'a·ro·chal'a·sis *pl.* -ses'
bleph'a·ro·chrom'hi·
 dro'sis
belph'a·roc'lo·nus
bleph'a·ro·con·junc'ti·vi'tis
bleph'a·ro·di·as'ta·sis
 pl. -ses'
bleph'a·ro·dys·chroi'a
bleph'a·ro·me·las'ma
bleph'a·ron' *pl.* -ra
bleph'a·ron'cus *pl.* -ci'
bleph'a·ro·pa·chyn'sis
bleph'a·ro·phi·mo'sis
 pl. -ses'
bleph'a·roph'ry·plas'tic
bleph'a·roph'ry·plas'ty
bleph'a·ro·phy'ma *pl.* -mas
 or -ma·ta
bleph'a·ro·plast'
bleph'a·ro·plas'tic
bleph'a·ro·plas'ty
bleph'a·ro·ple'gi·a
bleph'a·rop·to'sis *pl.* -ses'
bleph'a·ro·py'or·rhe'a
bleph'a·ror'rha·phy
bleph'a·ro·spasm
bleph'a·ro·sphinc'ter·ec'-
 to·my
bleph'a·ro·stat'
bleph'a·ro·ste·no'sis
 pl. -ses'

bleph'a·ro·sym'phy·sis
 pl. -ses'
bleph'a·ro·syn·ech'i·a
 pl. -i·ae'
bleph'a·rot'o·my
Bles'sig-I·van'ov cystoid
 degeneration
blind
blind'ness
blink
blis'ter
bloat
Bloch
 —equation
 —method
Bloch'-Sulz'ber'ger
 syndrome
block
block·ade', -ad'ed, -ad'ing
block'er
Blocq disease
Blond·lot' rays
blood
Blood'good' operation
blood'less
blood'let'ting
blood'shot'
blood'stream'
Bloom syndrome
blotch
blotch'i·ness
blotch'y
Blount'-Bar'ber syndrome
Blount disease
blow'fly'
blow'-in' fracture
blow'-out' fracture
blow'pipe'
Blum'berg' sign
Blu'me·nau'
 —nucleus
 —test
Blu'men·bach' clivus
Blu'mer shelf
blunt
Blyth test
board'like'
Bo·a'ri operation
Bo'as
 —point
 —reagent
 —sign
 —test

Bo'as-Op'pler bacillus
Bob'roff' operation
Boch'da·lek'
—foramen
—ganglion
—hernia
—triangle
Bock'hart' impetigo
Bo·dan'sky
—method
—unit
Bo'di·an staining method
bod'y
Boeck
—disease
—sarcoid
—scabies
Boehm
—anoscope
—proctoscope
—sigmoidoscope
Boer'haa've syndrome
Boer'ner-Lu'kens test
Boet'ti·ger method
bog'gy
Bo·gros' space
Böh'ler angle
Böh'mer hematoxylin
Bohr
—effect
—mag'ne·ton'
boil
Boi'vin antigen
bo·las'ter·one'
bol·de'none'
bol'dine'
bole
bol'e·nol'
Bo'len test
Bo'ley gauge
Bol'lin·ger granules
bol·man'ta·late'
bo·lom'e·ter
bol'ster
Bol'ton
—cranial base
—nasion plane
—point
Boltz'mann distribution
Boltz test
bo'lus pl. -lus·es
bom·bard'ment
Bom·bayz' blood

bom'be·sin
Bo·nanz'no test
bond
bon'duc'
Bon'dy operation
bone
bone'let'
bone'set'ter
Bon·jean' ergotin
Bonne·vie'-Ull'rich
  syndrome
Bon·nier' syndrome
Bon'will triangle
bon'y
Bo·oph'i·lus
—an'nu·la'tus
Boor'man cancer
  classification
boost'er
boot
bo·rac'ic
bo'rate'
bo'rax'
bor'bo·ryg'mus pl. -mi'
Bor·deaux' mixture
bor'der
bor'der·line'
Bor'de·tel'la
—bron'chi·sep'ti·ca
—par'a·per'tus'sis
—per'tus'sis
Bor·det'-Gen·gou' bacillus
Bor·det' test
Bord'ey-Rich'ards method
bor'er
bo'ric
bor'ism
Bör'je·son-Fors'man-
  Leh'mann syndrome
bor'nane'
bor'ne·ol'
Born'holm' disease
bor'nyl
bo'ro·cit'ric
bo'ro·glyc'er·ide'
bo'ro·glyc'er·in
bo'ron'
bo'ro·sal'i·cyl'ic
Bor'rel' body
Bor·rel'i·a
—buc'ca'le'
—dut'to'ni·i'
—no'vy·i'

—re'cur·ren'tis
—re·frin'gens
—vin·cen'ti·i'
bor·rel'i·din
boss
bos'se·lat'ed
bos'se·la'tion
boss'ing
Bos'ton sign
Bo·tal'lo duct
bo·tan'ic
bo·tan'i·cal
bot'a·nist
bot'a·ny
bot'fly'
bo·thrid'i·um pl. -i·a or
  -i·ums
Both'ri·o·ceph'a·lus
—a·ne'mi·a
both'ri·oid'
both'ri·on'
both'ri·um pl. -ri·a or -ri·ums
bo·throp'ic
Bo'throps'
—al'ter·na'ta
—at'rox'
—jar'a·ra'ca
—neu·wie'di·i'
—num'mi·fer
bo·tog'e·nin
bot'ry·oid'
bot'ry·o·my·co'sis pl. -ses'
bot'ry·o·my·cot'ic
Bo·try'tis
Bött'cher cells
bot'u·li·form'
bot'u·lin
bot'u·li'nal
bot'u·li'num
bot'u·lism
bou'ba
Bou·chard'
—disease
—nodes
bouche de ta·pir'
Bou'gain·ville'
  rheumatism
bou·gie'
—à boule
bou·gie·nage'
Bouil·laud' disease
bouil'lon
Bouin

—fixative
—solution
Bou·len'ge·ri'na
Boul'ton solution
bound
bound'a·ry
Bour·get' test
Bourne method
Bourne·ville' disease
Bour'quin-Sher'man unit
bou'stro·phe·don'ic
bout
bou·ton'
—de bis'kra
—d'o'ri·ent
bou·ton·neuse'
bou·ton·niere'
bou·tons' ter·mi·naux'
Bou·ve·ret'
—disease
—syndrome
Bo·ve'ri test
Bo'vie
—cautery
—coagulator
—unit
bo'vine'
bow, bowed; bow'ing
Bow'ditch'
—effect
—law
bow'el
Bo'wen disease
bow'ing reflex
bow'leg'
Bow'man
—capsule
—glands
—membrane
box'i·dine'
Boyce position
Boy'den
—sphincter
—test meal
Boyle law
Boz·zo'lo
—disease
—sign
brace
brace'let
bra'chi·a cer'e·bel'li'
bra'chi·al
bra'chi·al'gi·a

—stat'i·ca par'es·thet'i·ca
bra'chi·a'lis
bra'chi·a'tion
bra'chi·form'
bra'chi·o·ce·phal'ic
bra'chi·o·cru'ral
bra'chi·o·cu'bi·tal
bra'chi·o·cyl·lo'sis *pl.* -ses'
bra'chi·o·fa'ci·o·lin'gual
bra'chi·o·ra'di·a'lis
bra'chi·ot'o·my
bra'chi·um *pl.* -chi·a
—col·lic'u·li' in·fe'ri·o'ris
—colliculi su·pe'ri·o'ris
—con'junc·ti'vum
—conjunctivum cer'e·bel'li'
—pon'tis
—quad'ri·gem'i·num
in·fe'ri·us
—quadrigeminum
su·pe'ri·us
Brach'mann-de Lange'
syndrome
Bracht'-Wäch'ter bodies
brach'y·ba'si·a
brach'y·car'di·a
brach'y·ce·pha'li·a
brach'y·ce·phal'ic
brach'y·ceph'a·lism
brach'y·ceph'a·lous
brach'y·ceph'a·ly
brach'y·chei'li·a
brach'y·chei'rous
bra'chy·chi'li·a
bra·chych'i·ly
brach'y·cra'ni·al
brach'y·dac·tyl'i·a
brach'y·dac·tyl'ic
brach'y·dac'ty·lous
brach'y·dac'ty·ly
brach'y·fa'cial
brach'y·glos'sal
brach'y·glos'si·a
brach'yg·na'thi·a
brach·yg'na·thous
brach'y·ker'kic
brach'y·mei·o'sis *pl.* -ses'
brach'y·met'a·car'pi·a
brach'y·met'a·po'dy
brach'y·met'a·tar'si·a
brach'y·me·tro'pi·a
brach'y·mor'phic
brach'y·mor'phy

bra'chy·o·dont'
brach'y·pel'lic
brach'y·pel'vic
brach'y·pha·lan'gi·a
brach'y·pha·lan'gous
brach'y·pha·lan'gy
brach'y·po'dous
brach'y·pro·sop'ic
brach'y·rhi'ni·a
brach'y·rhyn'chus
brach'y·skel'ic
brach'y·sta'sis *pl.* -ses'
brach'y·stat'ic
brach'y·ther'a·py
brach'y·u·ran'ic
Brack'ett operation
Brack'in ureterointestinal
anastomosis
Brad'ley disease
brad'y·a·cu'si·a
brad'y·ar·rhyth'mi·a
brad'y·ar'thri·a
brad'y·aux·e'sis *pl.* -ses'
brad'y·car'di·a
brad'y·car'di·ac'
brad'y·car'dic
brad'y·crot'ic
brad'y·di·as'to·le
brad'y·di·as'to'li·a
brad'y·dys·rhyth'mi·a
brad'y·e·coi'a
brad'y·es·the'si·a
brad'y·glos'si·a
brad'y·ki·ne'si·a
brad'y·ki·ne'sis *pl.* -ses'
brad'y·ki·net'ic
brad'y·ki'nin
brad'y·ki·nin'o·gen
brad'y·laz'li·a
brad'y·lex'i·a
brad'y·pha'si·a
brad'y·phe'mi·a
brad'y·phra'si·a
brad'y·phre'ni·a
brad'y·pne'a
brad'y·pra'gi·a
brad'y·prax'i·a
brad'y·rhyth'mi·a
brad'y·sper'ma·tism
brad'y·sper'mi·a
brad'y·sphyg'mi·a
brad'y·tach'y·car'di·a
brad'y·tel'e·o·ki·ne'si·a

brad′y·tel′e·o·ki·ne′sis
  pl. -ses′
brad′y·u′ri·a
Brag′ard sign
braille
Brails′ford-Mor′qui·o
  syndrome
brain′case′
Brain reflex
brain′stem′
brain′wash′
branch′er
bran′chi·a *pl.* -ae′
bran′chi·al
bran′chi·o·gen′ic
bran′chi·og′e·nous
bran′chi·o′ma *pl.* -mas *or*
  -ma·ta
bran′chi·o·mere′
bran′chi·om′er·ism
bran′chi·o·mo′tor
Brandt syndrome
Bran′ha·mel′la cat′ar·rha′lis
Bran′ham sign
bran′ny
brash
Bras′si·ca
bras·siere′
Brat′ton and Mar′shall
  method
Brau′er operation
Braun anastomosis
Brau′ne ring
Braun test
Braun′wald′ sign
brawn′y
Brax′ton Hicks
  —contraction
  —sign
  —version
bra·ye′ra
bra·zal′um
break, broke, bro′ken,
  break′ing
break′through′
breast
breast′bone′
breast′-fed′
breath
breathe, breathed, breath′ing
breath′less
breath′less·ness
Bre′da disease

breech
breed, bred, breed′ing
bre·fel′din
breg′ma *pl.* -ma·ta
breg·mat′ic
breg′ma·to·dym′i·a
breg′ma·to·lamb′doid′
Breh and Gae′bler method
Brem′er test
bren′ner·o′ma *pl.* -mas *or*
  -ma·ta
Bren′ner tumor
breph′o·plas′tic
Bre′scia-Ci·mi′no
  arteriovenous fistula
bre·tyl′i·um tos′y·late′
Breu′er reflex
Breu′er·ton view
Breus mole
Breutsch disease
brev′i·col′is
brev′i·flex′or
brev′i·lin′e·al
brev′i·ra′di·ate′
Brew′er
  —infarcts
  —kidney
Brick′er ureteroileostomy
bridge, bridged, bridg′ing
bridge′work′
bri′dle
Briggs law
Bright
  —disease
  —murmur
Brill disease
Brill′-Sym′mers disease
Brill′-Zins′ser disease
brim′stone′
bri′nase ′
Bri·nell′
  —hardness test
  —number
Brin′ton disease
Bri·quet′
  —ataxia
  —syndrome
brise·ment′
Bris·saud′
  —disease
  —reflex
Bris·saud′-Ma·rie′
  syndrome

Bris′tow procedure
Brit′ish antilewisite
Brit′tain arthrodesis
brit′tle
broach
Broad′bent′
  —apoplexy
  —law
  —sign
Bro′ca
  —angle
  —aphasia
  —area
  —band
  —center
  —plane
  —point
Brock
  —operation
  —syndrome
Brock′en·brough sign
Brocq disease
bro·cre′sine′
Brö′del white line
Bro′ders
  —classification
  —index
Bro′die
  —abscess
  —bursa
  —knee
  —ligament
  —serocystic disease
  —tumor
Brod′mann
  —areas
  —map
bro′mate′
bro′ma·to·ther′a·py
bro′ma·to·tox′in
bro′ma·to·tox′ism
bro·ma′ze·pam′
bro′ma·zine′
brom·chlor′e·none′
brom·cre′sol′
bro′me·lain′
brom·eth′ol′
brom·hex′ine′
brom·hi·dro′sis *pl.* -ses′
bro′mic
bro′mide′
bro·mi·dro′si·pho′bi·a
bro′mi·dro′sis *pl.* -ses′

bro'min·ate'
brom'in·di'one'
bro'mine'
bro'min'ism
bro'mism
brom'i·so·val'um
bro'mo·ac'et·an'i·lid
bro'mo·cam'phor
bro'mo·cre'sol'
bro'mo·crip'tine'
bro'mo·de·ox'y·u'ri·dine'
bro'mo·der'ma
bro'mo·di'phen·hy'dra·
    mine'
bro'mo·form'
bro'mo·hy'per·hi·dro'sis
    pl. -ses'
bro'mo·hy'per·i·dro'sis
    pl. -ses'
bro'mo·i'o·dism
bro'mo·ma'ni·a
bro'mo·men'or·rhe'a
bro'mo·phe'nol'
bro'mo·thy'mol'
bro'mo·u'ra·cil
brom'phen·ir'a·mine'
bronch·ad'e·ni'tis
bron'chi·al
bron'chi·arc'ti·a
bron'chi·ec·ta'si·a
bron'chi·ec·ta·sis *pl.* -ses'
bron'chi·ec·tat'ic
bron'chi' lo·bar'es' et
    seg'men·ta'les'
bron'chil'o·quy
bron'chi·o·cele'
bron'chi·o·cri'sis
bron'chi·o·gen'ic
bron'chi·o'lar
bron'chi·ole'
bron'chi·o·lec'ta·sis *pl.* -ses'
bron'chi·o·li' res'pi·ra·to'ri·i'
bron'chi·o·li'tis
    —fi·bro'sa ob·lit'e·rans'
    —ob·lit'e·rans'
bron'chi·o'lus *pl.* -li'
bron'chi·o·spasm
bron·chit'ic
bron'chi'tis
    —con'vul·si'va
bron'chi·um *pl.* -chi·a
bron'cho·al·ve'o·lar
bron'cho·bil'i·ar'y

bron'cho·blas'to·my·co'sis
    pl. -ses'
bron'cho·can'di·di·a·sis
    pl. -ses'
bron'cho·cav'ern·ous
bron'cho·cele'
bron'cho·ceph'a·li'tis
bron'cho·con·stric'tion
bron'cho·con·stric'tor
bron'cho·dil'a·ta'tion
bron'cho·di·la'tor
bron'cho·e·de'ma
bron'cho·e·goph'o·ny
bron'cho·e·soph'a·ge'al
bron'cho·e·soph'a·gol'-
    o·gy
bron'cho·e·soph'a·gos'-
    co·py
bron'cho·gen'ic
bron·chog'e·nous
bron'cho·gram'
bron'cho·graph'ic
bron·chog'ra·phy
bron'cho·lith'
bron'cho·li·thi'a·sis *pl.* -ses'
bron·chol'o·gy
bron'cho·ma·la'ci·a
bron'cho·me'di·as·ti'nal
bron'cho·mon'i·li'a·sis
    pl. -ses'
bron'cho·mo'tor
bron'cho·my·co'sis *pl.* -ses'
bron·chop'a·thy
bron·choph'o·ny
bron'cho·plas'ty
bron'cho·ple'gi·a
bron'cho·pleu'ral
bron'cho·pneu·mo'ni·a
bron'cho·pneu'mo·ni·tis
bron'cho·pneu'mop'a·thy
bron'cho·pul'mo·nar'y
bron'chor·rha'gi·a
bron·chor'rha·phy
bron'chor·rhe'a
bron'chor·rhe'al
bron'cho·scope'
bron'cho·scop'ic
bron·chos'co·py
bron'cho·spasm
bron'cho·spi'ro·che·to'sis
    pl. -ses'
bron'cho·spi·rog'ra·phy
bron'cho·spi·rom'e·ter

bron'cho·spi·rom'e·try
bron'cho·stax'is
bron'cho·ste·no'sis *pl.* -ses'
bron·chos'to·my
bron·chot'o·my
bron'cho·tra'che·al
bron'cho·ve·sic'u·lar
bron'chus *pl.* -chi'
    —lin'gu·lar'is inferior
    —lingularis superior
    —lo·bar'is inferior dex'ter
    —lobaris inferior si·nis'ter
    —lobaris me'di·us dex'ter
    —lobaris superior dex'ter
    —lobaris superior si·nis'ter
    —prin'ci·pa'lis dex'ter et
      si·nis'ter
    —seg'men·ta'lis anterior
      lo'bi' su·pe'ri·o'ris dex'tri'
    —segmentalis anterior lobi
      superioris si·nis'tri'
    —segmentalis ap'i·ca'lis
      lo'bi' in·fe'ri·o'ris dex'tri'
    —segmentalis apicalis lobi
      inferioris si·nis'tri'
    —segmentalis apicalis lobi
      su·pe'ri·o'ris dex'tri'
    —segmentalis ap'i·co·pos·
      te'ri·or lo'bi' su·pe'ri·o'ris
      si·nis'tri'
    —segmentalis ba·sa'lis ante-
      rior lo'bi' in·fe'ri·o'ris
      dex'tri'
    —segmentalis basalis anter-
      ior lobi inferioris si·nis'tri'
    —segmentalis basalis car·
      di·a·cus lo'bi in·fe'ri·o'ris
      dex'tri'
    —segmentalis basalis cardia-
      cus lobi inferioris
      si·nis'tri'
    —segmentalis basalis
      lat'er·a'lis lo'bi' in·fe'ri·
      o'ris dex'tri'
    —segmentalis basalis later-
      alis lobi inferioris si·nis'-
      tri'
    —segmentalis basalis me'-
      di·a'lis lo'bi' in·fe'ri·o'ris
      dex'tri'
    —segmentalis basalis me-
      dialis lobi inferioris
      si·nis'tri'

—segmentalis basalis posterior lo'bi' in·fe'ri·o'ris dex'tri'

—segmentalis basalis posterior lobi inferioris si·nis'tri'

—segmentalis lat'er·a'lis lo'bi' mo'di·i' dex'tri'

—segmentalis me'di·a'lis lo'bi' mo'di·i' dex'tri'

—segmentalis posterior lo'bi' su·pe'ri·o'ris dex'tri'

—segmentalis sub·ap'i·ca'lis lo'bi' in·fe'ri·o'ris dex'tri

—segmentalis subapicalis lobi inferioris si·nis'tri'

—segmentalis sub'su·pe'ri·or lo'bi' in·fe'ri·o'ris dex'tri'

—segmentalis subsuperior lobi inferioris si·nis'tri'

—segmentalis superior lo'bi' in·fe'ri·o'ris dex'tri'

—segmentalis superior lobi inferioris si·nis'tri'

Brön'sted

—and Low'ry substance

—theory

bron'to·pho'bi·a

Brooke

—ileostomy

—tumor

Bro'phy operation

brow

Brown

—ataxia

—test

Browne sign

Brown'i·an motion

Brown'-Pearce' tumor

Brown'-Sé·quard' syndrome

bru·cel'la pl. -lae'

Bru·cel'la

—a·bor'tus

—mel'i·ten'sis

—su'is

—tu'la·ren'sis

Bru·cel·la'ce·ae'

bru·cel'lar

bru·cel·li'a·sis pl. -ses'

bru·cel'lin

bru'cel·lo'sis pl. -ses'

Bruce protocol

Bruch membrane

bru'cine'

Bruck disease

Brück'e

—line

—muscle

—tunic

Bru·dzin'ski signs

Brug'i·a

—ma·lay'i'

bru·gi'a·sis pl. -ses'

Brugsch syndrome

bruis'a·bil'i·ty

bruise, bruised, bruis'ing

bruisse·ment'

bruit

—d'ai·rain'

—de ca·non'

—de choc'

—de craque·ment'

—de cuir neuf

—de di·able'

—de frôle·ment'

—de frotte·ment'

—de ga·lop'

—de lime

—de mou·lin'

—de parche·min'

—de paiule·ment'

—de râpe

—de rap·pel'

—de Ro·ger'

—de scie

—de souf·flet'

—de ta·bour'ka

—de tam·bour'

Brun·hil'de virus

Brun'ner glands

brun'ner·o'ma pl. -mas or -ma·ta

Bruns

—ataxia

—law

—syndrome

Brun'schwig operation

Brun sign

Brun'ton rule

Brush'field' spots

Brush'field'-Wy'att syndrome

brush'ite'

Brush'y Creek fever

Bru'ton agammaglobulinemia

brux

brux'ism

brux'o·ma'ni·a

Bry'ant

—line

—operation

—sign

—traction

—triangle

bryg'mus

bry·o'ni·a

bu'bo

bu'bon·ad'e·ni'tis

bu'bon·al'gi·a

bu·bon'ic

bu·bon·o·cele'

bu·bon·u'lus pl. -lus·es or -li'

bu·car'di·a

buc'ca pl. -cae'

—ca'vi' o'ris

buc'cal

buc'ci·na'tor

buc'co·ax'i·al

buc'coc·clu'sion

buc'co·cer'vi·cal

buc'co·dis'tal

buc'co·fa'cial

buc'co·gin'gi·val

buc'co·la'bi·al

buc'co·lin'gual

buc'co·me'si·al

buc'co·na'sal

buc'co·pha·ryn'ge·al

buc'co·pha·ryn'ge·us

buc'co·pul'pal

buc'co·ver'sion

buc'cu·la pl. -lae'

bu'chu

Buck

—extension

—operation

Buck'y diaphragm

bu'cli·zine'

buc·ne'mi·a

Budd

—cirrhosis

—disease

—jaundice

Budd'-Chi·a'ri syndrome

Bü′din·ger-Lud′loff-
Lä′wen disease
Bueng′ner bands
Buer′ger
—bougie
—disease
Buer′gi hypothesis
bu′fa·gin
buff′er
buff′y coat
bu·for′min
bu·fo·ta′lin
bu·fo·ten′i·dine′
bu·fo·ten′in
bu·fo·tox′in
bug
bug′ger·y
Bu′ie
—operation
—position
Buist method
bulb
bul′bar
bul′bi·form′
bul·bi′tis
bul′bo·a′tri·al
bul′bo·cap′nine′
bul′bo·cav′er·no′sus *pl.* -si′
bul′bo·mem′bra·nous
bul′bo·nu′cle·ar
bul′bo·spi′nal
bul′bo·spon′gi·o′sus *pl.* -si′
bul′bo·u·re′thral
bul′bous
bul′bo·ven·tric′u·lar
bul′bus *pl.* -bi′
—a·or′tae′
—ar·te′ri·o′sus
—cor′dis
—cor′nus pos·te′ri·o′ris
—oc′u·li′
—ol′fac·to′ri·us
—pe′nis
—pi′li′
—u·re′thrae′
—ve′nae′ jug′u·lar′is
inferior
—venae jugularis superior
—ves·tib′u·li′ va·gi′nae′
bu·le′sis
bu·lim′i·a
bu·lim′ic
bu·lim′o·rex′i·a

Bu·li′nus
bulk
bul′la *pl.* -lae′
—eth′moi·da′lis ca′vi′ na′si′
—ethmoidalis os′sis ethmoidalis
—tym′pa·ni′
bul′late′
bul·la′tion
bul·lec′to·my
bul′lous
Bum′ke pupil
bump′er
bu·nam′i·dine′
bun′dle
—of His
—of Kent
Bun′ga·rus
—can′di·dus
—fas′ci·a′tus
Bun′ge amputation
bung′-eye′
Büng′ner band
bun′ion
bun′ion·ec′to·my
bun′ion·ette′
Bun′nell
—tendon repair
—test
bu′no·dont′
Bun′sen
—absorption coefficient
—solubility coefficient
Bun′sen-Ros′coe law
Bun′yam·ve′ra virus
bun′ya·vi′rus
buph·thal′mi·a
buph·thal′mos
bu·piv′a·caine′
bu′pre·nor′phine ′
bu·pro′pi·on′
bur *also* burr
bu′ra·mate′
bur′bot
Bur′chard test
Bur′dach′ nucleus
Burd′wan fever
bu·ret′ *also* burette
bu·rette′ *var. of* buret
Bur′kitt lymphoma
burn
Bur·nett′ milk′-al′ka·li
syndrome

bur′nish
bur′nish·er
burn′out′
Bu′row solution
burp
burr *var. of* bur
bur′sa *pl.* -sas *or* -sae′
—an′se·ri′na
—bi·cip′i·to·gas′troc·ne′mi·
a′lis
—bi·cip′i·to·ra′di·a′lis
—clo·a′ca
—cu′bi·ta′lis in′ter·os′se·a
—i·li′a·ca sub′ten·din′e·a
—il′i·o·pec·tin′e·a
—in′fra·hy·oi′de·a
—in′fra·pat′el·lar′is pro·
fun′da
—is′chi·ad′i·ca mus′cu·li′
glu′tae·i′ max′i·mi′
—ischiadica musculi
glu′te·i′ max′i·mi′
—ischiadica musculi ob·tu′-
ra·to′ri·i′ in·ter′ni′
—mu·co′sa
—mucosa sub′cu·ta′ne·a
—mucosa sub·fas′ci·a′lis
—mucosa sub·mus′cu·lar′is
—mucosa sub′ten·din′e·a
—mus′cu·li′ co′ra·co·bra′-
chi·a′lis
—musculi gas′troc·ne′mi·i′
lat′er·a′lis
—musculi gastrocnemii me′-
di·a′lis
—musculi la·tis′si·mi′
dor′si′
—musculi ob·tu′ra·to′ri·i′
in·ter′ni′
—musculi pop·lit′e·i′
—musculi sar·to′ri·i′ pro′-
pri·a
—musculi sem′i·mem′bra·
no′si′
—musculi ster′no·hy·oi′-
de·i′
—musculi sub·scap′u·lar′is
—of Fab·ri′ci·us
—o′men·ta′lis
—o·var′i·ca
—pha·ryn′ge·a
—prae·pat′el·lar′is sub′cu·
ta′ne·a

—praepatellaris sub·fas′ci·
a′lis
—praepatellaris sub′ten·
din′e·a
—sub′a·cro′mi·a′lis
—sub′cu·ta′ne·a a·cro′mi·
a′lis
—subcutanea o′le·cra′ni′
—subcutanea pre·pat′el·
lar′is
—subcutanea tro′chan·ter′i·ca
—sub′del·toi′de·a
—sub·fas′ci·a′lis pre·pat′el·
lar′is
—sub′ten·din′e·a i·li′a·ca
—subtendinea mus′cu·li′
gas′troc·ne′mi·i′ lat′er·a′lis
—subtendinea musculi
gastrocnemii me′di·a′lis
—subtendinea musculi
la·tis′si·mi′ dor′si′
—subtendinea musculi
ob·tu′ra·to′ri·i′ in·ter′ni′
—subtendinea musculi
sub·scap′u·lar′is
—subtendinea pre·pat′el·
lar′is
—sy·no′vi·a′lis
—synovialis sub′cu·ta′ne·a
—synovialis sub·fas′ci·a′lis
—synovialis sub·mus′-
cu·lar′is
—synovialis sub·ten·din′e·a
—ten′di·nis A·chil′lis
—tendinis cal·ca′ne·i′
—tro′chan·ter′i·ca mus′cu·
li′ glu′tae·i′ me′di·i′ anterior
—trochanterica musculi
glutaei min′i·mi′
—trochanterica musculi
glu′te·i′ max′i·mi′
—trochanterica musculi glutei
min′i·mi′
bur′sae′
—sub′ten·din′e·ae′
mus′cu·li′ sar·to′ri·i′
—tro′chan·ter′i·cae′ mus′-
cu·li′ glu′te·i′ me′di·i′
bur′sal
bur·sec′to·my
Bur′ser·a′ce·ae′
bur·si′tis

bur′so·cen·te′sis *pl.* -ses′
bur′so·lith′
bur·sop′a·thy
bur·sot′o·my
burst
bur′su·la
Bur′ton
—line
—sign
Bur′y disease
Busch′ke disease
bu′se·re·lin
bu·spi′rone′
Bus·quet′ disease
Bus′se-Busch′ke disease
bu·sul′fan′
bu′ta·bar′bi·tal′
bu′ta·caine′
bu·tac′e·tin
bu·tal′bi·tal′
bu·tam′ben
bu′tane′
bu·ta·no′ic
bu′ta·nol′
bu·ta·per′a·zine′
bu′tene′
bu′te·nyl
bu′te·thal′
bu·teth′a·mine′
bu·thi′a·zide′
Bu′thus
—co·ci′ta′nus
—i·tal′i·cus
—mar·ten′si′
But′ler
—and Tut′hill method
—solution
bu·to′py·ro·nox′yl
bu·tor′pha·nol′
bu·tox′a·mine′
bu·trip′ty·line′
butt
but′tock
but′ton
but′ton·hole′
but′ton·hook′
but′tress
bu′tyl
—hy·drox′y·ben′zo·ate′
—par′a·hy·drox′y·ben′zo·ate′
bu′tyl·ene′
bu·tyl′i·dene′
bu′tyl·par′a·ben

bu′ty·ra′ceous
bu′ty·rate′
bu·tyr′ic
bu′ty·rin
bu′ty·rin·ase′
bu′ty·roid′
bu′ty·ro·phe′none′
bu′ty·rous
bu′ty·ryl
bux′ine′
Buz′zard reflex
Bwam′ba
—fever
—virus
By′ler disease
by′pass′
bys′si·no′sis *pl.* -ses′
bys′soid′
bys′so·phthi′sis *pl.* -ses′
By′wa′ters syndrome

C

caa′pi
Cab′ot rings
cac·an′thrax′
cac·a′tion
cac′a·to′ry
cac′er·ga′si·a
cac′es·then′ic
cac′es·the′si·a
cac′es·the′sic
ca·chec′tic
ca·chec′tin
ca·chet′
ca·chex′i·a
—ex′oph·thal′mi·ca
—hy′po·phys′i·o·pri′va
—stru′mi·pri′va
—thy′ro·pri′va
cach′in·na′tion
cac′o·de′mo·no·ma′ni·a
cac′o·dyl
cac′o·dyl·ate′
cac′o·dyl′ic
cac′o·gen′e·sis
cac′o·gen′ic
cac′o·geu′si·a
ca·cos′mi·a
ca·dav′er
ca·dav′er·ic
ca·dav′er·ine′
ca·dav′er·ous

cad'mi·o'sis
cad'mi·um
ca·du'ca
ca·du'ce·us
caec-. See words spelled
    cec-.
caeci-. See words spelled
    ceci-.
cae·ci·tas
caeco-. See words spelled
    ceco-.
cae'cus
cae·sar'e·an *var. of* cesarean
ca·fard'
caf·fe'ic
caf·feine'
caf'fein·ism
Caf'fey disease
Caille test
cais'son'
Ca·jal'
  —cell
  —gold'-sub'li·mate' method
  —interstitial nucleus
  —silver method
caj'e·put
caj'e·pu·tol'
Cal'a·bar'
  —bean
  —swellings
cal'a·mine'
cal'a·mus *pl.* -mi'
  —scrip·to'ri·us
cal·ca'ne·al
cal·ca'ne·an
cal·ca'ne·i'tis
cal·ca'ne·o·a·poph'y·si'tis
cal·ca'ne·o·as·trag'a·lar
cal·ca'ne·o·a·strag'a·loid'
cal·ca'ne·o·ca'vus
cal·ca'ne·o·cla·vic'u·lar
cal·ca'ne·o·cu'boid'
cal·ca'ne·o·dyn'i·a
cal·ca'ne·o·fib'u·lar
cal·ca'ne·o·na·vic'u·lar
cal·ca'ne·o·plan'tar
cal·ca'ne·o·scaph'oid'
cal·ca'ne·o·tib'i·al
cal·ca'ne·o·val'gus
cal·ca'ne·um *pl.* -ne·a
cal·ca'ne·us *pl.* -ne·i'
cal·ca'no·dyn'i·a
cal'car' *pl.* cal·car'i·a

—a'vis
—fem'o·ra'le'
—pe'dis
cal'ca·rate'
cal·car'e·a
cal·car'e·ous
cal'ca·rine
cal·car'i·u'ri·a
cal·ce'mi·a
cal·ci·bil'i·a
cal'cic
cal'ci·co'sis *pl.* -ses'
cal·cif'a·mes'
cal·cif'er·ol'
cal·cif'er·ous
cal·cif'ic
cal'ci·fi·ca'tion
cal'ci·fy', -fied', -fy'ing
cal'cig'er·ous
cal·cim'e·ter
cal'ci·na'tion
cal'cine', -cined', -cin'ing
cal'ci·no'sis *pl.* -ses'
  —cu'tis cir'cum·scrip'ta
  —cutis u'ni·ver·sa'lis
  —universalis
cal'ci·pe'ni·a
cal'ci·pex'ic
cal'ci·pex'is
cal'ci·pex'y
cal'ci·phil'i·a
cal'ci·phy·lac'tic
cal'ci·phy·lax'is *pl.* -lax'es'
cal'ci·priv'i·a
cal'cite'
cal'ci·to'nin
cal'ci·um
cal'ci·u'ri·a
cal'co·glob'u·lin
cal'co·sphe'rite'
cal'co·spher'ule'
cal'cu·lar'y
cal'cu·lif'ra·gous
cal'cu·lo·gen'e·sis *pl.* -ses'
cal'cu·lo'sis *pl.* -ses'
cal'cu·lous *(pertaining to*
  calculi)
  ♦*calculus*
cal'cu·lus *(an abnormal*
  concretion in the body),
  pl. -li' *or* -lus·es
  ♦*calculous*
  —fel'le·us

Cal·da'ni ligament
Cald'well-Luc' operation
Cald'well projection
cal'e·fa'cient
ca·len'du·lin
cal'en·tu'ra
calf *pl.* calves
ca'li·ber *also* calibre
cal'i·brate', -brat'ed, -brat'ing
cal'i·bra'tion
cal'i·bra'tor
cal'i·bre *var. of* caliber
cal'i·ce'al *var. of* calyceal
ca'li·cec'ta·sis *pl.* -ses', *var.*
  of calycectasis
ca'li·cec'to·my *var. of*
  calycectomy
cal'i·for'ni·um
ca·lic'i·form' *var. of*
  calyciform
ca·lic'i·nal *var. of* calycinal
ca'li·cine' *var. of* calycine
ca·lic'u·lus *pl.* -li', *also*
  calyculus
  —gus'ta·to'ri·us
  —oph·thal'mi·cus
cal'i·per
cal'is·then'ics
ca'lix *pl.* ca'li·ces', *var. of*
  calyx
Cal'kins method
Cal'lan·der amputation
Cal'la·way' test
Cal·le'ja islands
Call'-Ex'ner bodies
cal'li·pe'di·a
Cal·liph'o·ra
  —vom'i·to'ri·a
Cal'li·pho'ri·dae'
cal'lo·ma'ni·a
cal'lo'sal
cal'lose'
cal·los'i·tas
cal·los'i·ty
cal'lo·so·mar'gi·nal
cal'lo·sum *pl.* -sa
cal'lous *(hard)*
  ♦*callus*
cal'lus *(a callosity)*
  ♦*callous*
calm'a·tive
Cal·mette'
  —test

—vaccine
cal·mod′u·lin
cal′o·mel′
cal′or
ca·lor′ic
cal′o·rie
ca·lor′i·fa′cient
cal′o·rif′ic
ca·lor′i·gen′ic
cal′o·rim′e·ter
cal′o·ri·met′ric
cal′o·rim′e·try
cal′o·ri·punc′ture
ca·lor′i·trop′ic
Ca·lot′ triangle
cal′pain′
ca·lum′ba
cal·var′i·a *pl.* -i·ae′
cal·var′i·al
cal·var′i·um
Cal·vé′
  —disease
  —ver′te·bra pla′na
Cal·vé′-Per′thes disease
cal·vi′ti·es′
calx *pl.* cal′ces′
cal′y·can′thine′
cal′y·ce′al *also* caliceal
cal′y·cec′ta·sis *pl.* -ses′, *also*
  calicectasis
cal′y·cec′to·my *also*
  calicectomy
cal′y·ces′
  —re·na′les′
  —renales ma·jo′res′
  —renales mi·no′res′
ca·lyc′i·form′ *also* caliciform
ca·lyc′i·nal *also* calicinal
cal′y·cine′ *also* calicine
ca·lyc′u·li′ gus′ta·to′ri·i′
ca·lyc′u·lus *pl.* -li′, *var. of*
  caliculus
cal′y·ec′ta·sis *also*
  cal′i·ec′ta·sis
Ca·lym′ma·to·bac·te′ri·um
  gran′u·lo′ma·tis
ca′lyx *pl.* -lyx·es *or*
  cal′y·ces′, *also* calix
cam·bi′um *pl.* -bi·ums *or*
  -bi·a
cam′er·a *pl.* -ae′
  —anterior bul′bi′
  —lu′ci·da

—oc′u·li′ anterior
—oculi posterior
—posterior bul′bi′
—sep′ti′ lu′ci·di′
—vit′re·a bul′bi′
cam′i·sole′
Cam′midge test
Camp′bell operation
Cam′per
  —chiasma
  —fascia
  —ligament
  —line
cam·pes′ter·ol′
cam′phene′
cam′phor
cam′phor·a′ceous
cam′phor·at′ed
cam′phor·ic
cam′phor·ism
cam·pim′e·ter
cam·pim′e·try
camp′to·cor′mi·a
camp′to·dac′ty·ly
camp′to·spasm
camp′to·the′cin
Cam′py·lo·bac′ter
  —co′li
  —fe′tus
  —je·ju′ni′
Cam·u·ra′ti-En′gel·mann
  disease
ca·nal′
  —of Cor′ti
  —of Her′ing
  —of Nuck
  —of Schlemm
ca·na′les′
  —al′ve·o·lar′es′ max·il′lae′
  —di·plo′i·ci′
  —lon′gi·tu′di·na′les′ mo·
    di′o·li′
  —pal·a·ti′ni′
  —palatini mi·no′res′
  —sem′i·cir′cu·lar′es′ os′se·i′
can′a·lic′u·lar
can′a·lic′u·la′tion
can′a·lic′u·li′
  —ca·rot′i·co·tym·pan′i·ci′
  —den′ta·les′
  —vas′cu·lo′si′
can′a·lic′u·li·za′tion
can′a·lic′u·lo·plas′ty

can′a·lic′u·lus *pl.* -li′
  —chor′dae′ tym′pa·ni′
  —coch′le·ae′
  —lac′ri·ma′lis
  —mas·toi′de·us
  —tym·pan′i·cus
can′a·line′
ca·na′lis *pl.* -les′
  —ad′duc·to′ri·us
  —al′i·men·tar′i·us
  —a·na′lis
  —ba·si·pha·ryn′ge·us
  —ca·rot′i·cus
  —car′pi′
  —cen·tra′lis
  —cer′vi·cis u′ter·i′
  —con·dy·lar′is
  —con·dy·loi′de·us
  —fa·ci·a′lis
  —fem′o·ra′lis
  —hy′a·loi′de·us
  —hy′po·glos′si′
  —in′ci·si′vus
  —in′fra·or′bi·ta′lis
  —in′gui·na′lis
  —man·dib′u·lae′
  —mus′cu·lo·tu·bar′i·us
  —na′so·lac′ri·ma′lis
  —nu·tri′ci·us
  —ob′tu·ra·to′ri·us
  —op′ti·cus
  —pal′a·ti′nus major
  —pal′a·to·vag′i·na′lis
  —pha·ryn′ge·us
  —pter′y·goi′de·us
  —pter′y·go·pal′a·ti′nus
  —pu′den·da′lis
  —py·lo′ri·cus
  —rad′i·cis den′tis
  —sa·cra′lis
  —sem′i·cir′cu·lar′is anterior
  —semicircularis lat′er·a′lis
  —semicircularis posterior
  —semicircularis superior
  —spi·na′lis
  —spi·ra′lis coch′le·ae′
  —spiralis mo·di′o·li′
  —ven·tric′u·li′
  —ver′te·bra′lis
  —vom′er·o·vag′i·na′lis
can′a·li·za′tion
can′al·ize′, -ized′, -iz′ing
ca·nal′o·plas′ty

ca·nals' of Pe·tit'
Can'a·van disease
can'a·van'ine'
can'cel·late'
can'cel·lat'ed
can'cel·lous
can'cer
—en cui·rasse'
—oc·cul'tus
can'cer·e'mi·a
can'cer·i·cid'al
can'cer·i·gen'ic
can'cer·i·za'tion
can'cer·o·gen
can'cer·o·gen'ic
can'cer·o·pho'bi·a
can'cer·ous
can'cer·pho'bi·a
can'cri·form'
can'croid'
can'crum
—na'si'
—o'ris
—pu·den'di'
can·del'a
can·di·ci'din
Can'di·da
—al'bi·cans'
can'di·dal
can'di·de'mi·a
can'di·di·di'a·sis *pl.* -ses'
can'di·did
can'di·do'sis *pl.* -ses'
can'di·ru'
can'dle
cane
Can'i·dae'
ca'nine'
ca·nin'i·form'
ca·ni'nus *pl.* -ni'
ca·ni'ti·es'
—un'gui·um
can'ker
can'na·bi·di·ol'
can·na·bin
can·nab'i·nol'
can·na·bis
can·na·bism
Can'niz·za'ro reaction
Can'non
—law of denervation
—point
—ring

—wave
can'nu·la *pl.* -las *or* -lae'
can'nu·lar
can'nu·late', -lat'ed, -lat'ing
can'nu·la'tion
can'nu·li·za'tion
can'nu·lize', -lized', -liz'ing
can're·none'
can'thal
can'tha·ri·a'sis *pl.* -ses'
can'thar'i·dal
can'thar'i·date'
can·thar'i·din
can·thar'i·dism
Can'tha·ris
—ves'i·ca·to'ri·a
can·thec'to·my
can·thi'tis
can·thol'y·sis *pl.* -ses'
can'tho·plas'ty
can·thor'rha·phy
can·thot'o·my
can'thus *pl.* -thi'
caou'tchouc'
cap
—of Zinn
ca·pac'i·tance
ca·pac'i·ta'tion
ca·pac'i·tor
ca·pac'i·ty
Cap·gras' syndrome
cap'il·lar'ec·ta'si·a
Cap'il·lar'i·a
—aer'o·phi'la
—he·pat'i·ca
—phil'ip·pi·nen'sis
cap'il·la·ri'a·sis *pl.* -ses'
cap'il·lar'i·o·mo'tor
cap'il·la·ri'tis
cap'il·lar'i·ty
cap'il·la·ros'co·py
cap'il·lar'y
cap'il·li·ti'um *pl.* -ti·a
cap'il·lo·ve'nous
ca·pil'lus *pl.* -li'
cap'i·stra'tion
cap'i·tate'
cap'i·ta'tum *pl.* -ta
cap'i·tel'lar
cap'i·tel'lum *pl.* -la
ca·pit'u·lar
ca·pit'u·lum *pl.* -la
—cos'tae'

—fib'u·lae'
—hu'mer·i'
—mal'le·i'
—man·dib'u·lae'
—os'si·um met'a·car·pa'-
li·um
—ossium met'a·tar·sa'-
li·um
—ra'di·i'
—San'to·ri'ni·i'
—sta'pe·dis
—ul'nae'
Ca'pi·vac'ci·us ulcer
Cap'lan syndrome
Capps pleural reflex
cap'rate'
cap're·o·late'
cap'ric
ca·pril'o·quism
cap'rin
cap'ro·ate'
ca·pro'ic
cap'ro·in
cap'ry·late'
ca·pryl'ic
cap·sa'i·cin
cap'sid
cap·sid'al
cap·si'tis
cap'so·mer'
cap·sot'o·my
cap'su·la *pl.* -lae'
—ad'i·po'sa re'nis
—ar·tic'u·lar'is
—articularis a·cro'mi·o·cla·
vic'u·lar'is
—articularis ar·tic'u·la'ti·o'-
nis ra'di·o·car'pe·ae'
—articularis articulationis
tar'si' trans·ver'sae'
—articularis articulationis
tem'po·ro·man·dib'u·
lar'is
—articularis ar·tic'u·la'ti·o'-
num ver'te·brar'um
—articularis at·lan'to·ax'i·
a'lis lat'er·a'lis
—articularis atlantoaxialis
me'di·a'na
—articularis at·lan'to·oc·
cip'i·ta'lis
—articularis cal·ca'ne·o·cu·
boi'de·ae'

—articularis cap'i·tis cos'-
tae'
—articularis car'po·met'a·
car'pe·a pol'li·cis
—articularis cos'to·trans'-
ver·sar'i·ae'
—articularis cox'ae'
—articularis cri'co·ar'y·tae·
noi'de·a
—articularis cri'co·ar'y·te·
noi'de·a
—articularis cri'co·thy're·
oi'de·a
—articularis cri'co·thy·roi'-
de·a
—articularis cu'bi·ti'
—articularis ge'nus
—articularis hu'mer·i'
—articularis man·dib'u·
lae'
—articularis ma'nus
—articularis os'sis pi'si·for'-
mis
—articularis ra'di·o·ul·nar'-
is dis·ta'lis
—articularis ster'no·cla·vic'-
u·lar'is
—articularis ster'no·cos·
ta'lis
—articularis sub'ta·lar'is
—articularis ta'lo·cal·ca'-
ne·a
—articularis ta'lo·cru·ra'lis
—articularis ta'lo·na·vic'u·
lar'is
—articularis tib'i·o·fib'u·
lar'is
—ex·ter'na
—fi·bro'sa glan'du·lae' thy·
roi'de·ae'
—fibrosa (Glis·so'ni')
—fibrosa per'i·vas'cu·lar'is
—fibrosa re'nis
—glo·mer'u·li'
—in·ter'na
—len'tis
—nu'cle·i' den·ta'ti'
cap'su·lae'
—ar·tic'u·lar'es' at'lan·to·
ep'i·stroph'i·cae'
—articulares ca·pit'u·li'
cos'tae'
—articulares car'po·met'a·

car'pe·ae'
—articulares dig'i·to'rum
ma'nus
—articulares digitorum
pe'dis
—articulares in'ter·met'a·
car'pe·ae'
—articulares in'ter·met'a·
tar'se·ae'
—articulares in'ter·pha·lan'-
ge·ar'um ma'nus
—articulares interphalangearum pe'dis
—articulares met'a·car'po·
pha·lan'ge·ae'
—articulares met'a·ter'so·
pha·lan'ge·ae'
—articulares tar'so·met'a·
tar'se·ae'
cap'su·lar
cap'sule'
cap'su·lec'to·my
cap'su·li'tis
cap'su·lo·len·tic'u·lar
cap'su·lo'ma pl. -mas or
  -ma·ta
cap'su·lo·per'i·os'te·al
cap'su·lo·plas'ty
cap'su·lor'rha·phy
cap'su·lo·tha·lam'ic
cap'su·lo·tome'
cap'su·lot'o·my
cap'ta·mine'
cap'ti·va'tion
cap'to·di'ame'
cap'to·di'a·mine'
cap'to·pril
cap'ture
cap'u·ride'
cap'ut pl. cap'i·ta
  —an'gu·lar'e' mus'cu·li'
  qua·dra'ti' la'bi·i'
  su·pe'ri·o'ris
  —brev'e' mus'cu·li'
  bi·cip'i·tis bra'chi·i'
  —breve musculi bicipitis
  fem'o·ris
  —cos'tae'
  —de'for·ma'tum
  —ep'i·dym'i·dis
  —fem'o·ris
  —fib'u·lae'
  —gal'e·a'tum

—hu·mer·a'le' mus'cu·li'
ex·ten'so·ris car'pi'
ul·nar'is
—humerale musculi
flex·o'ris car'pi' ul·nar'is
—humerale musculi flexoris
dig'i·to'rum sub·li'mis
—humerale musculi
pro·na'to·ris te·re'tis
—hu'mer·i'
—hu'mer·o·ul·nar'e' mus'-
cu·li' flex·o'ris dig'i·to'-
rum su'per·fi'ci·a'lis
—in'fra·or'bi·ta'le' mus'cu·
li' qua·dra'ti' la'bi·i'
—lat'er·a'le' mus'cu·li'
gas'troc·ne'mi·i'
—laterale musculi tri·cip'i·
tis bra'chi·i'
—lon'gum mus'cu·li'
bi·cip'i·tis bra'chi·i'
—longum musculi bicipitis
fem'o·ris
—longum musculi
tri·cip'i·tis bra'chi·i'
—mal'le·i'
—man·dib'u·lae'
—me'di·a'le' mus'cu·li'
gas'troc·ne'mi·i'
—mediale musculi tri·cip'i·
tis bra'chi·i'
—me·du'sae'
—mus'cu·li'
—nu'cle·i' cau·da'ti'
—ob·li'quum mus'cu·li'
ad·duc'to·ris hal'lu·cis
—obliquum musculi
adductoris pol'li·cis
—ob'sti·pum
—os'sis met'a·car'pa'lis
—ossis met'a·tar·sa'lis
—pan·cre'a·tis
—pha·lan'gis ma'nus
—phalangis pe'dis
—pro·fun'dum mus'cu·li'
flex·o'ris pol'li·cis brev'is
—qua·dra'tum
—ra'di·a'le' mus'cu·li' flex·
o'ris dig'i·to'rum su'per·
fi'ci·a'lis
—ra'di·i'
—sta'pe'dis
—suc'ce·da'ne·um

—su'per·fi'ci·a'le' mus'-
cu·li' flex·o'ris pol'li·cis
brev'is
—ta'li'
—trans·ver'sum mus·cu·li'
ad·duc·to'ris hal'lu·cis
—transversum musculi
adductoris pol'li·cis
—ul'nae'
—ul·nar'e' mus'cu·li' ex'-
ten·so'ris car'pi' ul·nar'is
—ulnare musculi flex·o'ris
car'pi' ul·nar'is
—ulnare musculi pro'na·to'-
ris te·re'tis
—zy'go·mat'i·cum mus'cu·
li' qua·dra'ti' la'bi·i'
su·pe·ri·o'ris
Car'a·bel'li cusp
car·am'i·phen
car'a·pace'
ca·ra'te
car'ba·chol'
car'ba·cryl'a·mine'
car'ba·cryl'ic
car'ba·dox'
car'ba·mate'
car'ba·maz'e·pine'
car·bam'ic
car'ba·mide'
car·bam'i·dine'
carb·a'mi·no
carb·a'mi·no·he'mo·
glo'bin
car·bam'o·yl·trans'fer·ase'
car'ba·myl
car'ba·myl·cho'line'
carb·an'i·on'
car·bar'sone'
car·ba·zide'
car·baz'o·chrome'
car·ba·zole'
car·ba·zot'ic
car·ben·i·cil'lin
car·ben·ox'o·lone'
car·be'ta·pen'tane'
car'bide'
car'bi·do'pa
car'bi·nol'
car'bin·ox'a·mine'
car'bi·phene'
car'bo
car·bo·ben·zox'y

car'bo·cho'line'
car'bo·clo'ral
car'bo·cy'clic
car'bo·he'mo·glo'bin
car'bo·hy'drase'
car'bo·hy'drate'
car'bo·hy'dra·tu'ri·a
car'bo·late', -lat'ed, -lat'ing
car'bol·fuch'sin
car·bol'ic
car'bo·li'gase'
car'bo·lism
car'bo·lize'
car'bo·lu'ri·a
car'bo·mer
car'bo·my'cin
car'bon
car'bo·na'ceous
car'bon·ate', -at'ed, -at'ing
car·bon'ic
car'bo·ni·um
car'bon·i·za'tion
car'bon·ize', -ized', -iz'ing
car'bon·u'ri·a
car'bon·yl
car·box'y·he'mo·glo'bin
car·box'y·he'mo·glo'bin·e'-
mi·a
car·box'yl
car·box'yl·ase'
car·box'yl·a'tion
car·box'yl'ic
car·box'yl·trans'fer·ase'
car·box'y·meth'yl·cel'lu·
lose'
car·box'y·my'o·glo'bin
car·box'y·pep'ti·dase'
car·box'y·pol'y·pep'ti·
dase'
car'bro·mal
car·bun'cle
car·bun'cu·lar
car·bun'cu·loid'
car·bun'cu·lo'sis pl. -ses'
car·bu'ta·mide'
car'byl·a·mine'
car'cass
Car'cas·sonne' ligament
car'ci·nec'to·my
car'ci·ne'mi·a
car'ci·no·em'bry·on'ic
car·cin'o·gen
car'ci·no·gen'e·sis

car'ci·no·ge·net'ic
car'ci·no·gen'ic
car'ci·no·ge·nic'i·ty
car'ci·noid'
car'ci·noi·do'sis pl. -ses'
car'ci·nol'y·sis
car'ci·no·lyt'ic
car'ci·no'ma pl. -mas or
-ma·ta
—bron'chi·o·lo'rum
—in si'tu
—mu'co·cel'lu·lar'e'
o·var'i·i'
—oc·cul'ta
—sim'plex'
—sub·stan'ti·ae' cor'ti·ca'lis
su'pra·re'na·lis
car'ci·no'ma·toid'
car'ci·no'ma·toi'des' al've·
o·gen'i·ca mul'ti·cen'-
tri·ca
car'ci·no'ma·to'sis pl. -ses'
car'ci·no'ma·tous
car'ci·no·pho'bi·a
car'ci·no·sar·co'ma pl. -mas
or -ma·ta
car'ci·no'sis pl. -ses'
Car'den amputation
car'di·a pl. -ae' or -as
—ven·tric'u·li'
car'di·ac'
car'di·al
car'di·al'gi·a
car'di·ant
car'di·as·the'ni·a
car'di·asth'ma
car'di·cen·te'sis pl. -ses'
car'di·ec'ta·sis pl. -ses'
car'di·ec'to·my
car'di·o·ac·cel'er·a'tor
car'di·o·ac'tive
car'di·o·an'gi·og'ra·phy
car'di·o·an'gi·ol'o·gy
car'di·o·a·or'tic
car'di·o·ar·te'ri·al
car'di·o·asth'ma
car'di·o·au'di·to'ry
car'di·o·cele'
car'di·o·cen·te'sis pl. -ses'
car'di·o·cha·la'si·a
car'di·o·cir·rho'sis pl. -ses'
car'di·o·cla'si·a
car'di·o·di'a·phrag·mat'ic

car′di·o·di·la′tor
car′di·o·di·o′sis *pl.* -ses′
car′di·o·dy·nam′ic
car′di·o·dy·nam′ics
car′di·o·dyn′i·a
car′di·o·e·soph′a·ge′al
car′di·o·fa′cial
car′di·o·gen′e·sis *pl.* -ses′
car′di·o·gen′ic
car′di·o·gram′
car′di·o·graph′
car′di·o·graph′ic
car′di·og′ra·phy
car′di·o·he·pat′ic
car′di·o·hep′a·to·meg′a·ly
car′di·oid′
car′di·o·in·hib′i·tor
car′di·o·in·hib′i·to′ry
car′di·o·ki·net′ic
car′di·o·ky′mo·graph′ic
car′di·o·ky·mog′ra·phy
car′di·o·lip′in
car′di·o·lith′
car′di·ol′o·gist
car′di·ol′o·gy
car′di·ol′y·sis *pl.* -ses′
car′di·o·ma·la′ci·a
car′di·o·me·ga′li·a gly′co·
  gen′i·ca dif·fu′sa
car′di·o·meg′a·ly
car′di·o·mel′a·no′sis *pl.* -ses′
car′di·o·men′su·ra′tor
car′di·o·men′to·pex′y
car′di·om·e′ter
car′di·o·met′ric
car′di·om′e·try
car′di·o·mo·til′i·ty
car′di·o·my′o·li·po′sis
  pl. -ses′
car′di·o·my′o·path′ic
car′di·o·my′o·op′a·thy
car′di·o·my′o·pex′y
car′di·o·my·ot′o·my
car′di·o·ne·cro′sis *pl.* -ses′
car′di·o·nec′tor
car′di·o·neph′ric
car′di·o·neu′ral
car′di·o·neu·ro′sis *pl.* -ses′
car′di·o-o·men′to·pex′y
car′di·o·pal′u′dism
car′di·o·path′
car′di·o·path′i·a
car′di·o·path′ic

car′di·o·pa·thol′o·gy
car′di·op′a·thy
car′di·o·per′i·car′di·o·
  pex′y
car′di·o·per′i·car·di′tis
car′di·o·pho′bi·a
car′di·o·phone′
car′di·o·phren′ic
car′di·o·plas′ty
car′di·o·ple′gi·a
car′di·o·ple′gic
car′di·o·pneu·mat′ic
car′di·o·pneu′mo·graph′
car′di·o·pneu·mog′ra·phy
car′di·o·pro·tec′tive
car′di·op·to′si·a
car′di·op·to′sis *pl.* -ses′
car′di·o·pul′mo·nar′y
car′di·o·pul·mon′ic
car′di·o·punc′ture
car′di·o·py·lor′ic
car′di·o·ra′di·o·log′ic
car′di·o·ra′di·ol′o·gy
car′di·o·re′nal
car′di·o·res′pi·ra·to′ry
car′di·or·rha·phy
car′di·or·rhex′is *pl.* -rhex′es′
car′di·os′chi·sis *pl.* -ses′
car′di·o·scope′
car′di·o·se·lec′tive
car′di·o·spasm
car′di·o·sphyg′mo·graph′
car′di·o·ste·no′sis *pl.* -ses′
car′di·o·sym′phy·sis
  pl. -ses′
car′di·o·ta·chom′e·ter
car′di·o·ta·chom′e·try
car′di·o·ther′a·py
car′di·o·tho·rac′ic
car′di·o·thy′ro·tox′i·co′sis
  pl. -ses′
car′di·ot′o·my
car′di·o·ton′ic
car′di·o·to·pog′ra·phy
car′di·o·to·pom′e·try
car′di·o·tox′ic
car′di·o·tox·ic′i·ty
car′di·o·val′vu·lar
car′di·o·val′vu·li′tis
car′di·o·val′vu·lo·tome′
car′di·o·val′vu·lot′o·my
car′di·o·vas′cu·lar
car′di·o·vec·tog′ra·phy

car′di·o·ver′sion
car′di·o·vert′
car′di·o·vert′er
car·di′tis
care′giv′er
Car′ey Coombs murmur
car′ies
  —sic′ca
ca·ri′na *pl.* -nas *or* -nae′
  —for′ni·cis
  —na′si′
  —tra′che·ae′
  —u′re·thra′lis
  —va·gi′nae′
ca·ri′nal
car′i·nate′
car′i·o·gen′e·sis *pl.* -ses′
car′i·o·gen′ic
car′i·o·stat′ic
car′i·ous
car·i′so·pro′dol′
Carl Smith disease
car·mal′um
Car′man
  —meniscus sign
  —tube
car·min′a·tive
car′mine
car·min′ic
car·min′o·phil
car′mus·tine′
car′ne·ous
car′ni·fi·ca′tion
car′ni·tine′
Car·niv′o·ra
car′ni·vore′
car·niv′o·rous
car′no·sine′
car′no·si·ne′mi·a
car′no·si·nu′ri·a
Car′noy fluid
ca′ro *pl.* car′nes′
  —qua·dra′ta ma′nus
  —quadrata syl′vi·i′
Car′o·li disease
car′o·tene′
car′o·te·ne′mi·a *also*
  carotinemia
ca·rot′e·no·der′mi·a *also*
  carotinodermia
ca·rot′e·noid′
car′o·te·no′sis *pl.* -ses′, *also*
  carotinosis

ca·rot'ic
ca·rot'i·co·cli'noid'
ca·rot'i·co·tym·pan'ic
ca·rot'id
ca·rot'i·dyn'i·a
car'o·tin
car'o·tin·ase'
car'o·tin·e'mi·a *var. of*
  carotenemia
ca·rot'i·no·der'mi·a *var. of*
  carotenodermia
car'o·ti·no'sis *pl.* -ses', *var.*
  of carotenosis
ca·rot'o·dyn'i·a
car'pa·ine'
car'pal
car·pec'to·my
Car'pen·ter syndrome
Car'pen·tier' annuloplasty
car·phen'a·zine'
car'pho·lo'gi·a
car'phol'o·gy
car·pi'tis
car'po·car'pal
car'po·met'a·car'pal
car'po·ped'al
car'po·pha·lan'ge·al
car'pop·to'sis *pl.* -ses'
car'pus *pl.* -pi'
car'ra·geen'
car'ra·gee'nan
Car·rel'-Da'kin treatment
car'ri·er
Car·ri·ón' disease
Carr'-Price' test
Carr'-Pur·cell'-Mei'boom'-
  Gill' sequence
car'sick'
car'sick'ness
Cars'well' grapes
Car'ter operation
Car·te'sian
car'tha·mus
car'ti·lage
  —of San'to·ri'ni
  —of Wris'berg'
car'ti·lag'i·nes'
  —a·lar'es' mi·no'res'
  —la·ryn'gis
  —na·sa'les' ac'ces·so'ri·ae'
  —na'si'
  —ses'a·moi'de·ae' na'si'
  —tra'che·a'les'

car'ti·la·gin'i·fi·ca'tion
car'ti·lag'i·noid'
car'ti·lag'i·nous
car'ti·la'go *pl.* -lag'i·nes'
  —a·lar'is major
  —ar·tic'u·lar'is
  —ar'y·tae·noi'de·a
  —ar'y·te·noi'de·a
  —au·ric'u·lae'
  —cor·nic'u·la'ta
  —cos·ta'lis
  —cri·coi'de·a
  —cu·ne'i·for'mis
  —ep'i·glot'ti·ca
  —ep'i·phys'i·a'lis
  —me·a'tus a·cu'sti·ci'
  —na'si' lat'er·a'lis
  —sep'ti' na'si'
  —ses'a·moi'de·a
  —thy're·oi'de·a
  —thy'roi'de·a
  —tri·tic'e·a
  —tu'bae' au'di·ti'vae'
  —vom'er·o·na'sa'lis
car'un'cle
ca·run'cu·la *pl.* -lae'
  —hy'me·na'les'
  —lac'ri·ma'lis
  —sub'lin·gua'lis
ca·run'cu·lar
ca·run'cu·late'
ca·run'cu·lat'ed
car'va·crol'
Car·val'lo sign
carv'er
car'vone'
Car'y-Blair' medium
car'y·o·phyl'lus
Ca·sal' collar
cas·an'thra·nol'
Ca·sa'res Gil stain
cas·cade', -cad'ed, -cad'ing
cas·car'a
  —a·mar'ga
  —sa·gra'da
case
ca'se·ase'
ca'se·ate', -at'ed, -at'ing
ca'se·a'tion
case'book'
ca'se·i·form'
ca'se·in
ca'se·in·ate'

ca'se·in'o·gen
ca'se·o·cal·cif'ic
ca'se·ous
Case pad sign
case'work'
Cas'i·mi·ro'a
  —ed'u·lis
Ca·so'ni test
Cas'sel·ber'ry
  —cannula
  —position
Cas'ser fontanel
cas·sette'
cast
Cas·taigne' method
Cas'ta·ne'da
  —rat'-lung' method
  —vaccine
cas'ta·no·sper'mine'
Cas'tel·la'ni
  —disease
  —paint
Cas'tel method
cast'like'
cas'trate', -trat'ed, -trat'ing
cas·tra'tion
cas'tro·phre'ni·a
cas'u·al·ty
cas'u·is'tics
cat'a·ba'si·al
ca·tab'a·sis *pl.* -ses'
cat'a·bat'ic
cat'a·bi·o'sis *pl.* -ses'
cat'a·bi·ot'ic
cat'a·bol'ic
ca·tab'o·lism
ca·tab'o·lite'
ca·tab'o·lize', -lized', -liz'ing
cat'a·caus'tic
cat'a·clei'sis *pl.* -ses'
cat'a·clon'ic
ca·tac'lo'nus
cat'a·crot'ic
ca·tac'ro·tism
cat'a·di·cro'tism
cat'a·did'y·mus *var. of*
  katadidymus
cat'a·di·op'tric
cat'a·gen
cat'a·gen'e·sis *pl.* -ses'
cat'a·ge·net'ic
cat'a·lase'
cat'a·lep'sis *pl.* -ses'

cat′a·lep′sy
cat′a·lep′tic
cat′a·lep′ti·form′
cat′a·lep′toid′
cat′a·lo′gi·a
ca·tal′y·sis *pl.* -ses′
cat′a·lyst
cat′a·lyt′ic
cat′a·ly·za′tion
cat′a·lyze′, -lyzed′, -lyz′ing
cat′a·lyz′er
cat′a·me′ni·a
cat′a·me′ni·al
cat′am·ne′sis *pl.* -ses′
cat′am·nes′tic
cat′a·pha′si·a
cat′a·pha′sis *pl.* -ses′
ca·taph′o·ra *(lethargy with periods of imperfect consciousness)*
  ♦*cataphoria*
cat′a·pho·re′sis *pl.* -ses′
cat′a·pho·ret′ic
cat′a·pho′ri·a *(double hypophoria)*
  ♦*cataphora*
cat′a·phor′ic
cat′a·phre′ni·a
cat′a·phy·lac′tic
cat′a·phy·lax′is
cat′a·pla′si·a *also* kataplasia
cat′a·pla′sis *pl.* -ses′
cat′a·plasm
cat′a·plec′tic
cat′a·plex′y
cat′a·ract′
cat′a·rac′ta
  —cen·tra′lis pul′ver·u·len′ta
  —co′ro·nar′i·a
  —neu′ro·der·mat′i·ca
cat′a·rac′to·gen′ic
cat′a·rac′tous
ca·ta·ri·a
ca·tarrh′
ca·tarrh′al
cat′ar·rhine′
cat′a·stal′sis
cat′a·stal′tic
ca·tas′ta·sis *pl.* -ses′
cat′a·state′
ca·tas′tro·phe
cat′a·stroph′ic
cat′a·to′ni·a

cat′a·ton′ic
cat′a·tri′cro·tism
cat′a·tro′pi·a
catch′ment area
cat′e·chin
cat′e·chol′
cat′e·chol′a·mine′
cat′e·chu
cat′e·chu′ic
cat′e·lec·trot′o·nus
cat′e·nat′ing
cat′e·noid′
ca·ten′u·late′
cat′gut′
Cath′a ed′u·lis
ca·thar′sis *pl.* -ses′
ca·thar′tic
ca·thect′
ca·thec′tic
ca·thep′sin
ca·ther′e·sis
cath′e·ret′ic
cath′e·ter
cath′e·ter·i·za′tion
cath′e·ter·ize′, -ized′, -iz′ing
cath′e·ter·o·stat′
ca·thex′is *pl.* -thex′es′
cath′i·so·pho′bi·a
cath′ode′
ca·thod′ic
ca·thol′i·con′
cat′i·on
cat′i·on′ic
cat′lin
ca·top′tric
Cat·tell′ Infant Intelligence Scale
Cau·ca′sian
cau′da *pl.* -dae′
  —cer′e·bel′li′
  —ep′i·di·dym′i·dis
  —e′qui·na
  —hel′i·cis
  —nu′cle·i′ cau·da·ti′
  —pan′cre·a′tis
  —stri·a′ti′
cau′dad′
cau′dal
cau′da·lis
cau′date′
cau·da′to·len·tic′u·lar
cau·da′tum *pl.* -ta
cau′do·ceph′a·lad′

caul
cau′lo·ple′gi·a
cau′mes·the′si·a
caus′al
cau·sal′gi·a
cau·sal′gic
caus′a·tive
cause
caus′tic
cau′ter·ant
cau′ter·i·za′tion
cau′ter·ize′, -ized′, -iz′ing
cau′ter·y
ca′va *pl.* -vae′
ca′val
cav′a·scope′
cave of Meck′el
ca·ver′na *pl.* -nae′
  —cor′po·ris spon′gi·o′si′ pe′nis
  —cor′po·rum cav′er·no·so′·rum pe′nis
cav′er·nil′o·quy
cav′er·ni′tis
cav′er·no′ma *pl.* -mas *or* -ma·ta
cav′er·no·si′tis
cav′er·no·sog′ra·phy
cav′er·no·som′e·try
cav′er·nos′to·my
cav′er·no′sum *pl.* -sa
cav′ern·ous
Ca′vi·a
Cav′i·i·dae′
cav′i·tar′y
cav′i·tas *pl.* cav′i·ta′tes′
  —glen′oi·da′lis
  —pul′pae′
cav′i·tate′, -tat′ed, -tat′ing
cav′i·ta′tion
Ca·vi′te
ca·vi′tis
cav′i·ty
ca′vo·gram′
ca·vog′ra·phy
ca′vo·sur′face
ca′vo·val′gus
ca′vum *pl.* -va
  —ab·dom′i·nis
  —ar·tic′u·lar′e′
  —con′chae′
  —co′ro·na′le′
  —den′tis

—ep'i‧du‧ra'le'
—hy'a‧loi'de‧um
—in'fra‧glot'ti‧cum
—la‧ryn'gis
—me'di‧as'ti‧na'le' an‧te'-
  ri‧us
—mediastinale pos‧te'ri‧us
—med'ul‧lar'e'
—Mon‧ro'i‧i'
—na'si'
—o'ris
—oris pro'pri‧um
—pel'vis
—per'i‧car'di‧i'
—per'i‧to‧nae'i'
—per'i‧to‧ne'i'
—pha‧ryn'gis
—pleu'rae'
—pleu'ro‧per'i‧car'di‧a'co‧
  per'i‧to‧ne‧a'le'
—pleu'ro‧per'i‧car'di‧a'le'
—psal‧te'ri‧i'
—sep'ti' pel‧lu'ci‧di'
—sub'a‧rach'noi‧de‧a'le'
—sub'du‧ra'le
—tho‧ra'cis
—tri‧gem'i‧na'le'
—tym'pa‧ni'
—u'ter‧i'
—ve'li' in‧ter‧pos'i‧ti'
—Ver'gae'
ca'vus
Ca‧ze‧nave' disease
ce‧as'mic
ce‧bo‧ce‧pha'li‧a
ce‧bo‧ce‧phal'ic
ce‧bo‧ceph'a‧lus
ce‧bo‧ceph'a‧ly
ce'cal
ce‧cec'to‧my
ce‧ci'tis
ce‧co‧cele'
ce‧co‧col'ic
ce‧co‧co'lon
ce‧co‧co'lo‧pex'y
ce‧co‧co‧los'to‧my
ce‧co‧fix‧a'tion
ce‧co‧il'e‧os'to‧my
ce‧co‧pex'y
ce‧co‧pli‧ca'tion
ce‧cor'rha‧phy
ce‧co‧sig'moid‧os'to‧my
ce‧cos'to‧my

ce‧cot'o‧my
ce'cum *pl.* -ca
—cu'pu‧lar'e'
—ves'tib'u‧lar'e'
cef'a‧clor'
cef'a‧drox'il
cef'a‧man'dole'
ce‧faz'o‧lin
cef‧met'a‧zole'
cef'o‧per'a‧zone'
ce‧for'a‧nide'
cef'o‧te'tan
ce‧fox'i‧tin
cef'ti‧zox'ime'
cef‧tri'a‧xone'
cef‧u'ro‧xime'
Ceg'ka sign
ce‧len'ter‧on'
Ce‧les'tin
—latex rubber tube
—prosthesis
ce‧li'ac'
ce‧li‧a‧del'phus
ce‧li‧ec‧ta'si‧a
ce‧li‧ec'to‧my
ce‧li‧o‧cen‧te'sis *pl.* -ses'
ce‧li‧o‧col‧pot'o‧my
ce‧li‧o‧en‧ter‧ot'o‧my
ce‧li‧o‧gas‧trot'o‧my
ce‧li‧o‧hys'ter‧ec'to‧my
ce‧li‧o'ma *pl.* -mas *or* -ma‧ta
ce‧li‧o‧my'o‧mec'to‧my
ce‧li‧o‧my'o‧si'tis
ce‧li‧o‧par'a‧cen‧te'sis
  pl. -ses'
ce‧li‧or'rha‧phy
ce‧li‧o‧sal'pin‧gec'to‧my
ce‧li‧o‧sal'pin‧got'o‧my
ce‧li‧o‧scope'
ce‧li‧os'co‧py
ce‧li‧ot'o‧my
ce‧li'tis
cell
—of Betz
cel'la *(an enclosure), pl.* -lae'
  ♦*sella*
cel‧loi'din
cells
—of Bött'cher
—of Ca'jal'
—of Clau'di‧us
—of Dei'ters
—of Gia‧nuz'zi

—of Hen'sen
—of Kult‧schitz'sky
—of Mey'nert
—of Pan'eth
—of Schwann
—of van Ge‧huch'ten
cel'lu‧la *pl.* -lae'
cel'lu‧lae'
—an‧te'ri‧o'res'
—eth'moi‧da'les'
—mas‧toi'de‧ae'
—me'di‧ae'
—pneu‧ma'ti‧cae'
—pneumaticae tu'bae'
  au'di‧ti'vae'
—pneumaticae tu‧bar'i‧ae'
—pos‧te'ri‧o'res'
—tym'pan'i‧cae'
cel'lu‧lar
cel'lu‧lar'i‧ty
cel'lu‧lase'
cel'lule'
—claire
cel'lu‧li‧cid'al
cel'lu‧lif'u‧gal
cel'lu‧lin
cel'lu‧lip'e‧tal
cel'lu‧li'tis
cel'lu‧lo‧ra‧dic'u‧lo‧neu‧
  ri'tis
cel'lu‧lose'
cel'lu‧lo'sic
ce'lom
ce‧los'chi‧sis
ce'lo‧scope'
ce‧lo‧so'ma *pl.* -mas *or*
  -ma‧ta
ce‧lo‧so'mi‧a
ce‧lo‧so'mus *pl.* -mi' *or*
  -mus‧es
ce‧lo‧the'li‧o'ma *pl.* -mas *or*
  -ma‧ta
ce‧lo‧zo'ic
Cel'si‧us
ce‧ment'
ce‧ment'i‧cle
ce‧ment'i‧fi‧ca'tion
ce‧men‧ta'tion
ce‧men'tin
ce‧men'to‧blast'
ce‧men'to‧blas'to‧ma
  pl. -mas *or* -ma‧ta
ce‧men'to‧cla'si‧a

ce·men′to·cyte′
ce·men′to·den′ti·nal
ce·men′to·e·nam′el
ce·men′to·gen′e·sis *pl.* -ses′
ce′men·to′ma *pl.* -mas *or*
  -ma·ta
ce·men′tome′
ce·men′to·path′i·a
ce·men′to·phyte′
ce·men′to·sis *pl.* -ses′
ce·men′tum *pl.* -ta
ce′nes·the′si·a
ce′nes·thet′ic
ce′nes·thop′a·thy
ce′no·gen′e·sis
ce′no·ge·net′ic
ce′no·site′
cen′sor
cen′tau·ry
cen′ter
cen·te′sis *pl.* -ses′
cen′ti·grade′
cen′ti·gram′
cen′ti·gray′
cen′ti·li′ter
cen′ti·me′ter
cen′ti·nor′mal
cen′ti·pede′
cen′ti·poise′
cen′ti·stokes′
cen′trad′
cen′trage
cen′tral
cen′tren·ce·phal′ic
cen′tric
cen·tri·cip′i·tal
cen·tric′i·put
cen·trif′u·gal
cen·trif·u·gal·i·za′tion
cen·trif′u·gal·ize′
cen·trif′u·ga′tion
cen′tri·fuge′
cen′tri·lob′u·lar
cen′tri·ole′
cen·trip′e·tal
cen′tro·ac′i·nar
cen′tro·cyte′
cen′tro·don′tous
cen′tro·dor′sal
cen′tro·ki·ne′si·a
cen′tro·lec′i·thal
cen′tro·me′di·an
cen′tro·mere′

cen′tro·phose′
cen′tro·plasm
cen′tro·scle·ro′sis
cen′tro·some′
cen′tro·sphere′
cen′tro·the′ca
cen′trum *pl.* -trums *or* -tra
  —me′di·a′num
  —o′va·le′
  —sem′i·o·va′le′
  —ten·din′e·um
  —tendineum per′i·ne′i′
Cen′tru·roi′des
ceph·a′e·line′
ceph′a·lad′
ceph·a·lal′gi·a
ceph·a·lal′gic
ceph·a·lal′gy
ceph·a·le′a
  —at·ton′i·ta
ceph′al·e·de′ma *pl.* -mas *or*
  -ma·ta
ceph·a·lex′in
ceph′al·he·mat′o·cele′
ceph′al·he·ma·to′ma
  pl. -mas *or* -ma·ta
ceph′al·hy′dro·cele′
ce·phal′ic
ceph′a·lin
ceph′a·li′tis
ceph·a·li·za′tion
ceph′a·lo·bra′chi·al
ceph′a·lo·cau′dad
ceph′a·lo·cau′dal
ceph′a·lo·cele′
ceph′a·lo·cen·te′sis *pl.* -ses′
ceph′a·lo·chord′
ceph′a·lo·di·pros′o·pus
ceph′a·lo·dyn′i·a
ceph′a·lo·gas′ter
ceph′a·lo·gen′e·sis *pl.* -ses′
ceph′a·lo·gly′cin
ceph′a·lo·gram′
ceph′a·log′ra·phy
ceph′a·lo·gy′mi·a
ceph′a·lo·gy′ric
ceph′a·lo·he·mat′o·cele′
ceph′a·lo·he·ma·to′ma
  pl. -mas *or* -ma·ta
ceph′a·loid′
ceph′a·lom′e·lus
ceph′a·lo·me·ni′a
ceph′a·lo·men·in·gi′tis

ceph′a·lom′e·ter
ceph′a·lo·met′ric
ceph′a·lo·met′rics
ceph′a·lom′e·try
ceph′a·lo·mo′tor
ceph′a·lone′
ceph′a·lo′ni·a
ceph′a·lo-or′bit·al
ceph′a·lop′a·gus
  —oc·cip′i·ta′lis
  —pa·ri′e·ta′lis
ceph′a·lop′a·thy
ceph′a·lo·pel′vic
ceph′a·lo·pha·ryn′ge·us
ceph′a·lo·ple′gi·a
ceph′a·lo·pod′
ceph′a·lor′i·dine′
ceph′a·los′co·py
ceph′a·lo·spo′rin
ceph′a·lo·spo·ri·o′sis
  pl. -ses′
Ceph′a·lo·spo′ri·um
ceph′a·lo·stat′
ceph′a·lo·thin
ceph′a·lo·tho·rac′ic
ceph′a·lo·tho·ra·co·il′i·op′-
  a·gus
ceph′a·lo·tho·ra·cop′a·gus
  —a·sym′me·tros′
  —di·bra′chi·us
  —di·sym′me·tros′
  —mon′o·sym′me·tros′
ceph′a·lo·tome′
ceph′a·lot′o·my
ceph′a·lo·trac′tor
ceph′a·lox′i·a
ceph′a·pir′in
ceph′ra·dine′
ce′ra
ce·ra′ceous
cer·am′i·dase′
cer·am′ide′
cer′a·sine′
ce′rate′
cer′a·to·cri′coid′
cer′a·to·hy′al
cer′a·to·pha·ryn′ge·us
Cer′a·toph·yl′lus
cer′a·to·po·gon′i·dae′
cer·car′i·a *pl.* -i·ae′
cer·car′i·al
cer·car′i·an
cer·clage′

Cer'co·mo'nas
—in·tes'ti·na'lis
Cer'co·pith'e·coi'de·a
Cer'co·pith'e·cus
cer'cus pl. -ci
ce're·al
ce're·a flex'i·bil'i·tas
cer'e·bel'lar
cer'e·bel·lif'u·gal
cer'e·bel·lip'e·tal
cer'e·bel·li'tis
cer'e·bel'lo·med'ul·lar'y
cer'e·bel'lo·pon'tile'
cer'e·bel'lo·pon'tine'
cer'e·bel'lo·ret'i·nal
cer'e·bel'lo·ru'bral
cer'e·bel'lo·ru'bro·spi'nal
cer'e·bel'lo·spi'nal
cer'e·bel'lo·tha·lam'ic
cer'e·bel'lo·ves·tib'u·lar
cer'e·bel'lum pl. -lums or -la
cer'e·bral
cer'e·bra'tion
cer'e·bric
ce·re'bri·form'
cer'e·brif'u·gal
cer'e·brin'ic
cer'e·brip'e·tal
cer'e·bri'tis
cer'e·bro·car'di·ac'
cer'e·bro·cen'tric
cer'e·bro·cer'e·bel'lar
cer'e·bro·cor'ti·cal
cer'e·bro·cu'pre·in
cer'e·broid'
cer'e·bro'ma pl. -mas or -ma·ta
cer'e·bro·mac'u·lar
cer'e·bro·ma·la'ci·a
cer'e·bro·med'ul·lar'y
cer'e·bro·me·nin'ge·al
cer'e·bro·men·in·gi'tis
cer'e·bron
cer'e·bron'ic
cer'e·bro·oc'u·lar
cer'e·bro·path'i·a psy'chi·
  ca tox·e'mi·ca
cer'e·brop'a·thy
cer'e·bro·phys'i·ol'o·gy
cer'e·bro·pon'tile'
cer'e·bro·pon'tine'
cer'e·bro·ret'i·nal
cer'e·bro·scle·ro'sis pl. -ses'
cer'e·brose'

cer'e·bro·side'
cer'e·bro·spi'nal
cer'e·bro·spi'nant
cer'e·bro·ten'di·nous
cer'e·brot'o·my
cer'e·bro·to'ni·a
cer'e·bro·vas'cu·lar
cer'e·brum pl. -brums or -bra
cere'cloth'
Ce·ren'kov radiation
ce'ric
ce'roid'
ce·ro'ma (waxy tumor),
  pl. -mas or -ma·ta
  ♦seroma
ce'ro·plas'ty
ce'rot'ic
ce'rous
cer'ti·fi'a·ble
cer'ti·fi·ca'tion
ce·ru'le·in
ce·ru'lo·plas'min
ce·ru'men
ce·ru'mi·nal
ce·ru'mi·nol'y·sis
ce·ru'mi·no'ma pl. -mas or
  -ma·ta
ce·ru'mi·no'sis pl. -ses'
ce·ru'mi·nous
cer'vi·cal
cer'vi·ca'lis as·cen'dens
cer'vi·cec'to·my
cer'vi·ci'tis
cer'vi·co·au'ral
cer'vi·co·au·ric'u·lar
cer'vi·co·ax'il·lar'y
cer'vi·co·bra'chi·al
cer'vi·co·bra'chi·al'gi·a
cer'vi·co·buc'cal
cer'vi·co·col·pi'tis
cer'vi·co·dor'sal
cer'vi·co·dyn'i·a
cer'vi·co·fa'cial
cer'vi·co·la'bi·al
cer'vi·co·lin'gual
cer'vi·co-oc·cip'i·tal
cer'vi·co·plas'ty
cer'vi·co·pu'bic
cer'vi·co·rec'tal
cer'vi·co·scap'u·lar
cer'vi·co·tho·rac'ic
cer'vi·co·tho'ra·co·lum'bo·
  sa'cral

cer'vi·co·tro'chan·ter'ic
cer'vi·co·u'ter·ine
cer'vi·co·vag'i·nal
cer'vi·co·vag'i·ni'tis
cer'vi·co·ves'i·cal
cer'vix pl. -vi·ces' or -vix·es
  —co·lum'nae' pos·te'ri·o'-
    ris gris'e·ae'
  —den'tis
  —ob·sti'pa
  —u'ter·i'
  —ve·si'cae'
ce'ryl
ce·sar'e·an also caesarean
Ce·sar'is-De·mel' bodies
Ces·tan'
  —sign
  —syndrome
Ces·tan'-Che·nais'
  syndrome
Ces·to'da
ces'tode'
ces·to·di'a·sis pl. -ses'
ces'toid'
Ces·toi'de·a
ces·toi'de·an
ces'tus
ce·ta'ce·um
cet'al·ko'ni·um
ce'tic
ce·tin'ic
ce'to·phen'i·col'
ce'tri·mide'
ce'tyl
  —ce'tyl·ate'
  —pal'mi·tate'
ce'tyl·pyr'i·din'i·um
ce·va'dil'la
cev'a·dine'
cev'i·tam'ic
Chad'dock
  —reflex
  —sign
Chad'wick sign
Chae·to'mi·um
chafe, chafed, chaf'ing
Cha'gas-Cruz' disease
Cha'gas disease
cha·go'ma
Cha'gres fever
cha·la'si·a (relaxation of a
  sphincter)
  ♦chalaza

cha·la′za (*spiral band of albumen extending from the end of an egg yolk to the shell*), *pl.* -zae′ *or* -zas
♦*chalasia*
cha·la′zi·on′ *pl.* -zi·a
cha·la′zo·der′mi·a
chal·ci′tis
chal·co′sis *pl.* -ses′
chal·i·co′sis *pl.* -ses′
chal′lenge
chal′one′
cha·lyb′e·ate′
cham′ber
Cham′ber·lain
—line
—projection
Cham′ber·lain-Towne′
technique
cham′e·ce·phal′ic
cham′e·ceph′a·lous
cham′e·ceph′a·lus *pl.* -li′
cham′e·ceph′a·ly
cham′e·cra′ni·al
cham′e·pro·so′pic
cham′fer
cham′o·mile′
chan′cre
—re′dux′
chan′cri·form′
chan′croid′
chan·croi′dal
change
chan′nel
Cha·os′ cha′os′
Cha′oul therapy
chap, chapped, chap′ping
Chap′man bag
Cha·put′ method
char′ac·ter
char′ac·ter·is′tic
char′ac·ter·i·za′tion
char′as
char′bon
char′coal′
Char·cot′
—arthritis
—arthropathy
—arthrosis
—cirrhosis
—disease
—foot
—intermittent fever

—joint
—laryngeal vertigo
—sign
—syndrome
—triad
—zone
Char·cot′-Bou·chard′
aneurysm
Char·cot′-Ley′den crystals
Char·cot′-Ma·rie′-Tooth′
disease
Char·cot′-Wil′brand′
syndrome
char′la·tin
char′la·tin·ism
Charles law
char′ley horse
Char′lin syndrome
Charl′ton blanching test
chart
char′ta *pl.* -tae′
char·treu′sin
char·tu·la *pl.* -lae′
Chas·sai·gnac′ tubercle
Chas′tek′ paralysis
Chauf·fard′-Min·kow′ski
syndrome
Chauf·fard′-Still′
—disease
—syndrome
Chausse view
Chaus·si·er′ line
Chea′dle disease
Chea′tle-Hen′ry operation
Chea′tle slit
check′bite′
check′er·ber′ry
check′up′
Ché′di·ak′-Hi·ga′shi
anomaly
cheek
cheek′bone′
chees′y
chei·lal′gi·a
chei·lec′to·my
chei′lec·tro′pi·on′
chei·li′tis
—ac·tin′i·ca
—ex·fo′li·a·ti′va
—glan′du·lar′is
—glandularis a·pos′te·ma·
to′sa
—ven′e·na′ta

chei′lo·an′gi·os′co·py
chei′lo·car′ci·no′ma
pl. -mas *or* -ma·ta
chei′lo·gnath′o·pal′a·tos′-
chi·sis *pl.* -ses′
chei′lo·gnath′o·pros′o·
pos′chi·sis *pl.* -ses′
chei′lo·gnath′o·u′ra·nos′-
chi·sis *pl.* -ses′
chei′lo·plas′ty
chei·lor′rha·phy
chei′los′chi·sis *pl.* -ses′
chei′lo′sis *pl.* -ses′
chei′lo·sto′ma·to·plas′ty
chei·lot′o·my
chei·rag′ra
chei·ral′gi·a
—par′es·thet′i·ca
cheir′ar·thri′tis
chei·rog·nos′tic
chei·ro·kin′es·the′si·a
chei·ro·kin′es·thet′ic
chei·rol′o·gy
chei·ro·meg′a·ly
chei·ro·plas′ty
chei·ro·pom′pho·lyx
chei′ro·scope′
chei′ro·spasm
che′late′
che·la′tion
chel′e·ryth′rine′
che·lic′er·a
chel′i·do·nine′
chem′a·bra′sion
chem′ex·fo·li·a′tion
chem′i·cal
chem′i·co·cau′ter·y
chem′i·lu′mi·nes′cence
che·mise′
chem′ist
chem′is·try
che′mo·au′to·troph′
che′mo·au′to·troph′ic
che′mo·bi·ot′ic
che′mo·cep′tor
che′mo·co·ag′u·la′tion
che′mo·dec·to′ma *pl.* -mas
or -ma·ta
che′mo·dif′fer·en′ti·a′tion
che′mo·im′mu·nol′o·gy
che′mo·ki·ne′sis *pl.* -ses′
che′mo·ki·net′ic
che′mo·lu′mi·nes′cence

che·mol′y·sis
che′mo·mor·pho′sis
pl. -ses′
che′mo·nu′cle·ol′y·sis
pl. -ses′
che′mo·pal′li·dec′to·my
che′mo·pro′phy·lac′tic
che′mo·pro′phy·lax′is
pl. -lax′es′
che′mo·psy′chi·at′ric
che′mo·psy·chi′a·try
che′mo·re·cep′tion
che′mo·re·cep′tive
che′mo·re·cep′tor
che′mo·re′flex′
che′mo·re·sis′tance
che′mo·sen′si·tive
che′mo·sen′si·tiv′i·ty
che′mo·sen′so·ry
che′mo·se′ro·ther′a·py
che·mo′sis *pl.* -ses′
che′mos·mo′sis *pl.* -ses′
che′mo·ster′i·lant
che′mo·ster′i·li·za′tion
che′mo·ster′i·lize′
che′mo·sur′ger·y
che′mo·sur′gi·cal
che′mo·syn′the·sis *pl.* -ses′
che′mo·syn·thet′ic
che′mo·tac′tic
che′mo·tax′is *pl.* -tax′es′
che′mo·thal′a·mot′o·my
che′mo·ther′a·peu′tic
che′mo·ther′a·peu′tics
che′mo·ther′a·pist
che′mo·ther′a·py
che·mot′ic
che′mo·trop′ic
che·mot′ro·pism
Che·nais′ syndrome
che′no·de
che′no·po′di·um
che·ro·pho′bi·a
Cher′ry and Cran′dall test
cher′ub·ism
Ches′el·den operation
Chev′a·lier′ Jack′son
operation
Chév′re·mont-Com·baire′
method
chev′ron
Cheyne′-Stokes′
respiration

Chi·a′ri
—malformation
—network
—syndrome
Chi·a′ri-From′mel
—disease
—syndrome
chi′asm
chi·as′ma *pl.* -ma·ta *or* -mas
—op′ti·cum
—ten′di·num
chi·as′mal
chi·as·mat′ic
chick′en·pox′
chi·cle′ro ulcer
chig′ger
chig′o
Chi′lai·di′ti syndrome
chil′blain
child
Child
—classification
—pancreatectomy
child′bear′ing
child′birth′
child′hood′
Chil′e
—ni′ter
—salt·pe′ter
Chi′lo·mas′tix
—mes·nil′i′
Chi′lop·o′da
chi·me′ra
chi·mer′ism
chin
chinch
Chi·nese′ res′tau·rant′
syndrome
chin′i·o·fon′
chi′o·na·blep′si·a
chi′o·na·blep′sy
chip′blow′er
chi·rap′si·a
chi′rap·sy
chi·rol′o·gy
chi′ro·meg′a·ly
chi·rop′o·dist
chi·rop′o·dy
chi′ro·pom′pho·lyx
chi′ro·prac′tic
chi′ro·prac′tor
chis′el
chi′tin

chi′tin·ous
chi′to·bi′ose′
chi·to′sa·mine′
Chi·tral′ fever
chla·my·de′mi·a
Chla·myd′i·a *pl.* -ae
—psit′ta·ci′
—tra·cho′ma·tis
Chla·myd′i·a′ce·ae′
chla·myd′i·o′sis *pl.* -ses′
chlam′y·do·spore′
chla·myd′o·spor′ic
Chla·myd′o·zo·a′ce·ae′
Chlam′y·do·zo′on
chlo·as′ma *pl.* -ma·ta
—grav′i·dar′um
—he·pat′i·cum
—pe′ri·o·ra′le vir′gin′i·um
—u′te·ri′num
chlo′phe·di′a·nol′
chlor·ac′ne
chlo′ral
chlo′ral·am′ide′
chlo′ral·form·am′ide′
chlo′ral·ism
chlo′ral·ize′
chlo′ra·lose′
chlo′ral·u′re·thane′
chlor·am′bu·cil
chlor′a·mine′
chlor′am·phen′i·col′
chlor′a·ne′mi·a
chlo′rate′
chlor·bu′tol′
chlor·cy′cli·zine′
chlor′dane′
chlor·dan′to·in
chlor·di·az′ep·ox′ide′
chlo·rel′lin
chlor·e′mi·a
chlor·gua′nide′
chlor·hex′i·dine′
chlor·hy′dri·a
chlo′ric
chlo′ride′
chlo′ri·dim′e·ter
chlo′ri·dim′e·try
chlo′ri·du′ri·a
chlo′ri·nat′ed
chlo′ri·na′tion
chlor·in′da·nol′
chlo′rine′
chlor′i·son′da·mine

chlo′rite′
chlor·mad′i·none′
chlor·mer′o·drin
chlor·mez′a·none′
chlo·ro·ac′e·to·phe′none′
chlo·ro·a·ne′mi·a
chlo·ro·az′o·din
chlo·ro·bu′ta·nol′
chlo·ro·cre′sol
chlo·ro·cru′o·rin
chlo·ro·form′
chlo·ro·for′mic
chlo·ro·form′ism
chlo·ro·form′i·za′tion
chlo·ro·gua′nide′
chlo·ro·leu·ke′mi·a
chlo·ro·lym·pho′ma
    pl. -mas *or* -ma·ta
chlo·ro·ma *pl.* -mas *or* -ma·ta
chlo·ro·meth′ane′
chlo·ro·my′e·lo′ma *pl.* -mas
    or -ma·ta
chlo·ro·per′cha
chlo·ro·pex′i·a
chlo·ro·phane′
chlo′ro·phe′nol′
chlo·ro·phen·o′thane′
chlo′ro·phyll
chlo′ro·phyl·lase′
Chlo·rop′i·dae′
chlo′ro·plast′
chlo′ro·plas′tin
chlo·ro·pro′caine′
chlo·rop′si·a
chlo′ro·pu′rine′
chlo′ro·quine′
chlo·ro·sar·co·ma *pl.* -mas
    or -ma·ta
chlo·ro′sis *pl.* -ses′
    —ru′bra
chlo·ro·then
chlo·ro·thi′a·zide′
chlo′ro·thy′mol′
chlo·rot′ic
chlo′ro·tri·an′i·sene′
chlo′rous
chlo·ro·vi′nyl·di·chlo′ro·
    ar′sine′
chlo′ro·xy′le·nol′
chlor·phen′e·sin
chlor′phen·ir′a·mine′
chlor′phe·nol′
chlor′phen·ox′a·mine′

chlor′phen′ter·mine′
chlor·pic′rin
chlor·pro′ma·zine′
chlor·pro′pa·mide′
chlor′pro·phen·py·rid′a·
    mine′
chlor′pro·thix′ene′
chlor′quin·al′dol′
chlor·tet′ra·cy′cline′
chlor·thal′i·done′
chlor·thy′mol′
chlor·u′re·sis
chlor·u′ri·a
chlor·zox′a·zone′
cho·a′na *pl.* -nae′
cho·a′nal
cho·a′nate′
choke, choked, chok′ing
cho′la·gog′ic
cho′la·gogue′
cho·lal′ic
chol′a·mine′
cho′lane′
cho′lan′e·re′sis
cho′lan·gei′tis
cho·lan′gi·ec′ta·sis *pl.* -ses′
cho·lan′gi·o·ad′e·no′ma
    pl. -mas *or* -ma·ta
cho·lan′gi·o·car′ci·no′ma
    pl. -mas *or* -ma·ta
cho·lan′gi·o·cath′e·ter
cho·lan′gi·o·en′ter·os′-
    to·my
cho·lan′gi·o·fi·bro′ma·to′-
    sis
cho·lan′gi·o·gas·tros′-
    to·my
cho·lan′gi·o·gram′
cho·lan′gi·o·graph′ic
cho·lan′gi·og′ra·phy
cho·lan′gi·o·hep′a·ti′tis
    pl. -tis·es *or* -tit′i·des′
cho·lan′gi·o·hep′a·to′ma
    pl. -mas *or* -ma·ta
cho·lan′gi·o·je′ju·nos′-
    to·my
cho·lan′gi·ole′
cho·lan′gi·o·lit′ic
cho·lan′gi·o·li′tis
cho·lan′gi·o′ma *pl.* -mas *or*
    -ma·ta
cho·lan′gi·o·pan′cre·a·tog′-
    ra·phy

cho·lan′gi·o·scope′
cho·lan′gi·o·scop′ic
cho·lan′gi·os′co·py
cho·lan′gi·os·to·my
cho·lan′gi·ot′o·my
cho′lan·git′ic
cho′lan·gi′tis
cho·lan′ic
cho·lan′o·poi·e′sis *pl.* -ses′
cho·lan′o·poi·et′ic
cho′late′
cho′le·bil′i·ru′bin
cho′le·cal′cif′er·ol′
cho′le·chro′me·re′sis
cho′le·chro′mo·poi·e′sis
cho′le·cy′a·nin
cho′le·cyst′
cho′le·cyst′a·gogue′
cho′le·cys·tal′gi·a
cho′le·cys·tec·ta′si·a
cho′le·cys·tec·to′my
cho′le·cys·ten·ter′ic
cho′le·cyst·en·ter·or′rha·
    phy
cho′le·cyst·en·ter·os·to′my
cho′le·cys′tic
cho′le·cys′tis
cho′le·cys·ti′tis *pl.* -tit′i·des′
cho′le·cys·to·cho·lan′gi·o·
    gram′
cho′le·cys·to·co·lon′ic
cho′le·cys·to·co·los′to·my
cho′le·cys·to·co·lot′o·my
cho′le·cys·to·cu·ta′ne·ous
cho′le·cys·to·du′o·de′nal
cho′le·cys·to·du′o·de·no·
    co′lic
cho′le·cys·to·du′o·de·nos′-
    to·my
cho′le·cys·to·e·lec′tro·co·
    ag′u·lec′to·my
cho′le·cys·to·en′ter·os′-
    to·my
cho′le·cys·to·gas′tric
cho′le·cys·to·gas·tros′-
    to·my
cho′le·cys·to·gram′
cho′le·cys·to·graph′ic
cho′le·cys·tog′ra·phy
cho′le·cys·to·il′e·os′to·my
cho′le·cys·to·je′ju·nos′-
    to·my
cho′le·cys·to·ki′nase′

cho'le·cys'to·ki·net'ic
cho'le·cys'to·ki'nin
cho'le·cys'to·li·thi'a·sis
cho'le·cys'to·li·thot'o·my
cho'le·cys'to·lith'o·trip'sy
cho'le·cys'to·ne·phros'-
   to·my
cho'le·cys'top'a·thy
cho'le·cys'to·pex'y
cho'le·cys'top·to'sis *pl.* -ses'
cho'le·cys·tor'rha·phy
cho'le·cys·tos'co·py
cho'le·cys·tos'to·my
cho'le·cys·tot'o·my
cho'le·doch'
cho·led'o·chal
cho·led'o·chec·ta'si·a
cho·led'o·chec'to·my
cho·led'o·chi'tis
cho·led'o·cho·cele'
cho·led'o·cho·cu·ta'ne·ous
cho·led'o·cho·cys·tos'-
   to·my
cho·led'o·cho·do·chor'rha·
   phy
cho·led'o·cho·du'o·de·
   nos'to·my
cho·led'o·cho·en'ter·os'-
   to·my
cho·led'o·cho·gas·tros'-
   to·my
cho·led'o·cho·gram'
cho·led'o·cho·il'e·os'to·my
cho·led'o·cho·je'ju·nos'-
   to·my
cho·led'o·cho·lith'
cho·led'o·cho·li·thi'a·sis
   pl. -ses'
cho·led'o·cho·li·thot'o·my
cho·led'o·cho·lith'o·trip'sy
cho·led'o·cho·plas'ty
cho·led'o·chor'rha·phy
cho·led'o·cho·scope'
cho·led'o·chos'co·py
cho·led'o·chos'to·my
cho·led'o·chot'o·my
cho·led'o·chus *pl.* -chi'
cho'le·glo'bin
cho'le·he'ma·tin
cho'le·ic
cho'le·lith'
cho'le·li·thi'a·sis *pl.* -ses'
cho'le·lith'ic

cho'le·li·thot'o·my
cho'le·lith'o·trip'sy
cho'le·li·thot'ri·ty
cho·lem'e·sis *pl.* -ses'
cho'le·mi·a
cho'le·mic
cho'le·per'i·to·ne'um
cho'le·poi·e'sis *pl.* -ses'
cho'le·poi·et'ic
cho'le·pra'sin
chol'er·a
—mor'bus
—nos'tras
—sic'ca
—sid'er·ans'
—vib'ri·o'
chol'er·a·gen
chol'er·a'ic
cho'le·re'sis *pl.* -ses'
cho'le·ret'ic
chol'er·ic
chol'er·i·form'
chol'er·ine'
chol'er·oid'
chol'er·o·ma'ni·a
chol'er·rha'gi·a
cho'le·scin'ti·gram'
cho'le·scin·tig'ra·phy
cho·les·tane'
cho·les'ta·nol'
cho·le·sta'sis *pl.* -ses'
cho'le·stat'ic
cho·les'te·a·to'ma *pl.* -mas
  or -ma·ta
cho·les'te·a·tom'a·tous
cho·les'te·a·to'sis *pl.* -ses'
cho·les'te·nol'
cho·les'ter·ase'
cho·les'ter·e'mi·a
cho·les'ter·in
cho·les'ter·in·e'mi·a
cho·les'ter·i·nu'ri·a
cho·les'ter·ol'
cho·les'ter·ol·e'mi·a
cho·les'ter·ol·er'e·sis
  pl. -ses'
cho·les'ter·ol·o·poi·e'sis
  pl. -ses'
cho·les'ter·ol·o'sis *pl.* -ses'
cho·les'ter·ol·u'ri·a
cho·les'ter·o'sis *pl.* -ses'
cho·les'ter·yl
cho'le·ther'a·py

cho'le·ver'din
chol'ic
cho'line'
cho'line·a·cet'y·lase'
cho'lin·er'gic
cho'lin·es'ter·ase'
cho'li·no·gen'ic
cho'li·no·lyt'ic
cho'li·no·mi·met'ic
chol'o·chrome'
cho'lo·he'mo·tho'rax'
cho'lo·lith'
cho'lo·li·thi'a·sis *pl.* -ses'
cho'lo·lith'ic
cho'lor·rhe'a
cho'lo·tho'rax'
cho·lu'ri·a
Cho'man method
chon'do·den'drine'
Chon'do·den'dron'
chon'dral
chon'dral'gi·a
chon'drec'to·my
chon'dric
chon'dri·fi·ca'tion
chon'dri·fy', -fied', -fy'ing
chon'dri·o·ki·ne'sis *pl.* -ses'
chon'dri·o'ma *pl.* -mas *or*
  -ma·ta
chon'dri'tis
chon'dro·ad'e·no'ma
  pl. -mas *or* -ma·ta
chon'dro·al·bu'mi·noid'
chon'dro·an'gi·o'ma
  pl. -mas *or* -ma·ta
chon'dro·blast'
chon'dro·blas'tic
chon'dro·blas·to'ma
  pl. -mas *or* -ma·ta
chon'dro·cal'ci·no'sis
  pl. -ses'
chon'dro·cal·syn'o·vi'tis
chon'dro·cla'sis *pl.* -ses'
chon'dro·clast'
chon'dro·cos'tal
chon'dro·cra'ni·um *pl.* -ni·a
chon'dro·cyte'
chon'dro·cyt'ic
chon'dro·der'ma·ti'tis
  —nod'u·lar'is hel'i·cis
chon'dro·dyn'i·a
chon'dro·dys·pla'si·a
  —punc·ta'ta

chon′dro·dys·tro′phi·a
—cal·cif′i·cans′ con·gen′i·ta
—fe·ta′lis
—fetalis cal·car′e·a
—fetalis cal·cif′i·cans′
—fetalis hy′po·plas′ti·ca
—hy′per·plas′ti·ca
—hy′po·plas′ti·ca
—ma·la′ci·a
chon′dro·dys·troph′ic
chon′dro·dys′tro·phy
chon′dro·ec′to·der′mal
chon′dro·en′do·the′li·o′ma
pl. -mas or -ma·ta
chon′dro·ep′i·phy·si′tis
chon′dro·ep′i·troch′le·ar′is
chon′dro·fi·bro′ma pl. -mas
or -ma·ta
chon′dro·fi′bro·sar·co′ma
pl. -mas or -ma·ta
chon′dro·gen
chon′dro·gen′e·sis pl. -ses′
chon′dro·ge·net′ic
chon′dro·gen′ic
chon·drog′e·nous
chon′dro·glos′sus
chon′dro·hu′mer·a′lis
chon′droid′
chon′dro·it′ic
chon′dro′i·tin
chon′dro·i′ti·nu′ri·a
chon′dro·li·po′ma pl. -mas
or -ma·ta
chon′dro·lip′o·sar·co′ma
pl. -mas or -ma·ta
chon·drol′o·gy
chon·drol′y·sis pl. -ses′
chon′dro′ma pl. -mas or
-ma·ta
chon′dro·ma·la′ci·a
chon·dro′ma·to′sis
chon·dro′ma·tous
chon′dro·mere′
chon′dro·met′a·pla′si·a
chon′dro·mu′cin
chon′dro·mu′coid′
chon′dro·my·o′ma pl. -mas
or -ma·ta
chon′dro·myx′o·fi·bro′ma
pl. -mas or -ma·ta
chon′dro·myx′oid′
chon′dro·myx·o′ma
pl. -mas or -ma·ta

chon′dro·myx′o·sar·co′ma
pl. -mas or -ma·ta
chon′dro·ne·cro′sis pl. -ses′
chon′dro-os′se·ous
chon′dro-os′te·o·dys′tro·
phy
chon′dro-os′te·o′ma
pl. -mas or -ma·ta
chon′dro-os′te·o·sar·
co′ma pl. -mas or -ma·ta
chon′dro·pa·thol′o·gy
chon′drop′a·thy
chon′dro·pha·ryn′ge·us
chon′dro·phyte′
chon′dro·pla′si·a
chon′dro·plast′
chon′dro·plas′tic
chon′dro·plas′ty
chon′dro·po·ro′sis pl. -ses′
chon′dro·pro′tein
chon′dro·sa·mine′
chon′dro·sar·co′ma pl. -mas
or -ma·ta
—myx′o′ma·to′des′
chon′dro·sar·co′ma·to′sis
chon′dro·sar·co′ma·tous
chon′dro·sin
chon·dro′sis pl. -ses′
chon′dro·skel′e·ton
chon·dros′te·o′ma pl. -mas
or -ma·ta
chon′dro·ster′nal
chon′dro·ster′no·plas′ty
chon′dro·tome′
chon·drot′o·my
chon′dro·xiph′oid′
cho′ne·chon′dro·ster′non′
Cho·part′
—amputation
—dislocation
—joint
Cho′pra test
chor′da pl. -dae′
—dor·sa′lis
—gu′ber·nac′u·lum
—o·bli′qua mem′bra′nae′
in′ter·os′se·ae′ an′te·bra′-
chi·i′
—sa·li′va
—tym′pa·ni′
chor′dae′
—ten·din′e·ae′
—Wil·lis′i·i′

chord′al (pertaining to
notochord)
♦cordal
chor′da·mes′o·blast′
chor′da·mes′o·derm′
Chor·da′ta
chor′date′
chor·dee′
chor·de′ic
chord′en·ceph′a·lon′
chor·di′tis
—fi′bri·no′sa
—no·do′sa
—tu′be·ro′sa
chor′do·blas·to′ma pl. -mas
or -ma·ta
chor′do·car·ci·no′ma
pl. -mas or -ma·ta
chor′do·ep′i·the′li·o′ma
pl. -mas or -ma·ta
chor′doid′
chor′do·ma pl. -mas or
-ma·ta
chor′do·skel′e·ton
chor·dot′o·my also
cordotomy
cho·re′a
—grav′i·dar′um
—in·sa′ni·ens
—nu′tans
cho·re′al
cho′re·at′ic
cho·re′ic
—a·bra′si·a
cho·re′i·form′
cho′re·o·ath′e·toid′
cho′re·o·ath′e·to′sis pl. -ses′
cho′re·oid′
cho′ri·al
cho′ri·o·ad′e·no′ma
pl. -mas or -ma·ta
—des′tru·ens
cho′ri·o·al′lan·to′ic
cho′ri·o·al·lan′to·is
cho′ri·o·am′ni·on′ic
cho′ri·o·am′ni·o·ni′tis
cho′ri·o·an′gi·o′ma
pl. -mas or -ma·ta
cho′ri·o·blas·to′sis pl. -ses′
cho′ri·o·cap′il·lar′is
cho′ri·o·car·ci·no′ma
pl. -mas or -ma·ta
cho′ri·o·cele′

cho'ri·o·ep'i·the'li·o'ma
pl. -mas *or* -ma·ta
cho'ri·o·ep'i·the'li·om'a·
tous
cho'ri·o·gen'e·sis *pl.* -ses'
cho'ri·oid'
cho'ri·oi'de·a
cho'ri·o'ma *pl.* -mas *or*
-ma·ta
cho'ri·o·men'in·gi'tis
cho'ri·on'
—al'lan·toi'de·um
—av'il·lo'sum
—fron·do'sum
—lae've'
—om'pha·loi'de·um
—vil·lo'sum
cho'ri·on·ep'i·the'li·o'ma
pl. -mas *or* -ma·ta
cho'ri·on·ic
cho'ri·o·ni'tis
cho'ri·o·ret'i·nal
cho'ri·o·ret'i·ni'tis
cho'ri·o·ret'i·nop'a·thy
chor'i·sis *pl.* -ses'
cho·ris'ta
cho·ris'to·blas·to'ma
pl. -mas *or* -ma·ta
cho'ris·to'ma *pl.* -mas *or*
-ma·ta
cho'roid'
cho·roi'dal
cho·roi'de·a
cho·roi·dec'to·my
cho'roid·e·re'mi·a
cho'roid·i'tis
—gut·ta'ta
cho·roi'do·cy·cli'tis
cho·roi'do·i·ri'tis
cho·roi'do·ret'i·ni'tis
Chot'zen syndrome
Chris·tel'ler method
Chris'ten·sen-Krab'be
disease
Chris'tian disease
Chris'tian-Web'er disease
Christ'mas
—disease
—factor
chro'maf·fin
chro'maf·fin'i·ty
chro·maf'fi·no·blas·to'ma
pl. -mas *or* -ma·ta

chro·maf'fi·no'ma *pl.* -mas
or -ma·ta
chro·maf'fi·nop'a·thy
chro'ma·phil'
chro'ma·phobe'
chro·ma'si·a
chro'mate'
chro'ma·te·lop'si·a
chro·mat'ic
chro'ma·tid
chro'ma·tin
chro'ma·tin-neg'a·tive
chro'ma·tin-pos'i·tive
chro'ma·tism
chro'ma·to·der'ma·to'sis
pl. -ses'
chro'ma·to·dys·o'pi·a
chro'ma·tog'e·nous
chro·mat'o·gram'
chro·mat'o·graph'
chro·mat'o·graph'ic
chro'ma·tog'ra·phy
chro'ma·toid'
chro'ma·to·ki·ne'sis
chro'ma·tol'o·gy
chro'ma·tol'y·sis *pl.* -ses'
chro'ma·to·lyt'ic
chro'ma·tom'e·ter
chro'ma·tom'e·try
chro·mat'o·path'y
chro'ma·to·phil'
chro'ma·to·phil'i·a
chro·mat'o·pho'bi·a
chro·mat'o·phore'
chro'ma·to·phor'ic
chro'ma·to·pho·ro'ma
pl. -mas *or* -ma·ta
chro'ma·to·pho'ro·troph'ic
chro'ma·to·pho'ro·trop'ic
chro'ma·toph'o·rous
chro·mat'o·plasm
chro·mat'o·plast'
chro·mat'o·pseu·dop'sis
pl. -ses'
chro'ma·top'si·a
chro'ma·top'sy
chro'ma·top·tom'e·ter
chro'ma·top·tom'e·try
chro'ma·to·sis *pl.* -ses'
chro'ma·tu'ri·a
chro'mes·the'si·a
chrom·het'er·o·tro'pi·a
chrom'hi·dro'sis *pl.* -ses'

chro'mic
chro'mi·cize', -cized',
-ciz'ing
chro'mid'i·al
chro'mid'i·um *pl.* -i·a
chro'mi·dro'sis *pl.* -ses'
chro'mi·um
Chro'mo·bac·te'ri·um
pl. -ri·a
chro'mo·blast'
chro'mo·blas'to·my·co'sis
pl. -ses'
chro'mo·cen'ter
chro'mo·crin'i·a
chro'mo·cys·tos'co·py
chro'mo·cyte'
chro'mo·dac'ry·or·rhe'a
chro'mo·der'ma·to'sis
pl. -ses'
chro'mo·gen
chro'mo·gen'e·sis *pl.* -ses'
chro'mo·gen'ic
chro'mo·lip'id
chro'mo·lip'oid'
chro·mol'y·sis *pl.* -ses'
chro'mo·mere'
chro'mo·my·co'sis *pl.* -ses'
chro'mo·nar'
chro'mo·ne'ma *pl.* -ma·ta
chro'mo·ne'mal
chro'mo·nu·cle'ic
chro'mo·nych'i·a
chro'mo·par'ic
chro'mo·pec'tic
chro'mo·pex'ic
chro'mo·pex'y
chro'mo·phage'
chro'mo·phane'
chro'mo·phil'
chro'mo·phile'
chro'mo·phil'ic
chro·moph'i·lous
chro'mo·phobe'
chro'mo·pho'bi·a
chro'mo·pho'bic
chro'mo·phore'
chro'mo·phor'ic
chro·moph'o·rous
chro'mo·phose'
chro'mo·phy·to'sis *pl.* -ses'
chro'mo·plasm
chro'mo·plast'
chro'mo·plas'tid

chro'mo·pro'tein
chro·mop'si·a
chro'mo·scop'ic
chro·mos'co·py
chro'mo·so'mal
chro'mo·some'
chro'mo·ther'a·py
chro'mo·tox'ic
chro'mo·trich'i·al
chro'mo·trope'
chro'mo·trop'ic
chro'mous
chro'nax·im'e·ter
chro·nax'i·met'ric
chro·nax·im'e·try
chro·nax'y
chron'ic
chro·nic'i·ty
chron'o·bi·ol'o·gy
chron'o·graph'
chron'o·log'ic or
    chron'o·log'i·cal
chron'o·met'ric
chro·nom'e·try
chron'o·pho'bi·a
chron'o·scope'
chron'o·ta·rax'is
chron'o·trop'ic
chro·not'ro·pism
chrys'a·ro'bin
chrys'a·zin
chrys'o·cy'a·no'sis pl. -ses'
chrys'o·der'ma pl. -ma·ta
Chrys'o·my'ia
    —bez'zi·a'na
chrys'o·pho·re'sis pl. -ses'
Chry'sops'
Chrys'o·spor'i·um
chrys'o·ther'a·py
chthon'o·pha'gi·a
chtho·noph'a·gy
chuck
Chur'chill-Cope' reflex
Churg'-Strauss' syndrome
Chvos'tek' sign
chy·lan'gi·o'ma pl. -mas or
    -ma·ta
chyle
chy'lec·ta'si·a
chy·le'mi·a
chy'li·dro'sis pl. -ses'
chy'li·fa'cient
chy'li·fac'tion

chy'li·fac'tive
chy·lif'er·ous
chy'li·fi·ca'tion
chy'li·form'
chy'lo·cele'
chy'lo·cyst'
chy'lo·cys'tic
chy'lo·der'ma
chy'loid'
chy·lol'o·gy
chy'lo·me·di'as·ti'num
chy'lo·mi'cron pl. -crons or
    -cra
chy'lo·mi'cron·e'mi·a
chy'lo·per'i·car'di·um
chy'lo·per'i·to·ne'um
chy'lo·phor'ic
chy'lo·poi·e'sis pl. -ses'
chy'lo·poi·et'ic
chy·lor·rhe'a
chy'lo·sis pl. -ses'
chy'lo·tho'rax'
chy'lous (pertaining to chyle)
    ♦chylus
chy·lu'ri·a
chy'lus (chyle)
    ♦chylous
chyme
chy'mi·fi·ca'tion
chy'mo·sin
chy'mo·sin·o'gen
chy'mo·tryp'sin
chy'mo·tryp·sin·o'gen
chy'mous
chy'mus
Ciac'ci·o fixatives
ci·bis'o·tome'
ci'bo·pho'bi·a
cic'a·trec'to·my
cic'a·tri'cial
cic'a·tric'u·la pl. -lae'
cic'a·trix' pl. cic'a·tri'ces' or
    -trix'es
cic'a·tri'zant
cic'a·tri·za'tion
cic'a·trize', -trized', -triz'ing
cic'lo·pir'ox'
cic'u·tism
cic'u·tox'in
Cie·szyn'ski rule
ci'gua·te'ra
ci'gua·tox'in
ci·la·stat'in

cil'i·a sing. -i·um
cil'i·ar'i·scope'
cil'i·ar'i·scop'ic
cil'i·a·rot'o·my pl. -mies
cil'i·ar'y
Cil'i·a'ta
cil'i·ate'
cil'i·at'ed
cil'i·ec'to·my
Cil'i·oph'o·ra
cil'i·o·ret'i·nal
cil'i·o·scle'ral
cil'i·o·spi'nal
cil'i·ot'o·my
cil'i·um in·ver'sum
cil·lo'sis
cil·lot'ic
ci·met'i·dine'
Ci'mex'
    —he·mip'ter·us
    —lec'tu·lar'i·us
    —ro'tun·da'tus
cim'i·cif'u·ga
cim'i·co'sis pl. -ses'
ci·nan'ser·in
cin·cham'i·dine'
cin·cho'na
cin·chon'a·mine'
cin·chon'ic
cin·chon'i·dine'
cin·cho·nine'
cin·cho·nism
cin·chon'i·za'tion
cin·chon·ize', -ized', -iz'ing
cin·cin'nat'i·en'sis
cin'e
cin'e·an'gi·o·car'di·o·
    gram'
cin'e·an'gi·o·car'di·og'-
    ra·phy
cin'e·an'gi·o·gram'
cin'e·an'gi·o·graph'
cin'e·an'gi·o·graph'ic
cin'e·an'gi·og'ra·phy
cin'e·den·sig'ra·phy
cin'e-e·soph'a·go·gram'
cin'e-e·soph'a·gos'co·py
cin'e-e·soph'a·gram'
cin'e·fluor'o·graph'ic
cin'e·fluo·rog'ra·phy
cin'e·fluo·ros'co·py
cin'e·mat'o·graph'ic
cin'e·ma·tog'ra·phy

cin′e·ma·to·ra′di·og′ra·phy
cin′e·mi·crog′ra·phy
cin′e·ole′
cin′e·phle·bog′ra·phy
cin′e·plas′tic
cin′e·plas′ty
cin′e·ra′di·og′ra·phy
cin′e·roent′gen·o·fluo·rog′-
ra·phy
cin′e·roent′ge·nog′ra·phy
cin′e·u·rog′ra·phy
cin′e·ven·tric′u·lo·gram′
cin′e·ven·tric′u·log′ra·phy
cin·ges′tol′
cin′gu·late′
cin′gu·lec′to·my
cin′gu·lot′o·my
cin′gu·lo·trac′to·my
cin′gu·lum *pl.* -la
—ex·trem′i·ta′tis in·fe′ri·o′-
ris
—extremitatis su·pe′ri·o′ris
—mem′bri′ in·fe′ri·o′ris
—membri su·pe′ri·o′ris
cin′na·mal′de·hyde′
cin′na·med′rine′
cin′na·mene′
cin·nam′ic
cin′na·mon
cin′na·myl
cin·nar′i·zine′
cin′per·ene′
cin′ta·zone′
cin·tri′a·mide′
cip′ro·flox′a·cin
cir·ca′di·an
cir′ci·nate′
cir′cle
—of diffusion
—of Hal′ler
—of Wil′lis
—of Zinn
Cir′con video camera
cir′cuit
cir′cu·lar
cir′cu·late′, -lat′ed, -lat′ing
cir′cu·la′tion
cir′cu·la·to′ry
cir′cu·lus *pl.* -li′
—ar·te′ri·o′sus cer′e·bri′
—arteriosus hal′ler·i′
—arteriosus i′ri·dis major
—arteriosus iridis minor

—arteriosus (Wil·lis′i·i′)
—ar·tic′u·lar′is vas′cu·lo′-
sus
—vas′cu·lo′sus ner′vi′
op′ti·ci′
cir′cum·a′nal
cir′cum·ar·tic′u·lar
cir′cum·cise′, -cised′, -cis′ing
cir′cum·ci′sion
cir′cum·cor′ne·al
cir′cum·duc′tion
cir′cum·fer·ence
cir′cum·fer·en′ti·a
—ar·tic′u·lar′is ra′di·i′
—articularis ul′nae′
cir′cum·fer·en′tial
cir′cum·fer·en′tial·ly
cir′cum·flex′
cir′cum·in′su·lar
cir′cum·len′tal
cir′cum·lo·cu′tion
cir′cum·loc′u·to′ry
cir′cum·ne′vic
cir′cum·nu′cle·ar
cir′cum·oc′u·lar
cir′cum·o′ral
cir′cum·or′bi·tal
cir′cum·pen′nate′
cir′cum·po·lar·i·za′tion
cir′cum·pul′par
cir′cum·re′nal
cir′cum·scribe′
cir′cum·stan′ti·al′i·ty
cir′cum·su′ture
cir′cum·ton′sil·lar
cir′cum·val′late′
cir′cum·vas′cu·lar
ci·ro′le·my′cin
cir·rho′sis *pl.* -ses′
cir·rhot′ic
cir′rus *pl.* -ri′
cir·sec′to·my
cir·sod′e·sis *pl.* -ses′
cir′soid′
cir·som′pha·los *pl.* -li
cis′pla·tin
cis′sa
cis′tern
cis·ter′na *pl.* -nae′
—am′bi·ens
—cer′e·bel′lo·med·ul′lar·is
—chi·as′ma·tis
—chy′li′

—cor′po·ris cal·lo′si′
—fos′sae′ lat·er·a′lis cer′e·
bri′
—in′ter·pe·dun′cu·lar′is
—lam′i·nae′ ter′mi·na′lis
—mag′na
—per′i·lym·phat′i·ca
—pon′tis
—ve′nae′ mag′nae′ cer′e·
bri′
cis·ter′nae′
—sub′a·rach′noi·da′les′
—sub′a·rach′noi·de·a′les′
cis·ter′nal
cis·ter′no·gram′
cis·ter′nog′ra·phy
cis′tron
cis·ves′ti·tism
cit′a·lo′pram′
Ci′tel′li angle
ci·ten′a·mide′
cit′ral
cit′rate′
cit′ric
cit′rin
cit′ri·nin
Cit′ro·bac′ter
—am′a·lo·nat′i·cus
—freun′di·i′
cit·ro·nel′la
cit·ro·nel′lal
ci·tro′vo·rum
ci·trul′lin
cit′rul·line′
cit′rul·lin·e′mi·a
cit′rul·li·nu′ri·a
cit·to′sis *pl.* -ses′
Ci·vatte′ poikiloderma
Ci′vi·ni′ni spine
Cla·do′ni·a
Cla′do point
clad′o·spo′ri·o′sis
Clad′o·spo′ri·um
Clag′ett-Bar′rett
esophagogastrostomy
clair·voy′ance
clam·ox′y·quin
clamp
clap
Clap′ton line
Clar′a cell
cla·rif′i·cant
clar′i·fi·ca′tion

clar'i·fy'
cla·rith'ro·my'cin
Clark
—classification
—electrode
—method
—rule
—sign
—test
Clarke
—column
—dorsal nucleus
Clarke'-Had'field'
  syndrome
clas·mat'o·cyte'
clas·mat'o·cyt'ic
clas·ma·to'sis *pl.* -ses'
clas·mo·cy·to'ma *pl.* -mas
  or -ma·ta
clasp
clas·si·fi·ca'tion
clas'si·fy'
clas'tic
clas'to·thrix
Clat'wor'thy sign
Claude syndrome
clau·di·cant'
clau·di·ca'tion
claus'tral
claus'tro·phil'i·a
claus'tro·pho'bi·a
claus'tro·pho'bic
claus'trum *pl.* -tra
clau·su'ra
cla'va *pl.* -vae'
cla'va·cin
cla'val
cla'vate'
Clav'i·ceps pur·pu're·a
clav'i·cle
clav'i·cot'o·my
cla·vic'u·la *pl.* -lae'
cla·vic'u·lar
cla·vic'u·late'
cla·vic'u·lec'to·my
clav'i·pec'to·ral
cla'vus *pl.* -vi'
claw'foot'
claw'hand'
claw'toe'
Clay'brook' sign
clear'ance
clear'ing

cleav'age
cleft
clei'do·cos'tal
clei'do·cra'ni·al
clei'do·hu'mer·al
clei'do·hy'oid'
clei'do·mas'toid'
clei'do·oc·cip'i·tal
clei'do·scap'u·lar
clei'do·ster'nal
clei·dot'o·my
Cle'land ligament
clem'as·tine'
clem'i·zole'
cle'oid'
Cle'ram·bault'-
  Kan·din'sky complex
click
click'-mur'mur syndrome
cli·din'i·um
cli'mac·ter'ic
cli'mac·te'ri·um *pl.* -ri·a
cli'mac'tic
cli'mate
cli·mat'ic
cli·ma·tol'o·gy
cli·ma·to·ther'a·py
cli'max'
clin'da·my'cin
clin'ic
clin'i·cal
cli·ni'cian
clin'i·co·path'o·log'ic
clin'i·co·pa·thol'o·gy
cli'no·ce·phal'ic
cli'no·ceph'a·lus *pl.* -li'
cli'no·ceph'a·ly
cli'no·dac'tyl·ism
cli'no·dac'ty·lous
cli'no·dac'ty·ly
cli'noid'
cli·nom'e·ter
cli·no·met'ric
cli'no·scope'
cli'o·quin'ol'
cli·ox'a·nide'
clip
clis'e·om'e·ter
clit'i·on'
clit'o·ral
clit'o·ral'gi·a
cli·tor'ic
clit'o·rid'e·an

clit'o·ri·dec'to·my
clit'o·ri·di'tis
clit'o·ri·dot'o·my
clit'o·ris *pl.* -ris·es *or*
  cli·to'ri·des'
clit'o·rism
clit'o·ri'tis
clit'o·ro·meg'a·ly
clit'o·rot'o·my
cli'vus *pl.* -vi'
  —mon·tic'u·li'
clo·a'ca *pl.* -cae'
clo·a'cal
clo'a·co·gen'ic
clo·cor'to·lone'
clo·faz'i·mine'
clo·fi'brate'
clo·ges'tone'
clo'ma·cran'
clo'me·ges'tone'
clo·meth'er·one'
clo·min'o·rex'
clo'mi·phene'
clo·mip'ra·mine'
clo'nal
clo·na'ze·pam'
clone, cloned, clon'ing
clon'ic
clo·nic'i·ty
clon'i·co·ton'ic
clon'ic-ton'ic
clon'i·dine'
clon'ism
clo·ni'trate'
clon·o'gen'ic
clon·o'graph'
clo'nor·chi'a·sis *pl.* -ses'
Clo·nor'chis
  —si·nen'sis
clon'o·spasm
clo'nus
clo·pam'ide'
clo'pen·thix'ol'
clo·per'i·done'
Clo·quet'
  —canal
  —ganglion
  —hernia
  —node
clo·raz'e·pate'
clor'a·zep'ic
clor·eth'ate'
clor·ex'o·lone'

clor'o·phene'
clor·pren'a·line'
clor·ter'mine'
clos·trid'i·al
Clos·trid'i·um
—bot'u·li'num
—chau·vo'ei'
—dif'fi·cile'
—his'to·lyt'i·cum
—no'vy·i'
—par'a·bot'u·li'num e'qui'
—per·frin'gens
—sep'ti·cum
—spo·rog'e·nes'
—ter'ti·um
—tet'a·ni'
—wel'chi·i'
clo'sure
clo'sy·late'
clot, clot'ted, clot'ting
clo·thi'a·pine'
clo·thix'a·mide'
clo·trim'a·zole'
clove
clove'-hitch'
clo'ver·leaf'
Clo'ward back fusion
clown'ism
clox'a·cil'lin
clo'za·pine'
clubbed
club'bing
club'foot'
club'hand'
clump'ing
clu'ne·al
clu'nes'
clu·pan'o·don'ic
clu'pein
clus'ter
clut'ter·ing
Clut'ton joints
clys'ma
cly'sis
clys'ter
cne'mi·al
cne'mic
cne'mis pl. cnem'i·des'
cni'do·blast'
co·ac'er·vate'
co·ac'er·va'tion
co'ad·ap·ta'tion
co·ag·glu'ti·na'tion

co·ag·glu'ti·nin
co·ag'u·la·bil'i·ty
co·ag'u·la·ble
co·ag'u·lant
co·ag'u·lase'
co·ag'u·late', -lat'ed, -lat'ing
co·ag'u·la'tion
co·ag'u·la'tive
co·ag'u·la'tor
co·ag'u·lop'a·thy
co·ag'u·lum pl. -la
Coak'ley
—cannula
—curette
—forceps
—operation
—trocar
co·a·lesce', -lesced', -lesc'ing
co'a·les'cence
co'a·les'cent
co·apt'
co'ap·ta'tion
co·a·
co·arc'tate'
co'arc·ta'tion
co'arc·tot'o·my
coarse
co'ar·tic'u·la'tion
coat
Coats disease
co·ax'i·al
co·bal'a·min
co'balt'
co·bal'tous
Co'ban'
—dressing
—wrap
Cobb syndrome
cob'ble·stone'
co'bra
co'ca
co·caine'
co·cain'ism
co·cain'i·za'tion
co'car·box'yl·ase'
co'car·cin'o·gen
co'car·cin'o·gen'e·sis
    pl. -ses'
coc'cal
Coc·cid'i·a
coc·cid'i·al
coc·cid'i·an
coc·cid'i·oi'dal

Coc·cid'i·oi'des'
—im·mi'tis
coc·cid'i·oi'din
coc·cid'i·oi·do'ma
coc·cid'i·oi·do·my·co'sis
    pl. -ses'
coc·cid'i·oi·do'sis pl. -ses'
coc·cid'i·o'sis pl. -ses'
coc·cid'i·o·stat'
coc·cid'i·o·stat'ic
coc·cid'i·um pl. -i·a
coc'ci·gen'ic
coc'ci·nel'la
coc'co·bac'il·lar'y
coc'co·ba·cil'li·form'
coc'co·ba·cil'lus pl. -li'
coc'coid'
coc'cu·lin
coc'cu·lus
coc'cus pl. -ci'
Coc'cus
coc'cy·al'gi·a
coc'cy·ceph'a·lus pl. -li'
coc'cy·dyn'i·a
coc·cyg'e·al
coc'cy·gec'to·my
coc·cyg'e·us pl. -e·i'
coc'cy·go·dyn'i·a
coc'cy·got'o·my
coc'cyx pl. coc'cy·ges' or
    -cyx·es
coch'i·neal'
coch'le·a pl. -ae' or -as
coch'le·ar
coch'le·ar'i·form'
coch'le·i'tis
coch'le·o·or·bic'u·lar
coch'le·o·pal'pe·bral
coch'le·o·ves·tib'u·lar
Coch'li·o·my'ia
—a·mer'i·ca'na
—hom'i·ni·vo'rax'
—mac'e·lar'i·a
Cock'ayne' syndrome
cock'roach'
coc'to·an'ti·gen
coc'to·im·mu'no·gen
coc'to·la'bile
coc'to·pre·cip'i·tin
coc'to·sta'bile
Code Blue
co'de·car·box'yl·ase'
co'de·hy'dro·gen·ase'

co'deine'
co'dex' *pl.* -di·ces'
Co·di·vil'la
—extension
—operation
Cod'man
—exercises
—triangle
—tumor
co·dom'i·nance
co·dom'i·nant
co'don'
co·dox'ime'
co·ef·fi'cient
coeli - See words spelled *celi-*.
coelio - See words spelled
celio-.
coe·lo·blas·to'ma *pl.* -mas
or -ma·ta
coe'lom *pl.* -loms *or*
coe·lo'ma·ta
coe·lom'ic
coe·los'chi·sis *pl.* -ses'
co·en'zyme'
coeur en sa·bot'
co·fac'tor
co·fer·ment
Cof'fey
—anastomosis
—operation
—technique
co·for'my·cin
Co'gan syndrome
cog'nate'
cog·ni'tion
cog'ni·tive
cog'wheel'
co·hab'i·ta'tion
co·here', -hered', -her'ing
co·her'ence
co·her'ent
co·he'sion
co·he'sive
Cohn'heim' theory
Cohn method
co·ho'ba
co'hort'
co'hosh'
coil
coi'no·site'
co·i'tal
co·i'tion
co·i·to·pho'bi·a

co'i·tus
—in'ter·rup'tus
—res'er·va'tus
co·la'tion
col·a·to'ri·um *pl.* -ri·a
col·a·ture
col'chi·cine'
col'chi·cin·i·za'tion
cold
cold'blood'ed
co·lec'to·my
Cole'man-Shaf'fer diet
co·le·o·cele'
Co'le·op'ter·a
co'le·op·to'sis *pl.* -ses'
co'le·ot'o·my
co'les'
—fem'i·ni'nus
co·les'ti·pol'
Co'ley toxin
co·li·bac·il'le'mi·a
co·li·bac·il·lo'sis *pl.* -ses'
co·li·bac·il·lu'ri·a
co'li·ba·cil'lus *pl.* -li'
col'ic
col'i·ca
col'i·cin
col'ick·y
col'i·cin'o·gen'ic
col'i·ci·nog'e·ny
col'i·co·ple'gi·a
co'li·form'
co'li·gran'u·lo'ma
co'li·phage'
co'li·punc'ture
co'li·sep'sis
co·lis'ti·meth'ate'
co·lis'tin
co·li'tis
—cys·ti·ca pro·fun'da
—cystica su·per·fi'ci·a'lis
—pol'y·po'sa
—ul'cer·a·ti'va
co'li·tox·e'mi·a
co'li·tox'i·co'sis
co'li·u'ri·a
col'la·gen
col'la·gen·ase'
col·lag'e·na'tion
col'la·gen'ic
col'la·gen·i·za'tion
col·lag'e·no·blast'
col·lag'e·no·cyte'

col'la·gen·o·gen'ic
col'la·gen·ol'y·sis
col·lag'e·no·lyt'ic
col'la·gen·o'sis *pl.* -ses'
col·lag'e·nous
col·lapse', -lapsed', -laps'ing
col'lar
col'lar·bone'
col'lar·ette'
col·lat'er·al
col·lat'er·al·i·za'tion
col·lect'
col·lec'tor
Col'les
—fascia
—fracture
—law
—ligament
Col·let' syndrome
col·lic'u·lec'to·my
col·lic'u·li'tis
col·lic'u·lus *pl.* -li'
—ab'du·cen'tis
—car'ti·lag'i·nis ar'y·te·
noi'de·ae'
—fa'ci·a'lis
—inferior
—sem'i·na'lis
—superior
—u're·thra'lis
col'li·dine'
Col'lier
—lid
—sign
col'li·ga'tive
col'li·mate', -mat'ed,
-mat'ing
col'li·ma'tion
col'li·ma'tor
Col'lin·so'ni·a
Col'lins solution
Col'lip unit
col'li·qua'tion
col·liq'ua·tive
Col'lis technique
col·lo·di'a·phys'e·al
col·lo'di·on'
col'loid'
col'loi·dal
col·loi'do·cla'si·a
col·loi'do·cla'sis *pl.* -ses'
col·loi'do·clas'tic
col·loi'do·pex'ic

col·loi′do·pex′y
col′loid·oph′a·gy
col′lum pl. -la
—an′a·tom′i·cum hu′mer·i′
—chi·rur′gi·cum hu′mer·i′
—cos′tae′
—den′tis
—dis·tor′tum
—fem′o·ris
—fol·lic′u·li′ pi′li′
—glan′dis
—mal′le·i′
—man·dib′u·lae′
—ra′di·i′
—scap′u·lae′
—ta′li′
—ve·si′cae′ fel′le·ae′
col′lu·to·ry
Col′lyer pelvimeter
col·lyr′i·um pl. -i·a or -i·ums
Col′o·bi′nae′
col′o·bine′
col′o·bo′ma pl. -ma·ta
—au′ris
—pal′pe·brae′
col′o·bo′ma·tous
co·lo·ce·cos′to·my
co·lo·cen·te′sis pl. -ses′
co·lo·cho·le′cys·tos′to·my
co·lo·cly′sis
co·lo·col′ic
co·lo·co·los′to·my
co·lo·cu·ta′ne·ous
col′o·cynth
co′lo·cyn′thin
co·lo·en·ter·i′tis
co·lo·fix·a′tion
co·lo·hep′a·to·pex′y
co·lo·il′e·al
co′lon pl. -lons or -la
—as·cen′dens
—de·scen′dens
—sig·moi′de·um
—trans·ver′sum
co·lon·al′gi·a
co·lo′ni·al
co·lon′ic
co·lon·op′a·thy
co·lon′o·scope′
co·lon′o·scop′ic
co·lon·os′co·py
col′o·ny
col′o·pex′y

co·loph′o·ny
co′lo·pli·ca′tion
co′lo·proc·tec′to·my
co′lo·proc·ti′tis
co′lo·proc·tos′to·my
co′lop·to′si·a
co′lop·to′sis
co′lo·punc′ture
col′or
col′or·a′tion
col′or·blind′
col′or·blind′ness
co′lo·rec′tal
co′lo·rec·ti′tis
co′lo·rec·tos′to·my
co′lo·rec′tum
col′or·im′e·ter
col′or·i·met′ric
col′or·im′e·try
co·lor′rha·phy
co′lo·sig′moid·os′to·my
co′los·to′my
co·los′tror·rhe′a
co·los′trous
co·los′trum
co·lot′o·my
co′lo·ty′phoid′
co′lo·vag′i·nal
co′lo·ves′i·cal
col·pal′gi·a
col′pa·tre′si·a
col′pec·ta′si·a
col′pec·to·my
col′pe·de′ma
col·peu′ry·sis pl. -ses′
col·pi′tis
col·po·clei′sis pl. -ses′
col′po·cele′
col′po·cys·ti′tis
col′po·cys′to·cele′
col′po·cys′to·gram′
col′po·cys′to·plas′ty
col′po·cys·tos′to·my
col′po·hy′per·pla′si·a
  cys′ti·ca
col′po·mi′cro·scope′
col′po·mi·cros′co·py
col′po·per′i·ne′o·plas′ty
col′po·per′i·ne·or′rha·phy
col′po·pex′y
col′po·plas′ty
col′po·pto′sis
col′por·rha′gi·a

col·por′rha·phy
col′por·rhex′is pl. -rhex·es′
col′po·scope′
col·po·scop′ic
col·pos′co·py
col·po·spasm
col′po·stat
col′po·ste·no′sis
col′po·ste·not′o·my
col·pot′o·my
col′po·xe·ro′sis
Colt cannula
colts′foot′
Co·lu′bri·dae′
Co·lum′bi·a-SK virus
co·lum′bin
co·lum′bi·um
col′u·mel′la pl. -lae′
col′umn
—of Ber′tin
—of Bur′dach′
—of Goll
—of Mor·ga′gni
co·lum′na pl. -nae′
—anterior me·dul′lae′
  spi·na′lis
—lat′er·a′lis me·dul′lae′
  spi·na′lis
—na′si′
—or′ni·cis
—posterior me·dul′lae′
  spi·na′lis
—ru·gar′um anterior
—rugarum posterior
—ver′te·bra′lis
co·lum′nae′
—a′na·les′
—car′ne·ae′
—gris′e·ae′
—rec·ta′les′
—re·na′les′
—ru·gar′um
co·lum′nar
col′umn·ing
co·lum′ni·za′tion
columns of Mor·ga′gni
co′ma
co′ma·tose′
Com′by sign
com′e·do′ pl. com′e·do′nes′
co·me·do·car′ci·no′ma
  pl. -mas or -ma·ta
co·me·do·mas·ti′tis

co′mes′ *pl.* com′i·tes′
com·men′sal
com·men′sal·ism
com′mi·nute′, -nut·ed,
 -nut′ing
com′mi·nu′tion
com′mis·su′ra *pl.* -rae′
—al′ba me·dul′lae′
 spi·na′lis
—anterior alba medullae
 spinalis
—anterior cer′e·bri′
—anterior gris′e·a me·dul′-
 lae′ spi·na′lis
—for′ni·cis
—ha·ben′u·lar′um
—hip′po·cam′pi′
—inferior (Gud·den′i′)
—la′bi·o′rum anterior
—labiorum o′ris
—labiorum posterior
—mol′lis
—pal′pe·brar′um lat′er·a′lis
—palpebrarum me′di·a′lis
—posterior cer′e·bri′
—posterior me·dul′lae′
 spi·na′lis
—superior (Mey′ner·ti′)
com′mis·su′rae′ su′pra·
 op′ti·cae′
com·mis′su·ral
com′mis·sure
—of Fo·rel′
com·mis′su·ror′rha·phy
com·mis′sur·ot′o·my
com·mit′ment
com·mode′
com′mon
com·mo′ti·o′
—cer′e·bri′
—ret′i·nae′
—spi·na′lis
com·mu′ni·ca·ble
com·mu′ni·ca·bil′i·ty
com·mu′ni·cans′
com·mu′ni·cate′, -cat·ed,
 -cat′ing
com·mu′ni·ca′tion
com·mu′nis
com′mu·ta′tor
Co·mol′li sign
com·pac′ta
com·pact′er

com·pac′tion
com·par′a·scope′
com·par′a·tive
com·part′ment
com′part·men′tal·i·za′tion
com·pat′i·bil′i·ty
com·pat′i·ble
com·pen·sate′, -sat·ed,
 -sat′ing
com·pen·sa′tion
com·pen·sa·to′ry
com′pe·tence
com′pe·ten·cy
com′pe·tent
com·pet′i·tive
com·plaint′
com′ple·ment
com′ple·men′ta·ry
com′ple·men·ta′tion
com′plex′
com·plex′ion
com·plex′ion·al
com·plex′ioned
com·plex′us
com·pli′ance
com′pli·cate′, -cat·ed,
 -cat′ing
com′pli·ca′tion
com·po′nent
com·pos′ite
com·po·si′tion
com′pos men′tis
com′pound′ *n.*
com·pound′ *v.*
com′press′ *n.*
com·press′ *v.*
com·pres′sion
com·pres′sor
—bul′bi′ pro′pri·us muscle
—hem′i·sphe′ri·cum bul′bi
 muscle
—la′bi·i′ muscle
—nar′is muscle
—na′si′
—rad′i·cis pe′nis
—u′re′thrae′
—va·gi′nae′
—ve′nae′ dor·sa′lis
com′pro·mise′
Comp′ton
—effect
—electron
com·pul′sion

com·pul′sive
com·put′er·ized′
com·pu·tro′ni·um
con′al·bu′min
co·na′tion
con′a·tive
con′ca·nav′a·lin
con·cat′e·na′tion
Con·ca′to disease
con′cave′
con·cav′i·ty
con·ca′vo-con′vex′
con·ceive′, -ceived′, -ceiv′ing
con′cen·tra′tion
con·cen′tric
con′cept′
con·cep′tion
con·cep′tion·al
con·cep′tive
con·cep′tu·al
con·cep′tus *pl.* -tus·es *or* -ti′
con′cha *pl.* -chae′
—au·ric′u·lae′
—na·sa′lis inferior
—nasalis me′di·a
—nasalis superior
—nasalis su·pre′ma
—nasalis suprema
 (San′to·ri′ni)
—sphe·noi·da′lis
con·chi′tis
con·choi′dal
con·cho·tome′
con′cli·na′tion
con·com′i·tant
con·cor′dance
con′cre·ment
con·cres′cence
con·cre′ti·o′
—cor′dis
—per′i·car′di·i′
con·cre′tion
con′cre·tiz′ing
con·cur′rent
con·cus′sion
con′den·sate′
con′den·sa′tion
con·dens′er
con·di′tion
con·di′tion·al
con·di′tion·al·ly
con′dom
con·duct′

con·duc'tance
con·duct'i·bil'i·ty
con·duc'tion
con'duc·tiv'i·ty
con'duc·tom'e·try
con·duc'tor
—so·no'rus of Berg'mann
con'du·it
con·du'pli·ca'to cor'po·re'
con'du·ran'go
con'dy·lar
con'dy·lar·thro'sis *pl.* -ses'
con'dyle'
con'dy·lec'to·my
con'dyl'i·on'
con'dy·loid'
con'dy·lo'ma *pl.* -mas *or*
  -ma·ta
—a·cu'mi·na'tum
—la'tum
con'dy·lo·ma·to'sis *pl.* -ses'
con'dy·lom'a·tous
con'dy·lot'o·my
con'dy·lus *pl.* -li'
—hu'mer·i'
—lat'er·a'lis fem'or·is
—lateralis tib'i·ae'
—me'di·a'lis fem'or·is
—medialis tib'i·ae'
—oc·cip'i·ta'lis
cone
coned'-down'
—appearance
—view
cone'-mon'o·chro'mat
co·nex'us *pl.* -us
con·fab'u·la'tion
con·fab'u·lo'sis *pl.* -ses'
con·fec'tion
con·fer'tus
con·fi·den'ti·al'i·ty
con·fig'u·ra'tion
con·fine'ment
con'flict'
con'flu·ence
con'flu·ens sin'u·um
con'flu·ent
con·fo'cal
con'for·ma'tion
con'for·ma'tion·al
con·form'er
con'fron·ta'tion
con'fron·ta'tion·al

con·fu'sion
con·fu'sion·al
con'ge·la'tion
con'gen'i·tal
con·gest'ed
con·ges'tin
con·ges'tion
con·ges'tive
con·glo'bate'
con'glo·ba'tion
con·glom'er·ate', -at'ed,
  -at'ing
con·glom'er·a'tion
con·glu'tin
con·glu'ti·nant
con·glu'ti·na'tion
con·glu'ti·nin
Con'go red test
con'gress
con·gru'ence
con·gru'ent
con·hy'drine'
co'ni'
—ep'i·di·dym'i·dis
—tu'bu·lo'si'
con'i·cal
co·nid'i·al
co·nid'i·o·phore'
co·nid'i·um *pl.* -i·a
co'ni·ine'
co·ni'om'e·ter
co·ni·o'sis *pl.* -ses'
co'ni·o·spo'ri·o'sis *pl.* -ses'
co·ni·ot'o·my
co'ni·um
con'i·za'tion
con'joined'
con'joint'
con'ju·gal
con'ju·gal'i·ty
con'ju·gant
con·ju·ga'ta *pl.* -tae'
—ve'ra
con'ju·gate', -gat'ed, -gat'ing
con'ju·ga'tion
con·junc·ti'va *pl.* -vas *or*
  -vae'
con'junc·ti'val
con·junc'ti·vi'tis
—cat'ar'rha'lis aes·ti'va
—gran'u·lo'sa
—med'i·ca·men·to'sa
—no·do'sa

con'junc·ti'vo·plas'ty
con·nec'tive
con·nec'tor
con·nex'us
—in'ter·ten·din'e·us
—in'ter·tha·lam'i·cus
Conn syndrome
co'noid'
Con·ol·ly system
con'qui·nine'
Con'rad'i disease
con·san·guin'e·ous
con·san·guin'i·ty
con'science
con'scious
con'scious·ly
con'scious·ness
con·sec'u·tive
con·sen'su·al
con·sen'su·al·ly
con·sent'
con·ser'va·tive
con·sis'tence
con·sis'ten·cy
con·sol'i·dant
con·sol'i·date', -dat'ed,
  -dat'ing
con·sol'i·da'tion
con·sol'i·da'tive
con·sper'gent
con'stant
con·stel·la'tion
con'sti·pate', -pat'ed,
  -pat'ing
con'sti·pa'tion
con'sti·tute', -tut'ed, -tut'ing
con'sti·tu'tion
con'sti·tu'tion·al
con'sti·tu'tive
con·strict'
con·stric'tion
con·stric'tive
con·stric'tor
—rad'i·cis pe'nis
—va·gi'nae'
con·sult'
con·sul'tant
con·sul·ta'tion
con·sume', -sumed',
  -sum'ing
con·sum'ma·to'ry
con·sump'tion
con·sump'tive

con·sump′tive·ly
con′tact′
con·tac′tant
con·tact·ol′o·gy
con·ta′gion
con·ta′gious
con·ta′gi·um *pl.* -gi·a
con·tain′er
con·tam′i·nant
con·tam′i·nate′, -nat′ed,
  -nat′ing
con·tam′i·na′tion
con·tem′pla·ti·o′
con·tem′pla·tive
con·tin′gen·cy
con·ti·gu′i·ty
con·tig′u·ous
con′ti·nence
con′ti·nent
con·tin′u·ous
con·tor′tion
con·tour′
con′tra-an′gles
con′tra-ap′er·ture
con′tra·cep′tion
con′tra·cep′tive
con·tract′
con·trac′tile
con′trac·til′i·ty
con·trac′tion
con·trac′tor
con·trac′ture
con′tra·fis′sure
con′tra·ges′tive
con′tra·in′di·cant
con′tra·in′di·cate′, -cat′ed,
  -cat′ing
con′tra·in′di·ca′tion
con′tra·in′su·lar
con′tra·lat′er·al
con·trar′i·ness
con′trast′
con′tra·stim′u·lant
con′tra·ver′sive
con′tre·coup′
con′trec·ta′tion
con·trol′
con·tuse′, -tused′, -tus′ing
con·tu′sion
co′nus *pl.* -ni
  —ar·te′ri·o′sus pul′mo·na′-
    lis
  —e′las′ti·cus la·ryn′gis

—med′ul·lar′is
—ter′mi·na′lis
—tu′bu·lo′si′
con·va·lesce′
con·va·les′cence
con·va·les′cent
con·val·lar′i·a
con·vec′tion
con·ver′gence
con·ver′gent
con·ver′sion
con·vert′er
con·ver′tin
con·vex′
con·vex′i·ty
con·vex′o-con′cave′
con·vex′o-con′vex′
con′vo·lut′ed
con′vo·lu′tion
con′vo·lu′tion·al
con·vul′sant
con·vul′sion
con·vul′si·o′ par·tic′u·lar′is
con·vul′sive
Con′way′
  —cell
  —method
Con′way-Byrne′ diffusion
  method
Cooke′-Pon′der method
cook′ie
Coo′ley
  —anemia
  —trait
Coombs
  —serum
  —test
Coons fluorescent
  antibody method
Coo′per
  —disease
  —fascia
  —ligament
  —method
Coo·pe′ri·a
coo′per·id
Coo′per·nail′ sign
co·or′di·na′tion
co·os·si·fi·ca′tion
co·os′si·fy′
co·pai′ba
cope, coped, cop′ing
co′pe·pod′

Co·pep′o·da
co·pol′y·mer
co·pol′y·mer·i·za′tion
cop′per·as
cop′per·head′
co′pre·cip′i·tin
co′pre·cip′i·tate′, -tat′ed,
  -tat′ing
co′pre·cip′i·ta′tion
cop·rem′e·sis
cop′ro·an′ti·bod′y
cop·roc′tic
cop′ro·lag′ni·a
cop′ro·la′li·a
cop′ro·lith′
cop·rol′o·gy
cop′ro·ma
cop′ro·pha′gi·a
cop·roph′a·gous
cop·roph′a·gy
cop′ro·phil′i·a
cop·roph′i·lous
cop′ro·pho′bi·a
cop′ro·phra′si·a
cop′ro·por·phyr′i·a
cop′ro·por′phy·rin
cop′ro·por·phy·rin′o·gen
cop′ro·por′phy·ri·nu′ri·a
cop·ros′ta·nol′
cop·ros′ta·sis
cop·ros′ter·ol′
cop′ro·zo′·a
cop′ro·zo′ic
cop′u·la *pl.* -las *or* -lae′
cop′u·late′, -lat′ed, -lat′ing
cop′u·la′tion
co·quille′
cor
  —bi′au·ric′u·lar′e′
  —bi·loc′u·lar′e′
  —bi·ven·tric′u·lar′e′
  —bo·vi′num
  —pseu′do·tri·loc′u·lar′e′
  —pul′mo·na′le′
  —tri·a′tri·a′tum
  —tri·au·ric′u·lar′e′
  —tri·loc′u·lar′e′
  —triloculare bi·a′tri·um
  —trioculare bi·ven·tric′u·
    lar′e′
  —trioculare mon·a′tri·a′tum
  —vil′lo′sum
cor′a·cid′i·um *pl.* -i·a

cor'a·co·a·cro'mi·al
cor'a·co·bra'chi·a'lis
   pl. -les'
   —brev'is
   —superior
cor'a·co·cla·vic'u·lar
cor'a·co·hu'mer·al
cor'a·coid'
cor'a·coi·di'tis
cor'al
cor·al'li·form'
cor'al·lin
cord
cord'al *(pertaining to vocal*
   cord)
   ♦*chordal*
cor'date'
cor·dec'to·my
cor'dial
cor'di·form'
cor·di'tis
   —no·do'sa
cor'do·pex'y
cor·dot'o·my *var. of*
   chordotomy
Cor'dy·lo'bi·a
   —an'thro·poph'a·ga
core
cor'e·cli'sis *pl.* -ses'
cor·ec'ta·sis *pl.* -ses'
cor·ec'tome'
co·rec'to·me'di·al'y·sis
co·rec'to·my
cor·ec·to'pi·a
cor'e·di·al'y·sis *pl.* -ses'
cor'e·di·as'ta·sis
co·rel'y·sis *pl.* -ses'
cor'e·mor·pho'sis *pl.* -ses'
cor'en·cli'sis
cor'e·om'e·ter
cor'e·om'e·try
cor'e·o·plas'ty
co'-re·pres'sor
cor'e·ste·no'ma
Co'ri
   —cycle
   —disease
   —ester
   —gly'co·ge·no'ses'
   —lim'it dex'tri·no'sis
co·ri·a'ceous
   —strep'i·tus
co·ri·an'der

co'ri·um *pl.* -ri·a
cork'screw'
cor'ne·a
   —gut·ta'ta
cor'ne·al
Cor·ne'li·a de Lange'
   syndrome
Cor·nell'
   —response
   —unit of riboflavin
Cor·nell'-Coxe' scale
cor'ne·o·bleph'a·ron'
cor'ne·o·i·ri'tis
cor'ne·o·man·dib'u·lar
cor'ne·o·oc'u·lo·gy'ric
cor'ne·o·pter'y·goid'
cor'ne·o·scle'ra
cor'ne·o·scle'ral
cor'ne·ous
cor'ne·um
cor·nic'u·late
cor·nic'u·lum *pl.* -la
   —la·ryn'gis
cor'ni·fi·ca'tion
cor'ni·fied'
cor'noid'
cor'nu *pl.* -nu·a
   —Am·mo'nis
   —an·te'ri·us me·dul'lae'
     spi·na'lis
   —anterius ven·tric'u·li'
     lat'er·a'lis
   —cer'vi'
   —coc·cyg'e·a
   —coc·cyg'e·um
   —cu·ta'ne·um
   —in·fe'ri·us car'ti·lag'i·nis
     thy're·oi'de·ae'
   —inferius cartilaginis
     thy·roi'de·ae'
   —inferius fos'sae' o·va'lis
   —inferius mar'gi·nis
     fal'ci·for'mis
   —inferius ven·tric'u·li'
     lat'er·a'lis
   —lat'er·a'le' me·dul'lae'
     spi·na'lis
   —ma'jus os'sis hy·oi'de·i'
   —mi'nus os'sis hy·oi'de·i'
   —pos·te'ri·us me·dul'lae'
     spi·na'lis
   —posterius ven·tric'u·li'
     lat'er·a'lis

   —sa·cra'le'
   —su·pe'ri·us car'ti·lag'i·nis
     thy're·oi'de·ae'
   —superius cartilaginis
     thy·roi'de·ae'
   —superius fos'sae' o·va'lis
   —superius mar'gi·nis
     fal'ci·for'mis
cor'nu·al
cor'nu·com·mis'sur·al
cor·o·clei'sis *pl.* -ses', *var. of*
   coroclisis
cor·o·cli'sis *pl.* -ses', *also*
   corocleisis
co·rol'la
co·rom'e·ter
co·ro'na *pl.* -nae'
   —cap'i·tis
   —cil'i·ar'is
   —clin'i·ca
   —den'tis
   —glan'dis pe'nis
   —ra·di·a'ta
   —seb'or·rhe'i·ca
   —ven'er·is
cor'o·nad'
co·ro'nal
cor'o·na'le'
cor'o·na'lis
cor'o·na·ri'tis
cor'o·nar'y
cor'o·na·vi'rus
co·ro'ne'
co·ro'ner
cor'o·net'
co·ro'ni·on' *pl.* -ni·a
co·ro'no·bas'i·lar
co·ro'no·fa'cial
cor'o·noid'
cor'o·noid·ec'to·my
co·ros'co·py
co·rot'o·my
Cor'per and Cohn method
cor·po'ra
   —al'bi·can'tes'
   —am'y·la'ce·a
   —A·ran'ti·i'
   —ar'e·na'ce·a
   —bi·gem'i·na
   —cav'er·no'sa
   —hem'or·rhag'i·ca
   —par'a·a·or'ti·ca
   —quad'ri·gem'i·na

—res'ti·for'mi·a
cor·po're·al
corpse
cor'pu·lence
cor'pu·lent
cor'pus *pl.* -po·ra
—ad'i·po'sum buc'cae'
—adiposum fos'sae'
  is'chi·o·rec·ta'lis
—adiposum in'fra·pat'el·
  lar'e'
—adiposum or'bi·tae'
—al'bi·cans'
—a·myg'da·loi'de·um
—a·tret'i·cum
—cal·ca'ne·i'
—cal·lo'sum
—can'di·cans'
—ca·ver·no'sum cli·to'ri·dis
—cavernosum pe'nis
—cavernosum u·re'thrae'
—cer'e·bel'li'
—cil'i·ar'e'
—cli·to'ri·dis
—coc·cyg'e·um
—cos'tae'
—de·lic'ti'
—ep'i·di·dym'i·dis
—fem'o·ris
—fi·bro'sum
—fib'u·lae'
—for'ni·cis
—ge·nic'u·la'tum
—geniculatum lat'er·a'le'
—geniculatum me'di·a'le'
—glan'du·lae' bul'bo·u're·
  thra'lis
—glandulae su'do·rif'er·ae'
—glan'du·lar'e' pros'ta·tae'
—hem'or·rhag'i·cum
—hu'mer·i'
—in·cu'dis
—lin'guae'
—lu'te·um
—Lu·y'si·i'
—mam'il·lar'e'
—mam'mae'
—man·dib'u·lae'
—max·il'lae'
—med'ul·lar'e' cer'e·bel'li'
—nu'cle·i' cau·da'ti'
—os'sis hy·oi'de·i'
—ossis il'i·i'

—ossis il'i·um
—ossis is'chi·i'
—ossis met'a·car·pa'lis
—ossis met'a·tar·sa'lis
—ossis pu'bis
—ossis sphe'noi·da'lis
—os'si·um met'a·car·pa'-
  li·um
—ossium met'a·tar·sa'li·um
—pan·cre'a·tis
—pap'il·lar'e' co'ri·i'
—pe'nis
—pha·lan'gis dig'i·to'rum
  ma'nus
—phalangis digitorum
  pe'dis
—pin'e·a'le'
—pon'to·bul'bar·e'
—quad'ri·gem'i·na
—ra'di·i'
—res'ti·for'me'
—re·tic'u·lar'e' co'ri·i'
—spon'gi·o'sum pe'nis
—spongiosum u·re'thrae'
  mu·li·e'bris
—ster'ni'
—stri·a'tum
—ta'li'
—tib'e·ae'
—trap'e·zoi'de·um
—ul'nae'
—un'guis
—u'ter·i'
—ven·tric'u·li'
—ver'te·brae'
—ves'i·cae' fel'le·ae'
—vesicae u'ri·nar'i·ae'
—ve·sic'u·lae' sem'i·na'lis
—vit're·um
—Wolf'fi'
cor'pus·cle
—of Gol'gi
cor'pus'cu·la
—ar·tic'u·lar'i·a
—bul·boi'de·a
—gen'i·ta'li·a
—lam'el·lo'sa
—ner'vo'rum ar·tic'u·lar'i·a
—nervorum gen'i·ta'li·a
—ner'vo'sa ter'mi·na'li·a
—re'nis
—tac'tus

cor·pus'cu·lar
cor·pus'cu·lum *pl.* -la
—ar·tic'u·lar'e' mo'bi·le'
cor·rect'
cor·rec'tion
cor·rec'tive
cor're·late', -lat'ed, -lat'ing
cor're·la'tion
cor·rel'a·tive
cor're·spon'dence
cor're·spond'ing
Cor'ri·gan
—cautery
—disease
—line
—pulse
—respiration
—sign
cor'rin
cor·rode', -rod'ed, -rod'ing
cor·ro'sion
cor·ro'sive
cor·ro'sive·ness
cor·ru'ga'tor
—cu'tis a'ni'
—su'per·cil'i·i'
cor'set
cor'tex' *pl.* -ti·ces'
—cer'e·bel'li'
—cer'e·bri'
—glan'du·lae' su'pra·re·
  na'lis
—len'tis
—no'di' lym·phat'i·ci'
—re'nis
Cor'ti
—arch
—canal
—cells
—ganglion
—membrane
—organ
—rods
—tunnel
cor'ti·cal
cor'ti·cate'
cor'ti·cec'to·my
cor'ti·cif'u·gal
cor'ti·cin
cor'ti·cip'e·tal
cor'ti·co·a·dre'nal
cor'ti·co·af'fer·ent
cor'ti·co·au'to·nom'ic

cor'ti·co·bul'bar
cor'ti·co·cer'e·bral
cor'ti·co·col·lic'u·lar
cor'ti·co·ef'fer·ent
cor'ti·co·ge·nic'u·late'
cor'ti·co·hy'po·tha·lam'ic
cor'ti·coid'
cor'ti·co·med'ul·lar'y
cor'ti·co·ni'gral
cor'ti·co·nu'cle·ar
cor'ti·co·pal'li·dal
cor'ti·co·pleu·ri'tis
cor'ti·co·pon'tile'
cor'ti·co·pon'tine'
cor'ti·co·pon'to·cer'e·
  bel'lar
cor'ti·co·ru'bral
cor'ti·co·spi'nal
cor'ti·co·ster'oid'
cor'ti·cos'ter·one'
cor'ti·co·stri'ate'
cor'ti·co·stri'a·to·spi'nal
cor'ti·co·stri'o·ni'gral
cor'ti·co·tha·lam'ic
cor'ti·co·troph'ic
cor'ti·co·trop'ic
cor'ti·co·tro'pin
cor'tin
Cor'ti·nar'i·us
cor'ti·sol'
cor'ti·sone'
cor'to·dox'one'
cor'tol'
cor'to·lone'
cor'us·ca'tion
Cor'vi·sart' disease
cor'vus
cor'y·ban'tism
co·rym'bi·form'
Cor'y·ne·bac·te'ri·um
  —diph·the'ri·ae'
  —hof'man'ni·i'
  —pseu'do·diph·the'rit'i·cum
  —xe·ro'sis
co·ry'ne·form'
co·ry'za
cos·me'sis
cos·met'ic
cos·met'i·cal·ly
cos'mid
cos'ta pl. -tae'
  —fluc'tu·an'tes'
  —spu'ri·ae'

  —ve'rae'
cos'tal
cos'tal'gi·a
cos·ta'lis
cos'tate'
cos·tec'to·my
Cos'ten syndrome
cos'ti·car'ti·lage
cos'ti·form'
cos'tive
cos'tive·ness
cos'to·ar·tic'u·lar
cos'to·car'ti·lage
cos'to·cen'tral
cos'to·cer'vi·cal
cos'to·cer'vi·ca'lis
cos'to·chon'dral
cos'to·chon·dri'tis
cos'to·cla·vic'u·lar
cos'to·col'ic
cos'to·cor'a·coid'
cos'to·di'a·phrag·mat'ic
cos'to·gen'ic
cos'to·in·fe'ri·or
cos'to·lum'bar'
cos'to·me'di·as·ti'nal
cos'to·phren'ic
cos'to·pleu'ral
cos'to·scap'u·lar
cos'to·ster'nal
cos'to·ster'no·plas'ty
cos'to·su·pe'ri·or
cos'to·tome'
cos·tot'o·my
cos'to·trans·verse'
cos'to·trans'ver·sec'to·my
cos'to·ver'te·bral
cos'to·xiph'oid'
co'syn·tro'pin
cot
co·tar'nine'
co·throm'bo·plas'tin
co'ti·nine' fu'ma·rate'
co'trans·am'i·nase'
co'trans·duc'tion
cot'ton
Cot'ton
  —fracture
  —procedure
co-twin'
cot'y·le'don
cot'y·loid'
couch'ing

cou·dé'
cough
cou'lomb
Coul'ter counter
cou'ma·din·i·za'tion
cou'ma·rin
Coun'cil·man
  —bodies
  —chisel
coun'sel
coun'sel·or
count
count'er
coun'ter·act' pl. -act'ed,
  -act'ing
coun'ter·ac'tion
coun'ter·bore'
coun'ter·ca·thex'sis
coun'ter·com·pul'sion
coun'ter·con·di'tion·ing
coun'ter·cur'rent
coun'ter·die'
coun'ter·ex·ten'sion
coun'ter·fis'sure
coun'ter·im'mu·no·e·lec'-
  tro·pho·re'sis pl. -ses'
coun'ter·in·ci'sion
coun'ter·in'di·ca'tion
coun'ter·in·vest'ment
coun'ter·ir'ri·tant
coun'ter·ir'ri·tate', -tat'ed,
  -tat'ing
coun'ter·ir'ri·ta'tion
coun'ter·o'pen·ing
coun'ter·pho'bi·a
coun'ter·pho'bic
coun'ter·poi'son
coun'ter·pres'sure
coun'ter·pul·sa'tion
coun'ter·punc'ture
coun'ter·shock'
coun'ter·sink'
coun'ter·stain'
coun'ter·stroke'
coun'ter·trac'tion
coun'ter·trans·fer'ence
coup
  —de fouet'
  —de sabre'
  —de sang'
  —de so·leil'
  —sur coup'
cou'ple

cou'plet
course
Cour·voi'si·er'
—gallbladder
—law
Cour·voi'si·er'-Ter·rier'
syndrome
cou·vade'
Cou've·laire' uterus
co·va'lence
co·va'lent
co·var'i·ance
Cow'dri·a ru'mi·nan'ti·um
Cow'en sign
Cow'ie test
Cow'ling rule
Cow'per
—cyst
—glands
—ligament
cow'per·i'tis
Cox
—vaccine
—yolk-sac method
cox'a *pl.* -ae'
—ad·duc'ta
—flex'a
—mag'na
—pla'na
—val'ga
—var'a
—var'a lux'ans
cox'al
cox·al'gi·a
cox·al'gic
cox·ar'thri·a
cox·ar'thri'tis
cox·ar'throc'a·ce
cox·ar'throp'a·thy
Cox'i·el'la
—bur·net'i·i'
cox·i'tis *pl.* -it'i·des'
—cot'y·loi'de·a
cox'o·dyn'i·a
cox'o·fem'o·ral
cox'o·tu·ber'cu·lo'sis
Cox·sack'ie
—disease
—virus
co·zy'mase'
Coz'zo·li'no zone
Crab'tree'
—dissector

—effect
cra'dle
Crä'mer method
cramp
Cramp'ton test
cramp'y
Cran'dall test
cra'ni·ad'
cra'ni·al
cra'ni·a'lis
cra'ni·ec'to·my
cra'ni·o·a·cro'mi·al
cra'ni·o·bas'al
cra'ni·o·buc'cal
cra'ni·o·car'po·tar'sal
cra'ni·o·cau'dad'
cra'ni·o·cau'dal
cra'ni·o·cele'
cra'ni·o·cer'e·bral
cra'ni·o·cer'vi·cal
cra'ni·oc'la·sis *pl.* -ses'
cra'ni·o·clast'
cra'ni·o·clas'ty
cra'ni·o·clei'do·dys·os·
to'sis *pl.* -ses'
cra'ni·o·did'y·mus *pl.* -mi'
cra'ni·o·fa'cial
cra'ni·o·fe·nes'tri·a
cra'ni·o·graph'
cra'ni·og'ra·phy
cra'ni·o·la·cu'ni·a
cra'ni·ol'o·gy
cra'ni·o·ma·la'ci·a
cra'ni·o·max'il·lar'y
cra'ni·o·me·nin'go·cele'
cra'ni·om'e·ter
cra'ni·o·met'ric
cra'ni·om'e·try
cra'ni·op'a·gus *pl.* -gi'
—fron'ta'lis
—oc·cip'i·ta'lis
—par'a·sit'i·cus
—pa·ri'e·ta'lis
cra'ni·op'a·thy
cra'ni·o·pha·ryn'ge·al
cra'ni·o·pha·ryn'gi·o'ma
pl. -mas *or* -ma·ta
cra'ni·o·phore'
cra'ni·o·plas'ty
cra'ni·o·ra·chis'chi·sis
pl. -ses'
—to·ta'lis
cra'ni·o·sa'cral

cra'ni·os'chi·sis *pl.* -ses'
cra'ni·o·scle·ro'sis *pl.* -ses'
cra'ni·os'co·py
cra'ni·o·spi'nal
cra'ni·o·ste·no'sis *pl.* -ses'
cra'ni·os·to'sis *pl.* -ses'
cra'ni·o·syn·os·to'sis
pl. -ses'
cra'ni·o·ta'bes'
cra'ni·o·ta·bet'ic
cra'ni·o·tome'
cra'ni·ot'o·my
cra'ni·o·trac'tor
cra'ni·o·tym·pan'ic
cra'ni·o·ver'te·bral
cra'ni·um *pl.* -ni·ums *or* -ni·a
—bif'i·dum
—cer'e·bra'le'
—vis'ce·ra'le'
crap'u·lous
craque·lé'
cra'ter
cra'ter'i·form'
cra'ter·i·za'tion
cra·vat'
craw'-craw'
Craw'ford-Ad'ams cup
arthroplasty
Craw'ford crutches
C'-re·ac'tive
creak
crease
cre·at'ic
cre·at'i·nase'
cre·a'tine'
cre·a'ti·ne'mi·a
cre·a'tine·phos·phor'ic
cre·at'i·nine'
cre·a'ti·nu'ri·a
cre·a'tor·rhe'a
Cre·dé'
—maneuver
—method
cre·mains'
cre·mas'ter
crem·as'ter·ic
cre·mate', -mat'ed, -mat'ing
cre·ma'tion
cre'ma·to'ri·um *pl.* -ri·ums
or -ri·a
crem·no·pho'bi·a
cre'na *pl.* -nae'
—a'ni'

—clu'ni·um
cre'nate'
cre'nat'ed
cre·na'tion
cre'no·cyte'
cre'no·cy·to'sis *pl.* -ses'
cre'o·sol'
cre'o·sote'
crep'i·tance
crep'i·tant
crep'i·tate', -tat'ed, -tat'ing
crep'i·ta'ti·o'
crep'i·ta'tion
crep'i·tus
cre·pus'cu·lar
cre·scen'do
cres'cent
   —of Gian·nuz'zi
cres·cen'tic
cres'co·graph'
cre'sol'
cre·sot'ic
cres'o·tin'ic
crest
cres'yl
cres'yl·ate'
cre·syl'ic
cre'tin
cre'tin·ism
Cré·tin' method
cre'tin·oid'
cre'tin·ous
Cré·tin'-Pou·yanne' method
Creutz'feldt-Ja'kob disease
crev'ice
cre·vic'u·lar
crib'bing
crib'rate'
crib·ra'tion
crib'ri·form'
crib'rose'
cri'brum *pl.* -bra
Cri·ce'ti·nae'
Cri·ce'tus
Crich'ton-Browne' sign
crick
cri'co·ar'y·te'noid'
cri'co·e·soph'a·ge'al
cri'coid'
cri'coi·dec'to·my
cri'coi·dyn'i·a
cri'co·pha·ryn'ge·al

cri'co·pha·ryn'ge·us
cri'co·thy'roid'
cri'co·thy·rot'o·my
cri·cot'o·my
cri'co·tra'che·al
cri'co·tra'che·ot'o·my
cri'co·vo'cal
cri'-du-chat'
Crig'ler-Naj·jar' syndrome
Crile
   —blade
   —clamp
   —forceps
   —head traction
   —hemostat
   —hook
   —knife
   —retractor
   —theory
crim'i·nol'o·gist
crim'i·nol'o·gy
cri'nis *pl.* -nes'
crin·o·gen'ic
cri·nos'i·ty
cri'nous
crip'ple
crise de dé·glo·bu·li·sa·tion'
cri'sis *pl.* -ses'
Crisp aneurysm
cris·pa'tion
cris'pa·tu'ra
   —ten'di·num
criss'cross'
cris'ta *pl.* -tae
   —a·cous'ti·ca
   —am'pul·lar'is
   —anterior fib'u·lae'
   —anterior tib'i·ae'
   —ar·cu·a'ta
   —bas'i·lar'is
   —buc'ci·na·to'ri·a
   —cap'i·tis cos'tae'
   —ca·pit'u·li' cos'tae'
   —col'li' cos'tae'
   —con·cha'lis max·il'lae'
   —conchalis os'sis pal·a·ti'ni'
   —div'i·dens
   —eth'moi·da'lis max·il'lae'
   —ethmoidalis os'sis pal·a·ti'ni'
   —fal'ci·for'mis
   —fe·nes'trae' coch'le·ae'

   —fron·ta'lis
   —gal'li'
   —i·li'a·ca
   —in'fra·tem'po·ra'lis
   —in'ter·os'se·a fib'u·lae'
   —interossea ra'di·i'
   —interossea tib'i·ae'
   —interossea ul'nae'
   —in'ter·tro'chan·ter'i·ca
   —lac'ri·ma'lis anterior
   —lacrimalis posterior
   —lat'er·a'lis fib'u·lae'
   —mar'gi·na'lis den'tis
   —me'di·a'lis fib'u·lae'
   —mus'cu·li' su'pi·na·to'ris
   —na·sa'lis max·il'lae'
   —nasalis os'sis pal·a·ti'ni'
   —ob'tu·ra·to'ri·a
   —oc·cip'i·ta'lis ex·ter'na
   —occipitalis in·ter'na
   —pal·a·ti'na
   —pu'bi·ca
   —sa·cra'lis in·ter·me'di·a
   —sacralis lat'er·a'lis
   —sacralis me'di·a
   —sacralis me'di·a'na
   —sep'ti' mar·gi·na'lis
   —sphe'noi·da'lis
   —su'pra·ven·tric'u·lar'is
   —ter'mi·na'lis a'tri·i' dex'tri'
   —trans·ver'sa
   —tu·ber'cu·li' ma·jo'ris
   —tuberculi mi·no'ris
   —u're·thra'lis u·re'thrae' fem'i·ni'nae'
   —urethralis urethrae mas'cu·li'nae'
   —urethralis urethrae mu'li·e'bris
   —urethralis urethrae vir'i·lis
   —ves·tib'u·li'
cris'tae'
   —cu'tis
   —ma·tri'cis un'guis
   —sa·cra'les' ar·tic'u·lar'es'
   —sacrales lat'er·a'les'
cris'tate'
crit
cri·te'ri·on *pl.* -i·a
crith
Cri·thid'i·a

cri·thid′i·al
crit′i·cal
crit′i·cal·ly
Crock′er tumor
Crocq disease
cro′cus
Crohn disease
cro′mo·lyn
Crooke
  —cells
  —change
Crookes tube
cross
cross′bite′
cross′breed′ing
cross′clamp′
cross′-eye′
cross′-eyed′
cross′fer′til·i·za′tion
cross′ing o′ver
cross′ match′ing
cross′-re·act′ing
cross sec′tion
cro·ta·lid
Cro·tal′i·dae′
crot′a·line′
cro·ta·lo·tox′in
Crot′a·lus
cro·tam′i·ton′
cro·taph′i·on′
crotch
cro′tin
cro′ton·ism
cro·tox′in
croup
croup′ous
croup′y
Crou·zon′-A′pert disease
Crou·zon′ disease
Crowe sign
crown
crown′ing
cru′ces′
  —pi·lo′rum
cru′cial
cru′ci·ate′
cru′ci·ble
cru′ci·form′
crude
cru·fo·mate′
cru′ra
  —am′pul·lar′i·a
  —ant·hel′i·cis

—mem′bra·na′ce·a
—membranacea am′pul·
  lar′i·a duc′tus sem′i·cir′-
  cu·lar′is
—os′se·a
—ossea am′pul·lar′i·a
cru′ral
cru′re·us
cru′ro·scro′tal
cru′ro·ves′i·cal
crus *pl.* cru′ra
—an·te′ri·us cap′su·lae′
  in·ter′nae′
—anterius sta·pe′dis
—brev′e′ in′cu·dis
—cer′e·bri′
—cli·to′ri·dis
—com·mu′ne′
—dex′trum di·a·phrag′-
  ma·tis
—fas·cic′u·li′ a·tri·o·ven·
  tric′u·lar′is dex′trum et
  si·nis′trum
—for′ni·cis
—hel′i·cis
—in·fe′ri·us an′nu·li′
  in′gui·na′lis sub·cu·ta′-
  ne·i′
—in·ter·me′di·um
  di·a·phrag′ma·tis
—lat′er·a′le′ an′u·li′
  in′gui·na′lis su′per·fi′-
  ci·a′lis
—laterale car′ti·lag′i·nis
  a·lar′is ma·jo′ris
—laterale di·a·phrag′ma·tis
—lon′gum in′cu·dis
—me′di·a′le′ an′u·li′
  in′gui·na′lis su′per·fi′-
  ci·a′lis
—mediale car′ti·lag′i·nis
  a·lar′is ma·jo′ris
—mediale di·a·phrag′ma·tis
—mem′bra·na′ce·um
  com·mu′ne′
—membranaceum sim′plex′
—os′se·um com·mu′ne′
—osseum sim′plex′
—pe·dun′cu·li′
—pe′nis
—pos·te′ri·us cap′su·lae′
  in·ter′nae′
—posterius sta·pe′dis

—sim′plex′
—si·nis′trum di·a′phrag′-
  ma·tis
—su·pe′ri·us an′nu·li′
  in′gui·na′lis sub·cu·ta′-
  ne·i′
crush
crus·ot′omy
crust
crus′ta *pl.* -tae′
  —lac′te·a
Crus·ta′ce·a
crutch
Cru′veil·hier′
  —disease
  —sign
  —ulcer
Cru′veil·hier′-
  Baum′gar′ten
  —cirrhosis
  —syndrome
crux *pl.* cru′ces′
Cruz disease
cry, cried, cry′ing
cry′al·ge′si·a
cry′an·es·the′si·a
cry′es·the′si·a
cry′mo·dyn′i·a
cry′mo·phil′ic
cry′o·ab·la′tion
cry′o·bi·o·log′i·cal
cry′o·bi·o·log′i·cal·ly
cry′o·bi·ol′o·gist
cry′o·bi·ol′o·gy
cry′o·cau′ter·y
cry′o·chem′
cry′o·crit′
cry′o·ex·trac′tion
cry′o·ex·trac′tor
cry′o·fi·brin′o·gen
cry′o·fi·brin′o·gen·e′mi·a
cry′o·gen
cry′o·gen′ic
cry′o·gen′i·cal·ly
cry′o·gen′ics
cry·og′e·ny
cry′o·glob′u·lin
cry′o·glob′u·lin·e′mi·a
cry′o·hy′drate′
cry′o·hy·poph′y·sec′to·my
cry′o·mag′net
cry·om′e·ter
cry′o·phake′

cry'o·phil'ic
cry'o·phy·lac'tic
cry'o·pre·cip'i·tate'
cry'o·pre·cip'i·ta'tion
cry'o·probe'
cry'o·pro'tein
cry'o·scope'
cry'o·scop'ic
cry·os'co·py
cry'o·stat'
cry'o·sur'geon
cry'o·sur'ger·y
cry'o·sur'gi·cal
cry'o·thal'a·mec'to·my
cry'o·thal'a·mot'o·my
cry'o·ther'a·py
cry'o·tol'er·ant
cry'o·tome'
crypt
cryp'ta *pl.* -tae'
cryp'tae'
—ton'sil·lar'es' ton·sil'lae'
  pal'a·ti'nae'
—tonsillares tonsillae
  pha·ryn'ge·ae'
crypt'am·ne'si·a
crypt·ec'to·my
cryp·ten'a·mine'
cryp'tic
cryp·ti'tis
cryp'to·bi·o'sis *pl.* -ses'
cryp'to·bi·ot'ic
cryp'to·coc·co'sis *pl.* -ses'
Cryp'to·coc'cus
—ne'o·for'mans'
cryp'to·did'y·mus
Cryp'to·gam'i·a
cryp'to·gen'ic
cryp'to·gli·o'ma
cryp'to·lith'
cryp'to·men·or·rhe'a
cryp'to·mere'
cryp'to·mer'o·ra·chis'-
  chi·sis *pl.* -ses'
cryp'tom·ne'si·a
cryp'toph·thal'mi·a
cryp'toph·thal'mos
cryp'to·po'rous
cryp'to·py'ic
cryp'to·pyr'role'
cryp·tor'chid
cryp'tor·chi·dec'to·my
cryp·tor'chid·ism

cryp'tor·chid'o·pex'y
cryp·tor'chis
cryp·tor'chism
cryp'to·spo·rid'i·o'sis
Cryp'to·spo·rid'i·um
cryp'to·xan'thin
cryp'to·zo'ite'
cryp'to·zy'gous
crys'tal
crys'tal·bu'min
crys'tal·fi'brin
crys'tal·lin *(a globulin of the
  crystalline lens)*
  ◆crystalline
crys'tal·line' *(similar to a
  crystal)*
  ◆crystallin
crys'tal·li·za'tion
crys'tal·lize', -lized', -liz'ing
crys'tal·lo·gram'
crys'tal·log'ra·phy
crys'tal·loid'
crys'tal·lo·pho'bi·a
crys'tal·lu'ri·a
Cte'no·ce·phal'i·des'
cte'noids'
cu'beb
cu'beb·ism
cu'bic
cu'bi·form'
cu'bi·tal
cu'bi·to·car'pal
cu'bi·to·ra'di·al
cu'bi·tus *pl.* -ti'
—val'gus
—var'us
cu'boid'
cu·boi'dal
cu·boi'de·o·na·vic'u·lar
cu·boi'do·dig'i·tal
Cu'cu·mis
cuff
cuff'ing
cui·rass'
cul'-de-sac'
cul'do·cen·te'sis *pl.* -ses'
cul'do·plas'ty
cul'do·scope'
cul'do·scop'ic
cul·dos'co·py
cul·dot'o·my
Cu'lex'
—fat'i·gans'

—pi'pi·ens
—quin'que·fas'ci·a'tus
cu'li·cide'
cu·lic'i·fuge'
Cu'li·coi'des'
Cul'len sign
cul'men *pl.* -mens *or* -mi·na
cul'ti·vate', -vat'ed, -vat'ing
cul'ti·va'tion
cul'tur·al
cul'ture, -tured, -tur·ing
cu'mic
cu'mu·la'tive
cu'mu·lus *pl.* -li'
—o'oph'o·rus
—o'vig'er·us
—pro·lig'er·us
cu'ne·ate'
cu'ne·i·form'
cu'ne·o·cu'boid'
cu'ne·o·na·vic'u·lar
cu'ne·o·scaph'oid'
cu'ne·us *pl.* -ne·i'
cu·nic'u·lar
cu·nic'u·lus *pl.* -li'
cun'ni·lin'gus
cun'nus *pl.* -ni'
cu'o·rin
cup, cupped, cup'ping
cu'po·la
cu'pram·mo'ni·a
cu'pre·a
cu'pre·ine
cu'pric
cu'prous
cu'pru·re'sis
cu'pru·ret'ic
cu'pu·la *pl.* -lae'
—coch'le·ae'
—cris'tae' am'pul·lar'is
—op'ti·ca
—pleu'rae'
cu'pu·lo·gram'
cu'rage
cu·ra're
cu·ra'ri·form'
cu·ra'ri·mi·met'ic
cu·ra'rine'
cu·ra'ri·za'tion
cu'ra·tive
curb
curd
cure, cured, cur'ing

cu·ret′ *var. of* curette
cu′ret·tage′
cu·rette′ *also* curet
cu·rette′ment
cu′rie
cu′ri·um
Cur′ling ulcer
Cur′rens formula
cur′rent
Cursch′mann spirals
cur·va′tor coc·cyg′e·us
cur·va·tu′ra *pl.* -rae′
—ven·tric′u·li′ major
—ventriculi minor
cur′va·ture
curve, curved, curv′ing
cur′vi·lin′e·ar
Cush′ing
—disease
—law
—syndrome
—ulcer
cush′ing·oid′
cush′ion
cusp
cus′pad
cus′pate′
cus′pid
cus′pi·dal
cus′pi·date′
cus′pis *pl.* -pi·des′
—anterior val′vae′ a′tri·o·
  ven·tric′u·lar′is dex′trae′
—anterior valvae atrioventricularis si·nis′trae′
—anterior val′vu·lae′
  bi·cus′pi·da′lis
—anterior valvulae
  tri·cus′pi·da′lis
—co·ro′nae′ den′tis
—me′di·a′lis val′vu·lae′
  tri·cus′pi·da′lis
—posterior val′vae′ a′tri·o·
  ven·tric′u·lar′is dex′trae′
—posterior valvae atrioventricularis si·nis′trae′
—posterior val′vu·lae′
  bi·cus′pi·da′lis
—posterior valvulae
  tri·cus′pi·da′lis
—sep·ta′lis val′vae′ a′tri·o·
  ven·tric′u·lar′is dex′trae′
cut, cut, cut′ting

cu·ta′ne·o·gas′tro·in·tes′ti·
  nal
cu·ta′ne·o·in·tes′ti·nal
cu·ta′ne·o·mu·co′sal
cu·ta′ne·ous
cut′down′
Cu·ter·e′bra
Cu′ter·e′bri·dae′
cu′ti·cle
cu′ti·col′or
cu·tic′u·la *pl.* -lae′
—den′tis
cu·tic′u·lar
cu·tic′u·lar·i·za′tion
cu′ti·dure
cu′tin
cu′tin·ase′
cu′tin·i·za′tion
cu′ti·re·ac′tion
cu′tis *pl.* -tes′ *or* -tis·es
—an′se·ri′na
—hy′per·e′las′ti·ca
—lax′a
—mar′mo·ra′ta
—pen′du·la
—rhom′boi·da′lis nu′chae′
—ve′ra
—ver′ti·cis gy·ra′ta
cu′ti·sec′tor
cu′ti·za′tion
Cut′ler-Beard′ technique
Cut′ler-Pow′er-Wil′der
  test
cut′ter
Cut′ting colloidal mastic
  test
cu·vette′
Cu·vier′
—canals
—ducts
cy·an′a·mide′
cy′a·nate′
cy′a·ne′mi·a
cy·an·he′ma·tin
cy·an·he′mo·glo′bin
cy·an·hi·dro′sis *pl.* -ses′
cy·an′ic
cy′a·nide′
cy·an·met·he′mo·glo′bin
cy·an·met·my′o·glo′bin
cy′a·no·ac′ry·late′
cy′a·no·co·bal′a·min
cy′a·no·der′ma

cy·an′o·gen
cy′a·no·ge·net′ic
cy′a·no·hy′drin
cy′a·nol′
cy′a·no·labe′
cy·an′o·phil′
cy′a·no·phil′ic
cy′a·noph′i·lous
cy·an′o·phose′
cy′a·no′pi·a
cy′a·nop′si·a
cy′a·nop′sin
cy′a·nosed′
cy′a·no′sis *pl.* -ses′
cy′a·not′ic
cy′a·nu′ric
cy·as′ma *pl.* -ma·ta
cy′ber·net′ic
cy′ber·net′ics
Cy′bex test
cy′cla·cil′lin
cy′cla·mate′
cy·clam′ic
cy·clan′de·late′
cy′clar·thro′sis *pl.* -ses′
cy′clase′
cy·claz′o·cine′
cy′cle
—of Gol′gi
—of Ross
cy·clec′to·my
cy′clen·ceph′a·lus *pl.* -li′
cy′clen·ceph′a·ly
cy′clic
cy′cli·cot′o·my
cy·clir′a·mine′
cy·clit′ic
cy·cli′tis
cy′cli·za′tion
cy′clize′, -clized′, -cliz′ing
cy′cli·zine′
cy′clo·bar′bi·tal′
cy′clo·ben′za·prine′
cy′clo·ceph′a·lus *pl.* -li′
cy′clo·ceph′a·ly
cy′clo·cho′roid·i′tis
cy′clo·cry·o·ther′a·py
cy′clo·cu′ma·rol′
cy′clo·di·al′y·sis *pl.* -ses′
cy′clo·di′a·ther′my
cy′clo·clog′e·ny
cy′clo·gram′
cy′clo·gua′nil

cy'clo·hex'ane'
cy'clo·hex'a·nol'
cy'clo·hex'i·mide'
cy'cloid'
cy'clo·i·som'er·ase'
cy'clo·ker'a·ti'tis
cy'clol'
cy'clo·mas·top'a·thy
cy'clo·meth'y·caine'
cy'clo·pen'ta·mine'
cy'clo·pen'tane'
cy'clo·pen·te'no·phe·nan'-
    threne'
cy'clo·pen·thi'a·zide'
cy'clo·pen'to·late'
cy'clo·phen'a·zine'
cy'clo·pho'rase'
cy'clo·pho'ri·a
cy'clo·phos'pha·mide'
Cy'clo·phyl·lid'e·a
cy'clo·phyl·lid'e·an
cy'clo'pi·a
cy'clo·ple'gi·a
cy'clo·ple'gic
cy'clo·pro'pane'
cy'clops'
cy'clo·scope'
cy'clo·ser'ine'
cy'clo·sis *pl.* -ses'
cy'clo·thi'a·zide
cy'clo·thy'mi·a
cy'clo·thy'mi·ac'
cy'clo·thy'mic
cy'clo·tome'
cy'clot'o·my
cy'clo·tron'
cy'clo·tro'pi·a
cy'cri·mine'
cy·do'ni·um
cy·e'sis *pl.* -ses'
cy·hep'ta·mide'
cyl'in·der
cy·lin'dric *or* cy·lin'dri·cal
cy·lin'dri·form'
cyl'in·droid'
cyl'in·dro'ma *pl.* -mas *or*
    -ma·ta
cyl'in·dru'ri·a
cy'ma·rin
cy·ma'rose'
cym'ba con'chae'
cym'bi·form'
cym'bo·ce·phal'ic

cym'bo·ceph'a·lous
cym'bo·ceph'a·ly
cy'mene'
cy'me·nyl
cy'mol'
cy·nan'che
cyn·an·thro'pi·a
cy·nan'thro·py
cyn'ic
cy'no·ceph'a·lus *pl.* -li
cy'no·ceph'a·ly
cy'no·dont'
cy'no·pho'bi·a
cy'no·rex'i·a
cy'o·pho'ri·a
cy·ot'ro·phy
cy·pen'a·mine'
cy·pra'ze·pam'
cy'pri·do·pho'bi·a
cy'pro·hep'ta·dine'
cy·pro'li·dol'
cy'pro·quin'ate'
cy·pro'ter·one'
cy·prox'i·mide'
cyr'to·graph'
cyr'toid'
cyr·tom'e·ter
cyr·tom'e·try
cyr·to'sis *pl.* -ses'
cyr'tu·ran'us
cyst
cyst·ad'e·no·car'ci·no'ma
    pl. -mas *or* -ma·ta
cyst·ad'e·no·fi·bro'ma
    pl. -mas *or* -ma·ta
cyst·ad'e·no'ma *pl.* -mas *or*
    -ma·ta
    —ad'a·man'ti·num
    —cy'lin·dro·cel'lu·lar'e'
        cel·loi'des' o·var'i·i'
    —pap'il·lif'er·um
cyst·ad'e·no·sar·co'ma
    pl. -mas *or* -ma·ta
cys·tal'gi·a
cys·ta·thi'o·nine'
cys·ta·thi'o·ni·nu'ri·a
cys·ta·tro'phi·a
cys'tec·ta'si·a
cys·tec'to·my
cys'te·ine'
cys'te·in'yl
cys'ten·ceph'a·lus
cys'tic

cys·ti·cer·ci'a·sis *pl.* -ses'
cys·ti·cer'coid'
cys·ti·cer·co'sis *pl.* -ses'
cys·ti·cer'cus *pl.* -ci'
cys·ti·form'
cys'tine'
cys·ti·ne'mi·a
cys·ti·no'sis *pl.* -ses'
cys·ti·nu'ri·a
cys·ti·stax'is
cys·ti'tis *pl.* -tit'i·des'
    —cys·ti·ca
    —em'phy·se'ma·to'sa
    —fol·lic'u·lar'is
    —glan'du·lar'is
cys·ti·tome'
cys·tit'o·my
cys·to·ad'e·no'ma *pl.* -mas
    or -ma·ta
cys·to·blast'
cys·to·bu·bon'o·cele'
cys·to·car'ci·no'ma *pl.* -mas
    or -ma·ta
cys·to·cele'
cys·to·co·los'to·my
cys·to·du·od'e·nos'to·my
cys·to·dyn'i·a
cys·to·e·lyt'ro·plas'ty
cys·to·en'ter·o·cele'
cys·to·ep'i·the'li·o'ma
    pl. -mas *or* -ma·ta
cys·to·fi·bro'ma *pl.* -mas *or*
    -ma·ta
    —pap'il·lar'e'
cys·to·gas'tros'to·my
cys·to·gen'e·sis *pl.* -ses'
cys·to·gram'
cys·to·graph'ic
cys·tog'ra·phy
cys'toid'
cys·to·je'ju·nos'to·my
cys'to·lith'
cys·to·li·thec'to·my
cys·to·li·thi'a·sis *pl.* -ses'
cys·to·lith'ic
cys·to·li·thot'o·my
cys·to'ma *pl.* -mas *or* -ma·ta
cys·to'ma·tous
cys·tom'e·ter
cys·to·met'ro·gram'
cys·to·me·trog'ra·phy
cys·tom'e·try
cys·to·mor'phous

cys'to·pa·ral'y·sis
cys'to·pex'y
cys'to·pho·tog'ra·phy
cys'to·plas'ty
cys'to·ple'gi·a
cys'to·proc·tos'to·my
cys'to·pros'ta·tec'to·my
cys'to·py'e·li'tis
cys'to·py'e·log'ra·phy
cys'to·py'e·lo·ne·phri'tis
cys'to·ra'di·og'ra·phy
cys'to·rec'to·cele'
cys·tor'rha·phy
cys'tor·rhe'a
cys'to·sar·co'ma *pl.* -mas *or*
  -ma·ta
  —phyl'lo'des'
  —phyl'loi'des'
cys'to·scope'
cys'to·scop'ic
cys·tos'co·py
cys'to·ste'a·to'ma *pl.* -mas
  or -ma·ta
cys·tos'to·my
cys'to·tome'
cys·tot'o·my
cys'to·u·re'ter·i'tis
cys'to·u·re'ter·o·cele'
cys'to·u·re·thri'tis
cys'to·u·re'thro·cele'
cys'to·u·re'thro·gram'
cys'to·u·re'thro·graph'ic
cys'to·u·re'throg'ra·phy
cys'to·u·re'thro·scope'
cys'tyl
cyt'ar·a·bine'
cy'tase'
cy·tas'ter
cyth'e·mol'y·sis *pl.* -ses'
cy'ti·dine'
cy'ti·dyl'ic
cy'to·al·bu'mi·no·log'ic
cy'to·an'a·lyz'er
cy'to·ar'chi·tec·ton'ic
cy'to·ar'chi·tec'tur·al
cy'to·ar'chi·tec'ture
cy'to·bi·ol'o·gy
cy'to·blast'
cy'to·blas·te'ma
cy'to·cen'trum
cy'to·chal'a·sin
cy'to·chem'i·cal
cy'to·chem'ism

cy'to·chem'is·try
cy'to·chrome'
cy'to·chy·le'ma
cy'to·cid'al
cy'to·cide'
cy·toc'la·sis *pl.* -ses'
cy'to·clas'tic
cy'to·crine
cy'to·crin'i·a
cy'tode'
cy'to·den'drite'
cy'to·derm'
cy'to·di'ag·no'sis *pl.* -ses'
cy'to·di·er'e·sis *pl.* -ses'
cy'to·dif'fer·en'ti·a'tion
cy'to·dis'tal
cy'to·gene'
cy'to·gen'e·sis *pl.* -ses'
cy'to·ge·net'ic
cy'to·ge·net'i·cist
cy'to·ge·net'ics
cy'to·gen'ic
cy·tog'e·nous
cy·tog'e·ny
cy'to·glob'u·lin
cy'to·gly'co·pe'ni·a
cy'to·his'to·gen'e·sis
cy'toid'
cy'to·ki'nin
cy'to·ki·ne'sis
cy'to·ki·net'ic
cy'to·lip'o·chrome'
cy'to·log'ic *or* cy'to·log'i·cal
cy·tol'o·gist
cy·tol'o·gy *(the branch of
  biology dealing with the cells)*
  ♦ sitology
cy'to·lymph'
cy·tol'y·sin
cy·tol'y·sis *pl.* -ses'
cy'to·ly'so·some'
cy'to·lyt'ic
cy'to·ma *pl.* -mas *or* -ma·ta
cy'to·me·gal'ic
cy'to·meg'a·lo·vi'rus
cy'to·mem'brane'
cy'to·met'a·pla'si·a
cy·tom'e·ter
cy'to·met'ric
cy·tom'e·try
cy'to·mi'tome'
cy'to·mor·phol'o·gy
cy'to·mor·pho'sis *pl.* -ses'

cy'to·my·co'sis *pl.* -ses'
cy'ton'
cy'to·path'ic
cy'to·path'o·gen'e·sis
cy'to·path'o·gen'ic
cy'to·path'o·ge·nic'i·ty
cy'to·pa·thol'o·gy
cy·top'a·thy
cy'to·pe'ni·a
cy'to·phag'o·cy·to'sis
cy·toph'a·gous
cy·toph'a·gy
cy'to·phil'
cy'to·pho·tom'e·ter
cy'to·pho'to·met'ric
cy'to·pho·tom'e·try
cy'to·phys'i·ol'o·gy
cy'to·plasm
cy'to·plas'mic
cy'to·plas'tin
cy'to·poi·e'sis *pl.* -ses'
cy'to·phy·lax'is
cy'to·phy·let'ic
cy'to·phys'ics
cy'to·pi·pette'
cy'to·prox'i·mal
cy'to·pyge'
cy'to·re·tic'u·lum
cy'tor·rhyc'tes'
cy'to·scop'ic
cy·tos'co·py
cy'to·sid'er·in
cy'to·sine'
  —ar'a·bin'o·side'
cy'to·skel'e·ton
cy'to·sol'
cy'to·some'
cy'tost'
cy'to·stat'ic
cy'to·ste·at'o·ne·cro'sis
cy'to·stome'
cy'to·tac'tic
cy'to·tax'is
cy'to·tech·nol'o·gist
cy'toth'e·sis *pl.* -ses'
cy'to·tox'ic
cy'to·tox·ic'i·ty
cy'to·tox'i·co'sis *pl.* -ses'
cy'to·tox'in
cy'to·troph'o·blast'
cy'to·trop'ic
cy·tot'ro·pism
cy'to·zo'ic

cy'to·zo'on' *pl.* -zo'a
ccy'to·zyme'
cy·tu'ri·a

D

Da Cos'ta syndrome
dac'ry·a·gog'a·tre'si·a
dac'ry·a·gog'ic
dac'ry·a·gogue'
dac'ry·o·ad'e·nal'gi·a
dac'ry·o·ad'e·nec'to·my
dac'ry·o·ad'e·ni'tis
dac'ry·o·a·gog'a·tre'si·a
dac'ry·o·blen'nor·rhe'a
dac'ry·o·cele'
dac'ry·o·cyst'
dac'ry·o·cys·tal'gi·a
dac'ry·o·cys·tec'to·my
dac'ry·o·cys·ti'tis
dac'ry·o·cys'to·blen'nor·
  rhe'a
dac'ry·o·cys'to·cele'
dac'ry·o·cys'to·gram'
dac'ry·o·cys'top·to'sis
dac'ry·o·cys'to·rhi'no·ste·
  no'sis *pl.* -ses'
dac'ry·o·cys'to·rhi·nos'-
  to·my
dac'ry·o·cys'to·ste·no'sis
  pl. -ses'
dac'ry·o·cys·tos'to·my
dac'ry·o·cys'to·tome'
dac'ry·o·cys·tot'o·my
dac'ry·o·hem'or·rhe'a
dac'ry·o·lin
dac'ry·o·lith'
dac'ry·o·li·thi'a·sis *pl.* -ses'
dac'ry·o'ma *pl.* -mas *or*
  -ma·ta
dac'ry·on' *pl.* -ry·a
dac'ry·ops'
dac'ry·op·to'sis
dac'ry·o·py·o'sis
dac'ry·or·rhe'a
dac'ry·o·so'le·ni'tis
dac'ry·o·ste·no'sis *pl.* -ses'
dac'ry·o·syr'inx
  pl. -sy·rin'ges' *or* -syr'inx·es
dac'ti·no·my'cin
dac'tyl
dac'ty·lar
dac'ty·late'

dac'tyl·e·de'ma *pl.* -mas *or*
  -ma·ta
dac'ty·lif'er·ous
dac'ty·li·tis
  —syph'i·lit'i·ca
dac'tyl·o·gram'
dac'tyl·o·graph'
dac'ty·log'ra·pher
dac'ty·lo·graph'ic
dac'ty·log'ra·phy
dac'ty·lo·gry·po'sis
dac'ty·lol'o·gy
dac'ty·lol'y·sis *pl.* -ses'
  —spon·ta'ne·a
dac'ty·lo·meg'a·ly
dac'ty·los'co·py
dac'ty·lo·spasm
dac'ty·lo·sym'phy·sis
  pl. -ses'
dac'ty·lus *pl.* -li'
Da·gni'ni ex·ten'sion-
  ad·duc'tion reflex
Da·gra'di classification
dah'lin
dahl'lite'
Da'kin solution
Dall'dorf' test
Dal'rym·ple sign
dal'ton
dal'ton·ism
Dal'ton law
dam
d-a·mi'no acid oxidase
da·min'o·zide'
dam'mar
Da·moi'seau' curve
Da'na operation
Da'na-Put'nam syndrome
dan'a·zol'
Dan'bolt-Closs' syndrome
Dance sign
dan'der
dan'druff
Dan'dy-Walk'er syndrome
Dane particle
Dan'iell cell
Dan'iels·sen-Boeck'
  disease
Dan'los syndrome
dan'thron'
D'An'to·ni stain
dan'tro·lene'
Da'nysz phenomenon

Dan'zer and Hook'er
  method
dap'sone'
Dar'i·er
  —abscess
  —disease
Dark·sche'witsch nucleus
Dar'ling disease
Dar'rach procedure
Dar'row
  —red
  —solution
d'Ar'son·val current
dar'tos'
dar'trous
dar·win'i·an
Dar'win tubercle
Das'y·proc'ta
da'ta *sing.* -tum
Da·tu'ra
da·tu'rism
dau·er·schlaf'
dau·no'my'cin
dau'no·ru'bi·cin
Da·vai'ne·a
  —for'mo·sa'na
  —mad'a·gas·car'i·en'sis
Dav'en·port'
  —method
  —stain
Da'vid·sohn
  —differential test
  —presumptive test
Da·vi·el' operation
Daw'barn' sign
Daw'son encephalitis
Day
  —attic cannula
  —operation
daz'zle reflex of Pei'per
de·a·cid'i·fi·ca'tion
de·ac'ti·vate', -vat'ed,
  -vat'ing
de·ac'ti·va'tion
de·ac'y·lase'
deaf
de·af'fer·en·ta'tion
deaf'-mute'
deaf·mut'ism
deaf'ness
de·air'
de·al'co·hol'i·za'tion
de·am'i·dase'

de·am'i·di·za'tion

de·am'i·nase'

de·am'i·nate', -nat'ed,
-nat'ing

de·am'i·na'tion

de·an'es·the'si·ant

dea'nol' ac'et·am'i·do·
ben'zo·ate'

de·a·qua'tion

De·Ba'key aortic dissection

de·band'ing

De·bar'y·o·my'ces'
ne'o·for'mans'

de Beur'mann-Gou·ge·rot'
disease

de·bil'i·tant

de·bil'i·tate', -tat'ed, -tat'ing

de·bil'i·ty

de·bond'

De·bove' disease

de·branch'er

De·bré'-de To'ni-Fan·co'ni
syndrome

De·bré'-Sé·mé·laigne'
syndrome

de·bride', -brid'ed, -brid'ing

de·bride·ment'

de·bris'

de·bri'so·quin

de·bulk'

dec'a·dence

de·cal'ci·fi·ca'tion

de·cal'ci·fy', -fied', -fy'ing

dec'a·gram'

dec'a·li'ter

dec'al'vant

dec'a·me'ter

dec'a·me·tho'ni·um

de·can'cel·la'tion

dec'ane'

de·can'nu·late'

de·can'nu·la'tion

dec'a·no'ic

dec'a·nor'mal

de·cant'

de·can·ta'tion

de·cap'i·tate', -tat'ed, -tat'ing

de·cap'i·ta'tion

de·cap'su·la'tion

de·car'bon·i·za'tion

de·car'bon·ize', -ized',
-iz'ing

de·car·box'yl·ase'

de·car·box'yl·ate', -at'ed,
-at'ing

de·car·box'yl·a'tion

de·ca·thec'tion

dec·a·vi·ta·min

de·cay'

de·cel'er·a'tion

de·cen'tered

de·cen·tra'tion

de·cer'e·bel·la'tion

de·cer'e·brate', -brat'ed,
-brat'ing

de·cer'e·bra'tion

de·cer'e·brize', -brized',
-briz'ing

de·chlo'ri·da'tion

de·chlo'ri·na'tion

de·chlor·u'ra'tion

de·cho·les'ter·ol'i·za'tion

dec'i·bel'

de·cid'u·a *pl.* -ae'
  —ba·sa'lis
  —cap'su·lar'is
  —mar'gi·na'lis
  —men'stru·a'lis
  —pa·ri'e·ta'lis
  —re·flex'a
  —se·rot'i·na
  —sub·cho'ri·a'lis
  —ve'ra

de·cid'u·al

de·cid'u·ate

de·cid'u·a'tion

de·cid'u·i'tis

de·cid'u·o'ma
  —ma·lig'num

de·cid'u·o'sis

de·cid'u·ous

dec'i·gram'

dec'i·li'ter

dec'i·me'ter

dec'i·nor'mal

de·ci'sion

dec'li·na'tion

de·clive'

de·co·ag'u·lant

de·coc'tion

de·col·la'tion

de·col·la'tor

de·com'pen·sate'

de·com'pen·sa'tion

de·com·pose', -posed',
-pos'ing

de·com'po·si'tion

de·com'press'

de·com·pres'sion

de·con·di'tion

de·con·di'tion·ing

de·con·ges'tant

de·con·ges'tive

de·con·tam'i·nate', -nat'ed,
-nat'ing

de·con·tam'i·na'tion

de·cor'ti·cate', -cat'ed,
-cat'ing

de·cor'ti·ca'tion

de·crease'

dec're·ment

dec're·men'tal

de·crep'i·ta'tion

de·cre·scen'do

de·cres'cent

de·cru·des'cence

de·cu·ba'tion

de·cu'bi·tal

de·cu'bi·tus *pl.* -ti'

de·cur'rent

de·cus'sate'

de·cus·sa'ti·o'
  pl. -sa'ti·o'nes'
  —bra'chi·i' con'junc'ti'vi'
  —lem'nis·co'rum
  —ner·vo'rum troch'le·ar'-
    i·um
  —pe·dun'cu·lo'rum cer'e·
    bel·lar'i·um su·pe'ri·o'-
    rum
  —py'ram'i·dum

de·cus·sa'tion
  —of Fo·rel'
  —of the bra'chi·a
    con'junc·ti'va
  —of the lem·nis'ci'

de·cus·sa'ti·o'nes'
  —teg'men'ti'
  —teg'men·to'rum

de·dif·fer·en'ti·ate'

de·dif·fer·en'ti·a'tion

deep

de-ep'i·car'di·al·i·za'tion

Dees
  —operation
  —suture needle

Deet'jen bodies

def'e·cate', -cat'ed, -cat'ing

def'e·ca'tion

def'e·ca·to'ry
def'e·co·gram'
de'fect'
de·fec'tive
de·fem'i·ni·za'tion
de·fem'i·nize', -nized',
  -niz'ing
de·fense'
def'er·ens
def'er·ent
def'er·en·tec'to·my
def'er·en'tial
def'er·en·ti·o·ves'i·cal
def'er·en·ti'tis
def'er·ox'a·mine'
def'er·vesce'
def'er·ves'cence
def'er·ves'cent
de·fib'ril·late', -lat'ed,
  -lat'ing
de·fib'ril·la'tion
de·fib'ril·la'tor
de·fi'bri·nate', -nat'ed,
  -nat'ing
de·fi'bri·na'tion
de·fi'cien·cy
de·fi'cient
def'i·cit
de·flec'tion
de·flec'tor
de'flo·ra'tion
de'flo·res'cence
de·flu'vi·um
  —cap'il·lo'rum
  —un'gui·um
de·flux'i·o'
de·flux'ion
de·form'
de·form'a·bil'i·ty
de'for·ma'tion
de·for'mi·ty
de·func'tion·al·i·za'tion
de·fu'sion
de·gan'gli·on·ate', -at'ed,
  -at'ing
de·gen'er·a·cy
de·gen'er·ate', -at'ed, -at'ing
de·gen'er·a'tion
de·gen'er·a·tive
de·germ'
de·glov'ing
de·glu'ti·ble
de'glu·ti'tion

de·glu'ti·tive
de·glu'ti·to'ry
De·gos'-De·lort'-Tri·cot'
  syndrome
De·gos' disease
deg'ra·da'tion
de·grade', -grad'ed, -grad'ing
de·gran'u·la'tion
de'gus·ta'tion
De'hi·o test
de·his'cence
de·hu'man·i·za'tion
de'hu·mid'i·fi·ca'tion
de'hu·mid'i·fi'er
de'hu·mid'i·fy'
de·hy'drant
de·hy'dra·tase'
de·hy'drate', -drat'ed,
  -drat'ing
de·hy·dra'tion
de·hy'dro·a·ce'tic
de·hy'dro·a·scor'bic
de·hy'dro·cho'late'
de·hy'dro·cho·les'ter·ol'
de·hy'dro·cho'lic
de·hy'dro·cor'ti·cos'ter·
  one'
de·hy'dro·ep'i·an·dros'ter·
  one'
de·hy'dro·gen·ase'
de·hy'dro·gen·ate', -at'ed,
  -at'ing
de·hy'dro·gen·a'tion
de·hy'dro·gen·ize', -ized',
  -iz'ing
de·hy'dro·i'so·an·dros'ter·
  one'
de·hy'dro·ret'i·nol'
de·hyp'no·tize'
de·i'on·ize', -ized', -iz'ing
Dei'ters
  —cells
  —nucleus
dé'jà pen·sé'
dé'jà vu'
de·jec'ta
de·jec'tion
De·je·rine'
  —anterior bulbar syndromes
  —cortical sensory syndrome
De·je·rine'-Klump'ke
  syndrome
De·je·rine'-Sot'tas disease

De·je·rine'-Thom'as atro-
  phy
de·lac'ri·ma'tion
de'lac·ta'tion
Del'a·field' hematoxylin
de·lam'i·na'tion
de Lange' syndrome
Del'a·so'a sore
de·lay'
Del·bet' splint
Del Cas·til'lo syndrome
de·lead'
del'e·te'ri·ous
de·le'tion
Delfft test
Del'hi boil
De Li'ma operation
de·lim'i·ta'tion
de·lim'it·ed
de·lin'e·ate'
de·lin'e·a'tion
de·lin'quen·cy
de·lin'quent
de·lip'i·da'tion
del'i·quesce', -quesced',
  -quesc'ing
del'i·ques'cence
del'i·ques'cent
de·liq'ui·um
  —an'i·mi'
de·lir'i·ant
de·lir'i·fa'cient
de·lir'i·ous
de·lir'i·um
  —cor'dis
  —gran'di·o'sum
  —mi'te'
  —mus'si·tans'
  —tre'mens
del'i·tes'cence
de·liv'er
de·liv'er·y
del'le pl. del'len
del'o·mor'phic
del'o·mor'phous
De·lor'me' operation
de·louse', -loused', -lous'ing
del'phi·nine'
Del·phin'i·um
del Ri'o Hor·te'ga silver
  method
del'ta
del'toid'

del'to·pec'to·ral
de·lu'sion
de·lu'sion·al
de·lu'sion·ar'y
de·lu'sive
de·mand'
de·mar'cate', -cat'ed, -cat'ing
de'mar·ca'tion
de·mas'cu·lin·i·za'tion
de·mas'cu·lin·ize'
De·ma'ti·um
dem'e·car'i·um
dem'e·clo·cy'cline'
dem'e·cy'cline'
de·ment'
de·ment'ed
de·men'ti·a
—ag'i·ta'ta
—par'a·lyt'i·ca
—par'a·noi'des'
—prae'cox'
—pre'cox'
—pu·gi·lis'ti·ca
de·meth'yl·ate', -at'ed,
   -at'ing
de·meth'yl·a'tion
de·meth'yl·chlor·tet'ra·cy'-
   cline'
dem'i·fac'et
dem'i·lune'
—of Gian·nuz'zi'
—of Hei'den·hain'
dem'i·mon·stros'i·ty
de·min'er·al·i·za'tion
de·min'er·al·ize', -ized',
   -iz'ing
dem'i·pen'ni·form'
de·mise'
dem'o·dec'tic
Dem'o·dex'
—fol·lic'u·lo'rum
de·mod'u·la'tor
de'mo·gram'
de·mog'ra·phy
de·mo'ni·ac'
de'mon·o·ma'ni·a
de'mon·o·ma'ni·ac'
de'mon·op'a·thy
de'mon·o·pho'bi·a
de'mo·pho'bi·a
De Mor'gan spot
de·mor'phin·i·za'tion
de'mu·co·sa'tion

de·mul'cent
de Mus·sy'
—point
—sign
de·my'e·lin·ate', -at'ed,
   -at'ing
de·my'e·lin·a'tion
de·my'e·lin·i·za'tion
de·my'e·lin·ize', -ized',
   iz'ing
de·nar'co·tize', -tized',
   -tiz'ing
de·na'tur·a'tion
de·na'ture, -tured, -tur·ing
de·na'tur·i·za'tion
den·drax'on
den'dri·form'
den'drite'
den·drit'ic
den'droid'
den'dron   pl. -drons' or -dra
den·dro·phag'o·cy·to'sis
den·dro·phil'i·a
de·ner'vate', -vat'ed, -vat'ing
de·ner'va'tion
den'gue
de·ni'al
den'i·da'tion
den'i·gra'tion
Den'is Browne
—operation
—splint
Den'is method
de·ni'tro·ge·na'tion
Den'nie-Mar'fan'
   syndrome
De'non·vil·liers' fascia
dens   pl. den'tes'
—ep'i·stro'phe·i'
—in den'te'
—se·rot'i·nus
den·sim'e·ter
den'si·met'ric
den'si·tom'e·ter
den'si·to·met'ric
den'si·tom'e·try
den'si·ty
den·sog'ra·phy
den'tal
den·tal'gi·a
den'ta·ry
den'tate'
den'ta·tec'to·my

den·ta'tion
den·ta'to·re·tic'u·lar
den·ta'to·ru'bral
den·ta'to·tha·lam'ic
den·ta'to-thal'a·mo-
   cor'ti·cal
den·ta'tum
den'te·la'tion
den'tes'
—a·cu'sti·ci'
—ca·ni'ni'
—de·cid'u·i'
—in·ci'si·vi'
—mo·lar'es'
—per'ma·nen'tes'
—pre·mo·lar'es'
den'ti·a
—prae'cox'
—tar'da
den'ti·cle
den·tic'u·late'
den'ti·fi·ca'tion
den'ti·form'
den'ti·frice
den·tig'er·ous
den·ti·la'bi·al
den·ti·lin'gual
den'tin
den'ti·nal
den'tine'
den·tin'i·fi·ca'tion
den'ti·no·blas·to'ma
   pl. -mas or -ma·ta
den'ti·no·ce·men'tal
den'ti·no·e·nam'el
den'ti·no·gen'e·sis   pl. -ses'
—im'per·fec'ta
den'ti·no·gen'ic
den'ti·noid'
den'ti·no'ma   pl. -mas or
   -ma·ta
den'ti·nos'te·oid'
den'ti·num
den'tip'a·rous
den'ti·phone'
den'tist
den'tis·try
den·ti'tion
den'to·al·ve'o·lar
den'to·al've·o·li'tis
den'to·fa'cial
den'toid'
den'tu·lous

den'ture
de·nu'cle·at'ed
de'nu·da'tion
de·nude', -nud'ed, -nud'ing
de·o'dor·ant
de·on·tol'o·gy
de·or'sum·duc'tion
de·or'sum·ver'gence
de·or'sum·ver'sion
de·os'si·fi·ca'tion
de·ox'i·da'tion
de·ox'i·dize'
de·ox'y·a·den'o·sine'
de·ox'y·cho'late'
de·ox'y·cho'lic
de·ox'y·co·for'my·cin
de·ox'y·cor'ti·cos'ter·one'
de·ox'y·cor'tone'
de·ox'y·cos'tone'
de·ox'y·cy'ti·dine'
de·ox'y·e·phed'rine
de·ox'y·gen·ate'
de·ox'y·gen·a'tion
de·ox'y·gua'nine'
de·ox'y·pen'tose'
de·ox'y·pen'tose·nu·cle'ic
de·ox'y·pyr'i·dox'ine'
de·ox'y·ri'bo·nu·cle·ase'
de·ox'y·ri'bo·nu·cle'ic
de·ox'y·ri'bo·nu·cle·o·side'
de·ox'y·ri'bo·nu·cle·o·tide'
de·ox'y·ri'bose'
de·ox'y·sug'ar
de·ox'y·u'ri·dine'
De·page'-Jane'way
  gastrostomy
de·pan'cre·a·tize'
de·par'af·fin·ize', -ized',
  -iz'ing
de·pend'ence
de·pend'ent
de·per'son·al·i·za'tion
de·per'son·i·fi·ca'tion
de·pig'ment
de·pig'men·ta'tion
dep'i·late' -lat'ed, -lat'ing
dep'i·la'tion
de·pil'a·to'ry
dep'i·lous
de·plete', -plet'ed, -plet'ing
de·ple'tion
de·plu·ma'tion
de·po'lar·i·za'tion

de·pol'y·mer·ase'
de'po·lym'er·i·za'tion
de'po·lym'er·ize', -ized',
  -iz'ing
de·pos'it
dep'o·si'tion
de'pot
dep're·nyl
de·press'
de·pres'sant
de·pres'sion
de·pres'sive
de·press'o·mo'tor
de·pres'sor
  —a'lae' na'si'
  —an'gu·li·o'ris
  —ep'i·glot'ti·dis
  —la'bi·i' in·fe'ri·o'ris
  —sep'ti' na'si'
  —su'per·cil'i·i'
dep'ri·va'tion
dep'side'
dep'u·rant
dep'u·rate'
dep'u·ra'tion
de Quer'vain disease
der'a·del'phus
de·range'ment
Der'cum disease
de·re·al·i·za'tion
de're·ism
de're·is'tic
der'en·ceph'a·lus
der'en·ceph'a·ly
de're·pres'sion
der'ic
der'i·va'tion
de·riv'a·tive
der'ma·brad'er
der'ma·bra'sion
Der'ma·cen'tor
  —an'der·so'ni'
  —var'i·a'bi·lis
Der'ma·cen·trox'e·nus
  —ak'a·ri'
  —pe·dic'u·li'
  —rick·ett'si'
  —rickettsi con·o'ri'
der'ma·he'mi·a
der'mal
der'ma·my·i'a·sis pl. -ses'
  —lin'e·ar'is mi'grans'
  oes·tro'sa

Der'ma·nys'sus
  —a'vi·um
  —gal·li'nae'
der'ma·tag'ra
der'ma·tal'gi·a
der'ma·tan
der'ma·ta·neu'ri·a
der'mat·he'mi·a
der'ma·therm'
der'mat'ic
der'ma·ti'tis pl. -tis·es or
  -tit'i·des'
  —ac·tin'i·ca
  —au'to·fac·ti'ti·a
  —ca·lor'i·ca
  —coc·cid'i·oi'des'
  —con'ge·la'ti·o'nis
  —con·ti·nu·ée'
  —con·tu'si·for'mis
  —dys'men·or·rhe'i·ca
  —es'cha·rot'i·ca
  —ex·fo'li·a·ti'va ne·o'na·
    to'rum
  —ex·sic'cans' pal·mar'is
  —fac·ti'ti·a
  —gan'gre·no'sa
  —gangrenosa in·fan'tum
  —her·pet'i·for'mis
  —hi'e·ma'lis
  —hy'po·stat'i·ca
  —med'i·ca·men·to'sa
  —nod·u'lar'is ne·crot'i·ca
  —pap'il·lar'is cap'il·li'ti·i'
  —pap'u·lo·squa·mo'sa
    a·troph'i·cans'
  —re'pens
  —rhus
  —seb'or·rhe'i·ca
  —trau·mat'i·ca
  —veg'e·tans'
  —ven'e·na'ta
  —ver·ru·co'sa
der'ma·to·au'to·plas'ty
Der'ma·to'bi·a
  —hom'i·nis
der'ma·to·bi·a'sis pl. -ses'
der'ma·to·cele'
der'ma·to·cel'lu·li'tis
der'ma·to·cha·la'sis
der'ma·to·co·ni·o'sis
  pl. -ses'
der'ma·to·cyst'
der'ma·to·dyn'i·a

der′ma·to·dys·pla′si·a

der′ma·to·fi·bro′ma
 pl. -mas *or* -ma·ta

der′ma·to·fi′bro·sar·co′ma
 pl. -mas *or* -ma·ta
 —pro·tu′ber·ans′

der·mat′o·gen

der′ma·to·glyph′ics

der′ma·to·graph′i·a

der′ma·tog′ra·phism

der′ma·tog′ra·phy

der′ma·to·het′er·o·plas′ty

der′ma·toid′

der′ma·tol′

der′ma·to·log′ic *or*
 der′ma·to·log′i·cal

der′ma·tol′o·gist

der′ma·tol′o·gy

der′ma·tol′y·sis

der′ma·tome′

der′ma·to·meg′a·ly

der′ma·tom′ic

der′ma·to·my′ces′

der′ma·to·my′cete′

der′ma·to·my·co′sis
 pl. -ses′

der′ma·to·my·o′ma
 pl. -mas *or* -ma·ta

der′ma·to·my·o′si·tis

der′ma·to·neu·rol′o·gy

der′ma·to·neu·ro′sis
 pl. -ses′

der′ma·to·path′i·a

der′ma·to·path′ic

der′ma·to·pa·thol′o·gy

der′ma·to·path′o·pho′bi·a

der′ma·top′a·thy

Der′ma·toph′a·goi′des
 pter′o·nys·si′nus

der′ma·to·phi·li′a·sis
 pl. -ses′

der′ma·to·phi·lo′sis *pl.* -ses′

Der′ma·toph′i·lus pen′e·
 trans′

der′ma·to·phyte′

der′ma·to·phy′tid

der′ma·to·phy·to′sis
 pl. -ses′

der′ma·to·plas′tic

der′ma·to·plas′ty

der′ma·to·pol′y·neu·ri′tis

der′ma·tor·rha′gi·a

der′ma·tor·rhex′is

der′ma·to·scle·ro′sis
 pl. -ses′

der′ma·tos′co·py

der′ma·to·si·o·pho′bi·a

der′ma·to′sis *pl.* -ses′
 —pap′u·lo′sa ni′gra

der′ma·to·some′

der′ma·to·ther′a·py

der′ma·to·thla′si·a

der′ma·tot′o·my

der′ma·to·trop′ic

der′ma·to·zo′on′ *pl.* -zo′a

der′ma·to·zo′o·no′sis
 pl. -ses′

der′ma·tro′phi·a

der′mic

der′mis

der′mo·blast′

der′mo·cy′ma

der′mo·ep′i·der′mal

der′mo·graph′i·a
 —al′ba
 —ru′bra

der′mo·graph′ic

der·mog′ra·phism

der·mog′ra·phy

der′mo·he′mi·a

der′moid′

der′moid·ec′to·my

der′mo·la′bi·al

der′mo·li·po′ma

der·mom′e·ter

der·mom′e·try

der′mo·my·co′sis *pl.* -ses′

der′mo·my′o·tome′

der′mo·ne·crot′ic

der·mop′a·thy

der′mo·phle·bi′tis

der′mo·plas′ty

der′mo·skel′e·ton

der′mo·ste·no′sis *pl.* -ses′

der′mo·syn′o·vi′tis

der′mo·trop′ic

der′mo·vas′cu·lar

der·o·did′y·mus

de·ro′tate′

de′ro·ta′tion

der′ren·ga·de′ra

der′rid

des·am′i·dase′

de·sat′u·ra′tion

des·ce·me·ti′tis

Des′ce·met′ membrane

des′ce·met′o·cele′

de·scend′

de·scen′dens
 —cer′vi·cis
 —hy′po·glos′si′

de·scen′sus *pl.* de·scen′sus
 —tes′tis
 —u′ter·i′
 —ven·tric′u·li′

des·cin′o·lone′ a·cet′o·
 nide′

de·sen′si·ti·za′tion

de·sen′si·tize′, -tized′,
 -tiz′ing

de·ser′pi·dine′

de·sex′u·al·i·za′tion

de·sex′u·al·ize′

des′ic·cant

des′ic·cate′, -cat′ed, -cat′ing

des′ic·ca′tion

des′ic·ca′tive

des′ic·ca′tor

de·sip′ra·mine′

Des′i·vac′

des·lan′o·side′

des·mal′gi·a

des·mec′ta·sis

des·mi′tis

des′mo·cra′ni·um

des′mo·cyte′

des′mo·cy′to·ma *pl.* -mas *or*
 -ma·ta

des·mog′e·nous

des·mog′ra·phy

des′moid′

des′mo·lase′

des·mol′o·gy

des·mo′ma *pl.* -mas *or* -ma·ta

des·mop′a·thy

des′mo·pla′si·a

des′mo·plas′tic

des′mo·pres′sin

des′mor·rhex′is

des·mo′sis *pl.* -ses′

des′mo·some′

des·mos′ter·ol′

des·mot′o·my

Des′nos′ pneumonia

de·so′cial·i·za′tion

des′o·mor′phine′

des′o·nide′

de·sorp′tion

des·ox′i·meth′a·sone′

des·ox'y·cor'ti·cos'ter·one'
des·ox'y·e·phed'rine
des·ox'y·pyr'i·dox'ine'
des·ox'y·ri'bose'
de·spe'ci·at'ed
de·spe'ci·a'tion
d'Es·pine' sign
de·spi'ral·i·za'tion
des'qua·mate', -mat'ed,
   -mat'ing
des'qua·ma'ti·o'
  —in·sen'sib'i·lis
  —ne'o·na'to'rum
des'qua·ma'tion
des·quam'a·tive
des·quam'a·to'ry
des·thi'o·bi'o·tin
de·stru'do
de·sul'fi·nase'
de·sul'fu·rase'
de·tach'ment
de·tec'tor
de·ter'gent
de·te'ri·o·rate'
de·te'ri·o·ra'tion
de·ter'mi·nant
de·ter'mi·na'tion
de·ter'min·ism
de·ter'sive
de To'ni-Fan·co'ni-De·bré'
  syndrome
de·tor'sion
de·tox'i·cant
de·tox'i·cate', -cat'ed, -cat'ing
de·tox'i·ca'tion
de·tox'i·fi·ca'tion
de·tox'i·fy', -fied', -fy'ing
Det're reaction
de·tri'tion
de·tri'tus *pl.* de·tri'tus
de'trun·ca'tion
de·tru'sion
de·tru'sor
  —u·ri'nae'
  —ve·si'cae'
de·tu·ba'tion
de·tu·mes'cence
deu'tan
deu'ter·a·nom'a·lous
deu'ter·a·nom'a·ly
deu'ter·an·ope'
deu'ter·an·o'pi·a
deu'ter·an·op'ic

deu'ter·an·op'si·a
deu'ter·a'tion
deu·te'ri·um
deu'ter·on'
deu'ter·o·path'ic
deu'ter·op'a·thy
deu'ter·o·plasm
deu'ter·os'to·ma *pl.* -mas *or*
  -ma·ta
deu'ter·ot'o·ky
deu·tom'er·ite'
deu'to·plasm
deu'to·plas·mol'y·sis
  pl. -ses'
deu'to·sco'lex
Deutsch'län'der disease
de·vas'cu·lar·i·za'tion
De Ve'ga annuloplasty
de·vel'op·ment
de·vel'op·men'tal
de'vi·ant
de'vi·ate', -at'ed, -at'ing
de'vi·a'tion
Dev'ic disease
de·vice'
de'vi·om'e·ter
de·vi'tal·i·za'tion
de·vi'tal·ize' -ized', -iz'ing
de·void'
dev'o·lu'tion
dex'a·meth'a·sone'
dex·brom'phen·ir'a·mine'
dex·chlor'phen·ir'a·mine'
dex'i·o·car'di·a
dex·iv'a·caine'
dex·ox'a·drol'
dex·pan'the·nol'
dex'pro·pan'o·lol'
dex'ter
dex'trad'
dex'tral
dex·tral'i·ty
dex'tran'
dex·tran·ase'
dex·tran'o·mer
dex'trase'
dex·trau'ral
dex'tri·fer'ron'
dex'trin
dex'tri·no'sis *pl.* -ses'
dex'tri·nu'ri·a
dex'tro·am·phet'a·mine'
dex'tro·car'di·a

dex'tro·car'di·o·gram'
dex'tro·cer'e·bral
dex'tro·cli·na'tion
dex'tro·con'dy·lism
dex·troc'u·lar
dex·troc'u·lar'i·ty
dex'tro·cy'clo·ver'sion
dex'tro·duc'tion
dex'tro·gas'tri·a
dex'tro·glu'cose'
dex'tro·gram'
dex'tro·gy'rate'
dex'tro·gy·ra'tion
dex'tro·man'u·al
dex'tro·meth'or'phan
dex'tro·mor·am'ide'
dex·trop'e·dal
dex'tro·po·si'tion
dex'tro·pro·pox'y·phene'
dex'tro·ro'ta·to'ry
dex'tro·ro'to·sco'li·o'sis
  pl. -ses'
dex'tro·sco'li·o'sis *pl.* -ses'
dex'trose'
dex'tro·sin'is·tral
Dex'tro·stix
dex'tro·su'ri·a
dex'tro·thy·rox'ine'
dex'tro·tor'sion
dex'tro·trop'ic
dex'trous
dex'tro·ver'sion
d-fruc'tose'
d-ga·lac'to·meth'yl·ose'
d-glu'cose'
dho'bie
di'a·be'tes'
  —de·cip'i·ens
  —in·sip'i·dus
  —mel·li'tus
di'a·bet'ic
di'a·be'to·gen'ic
di'a·be·tog'e·nous
di'a·brot'ic
di'a·caus'tic
di'ac·e·te'mi·a
di'a·ce'tic
di·ac'e·tin
di·ac'e·tu'ri·a
di·a·ce'tyl
di·ac'e·tyl·mor'phine'
di'a·cho·re'sis *pl.* -ses'
di·ac'id

di·a·cla·si·a
di·ac·la·sis *pl.* -ses'
di·a·clast'
di·a·clas'tic
di·a·con'dy·lar
di·ac'ri·sis *pl.* -ses'
di·a·crit'ic *or* di·a·crit'i·cal
di·ac·tin'ic
di'a·derm'
di'a·der'mic
di·ad'o·cho·ki·ne'si·a
di·ad'o·cho·ki·ne'sis
di·ad'o·cho·ki·net'ic
di'ag·nose', -nosed',
    -nos'ing
di'ag·no'sis *pl.* -ses'
di'ag·nos'tic
di'ag·nos'ti·cal·ly
di'ag·nos·ti'cian
di·ag'o·nal
di'a·ki·ne'sis *pl.* -ses'
Di·ak'i·o·gi·an'nis sign
di'al·kyl'a·mine'
di·al'lyl·bar'bi·tu'ric
di·al'y·sance
di·al'y·sate'
di·al'y·sis *pl.* -ses'
di'a·lyz'a·ble
di'a·lyze', -lyzed', -lyz'ing
di'a·lyz'er
di'a·mag·net'ic
di'a·mag·net·ism
di·am'e·ter
    —o·bli'qua pel'vis
    —trans·ver'sa pel'vis
di'a·met'ric *or* di'a·met'ri·cal
di'a·mide'
di·am'i·dine'
di'a·mine'
di·am'i·no·di·phen'yl·sul'-
    fone'
di·am'i·no·pu'rine'
di·am'i·no·pyr'i·dine'
di·am'i·nu'ri·a
Di'a·mond method
di·a·mor'phine'
di·am'tha·zole'
di·ap'a·mide'
di·a·pa'son
di'a·pause'
di'a·pe·de'sis *pl.* -ses'
di'a·pe·det'ic
di'a·per

di'a·phane'
di·aph'a·nom'e·ter
di·aph'a·no·met'ric
di·aph'a·nom'e·try
di·aph'a·no·scope'
di·aph'a·nos'co·py
di·aph'e·met'ric
di·aph'o·rase'
di'a·pho·re'sis *pl.* -ses'
di'a·pho·ret'ic
di'a·phragm'
di'a·phrag·ma *pl.* -ma·ta
    —pel'vis
    —sel'lae'
    —u'ro·gen'i·ta'le'
di'a·phrag·mat'ic
di'a·phrag·ma·ti'tis
di'a·phrag·mat'o·cele'
di'a·phrag·mi'tis
di·aph'y·se'al
di·aph'y·sec'to·my
di·aph'y·sis *pl.* -ses'
di'a·phy·si'tis
di·ap'la·sis *pl.* -ses'
di'a·poph'y·sis *pl.* -ses'
di'ar·rhe'a
di'ar·rhe'al
di'ar·rhe'ic
di'ar·rhe'mi·a
di'ar'thric
di'ar·thro'di·al
di'ar·thro'sis *pl.* -ses'
di'ar·tic'u·lar
di·as'chi·sis *pl.* -ses'
di'a·schis'tic
di'a·scope'
di'a·scop'ic
di·as'co·py
di'a·stal'sis *pl.* -ses'
di'a·stase'
di·as'ta·sis *pl.* -ses'
    —rec'ti' ab·dom'i·nis
di'a·stat'ic
di'a·ste'ma *pl.* -ma·ta
di'a·ste'ma·to·cra'ni·a
di'a·ste'ma·to·my·e'li·a
di'a·ste'ma·to·py·e'li·a
di'as·ter
di'a·ster'e·o·i'so·mer
di'a·ster'e·o·i'so·mer'ic
di·as'to·le
di'a·stol'ic
di'a·tax'i·a

di'a·ther'mal
di'a·ther'ma·nous
di'a·ther'mic
di'a·ther'mo·co·ag'u·la'-
    tion
di'a·ther'my
di·ath'e·sis *pl.* -ses'
di'a·thet'ic
di'a·tom
di'a·to·ma'ceous
di'a·tom'ic
di'a·tri·zo'ate'
di'a·tri·zo'ic
di·ax'on
di'az'e·pam'
di·a·zine'
di·az'o
di·az'o·re·sor'ci·nol'
di·az'o·tize'
di·az'ox'ide'
di·ba'sic
di·ben'ze·pin
di·ben·zyl·chlor·eth'a·
    mine'
di·both'ri·o·ceph'a·li·a·sis
di·brom'sa·lan
di·bu'caine'
di·bu'to·line'
di·cal'ci·um
di·car'box·yl'ic
di·cen'tric
di·ce·pha'li·a
di·ceph'a·lism
di·ceph'a·lous *(having two*
    heads)
    ♦*dicephalus*
di·ceph'a·lus *(an individual*
    with two heads), *pl.* -li'
    ♦*dicephalous*
    —di·auch'e·nos'
    —mon'auch'e·nos'
    —mon'o·so'mus
    —par'a·sit'i·cus
    —tet'ra·bra'chi·us
    —tri·bra'chi·us
di·ceph'a·ly
di·chei'lus
di·chei'rus
di·chlor'a·mine'
di·chlo'ro·a·ce'tic
di·chlo'ro·ben'zene'
di·chlo'ro·di·phen'yl·tri·
    chlo'ro·eth'yl· ene'

di′chlo′ro·hy′drin
di′chlo′ro·i′so·pro·ter′-
  e·nol′
di′chlo′ro·phen·ar′sine′
di′chlo′ro·phe′nol·in′do·
  phe′nol′
di′chlo′ro·phen·ox′y·a·ce′-
  tic
di′chlor·phen′a·mide′
di·cho′ri·al
di′cho·ri·on′ic
di·chot′o·mize′, -mized′,
  -miz′ing
di·chot′o·my
di·chro′ic
di·chro′ine′
di′chro′ism
di·chro′ma·sy
di′chro·mat′
di·chro′mate′
di′chro·mat′ic
di·chro′ma·tism
di·chro′ma·top′si·a
di′chro′mic
di′chro·mism
di′chro′mo·phil′
di′chro·moph′i·lism
Dick
  —test
  —toxin
di·clox′a·cil′lin
di′co·phane′
di·co′ri·a
di·cou′ma·rin
di·cou′ma·rol′
Di′cro·coe′li·um
  —den·drit′i·cum
di·crot′ic
di·cro′tism
di′cro′tous
Dic′ty·o·cau′lus
dic′ty·o·ki·ne′sis
dic′ty·o·some′
dic′ty·o·tene′
di·cu′ma·rol′
di·cy′clo·mine′
di·dac′tic
di·dac′tyl·ism
di·dan′o·sine′
di·del′phi·a
di·del′phic
Di·del′phis
di′de·ox′y·cy′ti·dine′

di′de·ox′y·in′o·sine′
Di′dot operation
did′y·mal′gi·a
did′y·mi′tis
did′y·mous
Di·e′go blood group
di·el′drin
di′e·lec′tric
di·em′bry·o·ny
di′en·ce·phal′ic
di′en·ceph′a·lon′
die′ner
di′en·es′trol′
Di·ent′a·moe′ba
  —frag′i·lis
di·es′ter·ase′
di·es′trum
di·es′trus
di′et
di′e·tar′y
di′e·tet′ic
di′e·tet′ics
di·eth′a·nol′a·mine′
Die′thelm method
di·eth′yl
di·eth′yl·bar·bi′tu·rate′
di·eth′yl·bar′bi·tu′ric
di·eth′yl·car·bam′a·zine′
di·eth′yl·ene′
di·eth′yl·ene·di′a·mine′
di·eth′yl·mal′o·nyl·u′re·a
di·eth′yl·pro′pi·on′
di·eth′yl·stil·bes′trol′
  —di·pro′pi·o·nate′
di·eth′yl·to·lu′a·mide′
di·eth′yl·tryp′ta·mine′
di′e·ti′cian var. of dietitian
di′e·ti′tian also dietician
Die′tl crisis
di′e·to·ther′a·py
Dieu′la·foy′
  —aspirator
  —disease
dif′fer·en′tial
dif′fer·en′ti·ate′, -at′ed,
  -at′ing
dif′fer·en′ti·a′tion
dif′flu·ence
dif′frac′tion
dif·fu′sate′
dif·fuse′
dif·fus′i·bil′i·ty
dif·fus′i·ble

dif·fu′si·om′e·ter
dif·fu′sion
di·flor′a·sone′
di·flu′a·nine′
di′flu·cor′to·lone′
di·flu′mi·done′
di·fluor′o·meth′yl·or′ni·
  thine′
di′ga·met′ic
di·gas′tric
Di·ge′ne·a
di·gen′e·sis pl. -ses′
di′ge·net′ic
di·gen′ic
Di George′ syndrome
di·gest′
di·ges′tant
di·gest′i·bil′i·ty
di·gest′i·ble
di·ges′tion
di·ges′tive
Digh′ton syndrome
dig′it
dig′i·tal
dig′i·tal′gi·a
  —par′es·thet′i·ca
dig′i·tal′in
dig′i·tal′is
dig′i·tal′i·za′tion
dig′i·tal·ize′
dig′i·tal′ose′
dig′i·tate′
dig′i·ta′tion
dig′i·ti′
  —ma′nus
  —pe′dis
dig′i·ti·form′
dig′i·ti·grade′
dig′i·to′nin
dig′i·to·plan′tar
dig′i·tox·ic′i·ty
dig′i·tox′i·gen′in
dig′i·tox′in
dig′i·tox′ose′
dig′i·tox′o·side′
dig′i·tus pl. -ti′
  —I
  —II
  —III
  —IV
  —V
  —an′u·lar′is

—me′di·us
—min′i·mus
—pri′mus
—quar′tus
—quin′tus
—se·cun′dus
—ter′ti·us
di·glos′si·a
di·glyc′er·ide′
dig·na′thus
di·gox′in
di Gu·gliel′mo syndrome
di·hex′y·ver′ine′
di·hy′brid
di·hy′drate′
di·hy′dric
di·hy′dro·cho·les′ter·ol′
di·hy′dro·co′deine′
di·hy′dro·co′dein·one′
di·hy′dro·co·en′zyme′
di·hy′dro·er′go·cor′nine′
di·hy′dro·er·got′a·mine′
di·hy′dro·mor′phi·none′
di·hy′dro·pyr′i·dine′
di·hy′dro·quin′ine′
di·hy′dro·ta·chys′ter·ol′
di·hy′dro·the′e·lin
di·hy·drox′y·a·ce′tic
di·hy·drox′y·ac′e·tone′
di·hy·drox′y·a·lu′mi·num
di·hy·drox′y·an′thra·nol′
di·hy·drox′y·ben′zene′
di·hy·drox′y·es′trin
di·hy·drox′y·phen′yl·al′a·
nine′
di′i·o′do·hy·drox′y·quin
di′i·o′do·hy·drox′y·quin′o·
line′
di′i·o′do·ty′ro·sine′
di′i·so·pro′pyl
—fluor′o·phos′phate′
—phos′pho·ro·fluor′i·date′
di·kar′y·on′
di·ke′to·pi·per′a·zine′
dik′ty·o′ma *pl.* -mas *or*
-ma·ta
di·lac′er·a′tion
di·lat′a·ble
di·la′tan·cy
dil′a·ta′tion
di·late′, -lat′ed, -lat′ing
di·la′tion
dil′a·tom′e·ter

dil′a·to·met′ric
di·la′tor
—i′ri·dis
—nar′is
—pu·pil′lae′
—tu′bae′
Dil′ling rule
dil·ti′a·zem
dil′u·ent
di·lute′, -lut′ed, -lut′ing
di·lu′tion
Di·mas′tig·a·moe′ba
di·mef′a·dane′
di′me·fline′
di·meg′a·ly
di′men·hy′dri·nate′
di·men′sion
di′mer
di′mer·cap′rol′
dim′er·ous
di·meth′i·cone′
di·meth·in′dene′
di·meth·i′so·quin
di·meth·is′ter·one′
di·meth·ox′a·nate′
di·meth′yl
di·meth′yl·am′ine
di·meth′yl·ar·sin′ic
di·meth′yl·ben′zene′
di·meth′yl·ni′tros·am′ine′
di·meth′yl·tryp′ta·mine′
di·me′tri·a
dim′i·nu′tion
Di·mi′tri disease
di·mor′phic
di·mor′phism
di·mor′phous
dim′pling
di·neu′ric
din′ic *or* din′i·cal
di′ni′tro·chlo′ro·ben′zene′
di′no·prost′
di′no·pros′tone′
di·nu′cle·o·tide′
Di·oc′to·phy′ma
—re·na′le
di·oc′tyl
di′o·done′
di·ol′a·mine′
di·op′ter
di·op′tom′e·ter
di·op′tom′e·try
di·op′tral

di·op′tric
di·op′trics
di·or·tho′sis *pl.* -ses′
di′ose′
di·os′ge·nin
di·o′vu·lar
di·o′vu·la·to′ry
di·ox′ane′
di·ox′ide′
di·ox′in
di·ox′y·ben′zone′
di·ox′y·line′
di·pen′tene′
di·pep′ti·dase′
di·pep′tide′
di·per′o·don′
Di·pet′a·lo·ne′ma
per′stans′
di·pet′a·lo·ne·mi′a·sis
pl. -ses′
di·phal′lic
di·phal′lus
di·pha′sic
di·pheb′u·zol′
di·phem′a·nil′
di·phen′a·di′one′
di·phen′an′
di′phen·hy′dra·mine′
di′phen·ox′yl·ate′
di′phen·yl·chlor·ar′sine′
di′phen·yl·hy·dan′to·in
di′phen·yl·pyr′a·line′
di·pho′ni·a
di·phos′gene′
di·phos′phate′
di′phos·pho·thi′a·min
diph·the′ri·a
diph·the′ri·al
diph·the′ri·a·phor′
diph·ther′ic
diph′the·rit′ic
diph′the·ri′tis
diph′the·roid′
diph′the·ro·tox′in
diph·thon′gi·a
di·phyl′lo·both·ri′a·sis
pl. -ses′
Di·phyl′lo·both·ri′i·dae′
Di·phyl′lo·both′ri·um
—er′i·na′ce·i′
—la′tum
di·phy′o·dont′
dip′la·cu′sis *pl.* -ses′

—bin′au·ra′lis
—u′ni·au·ra′lis
di′plas·mat′ic
di·ple′gi·a
—fa·ci·a′lis
di·ple′gic
dip′lo·al·bu′mi·nu′ri·a
dip′lo·ba·cil′lus *pl.* -li′
dip′lo·blas′tic
dip′lo·car′di·ac′
dip′lo·ce·pha′li·a
dip′lo·ceph′a·lus *pl.* -li′
dip′lo·ceph′a·ly
dip′lo·coc′cal
dip′lo·coc′coid′
dip′lo·coc′cus *pl.* -ci′
Dip′lo·coc′cus
—gon′or·rhoe′ae′
—in′tra·cel′lu·lar′is
men′in·git′i·dis
—pneu·mo′ni·ae′
dip′lo·co′ri·a
dip′lo·ë′
dip′lo·et′ic
dip′lo·gen′e·sis *pl.* -ses′
Dip′lo·go·nop′o·rus
—gran′dis
di·plo′ic
dip′loid′
dip′loi·dy
dip′lo·kar′y·on′
dip′lo·mate′
dip′lo·mel′li·tu′ri·a
dip′lo·my·e′li·a
dip′lo·ne′ma *pl.* -ma·ta *or* -mas
dip′lo·neu′ral
di·plop′a·gus *pl.* -gi′
di·plo′pi·a
di·plo′pi·om′e·ter
dip′lo·scope′
di·plo′sis *pl.* -ses′
dip′lo·so·ma′ti·a
dip′lo·some′
dip′lo·tene′
di·po′lar
di′pole′
di·po′tas′si·um
dip′ping
di·pros′o·pus
—dir·rhi′nus
—par′a·sit′i·cus
—tet′roph·thal′mus

—tetrophthalmus te·tro′tus
di′pro·tri·zo′ate′
dip·se′sis
dip′set′ic
dip′si·a
dip′so·gen
dip′so·gen′ic
dip′so·ma′ni·a
dip′so·ma′ni·ac′
dip′so·pho′bi·a
dip′so·sis
dip′so·ther′a·py
dip′stick′
Dip′ter·a
dip′ter·an
dip′ter·ous
di′pus′
di·py′gus
—par′a·sit′i·cus
—tet′ra·pus′
—tri′pus′
dip′y·li·di′a·sis *pl.* -ses′
Di′py·lid′i·um
—ca·ni′num
di′py·rid′a·mole′
di·rect′
di·rec′tion
di·rec′tor
di·rhi′nic
Di′ro·fi·lar′i·a
—con′junc·ti′vae′
—im′mi·tis
di′ro·fil·a·ri·a′sis *pl.* -ses′
dis′a·bil′i·ty
dis·a′ble
dis·a′ble·ment
di·sac′cha·ri·dase′
di·sac′cha·ride′
dis·ag′gre·ga′tion
dis·ar·tic′u·late′
dis·ar·tic′u·la′tion
dis·as·sim′i·la′tion
dis·as·so′ci·a′tion
dis·as·sort′a·tive
disc *var. of* disk
dis·cern′
dis·cern′a·ble
dis·charge′
dis′ci·form′
dis′ci·in′ter·ver′te·bra′les′
dis·cis′sion
dis·ci′tis
dis′cli·na′tion

dis·clos′ing
dis·co·blas′tu·la *pl.* -las *or* -lae′
dis·co·gas′tru·la *pl.* -las *or* -lae′
dis·co·gen′ic
dis·co·gram′
dis·cog′ra·phy
dis·coid′
dis·coi′dal
dis·col′or·a′tion
dis·cop′a·thy
dis·coph′o·rous
dis·co·pla·cen′ta
dis·cor′dance
dis·co·ri′a *var. of* dyscoria
dis·crep′an·cy
dis·crete′
dis·crim′i·nate′, -nat′ed, -nat′ing
dis·crim′i·na′tion
dis·crim′i·na′tor
dis′cus *pl.* -ci′
—ar·tic′u·lar′is
—articularis ar·tic′u·la′ti·o′nis a·cro′mi·o·cla·vic′u·lar′is
—articularis articulationis man·dib′u·lar′is
—articularis articulationis ra′di·o·ul′nar′is dis·ta′lis
—articularis articulationis ster′no·cla·vic′u·lar′is
—articularis articulationis tem′po·ro·man·dib′u·lar′is
—in′ter·pu′bi·cus
—ner′vi′ op′ti·ci′
—pro·lig′er·us
dis·cu′tient
dis·di′a·clast′
dis·ease′
dis·eased′
dis′en·gage′ment
dis·e·qui·lib′ri·um
dis·fig′ure
dis·fig′ure·ment
dis·ger′mi·no′ma *pl.* -mas *or* -ma·ta
dis·gre·gate′, -gat′ed, -gat′ing
dis·gre·ga′tion
dis·im·mune′
dis·im·mu′ni·ty

dis'im·pact'
dis'in·fect'
dis'in·fec'tant
dis'in·fec'tion
dis·in·fes·ta'tion
dis·in·hi·bi'tion
dis·in·sec'tion
dis·in·sec'ti·za'tion
dis·in·ser'tion
dis·in'te·grant
dis·in'te·grate', -grat'ed,
  -grat'ing
dis·in'te·gra'tion
dis·in'te·gra'tor
dis·in·vag'i·na'tion
dis·joint'
dis·junc'tion
dis·junc'tive
disk *also* disc
disk·ec'to·my
disk'i·form'
disk·i'tis
dis'ko·gram'
dis·kog'ra·phy
dis'lo·cate'
dis·lo·ca'tion
dis·mem'ber
dis·mem'ber·ment
dis'mu·ta'tion
dis'oc·clude', -clud'ed,
  -clud'ing
di·so'di·um
  —cro'mo·gly'cate'
  —e'dath'a·mil
  —ed'e·tate'
di·so'ma
di·so'mus *pl.* -mi' *or* -mus·es
di'so·pyr'a·mide'
dis·or'der
dis·or'ga·ni·za'tion
dis·o'ri·en·ta'tion
dis'par·ate'
dis'pa·ra'tion
dis·par'i·ty
dis·pen'sa·ry
dis·pen'sa·to'ry
dis·pense', -pensed',
  -pens'ing
di·sper'mine'
di·sper'my
dis'per·sate'
dis·perse', -persed', -pers'ing
dis·per'sion

dis·per'sive
dis·per'soid'
di·spi'reme'
dis·place'
dis·place'ment
dis'po·si'tion
dis'pro·por'tion
dis·rup'tion
dis·rup'tive
dis·sect'
dis·sec'tion
dis·sec'tor
dis·sem'i·nate', -nat'ed,
  -nat'ing
dis·sem'i·na'tion
dis·sep'i·ment
dis·sim'i·late', -lat'ed,
  -lat'ing
dis·sim'u·la'tion
dis'si·pate'
dis·so'ci·ant
dis·so'ci·ate', -at'ed, -at'ing
dis·so'ci·a'tion
dis·so'ci·a'tive
dis'so·lu'tion
dis·solve', -solved', -solv'ing
dis·sol'vent
dis'so·nance
dis'tad'
dis'tal
dis'tal·ly
dis'tal·ward
dis·tend'
dis·ten'si·bil'i·ty
dis·ten'si·ble
dis·ten'tion
dis·tich'i·a
dis·ti'chi·a·sis *pl.* -ses'
dis·till'
dis'til·land
dis'til·late'
dis'til·la'tion
dis'to·ax'i·o·gin'gi·val
dis'to·ax'i·o·oc·clu'sal
dis'to·buc'cal
dis'to·buc'co·oc·clu'sal
dis'to·buc'co·pul'pal
dis'to·cer'vi·cal
dis'to·clu'sion
dis'to·gin'gi·val
dis'to·in·ci'sal
dis'to·la'bi·al
dis'to·lin'gual

dis'to·lin'guo·in·ci'sal
dis'to·lin'guo·oc·clu'sal
dis'to·lin'guo·pul'pal
Dis·to'ma
  —hae'ma·to'bi·um
  —he·pat'i·cum
dis'to·ma·to'sis *pl.* -ses'
di·sto'mi·a
dis'to·mi'a·sis *pl.* -ses'
dis'to·mo'lar
Dis·to'mum
di·sto'mus
dis'to·oc·clu'sal
dis'to·pul'pal
dis'to·pul'po·la'bi·al
dis'to·pul'po·lin'gual
dis·tor'tion
dis'to·ver'sion
dis·tract'i·bil'i·ty
dis·trac'tion
dis·trac'tive
dis·tress'
dis·tri·bu'tion
dis·tri·chi'a·sis *pl.* -ses'
dis·trix
dis·turb'
dis·tur'bance
di·sul'fate'
di·sul'fide'
di·sul'fi·ram
dis·use'
di·thi'az'a·nine'
dith'ra·nol'
di·thy'mol' di·i'o·dide'
dit'o·kous
Ditt'rich stenosis
di'u·rese'
di'u·re'sis *pl.* -ses'
di'u·ret'ic
di·u'ri·a
di·ur'nal
di·ur'nule'
di·va·ga'tion
di·va'lent
di·var'i·ca'tion
di·ver'gence
di·ver'gent
di·ver'sion
di·ver'sion·ar'y
di'ver·tic'u·la am·pul'lae'
  duc'tus def'er·en'tis
di'ver·tic'u·lar
di'ver·tic'u·lec'to·my

di'ver·tic'u·li'tis
di'ver·tic'u·lo'sis
di'ver·tic'u·lum *pl.* -la
—il'e·i'
di·vi'nyl
di·vi'sion
Div'ry-van Bo'gaert
  disease
di·vulse', -vulsed', -vuls'ing
di·vul'sion
di·vul'sor
di'zy·got'ic
diz'zy
djen·kol'ic
Do·bell' solution
do·bu'ta·mine'
Do'chez serum
Docke murmur
dock'ing
do'co·sa·no'ic
doc'tor
doc'trine
Dö'der·lein' bacillus
Doeh'le bodies
Doer'fler-Stew'art test
dog'-ear'
Do'giel
—cells
—corpuscle
dog'ma·tist
doigts en lor·gnette'
dol'i·cho·ce·phal'ic
dol'i·cho·ceph'a·lus *pl.* -li'
dol'i·cho·ceph'a·ly
dol'i·cho·cne'mic
dol'i·cho·co'lon
dol'i·cho·cra'ni·al
dol'i·cho·de'rus
dol'i·cho·fa'cial
dol'i·cho·hi·er'ic
dol'i·cho·ker'kic
dol'i·cho·kne'mic
dol'i·cho·mor'phic
dol'i·cho·pel'lic
dol'i·cho·pel'vic
dol'i·cho·plat'y·ceph'a·lus
dol'i·cho·pro·sop'ic
dol'i·chor·rhine'
Dol'i·chos'
dol'i·cho·sig'moid'
dol'i·cho·sten'o·me'li·a
dol'i·cho·u·ran'ic
Do'lin method

Dol'man test
do'lor
—cap'i·tis
—cox'ae'
—va'gus
do·lo'res'
—prae·sa'gi·en'tes'
do'lor·if'ic
do'lo·rim'e·ter
do'lo·ri·met'ric
do'lo·rim'e·try
do'lo·ro·gen'ic
do·mat'o·pho'bi·a
dome
dom'i·nance
dom'i·nant
do'mi·phen'
dom·per'i·done'
Don'a·hue' syndrome
Do'nath-Land'stei'ner test
Don'der law
do·nee'
Don'nan equilibrium
Don·né' corpuscles
do'nor
Don'o·van
—bodies
—solution
Don'o·va'ni·a gran'u·lo'-
  ma·tis
don'o·va·ni·a·sis *pl.* -ses'
do'pa
do'pa·mine'
do'pa·mi·ner'gic
do'pa-ox'i·dase'
do'pase'
Dopp'ler
—blood flow detector
—echocardiography
—effect
—monitor
—operation
—phenomenon
—principle
—shift
—signal
—study
—ultrasound
—wave
Do·rel'lo canal
Dor'en·dorf' sign
dor'mant
Dor'ner spore stain

do'ro·ma'ni·a
Dor'rance operation
dor'sad'
dor'sal
dor·sal'gi·a
dor·sa'lis
—pe'dis
dor'sal·ly
dor'sal·ward
Dor'set egg medium
Dor'sey
—cannula
—punch
dor'si·flex'ion
dor'si·flex'or
dor'si·spi'nal
dor'so·an·te'ri·or
dor'so·ceph'a·lad'
dor'so·cu·boi'dal
dor'so·ep'i·troch'le·ar'is
dor'so·in·ter·cos'tal
dor'so·lat'er·al
dor'so·lum'bar
dor'so·me'di·ad'
dor'so·me'di·al
dor'so·me'di·an
dor'so·me'si·al
dor'so·na'sal
dor'so·nu'chal
dor'so·pla'nar
dor'so·pos·te'ri·or
dor'so·ra'di·al
dor'so·sa'cral
dor'so·scap'u·lar
dor'so·ul'nar
dor'so·ven'trad'
dor'so·ven'tral
dor'so·ver'te·bral
dor'sum *pl.* -sa
—lin'guae'
—ma'nus
—na'si'
—pe'dis
—pe'nis
—sel'lae'
dos'age
dose
do·sim'e·ter
do·si·met'ric
do·sim'e·try
do'sis *pl.* -ses'
—cu·ra'ti'va
—ef'fi·cax'

—re·frac′ta
—tol′er·a′ta
Dot′ter-Jud′kins technique
dou′ble-blind′ test
doub′let
douche
Doug′las
—bag
—septum
doug·las·i′tis
Do′ver powder
dove′tail′
dow′el
Dow′ney cells
down′go′ing
down′hill′
down′slop′ing
down′stream′
Down syndrome
down′ward
dox′a·cu′ri·um
dox′a·pram′
dox′e·pin
dox′o·ru′bi·cin
dox′y·cy′cline′
dox·yl′a·mine′
Doyne choroiditis
drachm *var. of* dram
drac′on·ti′a·sis *pl.* -ses′
dra·cun′cu·li′a·sis
Dra·cun′cu·lus
—med′i·nen′sis
draft *also* draught
dra·gée′
Drag′stedt operation
drain
drain′age
dram *also* drachm
dram′a·tism
drape, draped, drap′ing
drap′e·to·ma′ni·a
draught *var. of* draft
Draw′-a-Per′son test
dream′-work′
drench
drep′a·no·cyte′
drep′a·no·cy·the′mi·a
drep′a·no·cyt′ic
drep′a·no·cy·to′sis *pl.* -ses′
Dres′bach′ syndrome
dress′ing
Dress′ler
—beat

—syndrome
Drey′er formula
Driesch law
drill
Drin′ker-Col′lins
  resuscitation
Drin′ker method
drip
drive
driv′el·ing
driv′er
drom′o·graph′
drom′o·ma′ni·a
drom′o·pho′bi·a
dro·mo·stan′o·lone′
dro′mo·trop′ic
dro·per′i·dol′
drop′let
drop′per
drop′si·cal
drop′sy
drug
drug′gist
drug′-re·sis′tant
drum′head′
Drum′mond sign
drunk
drunk′en
drunk′en·ness
drunk·om′e·ter
dru′sen
Dry·op′ter·is
—fil′ix-mas′
—mar′gi·na′lis
D′-state′
du′al·ism
du′al·is′tic
Du·ane′ retraction
  syndrome
du·az′o·my′cin
Du·bi′ni chorea
Du′bin-John′son
  syndrome
Du′bin-Sprinz′ syndrome
Du·bois′ cyst
Du·boi′si·a
Du·bos′-Bra·chet′ method
Du·boscq′ colorimeter
Du′bo·witz′ syndrome
Du·chenne′
—attitude
—disease
—muscular dystrophy

—paralysis
Du·chenne′-A·ran′ disease
Du·chenne′-Erb′ palsy
Du·chenne′-Grie′sin·ger
  disease
Du·crey′ bacillus
duct
—of A·ran′ti·us
—of Bel·li′ni
—of Cu·vier′
—of San′to·ri′ni
—of Ste′no
—of Sten′sen
—of Wir′sung
duct′al *(pertaining to a tube or channel)*
♦ductile
duc′tile *(capable of being reshaped without breaking)*
♦ductal
duc′tion
duct′less
duc′tu·lar
duc′tule′
duc′tu·li′
—ab′er·ran′tes′
—al′ve·o·lar′es′
—bi·lif′er·i′
—ef′fe·ren′tes′ tes′tis
—ex′cre·to′ri·i′ glan′du·lae′
  lac′ri·ma′lis
—in′ter·lob′u·lar′es′
—pro·stat′i·ci′
—trans·ver′si′
  ep′o·oph′o·ri′
duc′tu·lus *pl.* -li′
—a·ber′rans′ superior
duc′tus *pl.* duc′tus
—ar·te′ri·o′sus
—arteriosus bi·lat′er·a′lis
—bi·lif′er·i′
—ca·rot′i·cus
—cho·led′o·chus
—coch′le·ar′is
—cys′ti·cus
—def′er·ens
—e·jac′u·la·to′ri·us
—en′do·lym·phat′i·cus
—ep′i·di·dym′i·dis
—ep′o·oph′o·ri′ lon′gi·
  tu′di·na′lis
—ex′cre·to′ri·us glan′du·
  lae′ bul′bo·u′re·thra′lis

—excretorius ve·sic′u·lae′
  sem′i·na′lis
—glan′du·lae′ bul′bo·u·re·
  thra′lis
—he·pat′i·cus com·mu′nis
—hepaticus dex′ter
—hepaticus si·nis′ter
—in′ci·si′vus
—in′ter·lob′u·lar′es′
—lac′ri·ma′les′
—lac·tif′er·i′
—lin·gua′lis
—lo′bi′ cau·da′ti′ dex′ter
—lobi caudati si·nis′ter
—lym·phat′i·cus dex′ter
—mes′o·neph′ri·cus
—Muel′ler·i′
—na′so·lac′ri·ma′lis
—pan′cre·at′i·cus
—pancreaticus ac′ces·so′-
  ri·us
—par′a·mes′o·neph′ri·cus
—par′a·u′re·thra′les′
—par′o·ti·de′us
—per′i·lym·phat′i·ci′
—per′i·lym·phat′i·cus
—pro·stat′i·ci′
—re·u′ni·ens
—sem′i·cir′cu·lar′es
—sem′i·cir′cu·lar′is anterior
—semicircularis lat′er·a′lis
—semicircularis posterior
—semicircularis superior
—sub·lin·gua′les′ mi·no′res′
—sub·lin·gua′lis major
—sub·man·dib′u·lar′is
—sub·max′il·lar′is
—su′do·rif′er·us
—tho·rac′i·cus
—thoracicus dex′ter
—thy′re·o·glos′sus
—thy′ro·glos′sus
—u·tric′u·lo·sac′cu·lar′is
—ve·no′sus
—Wolf′fi′
Duf′fy blood group
Du′gas test
Dug′be fever
Duhr′ing disease
Dukes
—classification
—disease
—staging

dul′ca·ma′ra
dul′cin
dul′cite′
dul′ci·tol′
dull′ness
Du·long′ and Pe·tit′ law
dump′ing
Dun′lop traction
du′o·chrome′
du′o·crin′in
du′o·de′nal
du′o·de·nec′ta·sis *pl.* -ses′
du′o·de·nec′to·my
du′o·de·ni′tis
du′o·de·no·chol′an·gi′tis
du′o·de·no·chol′e·cys·tos′-
  to·my
du′o·de·no·cho·led′o·chot′-
  o·my
du′o·de·no·col′ic
du′o·de·no·cys·tos′to·my
du′o·de·no·en′ter·os′to·my
du′o·de·no·gas′tric
du′o·de·no·gas·tros′co·py
du′o·de·no·gram′
du′o·de·nog′ra·phy
du′o·de·no·he·pat′ic
du′o·de·no·il′e·os′to·my
du′o·de·no·je·ju′nal
du′o·de·no·je′ju·nos′to·my
du′o·de·nol′y·sis
du′o·de·no·mes′o·col′ic
du′o·de·no·pan·cre′at′ic
du′o·de·no·pan·cre·a·tec′-
  to·my
du′o·de·no·plas′ty
du′o·de·no·py′lo·rec′to·my
du′o·de·nor′rha·phy
du′o·de·no·scope′
du′o·de·nos′co·py
du′o·de·nos′to·my
du′o·de·not′o·my
du′o·de·num *pl.* -na *or*
  -nums
Du·play′
—disease
—operation
du′plex
du·plex′i·ty
du·pli·ca′ta cru·ci·a′ta
du′pli·ca′tion
du′pli·ca·ture
du·plic′i·tas

—cru·ci·a′ta
du·plic′i·ty
Du·puys′-Du·temps′
  phenomenon
Du′puy·tren′
—contracture
—operation
du′ra
—ma′ter
—mater en·ceph′a·li′
—mater spi·na′lis
du′ral
Du·rand′ disease
Du·rand′-Ni·co·las′-Fa′vre
  disease
Du·ran′-Rey′nals factor
du′ra·plas′
du·ra′tion
Dürck nodes
Du·ret′ hemorrhages
du·ri′tis
du·ro·ar′ach·ni′tis
du·ro·sar·co′ma *pl.* -mas *or*
  -ma·ta
Du·ro·zi·ez′
—disease
—murmur
Du·temps′ sign
Dut′ton disease
Du·val′ bacillus
Du′ven·hage′
Du·ver·ney′ fracture
Du·Vries′ hammer toe
  repair
dwarf
dwarf′ism
dy′ad′
dy·ad′ic
dy·clo′nine′
dy·dro·ges′ter·one′
dye
dy·man′thine′
dy·nam′e·ter
dy·nam′ic
dy·nam′ics
dy′na·mo·gen′ic
dy′na·mog·e′ny
dy′na·mo·gen′e·sis *pl.* -ses′
dy′na·mo·graph′
dy′na·mog′ra·phy
dy′na·mom′e·ter
dy′na·mo·neure′
dy′na·moph′a·ny

dy·nam′o·scope′
dy′na·mos′co·py
dy′na·therm′
dyne
dy·phyl′line′
dys′a·cou′si·a
dys′a·cou′sis *pl.* -ses′
dys′a·cous′ma
dys·ad′ap·ta′tion
dys·an′ag·no′si·a
dys·an′ti·graph′i·a
dys·a′phi·a
dys′ap·ta′tion
dys·ar·te′ri·ot′o·ny
dys·ar′thri·a
dys·ar′thric
dys′ar·thro′sis *pl.* -ses′
dys·au′to·no′mi·a
dys′bar·ism
dys·ba′si·a
—lor′dot′i·ca pro′gres·si′va
—neu′ras·then′ic·a
in′ter·mit′tens
dys·be′ta·lip′o·pro′tein·e′-
mi·a
dys·bu′li·a
dys′ce·pha′li·a man·dib′u·
lo·oc′u·lo·fa′ci·a′lis
dys·ceph′a·ly
dys·che′zi·a
dys·che′zic
dys·chi′ri·a
dys·chon′dro·pla′si·a
dys·chro·a
dys·chroi′a
dys·chro′ma·to·der′mi·a
dys·chro′ma·tope′
dys·chro′ma·top′si·a
dys·chro′mi·a
dys·chro′mo·der′mi·a
dys·chro·na′tion
dys′chro·nous
dys·co′ri·a *also* discoria
dys·cra′si·a
dys·cra′sic
dys·crat′ic
dys′di·ad′o·cho·ki·ne′si·a
dys·e′coi′a
dys·em′bry·o′ma
dys·em′bry·o·pla′si·a
dys·e′me·si′a
dys·em′e·sis
dys·e′mi·a

dys·en′ce·pha′li·a
splanch′no·cys′ti·ca
dys·en′do·crin·ism
dys·en·te′ri·a
dys·en·ter′ic
dys·en·ter′y
dys′er·e·the′si·a
dys′er·ga′si·a
dys′er·ga′sy
dys·er′gi·a
dys·es·the′si·a
dys·es·thet′ic
dys·func′tion
dys·ga·lac′ti·a
dys·gam′ma·glob′u·lin·e′-
mi·a
dys·gen′e·sis *pl.* -ses′
dys·gen′ic
dys·gen′ics
dys·ger′mi·no′ma *pl.* -mas
or -ma·ta
dys·geu′si·a
dys·glan′du·lar
dys·glob′u·lin·e′mi·a
dys·gnath′ic
dys·gno′si·a
dys·gram′ma·tism
dys·graph′i·a
dys·he′mo·poi·e′sis *pl.* -ses′
dys·he′mo·poi·et′ic
dys·hid′ri·a
dys′hi·dro′sis *pl.* -ses′
dys·in′su·lin·ism
dys·kar′y·o′sis
dys·kar′y·ot′ic
dys·ker′a·to′ma *pl.* -mas *or*
-ma·ta
dys·ker′a·to′sis *pl.* -ses′
—con·gen′i·ta
dys·ker′a·tot′ic
dys′ki·ne′si·a
dys′ki·net′ic
dys·la′li·a
dys·lex′i·a
dys·lex′ic
dys·lo′gi·a
dys′ma·se′sis
dys′ma·tu′ri·ty
dys·me′li·a
dys·men′or·rhe′a
—in′ter·men′stru·a′lis
dys·men′ti·a
dys·mer′o·gen′e·sis

dys·me′tri·a
dys·mim′i·a
dys·mne′si·a
dys·mne′sic
dys·mor′phi·a
dys·mor′phic
dys·mor′pho·gen′e·sis
dys·mor′pho·pho′bi·a
dys·mo·til′i·ty
dys·my′e·lin·o·gen′ic
dys·my′e·lo·poi·et′ic
dys·no′mi·a
dys′o·don·ti′a·sis
dys·on′to·gen′e·sis *pl.* -ses′
dys·on′to·ge·net′ic
dys·o′pi·a
dys·o·rex′i·a
dys·os′mi·a
dys·os′te·o·gen′e·sis
pl. -ses′
dys·os′to·sis *pl.* -ses′
—clei′do·cra′ni·a′lis
—mul′ti·plex′
dys·pan′cre·a·tism
dys·par′a·thy′roid·ism
dys′pa·reu′ni·a
dys·pep′si·a
dys·pep′tic
dys·per′i·stal′sis *pl.* -ses′
dys·pha′gi·a
—con·stric′ta
—glo′bo·sa
—lu′so′ri·a
—spas′ti·ca
dys·phag′ic
dys·pha′si·a
dys·phe′mi·a
dys·phoi·te′sis *pl.* -ses′
—spas′ti·ca
dys·pho′ni·a
dys·phor′ic
dys·pho′ro·gen′ic
dys·phra′si·a
dys·phre′ni·a
dys·pig′men·ta′tion
dys·pi·tu′i·ta·rism
dys·pla′si·a
—ep′i·phys′i·a′lis mul′ti·
plex′
—epiphysialis punc·ta′ta
—epiphysialis punc·tic′u·
lar′is

dys·plas'tic
dysp·ne'a
dysp·ne'al
dysp·ne'ic
dys·po·ne'sis
dys·po·net'ic
dys·prac'tic
dys·pra'gi·a
dys·prax'i·a
dys·pro'si·um
dys·pro'tein·e'mi·a
dys·ra·phism
dys·rhyth'mi·a
dys·rhyth'mic
dys·se·cre·to'sis
dys·so'cial
dys·som'ni·a
dys·sper'ma·tism
dys·sper'mi·a
dys·splen'ism
dys·spon'dyl·ism
dys·sta'si·a
dys·stat'ic
dys·sym'me·try
dys·syn'chro·nous
dys·syn·er'gi·a
　—cer'e·bel·lar'is my'o·
　　clon'i·ca
　—cerebellaris pro'gres·si'va
dys·syn'er·gy
dys·tax'i·a
dys·tec'ti·a
dys·tec'tic
dys·tha·na'si·a
dys·the'si·a
dys·thet'ic
dys·thy'mi·a
dys·thy'mi·ac'
dys·thy'mic
dys·thy·roi'dal
dys·tim'bri·a
dys·tith'i·a
dys·to'ci·a
dys·to'cic
dys·to'ni·a
　—mus'cu·lo'rum
　　de·for'mans'
dys·ton'ic
dys·to'pi·a
dys·top'ic
dys·tro'phi·a
　—ad'i·po·so·gen'i·ta'is
　—brev'i·col'lis

—me'di·a'na ca·nal'i·for'-
　mis
—my'o·ton'i·ca
—per'i·os·ta'lis hy'per·
　plas'ti·ca fa·mil'i·ar'is
—un'gui·um
dys·troph'ic
dys·tro'phin
dys·troph'o·neu·ro'sis
　pl. -ses'
dys'tro·phy
dys·u'ri·a
dys·u'ric

E

Ea'gle
—media
—test
Ea'gle-Bar'rett syndrome
Eales disease
ear
ear'ache'
ear'drum'
Earle L fibrosarcoma
ear'lobe'
ear'plug'
ear'wax'
Ea'ton
—agent
—virus
Ea'ton-Lam'bert syndrome
Eb'ers pa·py'rus
E'ber·thel'la
—ty·pho'sa
Eb'ner
—fibrils
—glands
e'bo·na'tion
é·bran'le·ment'
e·bri'e·tas
e·bri'e·ty
e'bri·ose'
e'bri·ous
Eb'stein'
—anomaly
—disease
eb'ul·lism
e'bur
—den'tis
e'bur·nat'ed
e'bur·na'tion
Ec·bal'li·um

ec·bol'ic
ec·cen'tric *also* excentric
ec·cen'tri·cal·ly
ec·cen'tro·chon'dro·os'te·
　o·dys'tro·phy
ec·cen'tro·chon'dro·pla'-
　si·a
ec·cen'tro·os'te·o·chon'-
　dro·dys·pla'si·a
ec·ceph'a·lo'sis *pl.* -ses'
ec'chon·dro'ma *pl.* -mas *or*
　-ma·ta
ec'chon·dro'sis *pl.* -ses'
—phy'sa·liph'o·ra
ec·chon'dro·tome'
ec'chy·mo'ma *pl.* -mas *or*
　-ma·ta
ec'chy·mose'
ec'chy·mo'sis *pl.* -ses'
ec'chy·mot'ic
ec'crine
ec'cri·sis *pl.* -ses'
ec'cy·e'sis *pl.* -ses'
ec·dem'ic
ec'der·on'
ec'der·on'ic
ec'dy·sis *pl.* -ses'
ec·go·nine'
e·chid'nin
Ech'id·noph'a·ga
—gal·li·na'ce·a
e·chid'no·tox'in
Ech'i·na'ce·a
ech'i·nate'
e·chi'no·coc'cal
e·chi'no·coc·ci'a·sis *pl.* -ses'
e·chi'no·coc·co'sis *pl.* -ses'
E·chi'no·coc'cus
—gran'u·lo'sus
e·chi'no·derm'
E·chi'no·der'ma·ta
E·chi'no·rhyn'chus
ech'i·no'sis *pl.* -ses'
E·chi'no·sto'ma
e·chin'u·late'
E'chis
ech'o
ech'o·a·cou'si·a
ech'o·a·or·tog'ra·phy
ech'o·car'di·o·gram'
ech'o·car'di·og'ra·phy
é·cho' des pen·sées'
ech'o·en·ceph'a·lo·gram'

ech'o·en·ceph'a·lo·graph'
ech'o·en·ceph'a·log'ra·phy
ech'o·gen'ic
ech'o·ge·nic'i·ty
ech'o·gram'
ech'o·graph'i·a
e·chog'ra·phy
ech'o·ki·ne'si·a
ech'o·ki·ne'sis pl. -ses'
ech'o·la'li·a
ech'o·la'lic
ech'o·la'lus
ech'o·lo·ca'tion
e·cho'ma·tism
ech'o·mim'i·a
ech'o·mo'tism
ech·op'a·thy
ech·oph'o·ny
ech'o·phot'o·ny
ech'o·phra'si·a
ech'o·prax'i·a
ech'o·prax'is
ech'o·prax'y
ech'o·re'no·gram'
ech'o·son'o·gram'
ech'o·thi'o·phate'
ech'o·u'ter·o·gram'
ech'o·vi'rus
Eck'er
—fissure
—fluid
Eck fistula
Eck'hout gastroplasty
ec·la'bi·um
e·clamp'si·a
—grav'i·dar'um
—nu'tans'
—ro'tans'
e·clamp'sism
e·clamp'tic
e·clamp'to·gen'ic
e·clec'tic
e·clec'ti·cism
e·clipse'
ec'ly·sis pl. -ses'
ec·mne'si·a
e·coch'le·a'tion
e'coid'
ec·o·log'i·cal
e·col'o·gist
e·col'o·gy
e·co·ma'ni·a
E·con'o·mo disease

é'cor·ché'
e·cos'tate'
e'cos·ta'tion
e·cos'ta·tism
ec'o·sys'tem
ec'phy·lac'tic
ec'phy·lax'is pl. -lax'es'
é·crase·ment'
é·cra·seur'
ec'sta·sy
ec·stat'ic
ec'ta·co'li·a
ec'tad'
ec'tal
ec·ta'si·a
—ven·tric'u·li' par'a·dox'a
ec'ta·sis pl. -ses'
ec·tat'ic
ec·ten'tal
ect·eth'moid'
ec·thy'ma
—gan'gre·no'sum
ec·thy're·o'sis pl. -ses'
ec'to·an'ti·gen
ec'to·bat'ic
ec'to·blast'
ec'to·car'di·a
ec'to·cer'vi·cal
ec'to·cer'vix
ec'to·cho·roi'de·a
ec'to·ci·ne're·a
ec'to·ci·ne're·al
ec'to·co'lon
ec'to·con'dyle'
ec'to·cor'ne·a
ec'to·cra'ni·al
ec'to·cu·ne'i·form'
ec'to·cyst'
ec'to·derm'
ec'to·der'mal
ec'to·der'mic
ec'to·der·mo'sis pl. -ses'
—e'ro·si'va plu'ri·o'ri·fi'ci·
a'lis
ec'to·en'tad'
ec'to·en'zyme'
ec'to·eth'moid'
ec'to·gen'ic
ec·tog'e·nous
ec'to·glob'u·lar
ec·tog'o·ny
ec'to·hor·mo'nal
ec'to·hor'mone'

ec'to·men'inx
pl. -me·nin'ges'
ec'to·mere'
ec'to·morph'
ec'to·mor'phic
ec'to·mor'phy
ec'to·pa'gi·a
ec·top'a·gus pl. -gi'
ec'to·par'a·site'
ec'to·par'a·sit'ic
ec'to·pec'to·ra'lis pl. -les'
ec'to·per'i·to·ne'al
ec'to·per'i·to·ni'tis
ec'to·phyte'
ec'to·phyt'ic
ec·to'pi·a
—cor'dis
—len'tis
—pu·pil'lae'
—re'nis
—tes'tis
ec·top'ic
ec'to·pla·cen'ta
ec'to·pla·cen'tal
ec'to·plasm
ec'to·plas·mat'ic
ec'to·plas'mic
ec'to·plast'
ec'to·plas'tic
ec'to·pot'o·my
ec'to·pter'y·goid'
ec'to·py
ec'to·sarc'
ec·tos'te·al
ec'tos·to'sis pl. -ses'
ec'to·thrix'
ec'to·zo'on' pl. -zo'a
ec'tro·dac'tyl'i·a
ec'tro·dac'tyl·ism
ec'tro·dac'ty·ly
ec'tro·gen'ic
ec·trog'e·ny
ec'tro·me'li·a
ec'tro·mel'ic
ec·trom'e·lus pl. -li'
ec·trom'e·ly
ec'tro·pi·on'
ec'tro·pi·on·i·za'tion
ec'tro·pi·on·ize', -ized', -iz'ing
ec'tro·sis pl. -ses'
ec'tro·syn·dac'ty·ly
ec·trot'ic
ec'ty·lot'ic

ec′tyl·u·re′a
ec′ze·ma
—er′y·the′ma·to′sum
—fis′sum
—her·pet′i·cum
—hy′per·troph′i·cum
—mad′i·dans′
—mar′gi·na′tum
—num′mu·lar′is
—pap′u·lo′sum
—pus′tu·lo′sum
—ru′brum
—seb′or·rhe′i·cum
—so′lar′e′
—squa·mo′sum
—sy·co′ma·to′sum
—sy·co′si·for′me′
—ty·lot′i·cum
—vac′ci·na′tum
—ve·sic′u·lo′sum
ec·zem′a·ti·za′tion
ec·zem′a·to·gen′ic
ec·zem′a·toid′
ec·zem′a·to′sis pl. -ses′
ec·zem′a·tous
Ed′dowes disease
ed′dy
Ed′e·bohls′ operation
Ed′el·mann sign
e·de′ma pl. -mas or -ma·ta
e·dem′a·tous
e·den′tate′
e·den′tu·late′
e·den′tu·lous
e′de·ol′o·gy
ed′e·tate′
e·det′ic
edge
Ed′in·ger-West′phal
nucleus
e·dis′yl·ate′
Ed′mond·son grading
system
ed·ro′phon′i·um
ed′u·ca·ble
Ed′wards syndrome
ef·face′ment
ef·fect′
ef·fec′tor
ef·fem′i·na·cy
ef·fem′i·na′tion
ef′fer·ent (centrifugal)
 ♦afferent

ef′fer·vesce′
ef′fer·ves′cence
ef′fer·ves′cent
ef·fi·ca·cy
ef·fleu·rage′
ef′flo·resce′
ef′flo·res′cence
ef′flu·ent (flowing out)
 ♦affluent
ef·flu′vi·um pl. -vi·a or
 -vi·ums
ef′fort
ef·fuse′, -fused′, -fus′ing
ef·fu′sion
E′gan technique
e·ger′sis
e·ger′tic
e·ges′ta
e·ges′tion
egg
e′gi·lops′
e·glan′du·lar
e·glan′du·lose′
e·glan′du·lous
e′go
e′go·bron·choph′o·ny
e′go·cen′tric
e′go·cen·tric′i·ty
e′go·cen′trism
e′go-dys·to′ni·a
e′go-dys·ton′ic
e′go·ism
e′go·ist
e′go·is′tic
e′go·ma′ni·a
e′go·ma′ni·ac′ or
 e′go·ma·ni′a·cal
e′goph′o·ny
e′go-strength′
e′go-syn·to′ni·a
e′go-syn·ton′ic
e′go·tism
e′go·tist
e′go·tis′tic or e′go·tis′ti·cal
e′go·trop′ic
Eh′lers-Dan′los′ syndrome
Eh′ren·rit′ter ganglion
Ehr′lich
—hematoxylin
—reagent
—stain
—test
—tumor

Ehr′lich-Heinz′ granules
Ehr′mann test
ei′co·sa·pen′ta·e·no′ic
ei·det′ic
ei′dop·tom′e·try
ei′ko·nom′e·ter
ei′loid′
Ei·me′ri·a
Ein′horn test
ein′stein′
ein·stein′i·um
Ein′tho·ven
—equation
—law
—triangle
Ei·se′ni·a
Ei′sen·men′ger
—complex
—syndrome
—tetralogy
e′jac·u·late′, -lat′ed, -lat′ing
e′jac·u·la′ti·o′
—de·fi′ci·ens′
—prae′cox′
—re′tar·da′ta
e′jac·u·la′tion
e′jac′u·la·tor u·ri′nae′
e·jac′u·la·to′ry
e·jac′u·lum
e·ject′
e·jec′ta
e·jec′tion
e·jec′tor
e·lab·o′ra′tion
el′a·id′ic
e·la′i·din
e′lai·op′a·thy
el′a·pid
E·lap′i·dae′
e·las′mo·branch′ poisoning
e·las′tance
e·las′tase′
e·las′tic
e·las·ti′ca
e·las·tic′i·ty
e·las′tin
e·las′to·fi·bro′ma pl. -mas or
 -ma·ta
—dor′si′
e·las′toid′
e·las·toi·do′sis pl. -ses′
e·las′to·ma pl. -mas or -ma·ta
e·las′to·mer

e·las'to·mer'ic

e·las·tom'e·ter

e·las'to·met'ric

e·las·tom'e·try

e·las'to·mu'cin

E·las'to·plast' bandage

e·las'tor·rhex'is

e·las'tose'

e·las·to'sis

—se·ni'lis

e·lat'er·in

e·la'tion

el'bow

el'der

el'drin

e·lec'tive

E·lec'tra complex

e·lec'tric *or* e·lec'tri·cal

e·lec'tri·fy', -fied', -fy'ing

e·lec'tri·za'tion

e·lec'tro·a·nal'y·sis

e·lec'tro·an'es·the'si·a

e·lec'tro·bi·o·log'ic *or*
  e·lec'tro·bi·o·log'i·cal

e·lec'tro·bi·ol'o·gy

e·lec'tro·cap'il·lar'i·ty

e·lec'tro·car'di·o·gram'

e·lec'tro·car'di·o·graph'

e·lec'tro·car'di·o·graph'ic

e·lec'tro·car'di·og'ra·phy

e·lec'tro·car'di·o·pho·nog'-
  ra·phy

e·lec'tro·car'di·o·scan'ner

e·lec'tro·car'di·o·scope'

e·lec'tro·ca·tal'y·sis *pl.* -ses'

e·lec'tro·cau'ter·y

e·lec'tro·chem'is·try

e·lec'tro·co·ag'u·late'

e·lec'tro·co·ag'u·la'tion

e·lec'tro·co'ma

e·lec'tro·con·trac·til'i·ty

e·lec'tro·con·vul'sive

e·lec'tro·cor'ti·cal

e·lec'tro·cor'ti·co·gram'

e·lec'tro·cor'ti·co·graph'ic

e·lec'tro·cor'ti·cog'ra·phy

e·lec'tro·cute', -cut'ed,
  -cut'ing

e·lec'tro·cu'tion

e·lec'tro·cys'to·scope'

e·lec'tro·cys'to·scop'ic

e·lec'tro·cys·tos'co·py

e·lec'trode'

e·lec'tro·der'mal

e·lec'tro·der'ma·tome'

e·lec'tro·des'ic·cate'

e·lec'tro·des'ic·ca'tion

e·lec'tro·di'ag·no'sis
  pl. -ses'

e·lec'tro·di·al'y·sis *pl.* -ses'

e·lec'tro·di·a·lyz'er

e·lec'tro·di·aph'a·ke'

e·lec'tro·dy'na·mom'e·ter

e·lec'tro·en·ce·phal'ic

e·lec'tro·en·ceph'a·lo·
  gram'

e·lec'tro·en·ceph'a·lo·-
  graph'

e·lec'tro·en·ceph'a·lo·-
  graph'ic

e·lec'tro·en·ceph'a·log'ra·
  phy

e·lec'tro·end'os·mo'sis
  pl. -ses'

e·lec'tro·ex·ci'sion

e·lec'tro·fit'

e·lec'tro·gal'van·ic

e·lec'tro·gas'tro·gram'

e·lec'tro·gas'tro·graph'

e·lec'tro·gas·trog'ra·phy

e·lec'tro·gen'ic

e·lec'tro·gram'

e·lec'trog'ra·phy

e·lec'tro·he·mos'ta·sis

e·lec'tro·hys'ter·o·graph'

e·lec'tro·hys'ter·o·graph'ic

e·lec'tro·hys'ter·og'ra·phy

e·lec'tro·im'mu·no·dif·fu'-
  sion

e·lec'tro·ky'mo·gram'

e·lec'tro·ky'mo·graph'

e·lec'tro·ky·mog'ra·phy

e·lec'tro·lep'sy

e·lec'tro·li·thot'ri·ty

e·lec'trol'y·sis

e·lec'tro·lyte'

e·lec'tro·lyt'ic

e·lec'tro·lyze', -lyzed',
  -lyz'ing

e·lec'tro·lyz'er

e·lec'tro·mag'net

e·lec'tro·mag·net'ic

e·lec'tro·mag'net·ism

e·lec'tro·mas·sage'

e·lec'tro·me·chan'i·cal

e·lec·trom'e·ter

e·lec'tro·met'ric

e·lec'tro·mo'tive

e·lec'tro·my'o·gram'

e·lec'tro·my'o·graph'

e·lec'tro·my'o·graph'ic

e·lec'tro·my·og'ra·phy

e·lec'tron'

e·lec'tro·nar·co'sis *pl.* -ses'

e·lec'tro·neg'a·tive

e·lec'tro·neg'a·tiv'i·ty

e·lec'tro·neu'rog'ra·phy

e·lec'tro·neu'ro·my·og'ra·
  phy

e·lec·tron'ic

e·lec'tro·nys'tag·mog'ra·
  phy

e·lec'tro·oc'u·lo·gram'

e·lec'tro·os·mo'sis *pl.* -ses'

e·lec'tro·pa·thol'o·gy

e·lec'tro·phil'ic

e·lec'tro·pho·bi·a

e·lec'tro·pho·re'sis

e·lec'tro·pho·ret'ic

e·lec'tro·pho·ret'o·gram'

e·lec'tro·pho'rus *pl.* -ri

e·lec'tro·pho'to·ther'a·py

e·lec'tro·phren'ic

e·lec'tro·phys'i·o·log'ic

e·lec'tro·phys'i·o·log'i·cal

e·lec'tro·phys'i·ol'o·gy

e·lec'tro·plex'y

e·lec'tro·pos'i·tive

e·lec'tro·punc'ture

e·lec'tro·py·rex'i·a

e·lec'tro·re·sec'tion

e·lec'tro·ret'i·no·gram'

e·lec'tro·ret'i·no·graph'

e·lec'tro·ret'i·no·graph'ic

e·lec'tro·ret'i·nog'ra·phy

e·lec'tro·ro·ta'tion

e·lec'tro·scis'sion

e·lec'tro·scope'

e·lec'tro·sec'tion

e·lec'tro·shock'

e·lec'tro·sleep'

e·lec'tro·sol'

e·lec'tro·some'

e·lec'tro·stat'ic

e·lec'tro·stim'u·la'tion

e·lec'tro·stri·at'o·gram'

e·lec'tro·sur'ger·y

e·lec'tro·sur'gi·cal

e·lec'tro·syn'the·sis *pl.* -ses'

e·lec'tro·tax'is
e·lec'tro·thal'a·mo·gram'
e·lec'tro·tha·na'si·a
e·lec'tro·ther'a·peu'tics
e·lec'tro·ther'a·py
e·lec'tro·therm'
e·lec'tro·ther'mal
e·lec'tro·ther'mic
e·lec'tro·ther'my
e·lec'tro·tome'
e·lec·trot'o·my
e·lec'tro·ton'ic
e·lec·trot'o·nus
e·lec'tro·tro'pism
e·lec'tro·va'lence
e·lec'tro·ver'sion
e·lec'tro·vert'
e·lec'tu·ar'y
el'e·doi'sin
e·le'i·din
el'e·ment
el'e·men'tal
el'e·men'ta·ry
el'e·o'ma pl. -mas or -ma·ta
el'e·om'e·ter
el'e·op'tene'
el'e·o·ste'a·ric
el'e·o·ther'a·py
el'e·phan'ti·ac'
el'e·phan'ti·as'ic
el'e·phan·ti'a·sis pl. -ses'
—neu·ro'ma·to'sa
—nos'tras
el'e·phan'toid'
el'e·vate'
el'e·va'tion
el'e·va'tor
El'ford membrane
e·lim'i·nant
e·lim'i·nate', -nat'ed, -nat'ing
e·lim'i·na'tion
e·lin·gua'tion
el'i·nin
e·li'sion
e·lix'ir
El'kin operation
El'li·ot
—operation
—position
el·lipse'
el·lip'sin
el·lip'sis pl. -ses'
el·lip'soid'

el'lip·soi'dal
el·lip'tic or el·lip'ti·cal
el·lip'to·cyte'
el·lip'to·cy·to'sis pl. -ses'
el·lip'to·cy·tot'ic
El'lis curve
El'lis-van Crev'eld
  syndrome
Ells'worth-How'ard test
e·lon'gate', -gat'ed, -gat'ing
e'lon·ga'tion
e·lope'
e·lope'ment
El Tor cholera
el'u·ate'
e·lude'
el'u·ent
e·lu'sive
e·lute', -lut'ed, e·lut'ing
e·lu'tion
e·lu'tri·a'tion
E'ly sign
e·ma'ci·ate', -at'ed, -at'ing
e·ma'ci·a'tion
e·mac'u·la'tion
em'a·nate', -nat'ed, -nat'ing
em'a·na'tion
e·man'ci·pate', -pat'ed,
  -pat'ing
e·man'ci·pa'tion
em'a·no·ther'a·py
e·man'si·o'
  —men'si·um
e·mas'cu·late', -lat'ed,
  -lat'ing
e·mas'cu·la'tion
em·balm'
em·bar'rass
em·bar'rass·ment
Emb'den-Mey'er·hof' cycle
em·bed', -bed'ded,
  -bed'ding, also imbed
em'bo·le
em'bo·lec'to·my
em'bo·le'mi·a
em·bol'ic
em·bol'i·form'
em'bo·lism
em'bo·li·za'tion
em'bo·lo·la'li·a
em'bo·lo·phra'si·a
em'bo·loid'
em'bo·lo·ther'a·py

em'bo·lus pl. -li'
em'bo·ly
em'bouche·ment'
em·bra'sure
em·bro·ca'tion
em'bry·ec'to·my
em'bry·o'
em'bry·o·blast'
em'bry·o·blas'tic
em'bry·o·car'di·a
em'bry·o·chem'i·cal
em'bry·o·cid'al
em'bry·oc·ton'ic
em'bry·oc'to·ny
em'bry·o·gen'e·sis
em'bry·o·ge·net'ic
em'bry·o·gen'ic
em'bry·og'e·ny
em'bry·oid'
em'bry·o·log'ic or
  em'bry·o·log'i·cal
em'bry·ol'o·gist
em'bry·ol'o·gy
em'bry·o'ma pl. -mas or
  -ma·ta
em'bry·o·mor'phous
em'bry·on'
em'bry·o·nal
em'bry·on'ic
em'bry·on'i·form'
em'bry·on·i·za'tion
em'bry·o·noid'
em'bry·o·ny
em'bry·op'a·thy
em'bry·o·phore'
em'bry·o·plas'tic
em'bry·o·to'ci·a
em'bry·o·tome'
em'bry·ot'o·my
em'bry·o·tox·ic'i·ty
em'bry·o·tox'on'
em'bry·o·troph'
em'bry·o·troph'ic
em'bry·ot'ro·phy
em'bry·ul'ci·a
em'bry·ul'cus
e·med'ul·late'
e·mer'gen·cy
e·mer'gent
e·mer'o·gene'
e·mer'o·ge·net'ic
em'e·sis pl. -ses'
em'e·ta·tro'phi·a

e·met'ic
em'e·to·ca·thar'sis *pl.* -ses'
em'e·to·ca·thar'tic
em'e·to·ma'ni·a
em'e·to·pho'bi·a
e·mic'tion
e·mic'to·ry
em'i·grate', -grat'ed,
  -grat'ing
em'i·gra'tion
em'i·nec'to·my
em'i·nence
em'i·nen'ti·a
  —ar'cu·a'ta
  —car'pi' ra'di·a'lis
  —carpi ul'nar'is
  —cla'vae'
  —col·lat'er·a'lis
  —con'chae'
  —cru'ci·a'ta
  —cru'ci·for'mis
  —fa·ci·a'lis
  —fos'sae' tri·an'gu·lar'is
  —il'i·o·pec·tin'e·a
  —il'i·o·pu'bi·ca
  —in'ter·con'dy·lar'is
  —in'ter·con'dy·loi'de·a
  —me'di·a'lis
  —py·ram'i·da'lis
  —scaph'ae'
  —te'res'
em'i·o·cy·to'sis *pl.* -ses'
em'is·sar'i·um *pl.* -i·a
  —con'dy·loi'de·um
  —mas·toi'de·um
  —oc·cip'i·ta'le'
  —pa·ri·e·ta'le'
em'is·sar'y
e·mis'sion
em·men'a·gog'ic
em·men'a·gogue'
em·men'i·a
em·men'ic
em·men'i·op'a·thy
em'me·nol'o·gy
em'me·trope'
em'me·tro'pi·a
em'me·trop'ic
Em'mon·si·el'la
  cap'su·la'ta
em'o·din
e·mol'lient
e·mo'ti·o·met'a·bol'ic

e·mo'ti·o·mo'tor
e·mo'ti·o·mus'cu·lar
e·mo'tion
e·mo'tion·al
e·mo'ti·o·vas'cu·lar
e·mo'tive
e'mo·tiv'i·ty
em'pasm
em·pas'ma *pl.* -mas *or* -ma·ta
em·path'ic
em'pa·thize', -thized',
  -thiz'ing
em'pa·thy
em'per'i·po·le'sis
em'phly·sis *pl.* -ses'
em·phrac'tic
em·phrax'is *pl.* -phrax'es'
em'phy·se'ma
em'phy·sem'a·tous
em·pir'ic *or* em·pir'i·cal
em·pir'i·cism
em·plas'tic
em·plas'trum *pl.* -tra
em·po'ri·at'ric
em·pros·thot'o·nos
emp'ty
emp'ty·sis
em'py·e'ma *pl.* -ma·ta *or*
  -mas
  —ne·ces'si·ta'tis
em'py·em'a·tous
em'py·e'mic
em'py·e'sis *pl.* -ses'
e·mul'gent
e·mul'si·fi·ca'tion
e·mul'si·fi'er
e·mul'si·fy', -fied', -fy'ing
e·mul'sin (*amygdalase*)
  ♦emulsion
e·mul'sion (*a suspension of
  small globules of one liquid in a
  second*)
  ♦emulsin
e·mul'sive
e·mul'soid'
e·munc'to·ry
em'yl·cam'ate'
e·nal'a·pril
e·nam'el
e·nam'e·lo·blas·to'ma
  pl. -mas *or* -ma·ta
e·nam'e·lo'ma *pl.* -mas *or*
  -ma·ta

e·nam'e·lo·plas'ty
e·nam'e·lum
e·nan'thate'
en·an'them
en'an·the'ma *pl.* -ma·ta
en'an·them'a·tous
e·nan'thic
en·an'ti·o·mer
en·an'ti·o·morph'
en·an'ti·o·mor'phous
en'ar·thri'tis
en'ar·thro'di·al
en'ar·thro'sis *pl.* -ses'
en bloc'
en·cai'nide'
en·can'this *pl.* -thi·des'
en·cap'su·late', -lat'ed,
  -lat'ing
en·cap'su·la'tion
en·cap'sule, -suled, -sul·ing
en'car·di'tis
en·case'
en·ceinte'
en·ce'li·al·gi·a
en·ce'li·i'tis
en·ceph'a·lal'gi·a
en·ceph'a·lat'ro·phy
en·ceph'a·laux'e
en·ceph'a·le'mi·a
en'ce·phal'ic
en·ceph'a·lit'ic
en·ceph'a·li'tis *pl.* -lit'i·des'
  —le'thar'gi·ca
  —per'i·ax'i·a'lis con·cen'-
    tri·ca
  —periaxialis dif·fu'sa
en·ceph'a·li·to·gen'ic
en·ceph'a·li·tog'e·nous
En·ce·phal'i·to·zo'on'
en·ceph'a·lo·cele' (*hernia of
  brain*)
  ♦encephalocoele
en·ceph'a·lo·clas'tic
en·ceph'a·lo·coele' (*cranial
  cavity*)
  ♦encephalocele
en·ceph'a·lo·cys'to·cele'
en·ceph'a·lo·cys'to·me·
  nin'go·cele'
en·ceph'a·lo·di·al'y·sis
  pl. -ses'
en·ceph'a·lo·dys·pla'si·a
en·ceph'a·lo·gram'

en·ceph'a·log'ra·phy
en·ceph'a·loid'
en·ceph'a·lo·lith'
en·ceph'a·lol'o·gy
en·ceph'a·lo'ma *pl.* -mas *or*
  -ma·ta
en·ceph'a·lo·ma·la'ci·a
en·ceph'a·lo·men'in·gi'tis
en·ceph'a·lo·me·nin'go·
  cele'
en·ceph'a·lo·men'in·gop'a·
  thy
en·ceph'a·lo·mere'
en·ceph'a·lo·mer'ic
en·ceph'a·lom'e·ter
en·ceph'a·lo·my'e·li'tis
en·ceph'a·lo·my·el'o·cele'
en·ceph'a·lo·my'e·lo·neu·
  rop'a·thy
en·ceph'a·lo·my'e·lon'ic
en·ceph'a·lo·my'e·lop'a·
  thy
en·ceph'a·lo·my'e·lo·ra·
  dic'u·li'tis
en·ceph'a·lo·my'e·lo·ra·
  dic'u·lop'a·thy
en·ceph'a·lo·my'e·lo'sis
  pl. -ses'
en·ceph'a·lo·my'o·car·di'-
  tis
en·ceph'a·lon' *pl.* -la
en·ceph'a·lo·nar·co'sis
  pl. -ses'
en·ceph'a·lop'a·thy
en·ceph'a·lo·punc'ture
en·ceph'a·lo·py·o'sis
  pl. -ses'
en·ceph'a·lo·ra·chid'i·an
en·ceph'a·lo·ra·dic'u·li'tis
en·ceph'a·lor·rha'gi·a
en·ceph'a·lo·scle·ro'sis
  pl. -ses'
en·ceph'a·lo·scope'
en·ceph'a·los'co·py
en·ceph'a·lo·sep'sis *pl.* -ses'
en·ceph'a·lo'sis *pl.* -ses'
en·ceph'a·lo·spi'nal
en·ceph'a·lo·thlip'sis
  pl. -ses'
en·ceph'a·lo·tome'
en·ceph'a·lot'o·my
en·ceph'a·lo·tri·gem'i·nal
en·chon'dral

en'chon·dro'ma *pl.* -mas *or*
  -ma·ta
en·chon'dro·ma·to'sis
  pl. -ses'
en'chon·dro'ma·tous
en'chon'dro·sar·co'ma
  pl. -mas *or* -ma·ta
en'chon·dro'sis *pl.* -ses'
en'chy·ma
en·cir'cle
en'clave'
en·clit'ic
en·cod'ing
en'col·pi'tis
en'cop·re'sis *pl.* -ses'
en·coun'ter
en·cra'ni·us
en·croach'
en·croach'ment
en·crust'
en'crus·ta'tion
en·crust'ed
en'cy·e'sis *pl.* -ses'
en'cy'o·py'e·li'tis
en·cyst'
en'cys·ta'tion
en·cyst'ment
end'a·del'phus
En'da·moe'ba
end'an·gi·i'tis
end'a·or'tic
end'a·or·ti'tis
end'ar·ter·ec'to·mize',
  -mized', -miz'ing
end'ar·ter·ec'to·my
end'ar·te'ri·al
end'ar·te'ri·ec'to·my
end'ar·te·ri'tis
  —de·for'mans'
  —ob·lit'er·ans'
end'ar·te'ri·um
end'ar·ter·op'a·thy
end'au'ral
end'brain'
end'-bulb'
en·deic'tic
en·de'mi·a
en·dem'ic
en·de'mi·ol'o·gy
en'de·mo·ep'i·dem'ic
end'ep·i·der'mic
end'ep·i·der'mis
end'er·gon'ic

en·der'mic
en'der·mo'sis *pl.* -ses'
en'der·on'
en'der·on'ic
end'-feet'
en'do·ab·dom'i·nal
en'do·an'eu·rys·mor'rha·
  phy
en'do·an'gi·i'tis
en'do·a'or·ti'tis
en'do·ap·pen'di·ci'tis
en'do·ar'te·ri'tis
en'do·bi·ot'ic
en'do·blast'
en'do·blas'tic
en'do·bron'chi·al
en'do·bron·chi'tis
en'do·car'di·ac'
en'do·car'di·al
en'do·car'di·op'a·thy
en'do·car·di'tis
  —len'ta
en'do·car'di·um *pl.* -di·a
en'do·ce'li·ac'
en'do·cel'lu·lar
en'do·cer'vi·cal
en'do·cer'vi·ci'tis
en'do·cer'vix *pl.* -vi·ces'
en'do·cho·led'o·chal
en'do·chon'dral
en'do·chon·dro'ma *pl.* -mas
  or -ma·ta
en'do·cho'ri·on'
en'do·chrome'
en'do·co·li'tis
en'do·col·pi'tis
en'do·cra'ni·al
en'do·cra·ni'tis
en'do·cra'ni·um *pl.* -ni·a
en'do·crine
en'do·crin'ic
en'do·crin·ism
en'do·crin'o·log'ic
en'do·crin'o·log'i·cal
en'do·cri·nol'o·gist
en'do·cri·nol'o·gy
en'do·crin'o·path'ic
en'do·cri·nop'a·thy
en'do·cri·no'sis *pl.* -ses'
en'do·cri·nos'i·ty
en'do·crin'o·ther'a·py
en·doc'ri·nous
en'do·cyst'

en·do·cys·ti'tis
en'do·cyte'
en'do·cy·to'sis *pl.* -ses'
en'do·derm'
en'do·der'mal
en'do·di·as'co·py
en'do·don'ti·a
en'do·don'tic
en'do·don'tics
en'do·don'tist
en'do·don·ti'tis
en'do·don'ti·um
en'do·don·tol'o·gy
en'do·en·ter·i'tis
en'do·en'zyme'
en'do·ep'i·der'mal
en'do·ep'i·the'li·al
en'do·e·soph'a·gi'tis
en·dog'a·mous
en·dog'a·my
en'do·gas'tric
en'do·gas·tri'tis
en'do·ge·net'ic
en'do·gen'ic
en·dog'e·nous
en·dog'e·ny
en'dog·na'thi·on'
en'do·in·tox'i·ca'tion
en'do·la·ryn'ge·al
en'do·lar'ynx
En·do'li·max'
—na'na
en'do·lymph'
en'do·lym'pha
en'do·lym·phan'gi·al
en'do·lym·phat'ic
en'do·lym'phic
en·dol'y·sin
en'do·mas'toi·di'tis
en'do·men'inx
  pl. -me·nin'ges'
en'do·mes'o·derm'
en'do·me·trec'to·my
en'do·me'tri·al
en'do·me'tri·oid'
en'do·me'tri·o'ma *pl.* -mas
  or -ma·ta
en'do·me'tri·o'sis *pl.* -ses'
en'do·me'tri·ot'ic
en'do·me·tri'tis
  —ex·fo'li·a·ti'va
en'do·me'tri·um
en·dom'e·try

en'do·mi·to'sis *pl.* -ses'
en'do·morph'
en'do·mor'phic
en'do·mor'phy
en'do·my'o·car·di'tis
en'do·mys'i·um *pl.* -i·a
en'do·na'sal
en'do·neu'ri·al
en'do·neu·ri'tis
en'do·neu·ri·um *pl.* -ri·a
en'do·nu'cle·ar
en'do·nu'cle·ase'
en'do·nu·cle'o·lus *pl.* -li
en'do·par'a·site'
en'do·par'a·sit'ic
en'do·par'a·sit·ism
en'do·pel'vic
en'do·pep'ti·dase'
en'do·per'i·car'di·al
en'do·per'i·car·di'tis
en'do·per'i·my'o·car·di'tis
en'do·per'i·to·ne'al
en'do·per'i·to·ni'tis
en'do·pha·ryn'ge·al
en'do·phle·bi'tis
en'doph'thal·mi'tis
  —pha·co·an'a·phy·lac'ti·ca
en'do·phyte'
en'do·phyt'ic
en'do·plasm
en'do·plas'mic
en'do·plast'
en'do·plas'tic
en'do·pol'y·poid'
en'do·psy'chic
en'do·py'e·lot'o·my
en'do·re·du'pli·ca'tion
en'do·rhi·ni'tis
en·dor'phin
en'do·sal·pin'gi·o'sis
  pl. -ses'
en'do·sal'pin·gi'tis
en'do·sal'pinx
  pl. -sal·pin'ges'
en'do·sarc'
en'do·scope'
en'do·scop'ic
en·dos'co·pist
en·dos'co·py
en'do·se·cre'to·ry
en'do·sep'sis *pl.* -ses'
en'do·skel'e·ton
en'dos·mom'e·ter

en'dos·mose'
en'dos·mo'sic
en'dos·mo'sis *pl.* -ses'
en'dos·mot'ic
en'do·some'
en'do·spore'
en·dos'te·al
en·dos'te·i'tis
en·dos'te·o'ma *pl.* -mas *or*
  -ma·ta
en·dos'te·um *pl.* -te·a
en·dos'ti'tis
en·dos'to'ma *pl.* -mas *or*
  -ma·ta
en·dos'to'sis *pl.* -ses'
en'do·sur'ger·y
en'do·ten·din'e·um
en'do·ten'on
en'do·the'li·al
en'do·the'li·al·i·za'tion
en'do·the'li·i'tis
en'do·the'lin
en'do·the'li·o·an'gi·i'tis
en'do·the'li·o·blas'to·ma
  pl. -mas *or* -ma·ta
en'do·the'li·o·cho'ri·al
en'do·the'li·o·cyte'
en'do·the'li·o·cy·to'sis
  pl. -ses'
en'do·the'li·oid'
en'do·the'li·ol'y·sin
en'do·the'li·o'ma *pl.* -mas *or*
  -ma·ta
  —an'gi·o·ma·to'sum
  —cap'i·tis
en'do·the'li·o·ma·to'sis
  pl. -ses'
en'do·the'li·o·sar·co'ma
  pl. -mas *or* -ma·ta
en'do·the'li·o·sis *pl.* -ses'
en'do·the'li·o·tox'in
en'do·the'li·um *pl.* -li·a
  —cam'er·ae' an·te'ri·o'ris
    cor'ne·ae'
  —camerae anterioris i'ri·dis
  —camerae anterioris oc'u·li'
en'do·ther'mic
en'do·ther'my
en'do·tho·rac'ic
en'do·thrix'
en'do·tox·e'mi·a
en'do·tox'ic
en'do·tox'i·co'sis *pl.* -ses'

en'do·tox'in
en'do·tra'che·al
en'do·trach'el·i'tis
en'do·u·re'thral
en'do·u'ter·ine
en'do·vag'i·nal
en'do·vas'cu·li'tis
en'do·ve'nous
end'plate'
en'e·ma
en·er·get'ic
en·er·get'ics
en·er·gid
en·er·giz'er
en·er·gom'e·ter
en·er·gy
en·er·vate' (to weaken),
  -vat'ed, -vat'ing
  ♦innervate
en·er·va'tion
en face'
en·flag'el·la'tion
en·gage'ment
en·gas'tri·us
En'gel·mann disease
En'gel-Reck'ling·hau'sen
  disease
en·globe'
en·globe'ment
en·gorge', -gorged', -gorg'ing
en·gorge'ment
en'gram
en·graph'i·a
en·hance'
en·hance'ment
en·he'ma·to·spore'
en·hex'y·mal
en·large'
en·large'ment
e'nol'
e'no·lase'
e'no·li·za'tion
e'no·ma'ni·a
en'oph·thal'mos'
en·os'to·sis pl. -ses'
e·nox'a·cin
En'roth' sign
en·sheathe', -sheathed',
  -sheath'ing
en'si·form'
en·som'pha·lus pl. -li'
en'som·phal'ic
en'stro·phe

en'tad'
en'tal
en'ta·me·bi'a·sis pl. -ses'
En'ta·moe'ba
  —buc·ca'lis
  —co'li'
  —gin'gi·va'lis
  —his'to·lyt'i·ca
  —na'na
en'ta·moe·bi'a·sis pl. -ses'
en·ta'si·a
en'ta·sis pl. -ses'
en·tat'ic
en·tel'e·chy
en'ter·ad'e·ni'tis
en'ter·al
en'ter·al'gi·a
en'ter·al'gic
en'ter·ec'ta·sis pl. -ses'
en'ter·ec'to·my
en'ter·el·co'sis pl. -ses'
en'ter·e·pip'lo·cele'
en·ter'ic
en·ter'ic-coat'ed
en·ter'i·coid'
en'ter·i'tis
  —cam'py·lo·bac'ter
  —ne·crot'i·cans'
en'ter·o·a·nas'to·mo'sis
  pl. -ses'
En'ter·o·bac'ter
  —aer·og'e·nes
  —ag·glo'mer·ans
  —clo·a'cae'
  —haf'ni·ae'
  —liq'ui·fa'ciens
En'ter·o·bac·te'ri·a'ce·ae'
en'ter·o·bac·te'ri·al
en'ter·o·bac·te'ri·um
  pl. -ri·a
en'ter·o·bi'a·sis pl. -ses'
en'ter·o·bil'i·ar'y
En'ter·o'bi·us
  —ver·mic'u·lar'is
en'ter·o·cele'
en'ter·o·cen·te'sis pl. -ses'
en'ter·o·cep'tive
en'ter·o·chro'maf·fin
en'ter·o·clei'sis pl. -ses'
en'ter·oc'ly·sis pl. -ses'
en'ter·o·coc'cus pl. -ci'
en'ter·o·coele'
en'ter·o·coe'lic

en'ter·o·co·lec'to·my
en'ter·o·co'lic
en'ter·o·co·li'tis
en'ter·o·co·los'to·my
en'ter·o·crin'in
en'ter·o·cu·ta'ne·ous
en'ter·o·cyst'
en'ter·o·cys'to·cele'
en'ter·o·cys·to'ma pl. -mas
  or -ma·ta
en'ter·o·cys'to·plas'ty
en'ter·o·cyte'
en'ter·o·dyn'i·a
en'ter·o·en·ter'ic
en'ter·o·en'ter·os'to·my
en'ter·o·e·pip'lo·cele'
en'ter·o·gas'tric
en'ter·o·gas·tri'tis
en'ter·o·gas'tro·cele'
en'ter·o·gas'trone'
en'ter·og'e·nous
en'ter·o·gram'
en'ter·o·graph'
en'ter·og'ra·phy
en'ter·o·hep'a·ti'tis, -tis·es
  or -tit'i·des'
en'ter·o·hep'a·to·cele'
en'ter·o·hy'dro·cele'
en'ter·o·ki'nase'
en'ter·o·ki·ne'si·a
en'ter·o·ki·net'ic
en'ter·o·lith'
en'ter·o·li·thi'a·sis pl. -ses'
en'ter·ol'o·gist
en'ter·ol'o·gy
en'ter·ol'y·sis pl. -ses'
en'ter·o·meg'a·ly
en'ter·o·mer'o·cele'
En'ter·o·mo'nas
en'ter·o·my·co'sis pl. -ses'
en'ter·o·my·i'a·sis pl. -ses'
en'ter·on'
en'ter·o·pa·re'sis pl. -ses'
en'ter·o·path'ic
en'ter·o·path'o·gen·e'sis
  pl. -ses'
en'ter·o·path'o·gen'ic
en'ter·op'a·thy
en'ter·o·pep'ti·dase'
en'ter·o·pex'y
en'ter·o·plas'tic
en'ter·o·plas'ty
en'ter·o·ple'gi·a

en'ter·o·proc'ti·a
en'ter·op·to'sis *pl.* -ses'
en'ter·op·tot'ic
en'ter·or·rha'gi·a
en'ter·or·rha·phy
en'ter·or·rhe'a
en'ter·or·rhex'is *pl.* -rhex'es'
en'ter·o·scope'
en'ter·o·sep'sis *pl.* -ses'
en'ter·o·spasm
en'ter·o·sta'sis *pl.* -ses'
en'ter·o·stax'is
en'ter·o·ste·no'sis *pl.* -ses'
en'ter·o·sto'mal
en'ter·os'to·my
en'ter·o·tome'
en'ter·ot'o·my
en'ter·o·tox·e'mi·a
en'ter·o·tox'i·gen'ic
en'ter·o·tox'in
en'ter·o·tox'ism
en'ter·o·trop'ic
en'ter·o·vag'i·nal
en'ter·o·ves'i·cal
en'ter·o·vi'ral
en'ter·o·vi'rus
en'ter·o·zo'ic
en'ter·o·zo'on' *pl.* -zo'a
en'thal·py
en'the·sis *pl.* -ses'
en·thet'ic
en·ti'ris
en'ti·ty
en'to·blast'
en'to·cele'
en'to·cho·roi'de·a
en'to·cone'
en'to·co'nid
en'to·cor'ne·a
en'to·derm'
en'to·der'mal
en'to·ec'tad'
en'tome'
en'to·mere'
en'to'mi·on' *pl.* -mi·a
en'to·mog'e·nous
en'to·mol'o·gist
en'to·mol'o·gy
en'to·mo·pho'bi·a
En'to·moph'tho·ra
en'to·pe·dun'cu·lar
en'to·plasm
ent·op'tic

ent'op'to·scop'ic
ent'op·tos'co·py
en'to·ret'i·na
en'to·sarc'
en'to·zo'al
en'to·zo'on' *pl.* -zo'a
en·train'ment
en·trap'
en·trap'ment
en·tro'pi·on'
en·tro'pi·on·ize', -ized',
   -iz'ing
en'tro·py
en'ty·py
e·nu'cle·ate', -at'ed, -at'ing
e·nu'cle·a'tion
e·nu'cle·a'tor
en·u·re'sis *pl.* -ses'
en·u·ret'ic
en·ven'om
en·ven'om·a'tion
en·vi'ron·ment
en·vi'ron·men'tal
en·vi'ron·men'tal·ism
en·vi'ron·men'tal·ist
en·vi'ron·men'tal·ly
en'zy·got'ic
en·zy·mat'ic
en'zyme'
en·zy'mic
en·zy·mol'o·gist
en·zy·mol'o·gy
en·zy·mol'y·sis *pl.* -ses'
en·zy·mo·lyt'ic
en·zy·mop'a·thy
en·zy·mu'ri·a
e'on·ism
e'o·sin
e'o·sin'o·cyte'
e'o·sin'o·pe'ni·a
e'o·sin'o·pe'nic
e'o·sin'o·phil'
e'o·sin'o·phile'
e'o·sin'o·phil'i·a
e'o·sin'o·phil'ic
e'o·sin'o·tac'tic
e·pac'tal
ep'ar·sal'gi·a
ep'ar·te'ri·al
ep·ax'i·al
e·pen'dy·ma
e·pen'dy·mal
e·pen'dy·mi'tis

e·pen'dy·mo·blast'
e·pen'dy·mo·blas·to'ma
   pl. -mas *or* -ma·ta
e·pen'dy·mo·cyte'
e·pen'dy·mo'ma *pl.* -mas *or*
   -ma·ta
e·pen'dy·mop'a·thy
ep'e·ryth'ro·zo'o·no'sis *pl.*
   -ses'
eph'apse'
e·phe'bi·at'rics
e·phe'bic
eph'e·bol'o·gy
e·phed'rine
e·phe'lis *pl.* -li·des'
e·phem'er·a
   —ma·lig'na
e·phem'er·al
eph'i·dro'sis *pl.* -ses'
   —cru·en'ta
   —tinc'ta
ep'i·an·dros'ter·one'
ep'i·blast'
ep'i·blas'tic
ep'i·blas'to·trop'ic
ep'i·bleph'a·ron'
ep'i·bol'ic
e·pib'o·ly
ep'i·bran'chi·al
ep'i·bul'bar
ep'i·can'thal
ep'i·can'thic
ep'i·can'thus
ep'i·car'di·a
ep'i·car'di·al
ep'i·car'di·ec'to·my
ep'i·car'di·um *pl.* -di·a
ep'i·carp'
ep'i·chord'al
ep'i·cho'ri·al
ep'i·cho'ri·on'
ep'i·col'ic
ep'i·co'mus
ep'i·con'dy·lal'gi·a
ep'i·con'dy·lar
ep'i·con'dyle'
ep'i·con'dyl'i·an
ep'i·con'dyl'ic
ep'i·con'dy·li'tis
ep'i·con'dy·lus *pl.* -li'
   —lat'e·ra'lis fem'o·ris
   —lateralis hu'mer·i'
   —me'di·a'lis fem'o·ris

—medialis hu'mer·i'
ep'i·cor'a·coid'
ep'i·cos'tal
ep'i·cra'ni·al
ep'i·cra'ni·um
ep'i·cra'ni·us *pl.* -ni·i'
ep'i·cri'sis *pl.* -ses'
e·pic'ri·sis *pl.* -ses'
ep'i·crit'ic
ep'i·cys·ti'tis
ep'i·cys·tot'o·my
ep'i·cyte'
ep'i·dem'ic
ep'i·de·mic'i·ty
ep'i·de'mi·o·gen'e·sis
  pl. -ses'
ep'i·de'mi·og'ra·phy
ep'i·de'mi·o·log'ic
ep'i·de'mi·o·log'i·cal
ep'i·de'mi·ol'o·gist
ep'i·de'mi·ol'o·gy
ep'i·derm'
ep'i·der'mal
ep'i·der·mat'ic
ep'i·der'ma·to·plas'ty
ep'i·der'mic
ep'i·der·mic'u·la
ep'i·der'mi·dal·i·za'tion
ep'i·der'mi·do'sis
ep'i·der'mis
ep'i·der·mi'tis
ep'i·der·mi·za'tion
ep'i·der'mo·dys·pla'si·a
  —ver·ru'ci·for'mis
ep'i·der'moid'
ep'i·der'moid·o'ma *pl.*-mas
  or -ma·ta
ep'i·der'mol'y·sis *pl.* -ses'
  —bul·lo'sa
  —bullosa dys·troph'i·ca
  —bullosa he·red'i·tar'i·a
    le·ta'lis
  —bullosa sim'plex'
ep'i·der·mo'ma *pl.* -mas *or*
  -ma·ta
ep'i·der·mo·my'co·sis
ep'i·der·moph'y·tid
Ep'i·der·moph'y·ton'
  —floc'co'sum
  —in'gui·na'le'
ep'i·der·mo·phy·to'sis
  pl. -ses'
ep'i·der·mo'sis

ep'i·di·a·scope'
ep'i·did'y·mal
ep'i·did'y·mec'to·my
ep'i·did'y·mis *pl.* -mi·des'
ep'i·did'y·mi'tis
ep'i·did'y·mo·or·chi'tis
ep'i·did'y·mot'o·my
ep'i·did'y·mo·va·sec'to·my
ep'i·did'y·mo·va·sos'to·my
ep'i·du'ral
ep'i·du·rog'ra·phy
ep'i·es'tri·ol'
ep'i·fas'ci·al
ep'i·fol·lic'u·li'tis
ep'i·gas·tral'gi·a
ep'i·gas'tric
ep'i·gas'tri·o·cele'
ep'i·gas'tri·um *pl.* -tri·a
ep'i·gas'tri·us
  —par'a·sit'i·cus
ep'i·gas'tro·cele'
ep'i·gen'e·sis
ep'i·ge·net'ic
ep'i·glot'tal
ep'i·glot'tic
ep'i·glot'ti·dec'to·my
ep'i·glot'tis
ep'i·glot·ti'tis
e·pig'na·thus
e·pig'o·nal
ep'i·gua'nine'
ep'i·hy'al
ep'i·hy'oid'
ep'i·la·mel'lar
ep'i·la'tion
ep'i·lem'ma
ep'i·lep'si·a
  —ar'ith·met'i·ca
  —mi'tis
  —par'ti·a'lis con·tin'u·a
  —ver·tig'i·no'sa
ep'i·lep'sy
ep'i·lep'tic
ep'i·lep'ti·form'
ep'i·lep·to·gen'ic
ep'i·lep·tog'e·nous
ep'i·lep'toid'
ep'i·lep·tol'o·gist
ep'i·lep·tol'o·gy
ep'i·loi'a
ep'i·man·dib'u·lar
ep'i·men'or·rha'gi·a
ep'i·men'or·rhag'ic

ep'i·men'or·rhe'a
ep'i·mer
e·pim'er·ase'
ep'i·mere'
ep'i·mer'ic
e·pim'er·i·za'tion
ep'i·mor'phic
ep'i·mor·pho'sis *pl.* -ses'
ep'i·my'o·car'di·um
ep'i·mys'i·al
ep'i·mys'i·um *pl.* -i·a
ep'i·neph'rine
ep'i·neph'ri·ne·mi·a
ep'i·ne·phri'tis
ep'i·neph'ros'
ep'i·neu'ral
ep'i·neu'ri·al
ep'i·neu'ri·um
ep'i·os'ic
ep'i·pa·tel'lar
ep'i·per'i·car'di·al
ep'i·pha·ryn'ge·al
ep'i·phar'ynx
  pl. -pha·ryn'ges'
ep'i·phe·nom'e·non' *pl.* -na
e·piph'o·ra
ep'i·phre'nal
ep'i·phren'ic
ep'i·phy·lax'is *pl.* -lax'es'
e·piph'y·se'al *var. of*
  epiphysial
ep'i·phys'i·al *also*
  epiphyseal
ep'i·phys'i·o·de'sis *pl.* -ses'
ep'i·phys'i·oid'
ep'i·phys'i·o·lis'the·sis
  pl. -ses'
ep'i·phys'i·ol'y·sis *pl.* -ses'
ep'i·phys'i·o·ne·cro'sis
  pl. -ses'
e·piph'y·sis *pl.* -ses'
  —cer'e·bri'
e·piph'y·si'tis
ep'i·phyte'
ep'i·pi'al
ep'i·pleu'ral
e·pip'lo·cele'
e·pip'lo·ec'to·my
e·pip'lo·en'ter·o·cele'
ep'i·plo'ic
e·pip'lo·i'tis
e·pip'lom·phal'o·cele'
e·pip'lo·on' *pl.* -lo·a

e·pip'lo·pex'y
ep'i·plor'rha·phy
ep'i·pro'pi·dine'
ep'ip·ter'ic
ep'i·ru'bi·cin
ep'i·scle'ra pl. -ras or -rae'
ep'i·scle'ral
ep'i·scle·ri'tis
e·pis'i·o·cli'si·a
e·pis'i·o·el'y·tror'rha·phy
e·pis'i·o·per'i·ne'o·plas'ty
e·pis'i·o·per'i·ne·or'rha·
   phy
e·pis'i·o·plas'ty
e·pis'i·or·rha'gi·a
e·pis'i·or'rha·phy
e·pis'i·o·ste·no'sis pl. -ses'
e·pis'i·ot'o·my
ep'i·sode'
ep'i·sod'ic
ep'i·some'
ep'i·spa'di·a
ep'i·spa'di·ac'
ep'i·spa'di·al
ep'i·spa'di·as
ep'i·spas'tic
ep'i·sphe'noid'
ep'i·spi'nal
ep'i·sple·ni'tis
e·pis'ta·sis pl. -ses'
e·pis'ta·sy
ep'i·stat'ic
ep'i·stax'is
e·pis'te·mo·phil'i·a
ep'i·ster'nal
ep'i·ster'num pl. -nums or
   -na
ep'i·stro'phe·us
ep'i·stroph'ic
ep'i·tar'sus
ep'i·tax'y
ep'i·ten·din'e·um
ep'i·ten'on
ep'i·tha·lam'ic
ep'i·thal'a·mus pl. -mi'
ep'i·tha·lax'i·a
ep'i·the'li·al
ep'i·the'li·al·i·za'tion
ep'i·the'li·al·ize', -ized',
   -iz'ing
ep'i·the'li·i'tis
ep'i·the'li·o·cho'ri·al
ep'i·the'li·o·fi'bril

ep'i·the'li·o·ge·net'ic
ep'i·the'li·oid'
ep'i·the'li·ol'y·sin
ep'i·the'li·ol'y·sis pl. -ses'
ep'i·the'li·o'ma pl. -mas or
   -ma·ta
   —ad'e·noi'des' cys'ti·cum
   —ba'so·cel'lu·lar'e'
   —cho'ri·o·ep'i·der·ma'le'
   —con·ta'gi·o'sum
ep'i·the'li·o·ma·to'sis
ep'i·the'li·om·a'tous
ep'i·the'li·o·my·o'sis
   pl. -ses'
ep'i·the'li·tis
ep'i·the'li·um pl. -li·a
   —an·te'ri·us cor'ne·ae'
   —cor'ne·ae'
   —duc'tus sem'i·cir'cu·
      lar'is
   —len'tis
ep'i·the'li·za'tion
ep'i·the'lize', -lized', -liz'ing
e·pith'e·sis pl. -ses'
ep'i·thi'a·zide'
ep'i·tope'
ep'i·trich'i·al
ep'i·trich'i·um
ep'i·troch'le·a
ep'i·troch'le·ar
ep'i·troch'le·ar'is
ep'i·tu·ber'cu·lo'sis pl. -ses'
ep'i·tym·pan'ic
ep'i·tym'pa·num
ep'i·typh·li'tis
ep'i·zo'ic
ep'i·zo'on' pl. -zo'a
ep'i·zo·ot'ic
ep'i·zo·ot'i·ol'o·gy
ep'och·al
ep'o·nych'i·um
ep'o·nym
ep'o·nym'ic
e·pon'y·mous
ep'o·oph'o·rec'to·my
ep'o·oph'o·ron'
Ep'som salt
Ep'stein'
   —blade
   —pearls
   —syndrome
Ep'stein-Barr' virus
e·pu'lis pl. -li·des'

ep'u·lo·fi·bro'ma pl. -mas or
   -ma·ta
ep'u·loid'
ep'u·lo'sis
e'qual
e·qua'tion
e·qua'tion·al
e·qua'tor
   —bul'bi' oc'u·li'
   —len'tis
e'qua·to'ri·al
e'qui·ax'i·al
e'qui·dom'i·nant
e'qui·lat'er·al
e·quil'i·brate', -brat'ed,
   -brat'ing
e·quil'i·bra'tion
e'qui·lib'ra·to'ry
e'qui·lib'ri·um pl. -ri·ums or
   -ri·a
e'qui·lin
e'quine'
eq'ui·no·ca'vus
eq'ui·no·val'gus
eq'ui·no·var'us
e'qui·nus
e'qui·po·ten'tial
e·quiv'a·lence
e·quiv'a·len·cy
e·quiv'a·lent
e·quiv'o·cal
e·ra'sion
Er'a·ty'rus
   —cus'pi·da'tus
Erb
   —atrophy
   —palsy
   —paralysis
   —point
   —scapulohumeral juvenile
      muscular dystrophy
   —sign
   —spastic spinal paraplegia
   —syphilitic paralysis
Erb'-Char·cot' disease
Erb'-Du·chenne' paralysis
Er'ben sign
Erb'-Gold'flam' symptom
   complex
er'bi·um
Erb'-Lan·dou'zy disease
Erb'-Zim'mer·lin type
Erd'mann reagent

e·rect'
e·rec'tile
e·rec'tion
e·rec'tor
—cli·to'ri·dis
—pe'nis
—pi'li'
—spi'nae'
er'e·mo·pho'bi·a
e·rep'sin
er'e·thism
er'e·this'mic
er'e·this'tic
er'e·thit'ic
er'eu·tho·pho'bi·a
erg
er·ga'si·a
er·ga'si·a·try
er·ga'si·o·ma'ni·a
er·ga'si·o·pho'bi·a
er·gas'tic
er·gas'to·plasm
er·go·ba'sine'
er·go·ba'si·nine'
er·go·cal·cif'er·ol'
er·go·cor'nine'
er·go·cris'tine'
er·go·gen'ic
er·go·gram'
er·go·graph'
er·go·graph'ic
er·go·loid'
er·gom'e·ter
er·go·met'ric
er·go·met'rine'
er·go·met'ri·nine'
er·go·no·met'ric
er·go·nom'ic
er·go·nom'ics
er·go·no'vine'
er·go·phore'
er·go·plasm
er·go·sine'
er·go·si·nine'
er·go·some'
er·gos'ta·nol'
er·gos'ter·in
er·gos'ter·ol'
er·go·stet'rine'
er·got
er·got'a·mine'
er·go·tam'i·nine'
er·go·ther'a·py

er'go·thi'o·ne'ine'
er'got·in
er'got'i·nine'
er'got·ism
er'got·ized'
er'go·tox'ine'
er'go·trop'ic
Er'ich·sen disease
er'i·gens
Er'i·o·dic'ty·on'
er'i·om'e·ter
E·ris'ta·lis
Er'len·mey'er flask
  deformity
e·rode', e·rod'ed, e·rod'ing
er'o·gen'ic
e·rog'e·nous *(arousing sexual
  desire)*
  ◆*aerogenous*
er'o·ma'ni·a
e'ros' *(the sum of all self-
  preservative instincts)*
  ◆*erose*
e·rose' *(having an irregularly
  toothed edge)*
  ◆*eros*
e·ro'si·o' in'ter·dig'i·ta'lis
  blas'to·my·ce'ti·ca
e·ro'sion
e·ro'sive
e·rot'ic
e·rot'i·ca
e·rot'i·cism
e·rot'i·cize'
e·rot'i·co·ma'ni·a
er'o·tism
e·ro'ti·za'tion
e·ro'tize'
e·ro·to·gen'e·sis
e·ro·to·gen'ic
e·ro·to·ma'ni·a
e·ro·to·ma'ni·ac'
e·ro·to·path'
e·ro·to·path'ic
er'o·top'a·thy
e·ro·to·pho'bi·a
er'rhine'
er'u·bes'cent
e·ru'cic
e·ruc'tate', -tat'ed, -tat'ing
e·ruc·ta'tion
e·rup'tion
e·rup'tive

E·ryn'gi·um
er'y·sip'e·las
—am'bu·lans'
—bul·lo'sum
—chron'i·cum
—dif·fu'sum
—glab'rum
—med·i·ca·men·to'sum
—mi'grans'
—per'stans'
er'y·si·pel'a·tous
er'y·sip'e·loid'
Er'y·sip'e·lo·thrix'
—in·sid'i·o'sa
e·rys'i·phake'
er'y·the'ma
—ab ig'ne'
—an'nu·lar'e' cen·trif'u·
  gum
—ar·thrit'i·cum ep'i·dem'i·
  cum
—bru·cel'lum
—bul·lo'sum
—ca·lo'ri·cum
—chron'i·cum mi'grans'
—chronicum migrans
  Af·ze'li·us
—cir'ci·na'tum
—el'e·va'tum di·u'ti·num
—en·dem'i·cum
—ep'i·dem'i·cum
—fig'u·ra'tum per'stans'
—fu'gax'
—gan'gre·no'sum
—glu'te·a'le'
—gy·ra'tum mi'grans'
—hy'per·e'mi·cum
—in·du'ra·ti'vum
—in'du·ra'tum
—in·fec'ti·o'sum
—in'ter·tri'go
—i'ris
—mar'gi·na'tum
—mi'grans'
—mul'ti·for'me'
—no·do'sum
—nu'chae'
—pal·mar'e' he·red'i·tar'i·um
—pap'u·la'tum
—par'a·lyt'i·cum
—per'ni·o'
—per'stans'
—punc·ta'tum

—scar'la·ti'ni·for'me'
—sim'plex'
—simplex gy·ra'tum
—so·lar'e'
—tox'i·cum ne'o·na·to'rum
—trau·mat'i·cum
—tu·ber'cu·la'tum
—ur'ti·cans'
—ven'e·na'tum
—ve·sic'u·lo'sum
er'y·the'ma·toid'
er'y·the'ma·tous
er'y·the'moid'
er'y·ther·mal'gi·a
er'y·thral'gi·a
er'y·thras'ma
e·ryth're·de'ma
er'y·thre'mi·a
er'y·thre'mic
er'y·thre'moid'
Er'y·thri'na
e·ryth'rism
er'y·thris'tic
er'y·thrite'
e·ryth'ri·tol'
e·ryth'ri·tyl
e·ryth'ro·blast'
e·ryth'ro·blas·te'mi·a
e·ryth'ro·blas'tic
e·ryth'ro·blas·to'ma
   pl. -mas *or* -ma·ta
e·ryth'ro·blas·to·pe'ni·a
e·ryth'ro·blas·to'sis *pl.* -ses'
   —fe·ta'lis
   —ne'o·na·to'rum
e·ryth'ro·blas·tot'ic
e·ryth'ro·chlo·ro'pi·a
e·ryth'ro·chlo·rop'si·a
e·ryth'ro·chlo'ro·py
e·ryth'ro·chro'mi·a
er'y·throc'la·sis
e·ryth'ro·clas'tic
e·ryth'ro·conte'
e·ryth'ro·cu'prein
e·ryth'ro·cy·a'no·sis
   pl. -ses'
e·ryth'ro·cyte'
e·ryth'ro·cy·the'mi·a
e·ryth'ro·cyt'ic
e·ryth'ro·cy'to·blast'
e·ryth'ro·cy·tol'y·sin
e·ryth'ro·cy·tol'y·sis
   pl. -ses'

e·ryth'ro·cy·tom'e·ter
e·ryth'ro·cy·tom'e·try
e·ryth'ro·cy'to·op'so·nin
e·ryth'ro·cy'to·pe'ni·a
e·ryth'ro·cy'to·poi·e'sis
   pl. -ses'
e·ryth'ro·cy'to·poi·et'ic
e·ryth'ro·cy'tor·rhex'is
e·ryth'ro·cy·tos'chi·sis
e·ryth'ro·cy·to'sis *pl.* -ses'
   —meg'a·lo·splen'i·ca
e·ryth'ro·cy'to·trop'ic
e·ryth'ro·de·gen'er·a·tive
e·ryth'ro·der'ma
   —des·quam'a·ti'vum
   —ich'thy·o·si·for'me'
      con·gen'i·tum
   —mac'u·lo'sa per'stans'
   —pso·ri·at'i·cum
e·ryth'ro·der·mi·a
e·ryth'ro·dex'trin
e·ryth'ro·don'ti·a
e·ryth'ro·gen
e·ryth'ro·gen'e·sis *pl.* -ses'
e·ryth'ro·gen'ic
e·ryth'ro·gone'
e·ryth'ro·go'ni·um
er'y·throid'
e·ryth'ro·ker'a·to·der'mi·a
e·ryth'ro·ki·net'ics
er'y·throl'
e·ryth'ro·leu·ke'mi·a
e·ryth'ro·leu·ko·blas·to'sis
e·ryth'ro·leu·ko'sis *pl.* -ses'
e·ryth'ro·leu'ko·throm·bo·
      cy·the'mi·a
er'y·throl'y·sin
er'y·throl'y·sis *pl.* -ses'
e·ryth'ro·ma'ni·a
e·ryth'ro·me·lal'gi·a
e·ryth'ro·me'li·a
er'y·throm'e·ter
e·ryth'ro·my'cin
e·ryth'ro·my'e·lo'sis
   pl. -ses'
er'y·thron'
e·ryth'ro·ne'o·cy·to'sis
   pl. -ses'
e·ryth'ro·pe'ni·a
e·ryth'ro·phage'
e·ryth'ro·pha'gi·a
e·ryth'ro·phag'o·cy·to'sis
   pl. -ses'

e·ryth'ro·phe·re'sis *pl.* -ses'
e·ryth'ro·phil'
er'yth·roph'i·lous
e·ryth'ro·phle'ine'
e·ryth'ro·pho'bi·a
e·ryth'ro·phore'
e·ryth'ro·phose'
er'y·thro'pi·a
e·ryth'ro·pla'si·a of
   Quey·rat'
e·ryth'ro·plas'tid
e·ryth'ro·poi·e'sis *pl.* -ses'
e·ryth'ro·poi·et'ic
e·ryth'ro·poi·e'tin
e·ryth'ro·pros'o·pal'gi·a
er'y·throp'si·a
er'y·throp'sin
e·ryth'ror·rhex'is
er'y·throse'
   —per'i·buc·ca'le pig'men·
      taire'
e·ryth'ro·sed'i·men·ta'tion
e·ryth'ro·sin
e·ryth'ro·sin'o·phil'
er'y·thro'sis *pl.* -ses'
e·ryth'ro·sta'sis *pl.* -ses'
e·ryth'ro·tox'in
er'y·throx'y·lon'
e·ryth'ru·lose'
er'y·thru'ri·a
Es'bach'
   —method
   —reagent
es·cape', -caped', -cap'ing
es·cap'ism
es'char'
es·cha·ro'sis
es·cha·rot'ic
Esch'e·rich'i·a
   —co'li'
es·chro·la'li·a
es·cor'cin
es·cu·le'tin
es·cu'lin
es·cutch'eon
es·er'a·mine'
es·er'i·dine'
es·er'ine'
Es'march'
   —bandage
   —operation
   —tourniquet
es'mo·lol'

e·sod'ic
es'o·eth'moi·di'tis
es'o·gas·tri'tis
e·soph'a·gal'gi·a
e·soph'a·ge'al
e·soph'a·gec·ta'si·a
e·soph'a·gec'ta·sis *pl.* -ses'
e·soph'a·gec'to·my
e·soph'a·gism
e·soph'a·gis'mus
e·soph'a·gi'tis
e·soph'a·go·bron'chi·al
e·soph'a·go·cele'
e·soph'a·go·du'o·de·nos'-
     to·my
e·soph'a·go·dyn'i·a
e·soph'a·go·en'ter·os'to·my
e·soph'a·go·e·soph'a·gos'-
     to·my
e·soph'a·go·gas'trec'to·my
e·soph'a·go·gas'tric
e·soph'a·go·gas'tro·du'o·
     de·nos'co·py
e·soph'a·go·gas'tro·plas'ty
e·soph'a·go·gas'tro·scope'
e·soph'a·go·gas'tros'co·py
e·soph'a·go·gas·tros'to·my
e·soph'a·go·gram'
e·soph'a·gog'ra·phy
e·soph'a·go·hi·a'tal
e·soph'a·go·je'ju·nos'to·my
e·soph'a·go·lar'yn·gec'-
     to·my
e·soph'a·go·ma·la'ci·a
e·soph'a·gom'e·ter
e·soph'a·go·my·co'sis
     pl. -ses'
e·soph'a·go·my·ot'o·my
e·soph'a·gop'a·thy
e·soph'a·go·pha·ryn'ge·al
e·soph'a·go·plas'ty
e·soph'a·go·pli·ca'tion
e·soph'a·gop·to'sis *pl.* -ses'
e·soph'a·go·res'pi·ra·to'ry
e·soph'a·go·sal'i·var'y
e·soph'a·go·scope'
e·soph'a·gos'co·py
e·soph'a·go·spasm
e·soph'a·go·ste·no'sis
     pl. -ses'
e·soph'a·gos'to·ma
e·soph'a·go·sto·mi'a·sis
     pl. -ses'

e·soph'a·gos'to·my
   —ex·ter'na
   —in·ter'na
e·soph'a·go·tome'
e·soph'a·got'o·my
e·soph'a·go·tra'che·al
e·soph'a·gus *pl.* -gi'
e·soph'o·gram'
es'o·pho'ri·a
es'o·phor'ic
es'o·tro'pi·a
es·pun'di·a
es'sence
es·sen'tial
Es'ser inlay graft
Es'sick cell band
es'ter
es'ter·ase'
es·ter'i·fi·ca'tion
es·ter'i·fy', -fied', -fy'ing
es·the'ma·tol'o·gy
es·the'si·a
es·the'si·ol'o·gy
es·the'si·om'e·ter
es·the'si·om'e·try
es·the'si·o·neu'ro·blas·to'-
     ma *pl.* -mas *or* -ma·ta
es·the'si·o·neu'ro·ep'i·the'-
     li·o'ma *pl.* -mas *or* -ma·ta
es·the'si·o·neu·ro'ma
     pl. -mas *or* -ma·ta
es·the'si·o·phys'i·ol'o·gy
es'the·sod'ic
es·thet'ic
es'thi·om'e·ne
es'ti·mate'
es'ti·ma'tion
es'ti·val
es'ti·va'tion
es'ti·vo-au·tum'nal
Est'lan'der operation
es'to·late'
es'tra·di·ol'
es'trane
es'tra·zi·nol'
es·tri'a·sis *pl.* -ses'
es'trin
es'trin·i·za'tion
es'tri·ol'
es'tro·gen
es'tro·gen'ic
es'trone'
es·tro'pi·pate'

es'trous
es'tru·al
es·tru·a'tion
es'trus
es'y·late'
et'a·fed'rine'
é·tat'
   —la·cu'naire'
   —ma·me·lon·ne'
   —mar·bre'
etch
eth'a·cry'nate'
eth'a·cry'nic
e·tham'bu·tol'
e·tham'i·van'
e·tham'syl·ate'
eth'a·nal'
eth'ane'
eth'a·no'ic
eth'a·nol'
eth'a·nol'a·mine'
eth'a·nol'ism
eth'a·ver'ine'
eth·chlor'vy·nol'
eth'ene'
eth'e·noid'
eth'e·none'
e'ther
e·the're·al
e·ther'i·fi·ca'tion
e·ther·i·za'tion
eth'i·cal
eth'i·cal'i·ty
eth'i·cal·ly
eth'i·cal·ness
eth'ics
eth'i·dene'
eth'i·nam'ate'
eth'ine'
e·thi'nyl *var. of* ethynyl
e·thi'on·a·mide'
e·thi'o·nine'
e·this'ter·one'
eth'mo·car·di'tis
eth'mo·ceph'a·lus *pl.* -li'
eth'mo·fron'tal
eth'moid'
eth'moi·dal
eth'moid·ec'to·my
eth'moid·i'tis
eth'moid·ot'o·my
eth'mo·lac'ri·mal
eth'mo·max'il·lar'y

eth′mo·na′sal
eth′mo·pal′a·tal
eth′mo·sphe′noid′
eth′mo·tur′bi·nal
eth′mo·vo′mer·ine
eth′nic
eth′no·graph′ic *or*
  eth′no·graph′i·cal
eth·nog′ra·phy
eth′no·log′ic *or*
  eth′no·log′i·cal
eth·nol′o·gy
eth′o·caine
eth′o·hep′ta·zine′
eth′o·hex′a·di′ol′
e·thol′o·gy
eth′o·nam′
eth′o·pro′pa·zine′
eth′o·sux′i·mide′
eth′o·to′in
eth·ox′a·zene′
eth·ox′y
eth′ox·zol′a·mide′
eth′y·benz·tro′pine′
eth′yl
eth′yl·al′de·hyde′
eth′yl·ate′
eth′yl·a′tion
eth′yl·cel′lu·lose′
eth′yl·ene′
eth′yl·ene·di′a·mine′
eth′yl·ene·di′a·mine·tet′ra·
  a·ce′tic
eth′yl·e′nic
eth′yl·e·phed′rine
eth′yl·es′tren·ol′
eth′yl·hy′dro·cu′pre·ine′
eth′yl·i·dene′
eth′yl·mor′phine′
eth′yl·nor·ep′i·neph′rine
eth′yl·stib′a·mine′
eth′yne′
e·thy′ner·one′
e·thy′no·di′ol′
e·thy′nyl *also* ethinyl
e·thy′nyl·es′tra·di·ol′
e′ti·o·cho·lan′o·lone′
e′ti·o·la′tion
e′ti·o·log′ic
e′ti·o·log′i·cal
e′ti·ol′o·gy
e′ti·o·path′o·gen′e·sis
  pl. -ses′

e′ti·o·por′phy·rin
e′to·do′lac
e·tret′i·nate′
e·trot′o·my
Eu′bac·te′ri·a′les′
eu·bac·te′ri·um *pl.* -ri·a
eu·bi·ot′ics
eu′caine′
eu·ca·lyp′tol′
eu·ca·lyp′tus *pl.* -ti
eu·cat′ro·pine′
Eu·ces·to′da
eu·chlor·hy′dri·a
eu·cho′li·a
eu·chro·mat′ic
eu·chro′ma·tin
eu·chro′ma·top′si·a
eu·chro′ma·top′sy
eu·chro′mo·some′
eu·cra′si·a
eu′di·e·mor′rhy·sis
eu′di·om′e·ter
eu′di·om′e·try
eu·dip′si·a
eu·es·the′si·a
eu·gen′ic
eu·gen′ics
eu′ge·nol′
Eu·gle′na
eu·glob′u·lin
eu·gnath′ic
eu·gly·ce′mi·a
eu·gon′ic
eu·kar′y·on′
eu·kar′y·ote′
eu·kar′y·ot′ic
eu·ker′a·tin
eu·ki·ne′si·a
eu·ki·ne′sis
eu·lam′i·nate′
Eu′len·burg′ disease
eu·me′tri·a
eu·mor′phic
Eu′my·ce′tes′
eu·noi′a
eu′nuch
eu′nuch·ism
eu′nuch·oid′
eu′nuch·oid·ism
eu·pan′cre·a·tism
eu′par·al
eu·pa·to′rin
eu·pep′si·a

eu·pep′tic
eu·pho′ni·a
Eu·phor′bi·a pil′u·lif′er·a
eu′pho·ret′ic
eu·pho′ri·a
eu·pho′ri·ant
eu·phor′ic
eu·phys′i·o·log′ic
eu·plas′tic
eu′ploid′
eu′ploi′dy
eup·ne′a
eu·prac′tic
eu′prax′i·a
eu′pro·cin
Eu·proc′tis chrys·or·rhoe′a
eu·py′rene′
eu·rhyth′mi·a
eu·ro·pis′o·ceph′a·lus
  pl. -li′
eu·ro′pi·um
eu′ro·pro·ceph′a·lus *pl.* -li′
Eu·ro′ti·a′les
eu′ry·ce·phal′ic
eu′ry·ceph′a·lous
eu′ry·cne′mic
eu′ryg·nath′ic
eu′ryg·na′thism
eu′ryg·na′thous
eu′ry·on′
eu′ry·so·mat′ic
eu′ry·ther′mal
eu′ry·ther′mic
Eu·scor′pi·us i·tal′i·cus
eu·sta′chi·an
eu·sta′chi·um
eu·stron′gy·loid′
eu·sys′to·le
eu·tha·na′si·a
eu·then′ics
Eu·the′ri·a
eu·ther′mic
eu·thy′mic
eu·thy′roid′
eu·thy′roid·ism
eu·top′ic
Eu·tri·at′o·ma
Eu·trom·bic′u·la
eu·tro′phi·a
eu·troph′ic
eu′tro·phy
e·vac′u·ant
e·vac′u·ate′, -at′ed, -at′ing

e·vac'u·a'tion
e·vac'u·a'tor
e·vag'i·nate', -nat'ed, -nat'ing
e·vag'i·na'tion
ev'a·nes'cent
Ev'ans blue
e·ven·tra'tion
Ev'ers·busch' operation
e·ver'sion
e·vert'
e·ver'tor
ev'i·ra'tion
e·vis'cer·ate', -at'ed, -at'ing
e·vis'cer·a'tion
ev'o·ca'tion
ev'o·ca'tor
e·voke', e·voked', e·vok'ing
ev'o·lu'tion
ev'o·lu'tion·ar'y
e·vul'si·o'
e·vul'sion
E'wald node
Ew'art sign
E wave
Ew'ing
—sarcoma
—tumor
ex·ac'er·bate', -bat'ed, -bat'ing
ex·ac'er·ba'tion
ex'al·ta'tion
ex·am'i·na'tion
ex·am'ine, -ined, -in·ing
ex·am'in·ee'
ex·an'them
—su'bi·tum
ex·an·the'ma pl. -ma·ta or -mas
ex·an·the·mat'ic
ex·an·them'a·tous
ex'ar·tic'u·la'tion
ex'ca·la'tion
ex'ca·vate'
ex·ca·va'ti·o' pl. -va'ti·o'nes'
—dis·ci'
—pa·pil'lae' ner'vi' op'ti·ci'
—rec'to·u'ter·i'na
—rec'to·ves'i·ca'lis
—ves·i'co·u'ter·i'na
ex'ca·va'tion
ex'ca·va'tor
ex·cen'tric var. of eccentric

ex·cer'e·bra'tion
ex·cer'nent
ex'ci·mer
ex·cip'i·ent
ex·cise', -cised', -cis'ing
ex·ci'sion
ex·cit'a·bil'i·ty
ex·cit'a·ble
ex·ci'tant
ex'ci·ta'tion
ex·cit'a·to'ry
ex·cite', -cit'ed, -cit'ing
ex·cite'ment
ex·ci'to·mo'tor
ex·ci'tor
ex·ci'to·se·cre'to·ry
ex·ci'to·vas'cu·lar
ex'clave'
ex·clu'sion
ex·coch'le·a'tion
ex·con'ju·gant
ex·co'ri·ate', -at'ed, -at'ing
ex·co'ri·a'tion
ex'cre·ment
ex'cre·men'tal
ex'cre·men·ti'tious
ex·cres'cence
ex·cres'cent
ex·cre'ta
ex·crete', -cret'ed, -cret'ing
ex·cret'er
ex·cre'tion
ex'cre·to'ry
ex·cur'sion
ex·cur'sive
ex'cur·va'tion
ex'cur·va·ture
ex·cy'clo·pho'ri·a
ex·cy'clo·tro'pi·a
ex'cys·ta'tion
ex·ec'u·tant
ex'e·dens
ex'el·cy·mo'sis pl. -ses'
ex·e'mi·a
ex'en·ce·pha'li·a
ex'en·ce·phal'ic
ex'en·ceph'a·lus pl. -li'
ex'en·ceph'a·ly
ex·en'ter·ate', -at'ed, -at'ing
ex·en'ter·a'tion
ex·en'ter·a·tive
ex·en'ter·i'tis
ex'er·cise', -cised', -cis'ing

ex·er·cis'er
ex·er'e·sis pl. -ses'
ex·er'gon'ic
ex·er'tion
ex·er'tion·al
ex'fe·ta'tion
ex·flag'e·la'tion
ex·fo'li·ate', -at'ed, -at'ing
ex·fo'li·a'tion
ex·fo'li·a·tive
ex·ha·la'tion
ex·hale', -haled', -hal'ing
ex·haus'tion
ex·haus'tive
ex·hib'it
ex·hi·bi'tion
ex·hi·bi'tion·ism
ex·hi·bi'tion·ist
ex·hi·bi'tion·is'tic
ex·hil'a·rant
ex·hil'a·rate', -rat'ed, -rat'ing
ex·hil'a·ra'tion
ex·hu·ma'tion
ex·hume', -humed', -hum'ing
ex·is·ten'tial
ex·is·ten'tial·ism
ex'i·tus
Ex'ner plexus
ex'o·bi·ol'o·gy
ex'o·car'di·a
ex'o·car'di·ac'
ex'o·car'di·al
ex'o·cat'a·pho'ri·a
ex'oc·cip'i·tal
ex'o·cer'vi·cal
ex'o·cer'vix pl. -vi·ces' or -vix·es
ex'o·cho'ri·on' pl. -ri·a
ex'o·coe'lom
ex'o·coe·lom'ic
ex'o·co·li'tis
ex'o·crine
ex'o·cri·nol'o·gy
ex'o·cy·to'sis pl. -ses'
ex'o·de·ox'y·ri'bo·nu'cle·ase'
ex'o·de·vi·a'tion
ex'o·don'ti·a
ex'o·don'tics
ex'o·don'tist
ex'o·en'zyme'
ex'o·er'gic

ex'o·e·ryth'ro·cyt'ic
ex·og'a·mous
ex·og'a·my
ex'o·gas'tru·la
ex'o·gas'tru·la'tion
ex'o·ge·net'ic
ex'o·gen'ic
ex·og'e·nous (*derived from external causes*)
♦axogenous
ex'o·hys'ter·o·pex'y
ex'o·me·tri'tis
ex·om'pha·los
ex'o·nu'cle·ase'
ex'o·pep'ti·dase'
Ex'o·phi'a·la
ex'o·pho'ri·a
ex'o·phor'ic
ex'oph·thal'mic
ex'oph·thal·mom'e·ter
ex'oph·thal·mom'e·try
ex'oph·thal'mos
ex'o·phyt'ic
ex'o·plasm
ex'o·psy'chic
ex'o·se·ro'sis
ex'o·skel'e·ton
ex'os·mose'
ex'os·mo'sis
ex'os·mot'ic
ex'o·so'mes·the'si·a
ex'o·spore'
ex'o·spo'ri·um *pl.* -ia
ex·os'to·sec'to·my
ex·os'tosed'
ex·os'to'sis *pl.* -ses'
  —car'ti·la·gin'e·a
ex·os'tot'ic
ex'o·ther'mal
ex'o·ther'mic
ex'o·tox'ic
ex'o·tox'in
ex'o·tro'pi·a
ex'o·trop'ic
ex·pand'er
ex·pan'sile
ex·pan'sive
ex·pec'tan·cy
ex·pect'ant
ex·pec'to·rant
ex·pec'to·rate', -rat'ed, -rat'ing
ex·pec'to·ra'tion

ex·pel', -pelled', -pel'ling
ex·pe'ri·en'tial
ex·per'i·ment
ex·per'i·men'tal
ex·per'i·men·ta'tion
ex·pert'
ex'pi·ra'tion
ex·pi'ra·to'ry
ex·pire', -pired', -pir'ing
ex·plain'
ex'pla·na'tion
ex'plant'
ex·plic'it
ex·plode', -plod'ed, -plod'ing
ex'plo·ra'tion
ex·plo'ra·to'ry
ex·plore'
ex·plor'er
ex·plo'sion
ex·plo'sive
ex'po·nen'tial
ex·pose', -posed', -pos'ing
ex·po'sure
ex·press'
ex·pres'sion
ex·pres·siv'i·ty
ex·pres'sor
ex·pul'sion
ex·pul'sive
ex'quis·ite
ex'quis·ite·ly
ex·san'gui·nate', -nat'ed, -nat'ing
ex·san'gui·na'tion
ex·san'guine
ex·san·guin'i·ty
ex·sect'
ex·sec'tion
ex·sic'cant
ex·sic'cate', -cat'ed, -cat'ing
ex·sic·ca'tion
ex·sic'ca·tive
ex·sic'ca·tor
ex·sorp'tion
ex'stro·phy
ex'suf·fla'tion
ex'suf·fla'tor
ex·tend'er
ex·ten'sion
ex·ten'sor
  —car'pi ra'di·a'lis ac'ces·so'ri·us

  —carpi radialis brev'i·or'
  —carpi radialis brev'is
  —carpi radialis in'ter·me'·di·us
  —carpi radialis lon'gi·or'
  —carpi radialis lon'gus
  —carpi ul·nar'is
  —carpi ulnaris dig'i·ti' min'·i·mi'
  —coc·cyg'e·us
  —com·mu'nis pol'li·cis et in'di·cis
  —dig'i·ti' an'nu·lar'is
  —digiti me'di·i'
  —digiti min'i·mi'
  —digiti quin'ti' pro'pri·us
  —dig'i·to'rum
  —digitorum brev'is
  —digitorum brevis ma'nus
  —digitorum com·mu'nis
  —digitorum lon'gus
  —hal'lu·cis brev'is
  —hallucis lon'gus
  —hallucis pro'pri·us
  —in'di·cis
  —indicis pro'pri·us
  —os'sis met'a·car'pi' pol'li·cis
  —ossis met'a·tar'si' hal'lu·cis
  —pol'li·cis brev'is
  —pollicis lon'gus
  —pri'mi' in'ter·no'di·i' lon'gus hal'lu·cis
  —primi internodii pol'li·cis
  —se·cun'di' in'ter·no'di·i' pol'li·cis
ex·te'ri·or
ex·te'ri·or·ize'
ex·te'ri·or·i·za'tion
ex'tern'
ex·ter'nad'
ex·ter'nal
ex·ter'nal·i·za'tion
ex·ter'nal·ize', -ized', -iz'ing
ex'ter·o·cep'tive
ex'ter·o·cep'tor
ex'ter·o·fec'tive
ex·tinc'tion
ex·tin'guish
ex'tir·pate', -pat'ed, -pat'ing
ex'tir·pa'tion
Ex'ton

—and Rose test
—method
—quantitative reagent
—test
ex·tor'sion
ex'tra·ar·tic'u·lar
ex'tra·buc'cal
ex'tra·bul'bar
ex'tra·cap'su·lar
ex'tra·car'di·ac'
ex'tra·car'di·al
ex'tra·car'pal
ex'tra·cel'lu·lar
ex'tra·cer'e·bral
ex'tra·chro'mo·so'mal
ex'tra·cor'po·ral
ex'tra·cor·po're·al
ex'tra·cor·pus'cu·lar
ex'tra·cor'ti·co·spi'nal
ex'tra·cra'ni·al
ex·tract'*v.*
ex·tract'*n.*
ex·tract'a·ble
ex·tract'ant
ex·trac'tion
ex·trac'tive
ex·trac'tor
ex'tra·cys'tic
ex'tra·du'ral
ex'tra·em'bry·on'ic
ex'tra·ep'i·phys'e·al
ex'tra·e·ryth'ro·cyt'ic
ex'tra·e·soph'a·ge'al
ex'tra·fas'ci·al
ex'tra·gen'i·tal
ex'tra·gin'gi·val
ex'tra·he·pat'ic
ex'tra·lig'a·men'tous
ex'tra·mam'ma·ry
ex'tra·mas'toid·i'tis
ex'tra·med'ul·lar'y
ex'tra·mu'ral
ex'tra·ne'ous
ex'tra·nu'cle·ar
ex'tra·oc'u·lar
ex'tra·o'ral
ex'tra·os'se·ous
ex'tra·pa·ren'chy·mal
ex'tra·pel'vic
ex'tra·per'i·car'di·al
ex'tra·per'i·ne'al (*outside the perineum*)
♦*extraperitoneal*

ex'tra·per'i·os'te·al
ex'tra·per'i·to·ne'al (*outside the peritoneum*)
♦*extraperineal*
ex'tra·pla·cen'tal
ex'tra·pleu'ral
ex·trap'o·late', -lat'ed, -lat'ing
ex·trap'o·la'tion
ex'tra·pros·tat'ic
ex'tra·psy'chic
ex'tra·pul'mo·nar'y
ex'tra·py·ram'i·dal
ex'tra·rec'tus
ex'tra·re'nal
ex'tra·sen'so·ry
ex'tra·sphinc·ter'ic
ex'tra·spi'nal
ex'tra·sys'to·le
ex'tra·tho·rac'ic
ex'tra·thy·roi'dal
ex'tra·tu'bal
ex'tra·u'ter·ine
ex'tra·vag'i·nal
ex·trav'a·sate', -sat'ed, -sat'ing
ex·trav'a·sa'tion
ex'tra·vas'cu·lar
ex'tra·ven·tric'u·lar
ex'tra·ver'sion
ex'tra·vis'u·al
ex·tre'mis
ex·trem'i·tas *pl.* -trem'i·ta'tes'
—a·cro'mi·a'lis cla·vic'u·lae'
—anterior li·e'nis
—inferior
—inferior li·e'nis
—inferior re'nis
—inferior tes'tis
—posterior li·e'nis
—ster·na'lis cla·vic'u·lae'
—superior
—superior li·e'nis
—superior re'nis
—superior tes'tis
—tu·bar'i·a o·var'i·i'
—u'ter·i'na o·var'i·i'
ex·trem'i·ty
ex·trin'sic
ex'tro·gas'tru·la'tion
ex'tro·spec'tion

ex'tro·ver'sion
ex'tro·vert'
ex·trude', -trud'ed, -trud'ing
ex·tru'do·clu'sion
ex·tru'sion
ex·tu'bate', -bat'ed, -bat'ing
ex·tu·ba'tion
ex·u'ber·ance
ex·u'ber·ant
ex·u'date'
ex·u'da'tion
ex·u'da·tive
ex·ude', -ud'ed, -ud'ing
ex'um·bil'i·ca'tion
ex·u'vi·a'tion
eye
eye'ball'
eye'brow'
eye'cup'
eyed'ness
eye'glass'es
eye'ground'
eye'lash'
eye'lid'
eye'piece'
eye'point'
eye'sight'
eye'spot'
eye'strain'
eye'tooth'
eye'wash'

F

fa·bel'la *pl.* -lae'
Fa'ber anemia
Fab fragment
fab'ri·ca'tion
Fa·bri'cus-Mol'ler test
Fa'bry disease
fab·u'la'tion
face
face'bow'
face'-lift'
fac'et
fac'e·tec'tomy
fa'cial
fa·ci·a'lis
fa·ci·es' *pl.* fa·ci·es'
—ab·dom'i·na'lis
—anterior an'te·bra'chi·i'
—anterior bra'chi·i'

—anterior cor′ne•ae′
—anterior cru′ris
—anterior den′ti•um prae′-
mo•lar′i•um et mo•lar′-
i•um
—anterior fem′o•ris
—anterior glan′du•lae′
su′pra•re•na′lis
—anterior i′ri•dis
—anterior lat′er•a′lis
hu′mer•i′
—anterior len′tis
—anterior max•il′lae′
—anterior me′di•a′lis
hu′mer•i′
—anterior pal′pe•brar′um
—anterior pan•cre′a•tis
—anterior par′tis pe•tro′sae′
os′sis tem′po•ra′lis
—anterior pa•tel′lae′
—anterior pros′ta•tae′
—anterior py′ram′i•dis
os′sis tem′po•ra′lis
—anterior ra′di•i′
—anterior re′nis
—anterior ul′nae′
—an′ter•o•lat′er•a′lis car′ti•
lag′i•nis ar′y•te•noi′de•ae′
—ar•tic′u•lar′es′ in•fe′ri•o′-
res′ at•lan′tis
—articulares inferiores
ver′te•brae′
—articulares su•pe′ri•o′res′
ver′te•brae′
—ar•tic′u•lar′is
—articularis a•cro′mi•a′lis
cla•vic′u•lae′
—articularis a•cro′mi•i′
—articularis anterior ax′is
—articularis anterior
cal•ca′ne•i′
—articularis anterior
ep′i•stro′phe•i′
—articularis ar′y•tae•noi′-
de•a car′ti•lag′i•nis
cri•coi′de•ae′
—articularis ar′y•te•noi′de•a
car′ti•lag′i•nis
cri•coi′de•ae′
—articularis cal•ca′ne•a
anterior ta′li′
—articularis calcanea
me′di•a ta′li′

—articularis calcanea
posterior ta′li′
—articularis cap′i•tis
cos′tae′
—articularis capitis
fib′u•lae′
—articularis ca•pit′u•li′
cos′tae′
—articularis capituli
fib′u•lae′
—articularis car′pe•a ra′di•i′
—articularis car′ti•lag′i•nis
ar′y•tae•noi′de•ae′
—articularis cartilaginis
ar′y•te•noi′de•ae′
—articularis cu•boi′de•a
cal•ca′ne•i′
—articularis fib′u•lar′is
tib′i•ae′
—articularis inferior tib′i•ae′
—articularis mal′le•o•lar′is
fib′u•lae′
—articularis malleolaris
tib′i•ae′
—articularis me′di•a
cal•ca′ne•i′
—articularis na•vic′u•lar′is
ta′li′
—articularis os′sis
tem′po•ra′lis
—articularis os′si•um
—articularis pa•tel′lae′
—articularis posterior ax′is
—articularis posterior
cal•ca′ne•i′
—articularis posterior
ep′is•tro′phe•i′
—articularis ster•na′lis
cla•vic′u•lae′
—articularis superior
tib′i•ae′
—articularis ta•lar′is
anterior cal•ca′ne•i′
—articularis talaris me′di•a
cal•ca′ne•i′
—articularis talaris posterior
cal•ca′ne•i′
—articularis thy′re•oi′de•a
car′ti•lag′i•nis cri•coi′-
de•ae′
—articularis thy•roi′de•a
car′ti•lag′i•nis cri•coi′-
de•ae′

—articularis tu•ber′cu•li′
cos′tae′
—au•ric′u•lar′is
—auricularis os′sis il′i•i′
—auricularis ossis il′i•um
—auricularis ossis sa′cri′
—bo•vi′na
—buc•ca′lis den′tis
—cer′e•bra′lis
—cerebralis a′lae′ mag′nae′
—cerebralis alae ma•jo′ris
—cerebralis os′sis fron•ta′lis
—cerebralis ossis pa•ri•e•ta′-
lis
—cerebralis par′tis squa•
mo′sae′ os′sis tem′po•ra′-
lis
—cerebralis squa′mae′
tem′po•ra′is
—co′li•ca li•e′nis
—con•tac′tus den′tis
—con•vex′a cer′e•bri′
—cos•ta′lis
—costalis pul•mo′nis
—costalis scap′u•lae′
—di•a•phrag•mat′i•ca
—diaphragmatica cor′dis
—diaphragmatica hep′a•tis
—diaphragmatica li•e′nis
—diaphragmatica pul•mo′-
nis
—dis•ta′lis den′tis
—dor•sa′les′ dig′i•to′rum
ma′nus
—dorsales digitorum pe′dis
—dor•sa′lis an′ti•bra′chi•i′
—dorsalis os′sis sa′cri′
—dorsalis ra′di•i′
—dorsalis scap′u•lae′
—dorsalis ul′nae′
—ex•ter′na os′sis fron•ta′lis
—externa ossis pa•ri•e•ta′lis
—fa′ci•a′lis den′tis
—fib′u•lar′is cru′ris
—fron•ta′lis
—frontalis os′sis fron•ta′lis
—gas′tri•ca
—gastrica li•e′nis
—glu′te•a os′sis il′i•i′
—hip′po•crat′i•ca
—inferior cer′e•bri′
—inferior hem′is•phae′ri•i′
cer′e•bel′li′

—inferior hem'is·phe'ri·i' cer'e·bel'li'
—inferior hemispherii cer'e·bri'
—inferior hep'a·tis
—inferior lin'guae'
—inferior mes'en·ceph'a·li'
—inferior pan·cre'a·tis
—inferior par'tis pe·tro'sae' os'sis tem'po·ra'lis
—inferior py·ram'i·dis os'sis tem'po·ra'lis
—in'fer·o·lat'er·a'lis pros'ta·tae'
—in'fra·tem'po·ra'lis max·il'lae'
—in'ter·lo·bar'es' pul'mo'-nis
—in·ter'na os'sis fron·ta'lis
—interna ossis pa·ri'e·ta'lis
—in·tes'ti·na'lis
—intestinalis u'ter·i'
—la'bi·a'lis den'tis
—lat'er·a'les' dig'i·to'rum ma'nus
—laterales digitorum pe'dis
—lat'er·a'lis
—lateralis bra'chi·i'
—lateralis cru'ris
—lateralis den'ti·um in'ci·si·vo'rum et ca'ni·no'rum
—lateralis fem'o·ris
—lateralis fib'u·lae'
—lateralis os'sis zy'go·mat'-i·ci'
—lateralis o·var'i·i'
—lateralis ra'di·i'
—lateralis tes'tis
—lateralis tib'i·ae'
—le'on·ti'na
—lin'gua'lis
—lingualis den'tis
—lu·na'ta ac'e·tab'u·li'
—ma·lar'is
—malaris os'sis zy·go·mat'-i·ci'
—mal'le·o·lar'is
—malleolaris lat'er·a'lis ta'li'
—malleolaris me'di·a'lis ta'li'
—mas'ti·ca·to'ri·a den'tis
—max'il·lar'is

—maxillaris a'lae' ma·jo'ris
—maxillaris lam'i·nae' per'-pen·dic'u·lar'is os'sis pal'a·ti'ni'
—maxillaris par'tis per'-pen·dic'u·lar'is os'sis pal'a·ti'ni'
—me'di·a'les' dig'i·to'rum ma'nus
—mediales digitorum pe'dis
—me'di·a'lis
—medialis bra'chi·i'
—medialis car'ti·lag'i·nis ar'y·te·noi'de·ae'
—medialis cer'e·bri'
—medialis cru'ris
—medialis den'ti·um in'ci·si·vo'rum et ca'ni·no'rum
—medialis fem'o·ris
—medialis fib'u·lae'
—medialis hem'is·phe'ri·i' cer'e·bri'
—medialis o·var'i·i'
—medialis pul·mo'nis
—medialis tes'tis
—medialis tib'i·ae'
—medialis ul'nae'
—me'di·as·ti·na'lis
—mediastinalis pul·mo'nis
—me'si·a'lis den'tis
—my'o·path'i·ca
—na·sa'lis lam'i·nae' ho'ri·zon·ta'lis os'sis pal'a·ti'ni'
—nasalis laminae per'pen·dic'u·lar'is os'sis pal'a·ti'ni'
—nasalis max·il'lae'
—nasalis par'tis ho'ri·zon·ta'lis os'sis pal'a·ti'ni'
—nasalis partis per'pen·dic'u·lar'is os'sis pal'a·ti'ni'
—oc'clu·sa'lis den'tis
—or'bi·ta'lis a'lae' mag'nae'
—orbitalis alae ma·jo'ris
—orbitalis max·il'lae'
—orbitalis os'sis fron·ta'lis
—orbitalis ossis zy'go·mat'-i·ci'
—os'se·a
—(ossea) cra'ni·i'
—pal'a·ti'na

—palatina lam'i·nae' ho'ri·zon·ta'lis os'sis pal'a·ti'ni'
—palatina par'tis ho'ri·zon·ta'lis os'sis pal'a·ti'ni'
—pal·mar'es' dig'i·to'rum ma'nus
—pa·ri'e·ta'lis
—parietalis os'sis parietalis
—pat'el·lar'is
—patellaris fem'o·ris
—pel'vi·na
—pelvina os'sis sa'cri'
—plan·tar'es' dig'i·to'rum pe'dis
—pop·lit'e·a
—posterior an'te·bra'chi·i'
—posterior bra'chi·i'
—posterior car'ti·lag'i·nis ar'y·te·noi'de·ae'
—posterior cor'ne·ae'
—posterior cru'ris
—posterior den'ti·um prae·mo'lar'i·um et mo·lar'i·um
—posterior fem'o·ris
—posterior fib'u·lae'
—posterior glan'du·lae' su'pra·re·na'lis
—posterior hep'a·tis
—posterior hu'mer·i'
—posterior i'ri·dis
—posterior len'tis
—posterior pal'pe·brar'um
—posterior pan·cre'a·tis
—posterior par'tis pe·tro'-sae' os'sis tem'po·ra'lis
—posterior pros'ta·tae'
—posterior py·ram'i·dis os'sis tem'po·ra'lis
—posterior ra'di·i'
—posterior re'nis
—posterior tib'i·ae'
—posterior ul'nae'
—pul'mo·na'lis cor'dis
—ra'di·a'les' dig'i·to'rum ma'nus
—re'na'lis glan'du·lae' su'pra·re·na'lis
—renalis li·e'nis
—sa'cro·pel·vi'na os'sis il'i·i'

—sphe′no•max′il•lar′is
—sphenomaxillaris a′lae′
mag′nae′
—ster′no•cos′ta′lis cor′dis
—superior he′mis•phae′ri•i′
cer′e•bel′li′
—superior he′mis•phe′ri•i′
cer′e•bel′li′
—superior hep′a•tis
—superior troch′le•ae′ ta′li′
—su′per•o•lat′er•a′lis
cer′e•bri′
—sym•phys′e•os′ os′sis
pu′bis
—sym•phys′i•a′lis
—tem′po•ra′lis a′lae′
mag′nae′
—temporalis alae ma•jo′ris
—temporalis os′sis fron•ta′-
lis
—temporalis ossis zy′go•
mat′i•ci′
—temporalis par′tis
squa•mo′sae
—temporalis squa′mae′
tem′po•ra′lis
—tib′i•a′lis cru′ris
—ul•nar′es′ dig′i•to′rum
ma′nus
—u′re•thra′lis pe′nis
—ves′i•ca′lis u′ter•i′
—ves•tib′u•lar′is den′tis
—vis•ce•ra′lis hep′a•tis
—visceralis li•e′nis
—vo•lar′es′ dig′i•to′rum
ma′nus
—vo•lar′is
—volaris an′ti•bra′chi•i′
—volaris ra′di•i′
—volaris ul′nae′
fa•cil′i•ta′tion
fa•cil′i•ty
fac′ing
fa•ci•o•bra′chi•al
fa•ci•o•cer′vi•cal
fa•ci•o•lin′gual
fa•ci•o•plas′ty
fa•ci•o•ple′gic
fa•ci•o•scap′u•lo•hu′mer•al
fa•ci•o•ste•no′sis *pl.* -ses′
F-ac′tin
fac•ti′tious
fac′tor

fac•to′ri•al
fac′ul•ta′tive
fac′ul•ty
faex
—me•dic′i•na′lis
Fah′rae•us sedimentation
test
Fahr disease
Fahr′en•heit′
fail′ure
faint
Fair′ley pigment
Fa•jer′sztajn′
—crossed sciatic sign
—test
fal′cate′
fal′cial
fal′ci•form′
fal′cine′
fal•cip′a•rum ma•lar′i•a
fal′cu•la
fal′cu•lar
fal•lo′pi•an
Fal•lot′
—pen•tal′o•gy
—te•tral′o•gy
fall′-out′
Falls test
Fal•ret′ disease
false
fal′si•fi•ca′tion
fal′si•fy
falx *pl.* fal′ces′
—ap′o•neu•rot′i•ca
—cer′e•bel′li′
—cer′e•bri′
—in′gui•na′lis
—sep′ti′
fa′mes′
fa•mil′i•al
fam′i•ly
fam′ine
fam′o•tide′
fa•mot′i•dine′
Fan•co′ni
—anemia
—syndrome
fang
fan′go
Fan′ni•a
fan′ning
fan′ta•size′
fan′ta•sy

fan′tri•done′
Fa′ra•beuf′
—elevator
—triangle
far′ad′
far′a•day′
Far′a•day′ shield
fa•rad′ic
far′a•dim′e•ter
far′a•dism
far′a•di•za′tion
far′a•dize′
far′a•do•con′trac•til′i•ty
far′a•do•mus′cu•lar
far′a•do•ther′a•py
Far′ber disease
far′cy
fa•ri′na
far′i•na′ceous
Far′ley, St. Clair′, and
Rei′sin•ger method
Far′mer and Abt method
far′ne•sol′
far′ne•syl
Farre white line
far′-sight′ed
far′-sight′ed•ness
fas′ci•a *pl.* -ae′ *or* -as
—an′te•bra′chi•i′
—ax′il•lar′is
—bra′chi•i′
—buc′co•pha•ryn′ge•a
—bul′bi′ (Te′no′ni)
—cer′vi•ca′lis
—clav′i•pec′to•ra′lis
—cli•to′ri•dis
—col′li′
—co′ra•co•cla•vic′u•lar′is
—cre′mas•te′ri•ca
—cri•bro′sa
—cru′ris
—den•ta′ta hip′po•cam′pi′
—di′a•phrag′ma•tis pel′vis
inferior
—diaphragmatis pelvis
superior
—diaphragmatis u′ro•gen′i•
ta′lis inferior
—diaphragmatis urogenita-
lis superior
—dor•sa′lis ma′nus
—dorsalis pe′dis
—en′do•tho•ra′ci•ca

—i·li′a·ca
—il′i·o·pec·tin′e·a
—in′fra·spi·na′ta
—la′ta
—lum′bo·dor·sa′lis
—lu·na′ta
—mas·se′ter′i·ca
—nu′chae′
—ob′tu·ra·to′ri·a
—par·o·tid′e·a
—par′o·tid′e·o·mas′se·ter′i·ca
—pec·tin′e·a
—pec′to·ra′lis
—pel′vis
—pelvis pa·ri′e·ta′lis
—pelvis vis′ce·ra′lis
—pe′nis
—penis pro·fun′da
—penis su′per·fi′ci·a′lis
—per′i·ne′i′ su′per·fi′ci·a′lis
—pha·ryn′go·bas′i·lar′is
—phren′i·co·pleu·ra′lis
—prae·ver′te·bra′lis
—pros′ta·tae′
—sper·mat′i·ca ex·ter′na
—spermatica in·ter′na
—sub·per′i·to·ne·a′lis
—sub·scap′u·lar′is
—su′per·fi′ci·a′lis
—superficialis per′i·ne′i′
—su′pra·spi·na′ta
—tem′po·ra′lis
—tho′ra·co·lum·ba′lis
—trans′ver·sa′lis
fas′ci·ae′
—mus′cu·lar′es′ bul′bi′
—musculares oc′u·li′
—or′bi·ta′les′
fas′ci·al
fas′ci·a·tome′
fas′ci·cle
fas·cic′u·lar
fas·cic′u·late′
fas·cic′u·la′tion
fas·cic′u·li′
—cor′po·ris res′ti·for′mis
—cor′ti·co·tha·lam′i·ci′
—in·ter′seg′men·ta′les′
—lon′gi·tu′di·na′les′
lig′a·men′ti′
cru′ci·for′mis at·lan′tis
—longitudinales pon′tis
—ma·mil′lo·teg′men·ta′les′

—pe·dun′cu·lo·mam′il·lar′es′
—pro′pri·i′ me·dul′lae′
spi·na′lis
—py′ram′i·da′les′
—ru′bro·re·tic′u·lar′es′
—thal′a·mo·cor′ti·ca′les′
—trans·ver′si′ ap′o·neu·ro′-
sis pal·mar′is
—transversi aponeurosis
plan·tar′is
fas·cic′u·li′tis
fas·cic′u·lus pl. -li′
—anterior pro′pri·us
(Flech′sig·i′)
—an′ter·o·lat′er·a′lis su′-
per·fi′ci·a′lis (Go·wer′si′)
—a′tri·o·ven·tric′u·lar′is
—cer′e·bel′lo·spi·na′lis
—cer′e·bro·spi·na′lis
anterior
—cerebrospinalis lat′er·a′lis
—cu′ne·a′tus (Bur·da′chi′)
—cuneatus me·dul′lae′
ob′lon·ga′tae′
—cuneatus medullae
spi·na′lis
—dor′so·lat′er·a′lis
—grac′i·lis me·dul′lae′
ob′lon·ga′tae′
—gracilis medullae
spi·na′lis
—in′ter·fas·cic′u·lar′is
—lat′er·a′lis plex′us
bra′chi·a′lis
—lateralis pro′pri·us
—lon′gi·tu′di·na′lis
dor·sa′lis
—longitudinalis dorsalis
me·dul′lae′ ob′lon·ga′tae′
—longitudinalis dorsalis
mes′en·ceph′a·li′
—longitudinalis dorsalis
pon′tis
—longitudinalis inferior
cer′e·bri′
—longitudinalis me·di·a′lis
—longitudinalis medialis
me·dul′lae′ ob′lon·ga′tae′
—longitudinalis medialis
mes′en·ceph′a·li′
—longitudinalis medialis
pon′tis
—longitudinalis superior

—ma·mil′lo·teg′men·ta′lis
—ma·mil′lo·tha·lam′i·cus
—me′di·a′lis plex′us
bra′chi·a′lis
—ob·li′quus pon′tis
—of Türck
—posterior plex′us
bra′chi·a′lis
—pro′pri·us
—ret′ro·flex′us
—sem′i·lu·nar′is
—sep′to·mar′gi·na′lis
—sol′i·tar′i·us
—sub′cal·lo′sus
—thal′a·mo·mam′il·lar′is
—un′ci·na′tus
fas′ci·ec′to·my
fas′ci·i′tis
fas′ci·num
fas·ci·od′e·sis pl. -ses′
fas·ci′o·la pl. -lae′
—ci·ne′re·a
Fas·ci′o·la
—gi·gan′ti·ca
—he·pat′i·ca
fas·ci′o·lar
fas·ci·o·li′a·sis pl. -ses′
fas·ci·o·lop′si·a·sis
Fas·ci·o·lop′sis
—bus′ki′
fas·ci·o·plas′ty
fas·ci·or′rha·phy
fas·ci·o·scap′u·lo·hu′-
mer·al
fas·ci·ot′o·my
fast
fast′-Fou′ri·er′ transform
fas·tid′i·ous
fas·tid′i·um
fas·tig′i·al
fas·tig′i·o·bul′bar
fas·tig′i·um
fast′ness
fat
fa′tal
fa·tal′i·ty
fat′i·ga·bil′i·ty
fat′i·ga·ble
fa·tigue′, -tigued′, -tigu′ing
fat′ty
fau′ces′
fau′cial
fau′na pl. -nas or -nae′

Faust method
fa·ve′o·late′
fa·ve′o·lus *pl.* -li′
fa′vid
fa′vi·des′
fa′vism
Fa′vre disease
fa′vus
Fa′zi·o-Londe′ atrophy
fear
fea′ture
feb′ri·cide′
fe·bric′u·la
feb′ri·fa′cient
fe·brif′ic
fe·brif′u·gal
feb′ri·fuge′
feb′rile
fe′bris
fe′cal
fe·ca·lith′
fe′cal·oid′
fe·ca·lo′ma *pl.* -mas *or* -ma·ta
fe·cal·u′ri·a
fe′ces′
Fech′ner law
fec′u·la *pl.* -lae′
fec′u·lence
fec′u·lent
fe′cund
fe′cun·date′, -dat′ed, -dat′ing
fe′cun·da′tion
fe·cun′di·ty
Fe·de·ri′ci sign
Fe′de-Ri′ga disease
feed′back′
feed′ing
feel, felt, feel′ing
Feer disease
Feh′ling
  —reagent
  —test
Feil′-Klip′pel syndrome
fel
fe′line′
fel·la′ti·o′
fel·la′tion
fel′la·tor
fel′la·trice′
Fell′-O′Dwy′er method
fel′low
fe·lod′i·pine′
fel′on

fe·lo′ni·ous
fel′o·ny
felt
felt′work′
Fel′ty syndrome
fel′y·pres′sin
fe′male′
fem′i·nine
fem′i·ni·za′tion
fem′i·nize′, -nized′, -niz′ing
fem′o·ral
fem′o·ro·cele′
fem′o·ro·il′i·ac′
fem′o·ro·pop′lit′e·al
fem′o·ro·tib′i·al
fem′to·chem′is·try
fem′to·li′ter
fe′mur *pl.* fem′o·ra
fen·al′a·mide′
fen′a·mole′
fen·clo′nine′
fe·nes′tra *pl.* -trae′
  —coch′le·ae′
  —o·va′lis
  —ro·tun′da
  —ves·tib′u·li′
fe·nes′tral
fen′es·trate′
fen′es·tra′tion
fen·eth′yl·line′
fen·flu′ra·mine′
fen′i·mide′
fen′met′ra·mide′
fen′nel
fe′no·pro′fen
fen′o·ter′ol′
fen′ta·nyl
Fen′wick disease
fen·yr′i·pol′
fer′-de-lance′
Fé′ré·ol′ node
fer′ment *n.*
fer·ment′ *v.*
fer′men·ta′tion
fer′men·ta·tive
fer′mi
fer′mi·um
fern
fern′ing
fer′rat′ed
fer′re·dox′in
fer′ric
fer′ri·heme′

fer′ri·he′mo·glo′bin
fer′ri·por′phy·rin
fer′ri·tin
fer′ro·cho′li·nate′
fer′ro·cy′a·nide′
fer′ro·heme′
fer′ro·he′mo·glo′bin
fer′ro·ki·net′ics
fer′ro·mag·net′ic
fer′ro·por′phy·rin
fer′ro·pro′tein′
fer′ro·pro′to·por′phy·rin
fer′ro·ther′a·py
fer′rous
fer·ru′gi·nous
fer′rule′
fer′rum
fer′tile
fer·til′i·ty
fer′til·i·za′tion
fer′til·ize′, -ized′, -iz′ing
fer·til′i·zin
Fer′u·la
fer·ves′cence
fes′ter
fes′ti·nate′, -nat′ed, -nat′ing
fes′ti·na′tion
fes·toon′
fe′tal
fe·ta′tion
fe′ti·cide′
fet′id
fet′ish
fet′ish·ism
fet′ish·ist
fe′to·am′ni·ot′ic
fe′to·glob′u·lin
fe·tog′ra·phy
fe·tol′o·gist
fe·tol′o·gy
fe·tom′e·try
fe′to·pla·cen′tal
fe′to·pro′tein′
fe′tor
  —ex o′re′
  —he·pat′i·cus
fe·tox′y·late′
fe′tus
  —com·pres′sus
  —cy·lin′dri·cus
  —in fe′tu′
  —pap′y·ra′ce·us
Feul′gen

—method
—reaction
fe'ver
fe'ver·ish
fi'at'
fi'ber
fi'ber·co·lon'o·scope'
fi'ber·gas'tro·scope'
fi'ber·op'tic
fi'ber·op'tics
fi'ber·ot'o·my
fi'ber·scope'
fi'bra pl. -brae'
fi'brae'
　—ar'cu·a'tae cer'e·bri'
　—arcuatae ex·ter'nae'
　—arcuatae externae
　　dor·sa'les'
　—arcuatae externae
　　ven·tra'les'
　—arcuatae in·ter'nae'
　—cer'e·bel'lo·ol'i·var'es'
　—cir'cu·lar'es' mus'cu·li'
　　cil'i·ar'is
　—cor'ti·co·nu'cle·ar'es'
　—cor'ti·co·pon·ti'nae'
　—cor'ti·co·re·tic'u·lar'es'
　　mes'en·ceph'a·li'
　—corticoreticulares pon'tis
　—cor'ti·co·spi'na'les'
　—in'ter·cru·ra'les'
　—len'tis
　—me·rid'i·o·na'les' mus'-
　　cu·li' cil'i·ar'is
　—ob·li'quae' ven·tric'u·li'
　—per'i·ven·tric'u·lar'es'
　—pon'tis pro·fun'dae'
　—pontis su'per·fi'ci·a'les'
　—pontis trans·ver'sae'
　—py'ram'i·da'les' me·dul'-
　　lae' ob'lon·ga'tae'
　—zon'u·lar'es'
fi'bri·form'
fi'bril
fi·bril'la pl. -lae'
fi'bril·lar
fi'bril·lar'y
fi'bril·late', -lat·ed, -lat·ing
fi'bril·la'tion
fi'bril·la·to'ry
fi'bril·lo·gen'e·sis pl. -ses'
fi'brin
fi'brin·ase'

fi'bri·no·cel'lu·lar
fi·brin'o·gen
fi'brin·o'gen·e'mi·a
fi'bri·no·gen'e·sis
fi'bri·no·gen'ic
fi'bri·no·ge·nol'y·sis
fi'brin·o'gen·o·pe'ni·a
fi'bri·nog'e·nous
fi'bri·no·hem'or·rhag'ic
fi'brin·oid'
fi'bri·no·ki'nase'
fi'bri·nol'y·sin
fi'bri·nol'y·sis pl. -ses'
fi'bri·no·lyt'ic
fi'bri·no·pe'ni·a
fi'bri·no·pep'tide'
fi'bri·no·pu'ru·lent
fi'bri·nous
fi'bri·nu'ri·a
fi'bro·ad'e·no'ma pl. -mas or
　-ma·ta
　—xan'tho·ma·to'des'
fi'bro·ad'e·no'sis pl. -ses'
fi'bro·ad'i·pose'
fi'bro·am'e·lo·blas·to'ma
　pl. -mas or -ma·ta
fi'bro·an'gi·o·li·po'ma
　pl. -mas or -ma·ta
fi'bro·an'gi·o'ma pl. -mas or
　-ma·ta
fi'bro·a·re'o·lar
fi'bro·blast'
fi'bro·blas'tic
fi'bro·blas·to'ma pl. -mas or
　-ma·ta
fi'bro·bron·chi'tis
fi'bro·cal·car'e·ous
fi'bro·cal·cif'ic
fi'bro·car·ci·no'ma pl. -mas
　or -ma·ta
fi'bro·car'ti·lage
fi'bro·car'ti·lag'i·nes'
　in'ter·ver'te·bra'les'
fi'bro·car'ti·lag'i·nous
fi'bro·car'ti·la'go
　pl. -lag'i·nes'
　—ba'sa'lis
　—na·vic'u·lar'is
fi'bro·ca'se·ous
fi'bro·cav'i·tar'y
fi'bro·cel'lu·lar
fi'bro·ce'men·to'ma
　pl. -mas or -ma·ta

fi'bro·chon·dri'tis
fi'bro·chon·dro'ma pl. -mas
　or -ma·ta
fi'bro·chon'dro-os'te·o'ma
　pl. -mas or -ma·ta
fi'bro·col·lag'e·nous
fi'bro·cyst'
fi'bro·cys'tic
fi'bro·cys·to'ma pl. -mas or
　-ma·ta
fi'bro·cyte'
fi'bro·cy'to·gen'e·sis
　pl. -ses'
fi'bro·dys·pla'si·a
fi'bro·e·las'tic
fi'bro·e·las'to·sis pl. -ses'
fi'bro·en'chon·dro'ma
　pl. -mas or -ma·ta
fi'bro·en'do·the'li·o'ma
　pl. -mas or -ma·ta
fi'bro·ep'i·the'li·o'ma
　pl. -mas or -ma·ta
fi'bro·fat'ty
fi'bro·gen'e·sis pl. -ses'
fi'bro·gen'ic
fi·brog'li·a
fi'bro·gli·o'ma pl. -mas or
　-ma·ta
fi'bro·hem'or·rhag'ic
fi'bro·he'mo·tho'rax'
fi'broid'
fi'broid·ec'to·my
fi'bro·lam'i·nar
fi'bro·lei'o·my·o'ma
　pl. -mas or -ma·ta
fi'bro·li·po'ma pl. -mas or
　-ma·ta
fi'bro·li·pom'a·tous
fi'bro·lip'o·sar·co'ma
　pl. -mas or -ma·ta
fi'bro·lym'pho·an'gi·o·
　blas·to'ma pl. -mas or
　-ma·ta
fi·brol'y·sis pl. -ses'
fi·bro'ma pl. -mas or -ma·ta
　—du'rum
　—fun·goi'des'
　—li·po'ma·to'des'
　—mol'le'
　—mol·lus'cum
　—pen'du·lum
　—sim'plex'
fi·bro'ma·to·gen'ic

fi·bro'ma·toid'
fi·bro'ma·to'sis *pl.* -ses'
  —gin·gi'vae'
fi·bro'ma·tous
fi·bro·mec'to·my
fi·bro·mem'bra·nous
fi·bro·mus'cu·lar
fi·bro·my·al'gi·a
fi·bro·my·i'tis
fi·bro·my·o'ma *pl.* -mas or
  -ma·ta
fi·bro·my'o·mec'to·my
fi·bro·my'o·si'tis *pl.* -ses'
fi·bro·myx·o'li·po'ma
  pl. -mas or -ma·ta
fi·bro·myx·o'ma *pl.* -mas or
  -ma·ta
fi·bro·myx'o·sar·co'ma
  pl. -mas or -ma·ta
fi·bro·nec'tin
fi·bro·neu·ro'ma *pl.* -mas or
  -ma·ta
fi·bro·os'te·o·chon·dro'ma
  pl. -mas or -ma·ta
fi·bro·os'te·o'ma *pl.* -mas or
  -ma·ta
fi·bro·os'te·o·sar·co'ma
  pl. -mas or -ma·ta
fi·bro·pap'il·lo'ma *pl.* -mas
  or -ma·ta
fi·bro·pla·si'a
fi·bro·plas'tic
fi·bro·plate'
fi·bro·pu'ru·lent
fi·bro·sar·co'ma *pl.* -mas or
  -ma·ta
  —myx'o·ma·to'des'
  —phyl·lo'des'
fi·bro·sar·com'a·tous
fi·bro·scle·ro'sis *pl.* -ses'
fi·brose'
fi·bro·se'rous
fi·bro'sis *pl.* -ses'
fi·bro·sit'ic
fi·bro·si'tis
  —os·sif'i·cans' pro'gres·
   si'va
fi·bro·tho'rax'
fi·brot'ic
fi'brous
fi·bro·vas'cu·lar
fi·bro·xan·tho'ma *pl.* -mas
  or -ma·ta

fi'bro·xan·thom'a·tous
fib'u·la *pl.* -lae' or -las
fib'u·lar
fib'u·lar'is
fib'u·lo·cal·ca'ne·al
fib'u·lo·cal·ca'ne·us
fib'u·lo·tib'i·a'lis
Fick
  —formula
  —method
  —principle
Fied'ler
  —disease
  —myocarditis
field
fi·èv're bou·ton·neuse'
fig'ure
fig'ure-ground'
fi'la
  —a·nas'to·mot'i·ca ner'vi'
   a·cus'ti·ci'
  —cor'o·nar'i·a
  —lat'er·a'li·a pon'tis
  —ol'fac·to'ri·a
  —ra·dic'u·lar'i·a
  —radicularia ner·vo'rum
   spi·na'li·um
fi·la'ceous
fil'a·ment
fil'a·men'ta·ry
fil'a·men·ta'tion
fil'a·men'tous
fil'a·men'tum
fi'lar
fi·lar'i·a *pl.* -ae'
fi·lar'i·al
fil'a·ri'a·sis *pl.* -ses'
fi·lar'i·cid'al
fi·lar'i·cide'
fi·lar'i·form'
Fi·lar'i·oi'de·a
Fil'a·tov'
  —disease
  —spots
Fil'a·tov-Dukes' disease
file
fil'i·al
fil'i·cin
fil'i·form'
fil'i·pin
Fi·lip'o·wicz' sign
fil'let
fill'ing

film
film'y
Fi'lo·ba·sid'i·el'la
  ne'o·for'mans'
fi'lo·po'di·um *pl.* -di·a
fi'lo·pres'sure
fil'ter
fil'ter·a·ble
fil'trate'
fil'tra'tion
fil'trum *pl.* -tra
  —ven·tric'u·li'
fi'lum *pl.* -la
  —du'rae' ma'tris spi·na'lis
  —lat'er·a'lis pon'tis
  —ter'mi·na'le'
fim'bri·a *pl.* -ae'
  —hip'po·cam'pi'
  —o·var'i·ca
fim'bri·ae' tu'bae' u'ter·i'-
  nae'
fim'bri·al
fim'bri·ate'
fim'bri·at'ed
fim'bri·a'tion
fim'bri·ec'to·my
fim'bri·o·cele'
fim'bri·o·den'tate'
Find'lay operation
fin'ger
fin'ger·breadth'
fin'ger·nail'
fin'ger·print'
fin'ger·print'ing
fin'ger·tip'
Fin'kel·stein'
  —sign
  —test
Fin'ney
  —operation
  —pyloroplasty
Fin'ney-von Ha'ber·er
  operation
Fi·no·chet'ti stirrup
fire'damp'
first'-aid' kit
first'-de·gree'
  —burn
  —heart block
Fish'berg' test
fis'sile
fis'sion
fis'sion·a·ble

fis·su·la *pl.* -lae'
—an'te fe·nes'tram'
fis·su·ra *pl.* -rae'
—an'ti·tra·go·hel'i·ci'na
—cal'ca·ri'na
—cer'e·bri' lat·er·a'lis
  (Syl'vi·i')
—cho·roi'de·a
—col·lat'er·a'lis
—hip'po·cam'pi'
—ho'ri·zon·ta'lis
  cer'e·bel'li'
—horizontalis pul·mo'nis
  dex'tri'
—lig'a·men'ti' ter'e·tis
—ligamenti ve·no'si'
—lon'gi·tu'di·na'lis
  cer'e·bri'
—me'di·a'na anterior
  me·dul'lae' ob'lon·ga'tae'
—mediana anterior
  medullae spi·na'lis
—mediana posterior
  medullae ob'lon·ga'tae'
—ob·li'qua pul·mo'nis
—or'bi·ta'lis inferior
—orbitalis superior
—pa·ri'e·to·oc·cip'i·ta'lis
—pet'ro·oc·cip'i·ta'lis
—pet'ro·squa·mo'sa
—pet'ro·tym·pan'i·ca
—pos'ter·o·lat'er·a'lis
  cer'e·bel'li'
—pri'ma
—pter'y·goi'de·a
—pter'y·go·max'il·lar'is
—pter'y·go·pal'a·ti'na
—se·cun'da
—sphe'no·oc·cip'i·ta'lis
—sphe'no·pe·tro'sa
—ster'ni'
—trans·ver'sa cer'e·bel'li'
—transversa cer'e·bri'
—tym'pa·no·mas·toi'de·a
—tym'pa·no·squa·mo'sa
fis·su'rae' cer'e·bel'li'
fis'su·ral
fis·su·ra'tion
fis'sure
—in a'no'
—of Ro·lan'do
—of Syl'vi·us
fis·tu·la *pl.* -las *or* -lae'

—au'ris con·gen'i·ta
—in a'no'
fis'tu·lar
fis'tu·late'
fis'tu·la·tion
fis'tu·la·tome'
fis'tu·lec'to·my
fis'tu·li·za'tion
fis'tu·lize', -lized', -liz'ing
fis'tu·lo·en'ter·os'to·my
fis'tu·lo·gram'
fis'tu·lot'o·my
fis'tu·lous
fit
Fitz·ger'ald-Gard'ner
  syndrome
Fitz-Hugh'-Cur'tis
  syndrome
fix'ate', -at'ed, -at'ing
fix·a'tion
fix'a·tive
fix'a·tor
flab'by
flac'cid
flac·cid'i·ty
Flack node
flag'el·lant
flag'el·lant·ism
fla·gel'lar
flag'el·late', -lat'ed, -lat'ing
flag'el·la'tion
fla·gel'li·form'
flag'el·lo·ma'ni·a
flag'el·lo'sis *pl.* -ses'
fla·gel'lum *pl.* -la
Flagg resuscitation
flail
Fla·ja'ni disease
flam'ma·ble
flange
flank
flap
flare
flare'up'
flask
flat'ness
Fla'tau' law
Fla'tau'-Schil'der disease
flat'foot'
flat'ten
flat'u·lence
flat'u·lent
fla'tus

—vag'i·na'lis
flat'worm'
fla·ve'do
fla'vin
fla'vine'
Fla'vi·vi'rus
Fla'vo·bac·te'ri·um
fla'vo·ki'nase'
fla'vone'
fla'vo·noid'
fla'vo·nol'
fla'vo·pro'tein'
fla'vor
fla'vo·xan'thin
fla·vox'ate'
flea
Flech'sig tract
fle·cai'nide'
fleck'fie'ber
fleck'milz'
Fleck test
Flei'scher-Kay'ser ring
Fleisch'mann bursa
flesh
flex
flex'i·bil'i·tas ce're·a
flex'i·bil'i·ty
flex'i·ble
flex'ile
flex·im'e·ter
flex'ion
Flex'ner
—bacillus
—report
Flex'ner-Job'ling
  carcinosarcoma
flex'or
—ac'ces·so'ri·us
—car'pi' ra'di·a'lis
—carpi radialis brev'is
—carpi ul·nar'is
—carpi ulnaris brev'is
—dig'i·ti' min'i·mi' brev'is
—digiti quin'ti' brev'is
—dig'i·to'rum ac'ces·so'-
  ri·us
—digitorum brev'is
—digitorum lon'gus
—digitorum pro·fun'dus
—digitorum sub·li'mis
—digitorum su'per·fi'ci·
  a'lis
—hal'lu·cis brev'is

—hallucis lon'gus
—os'sis met'a·car'pi·
pol'li·cis
—pol'li·cis brev'is
—pollicis lon'gus
flex'or·plas'ty
flex'u·ous
flex·u'ra *pl.* -rae'
—co'li' dex'tra
—coli si·nis'tra
—du'o·de'ni' inferior
—duodeni superior
—du'o·de'no·je'ju·na'lis
—per'i·ne·a'lis rec'ti'
—sa·cra'lis rec'ti'
flex'ur·al
flex'ure
flick'er
Flindt spots
Flint murmur
float'ers
floc
floc'cil·la'tion
floc'cose'
floc'cu·lar
floc'cu·late', -lat'ed, -lat'ing
floc'cu·la'tion
floc'cu·lence
floc'cu·lent
floc'cu·lo·nod'u·lar
floc'cu·lus *pl.* -li'
—sec'on·dar'i·i'
flop'py
flo'ra *pl.* -ras *or* -rae'
flor·an'ty·rone'
Flo'rence
—flask
—test
flo'res'
Flo'rey unit
flo'rid
flo'ri·form'
floss
flo·ta'tion
flow
flow'er bas'ket of
Boch'da·lek'
Flow'er index
flow'me'ter
flox·u'ri·dine'
flu
flu·ban'i·late'
flu·cin'o·nide'

fluc'tu·ance
fluc'tu·ant
fluc'tu·ate', -at'ed, -at'ing
fluc'tu·a'tion
flu·cy'to·sine'
flu·dar'a·bine'
flu'do·rex'
flu'dro·cor'ti·sone'
flu'fen·am'ic
Fluh'mann test
flu'id
flu'id·ex'tract'
flu'id·glyc'er·ate'
flu·id'i·ty
flu'id·ounce'
flu'i·dram'
fluke
flu'like'
flu·ma'ze·pil
flu'men *pl.* -mi·na
flu·meth'a·sone'
flu·met'ra·mide'
flu'mi·na
—pi·lo'rum
flu·min'o·rex'
flu·nar'i·zine'
flu·nid'a·zole'
flu'o·cin'o·lone' a·cet'o·
nide'
flu'o·cin'o·nide'
flu'o·cor'to·lone'
flu'or'
—al'bus
flu'or·chrome'
fluo·res'ce·in
fluo·res'cence
fluo·res'cent
fluo·res'cin
fluor'i·date', -dat'ed, -dat'ing
fluor'i·da'tion
fluor'ide'
fluor'i·di·za'tion
fluor'i·dize', -dized', -diz'ing
fluor'ine'
fluor'o·a·ce'tic
fluor'o·car'di·o·gram'
fluor'o·car'di·o·graph'
fluor'o·car'di·og'ra·phy
fluor'o·chrome'
fluor'o·graph'ic
fluo·rog'ra·phy
fluo·rom'e·ter
fluor'o·met'ric

fluo·rom'e·try
fluor'o·meth'o·lone'
fluor'o·phos'phate'
fluor'o·pho'to·met'ric
fluor'o·pho·tom'e·try
fluor'o·roent'ge·nog'ra·
phy
fluor'o·sal'an
fluor'o·scope'
fluor'o·scop'ic
fluo·ros'co·py
fluo·ro'sis *pl.* -ses'
fluor'o·u'ra·cil
flu·ox'e·tine'
flu·ox·y·mes'ter·one'
flu·per'o·lone'
flu·phen'a·zine'
flu'pred·nis'o·lone'
flu'ran·dren'o·lide'
flu·raz'e·pam'
flur·bip'ro·fen
flu·ro·ges'tone'
flu·ro'thyl
flu·rox'ene'
Flu'ry strain
flush
flu'ta·mide'
flut'ter
flux
fly
Fo·à-Kur'lov' cell
foam
foam'y
fo'cal
fo'cal·i·za'tion
fo'cal·ize', -ized', -iz'ing
fo·cim'e·ter
fo'cus *pl.* -cus·es *or* -ci'
Foer'ster
—cutaneous numeral test
—forceps
—operation
—sign
Foer'ster-Pen'field'
operation
fog'ging
fo'go sel·va'gem
foil
Foix
—sign
—syndrome
Foix'-Al'a·jou·a·nine'
syndrome

fo'late'
fold
Fo'ley Y'-plas'ty
fo'li·a'ceous
fo'li·a cer'e·bel'li
fo'li·ate'
fol'ic
fo·lie'
—à deux
—des per·sé·cu·tions'
—du doute
—du pour·quoi'
—mo·rale'
Fo'lin
—and Sved'berg' method
—and Wu method
—and Young'burg' method
—method
—reagent
—theory
Fo'lin, Can'non, and Den'is
method
Fo'lin-Cio·cal'teu reagent
Fo'lin-Far'mer method
fo·lin'ic
Fo'lin-Mc'Ell·roy' test
Fo'lin-Schaf'fer method
Fo'lin-Wu' test
fo'li·ose'
fo'li·um pl. -li·a
—cer'e·bel'li'
—ver'mis
fol'li·cle
fol·lic'u·lar
fol·lic'u·li'
—glan'du·lae' thy·roi'de·ae'
—lin·gua'les'
—lym·phat'i·ci'
ag'gre·ga'ti'
ap·pen'di·cis
ver'mi·for'mis
—lymphatici aggregati
in'tes·ti'ni' ten'u·is
—lymphatici gas'tri·ci'
—lymphatici la·ryn'ge·i'
—lymphatici li'e·na'les'
—lymphatici rec'ti'
—lymphatici sol'i·tar'i·i'
co'li'
—lymphatici solitarii
in'tes·ti'ni' ten'u·is
—o·oph'o·ri' pri·mar'i·i'
—oophori ve·sic'u·lo'si'

—o·var'i·ci' pri·mar'i·i'
—ovarici ve·sic'u·lo'si'
fol·lic'u·lin
fol·lic'u·li'tis
—ab·sce'dens et
suf·fo'di·ens
—ag'mi·na'ta
—bar'bae'
—de·cal'vans'
—ke'loi·da'lis
—sim'plex'
—u·ler'y·the'ma·to'sa
re·tic'u·la'ta
fol·lic'u·loid'
fol·lic'u·lo'ma pl. -mas or
-ma·ta
fol·lic'u·lo'sis pl. -ses'
fol·lic'u·lus pl. -li'
—lym·phat'i·cus
—pi'li'
fol'li·tro'pin
fol'low-up'
fo'men·ta'tion
fo'mes' pl. fom'i·tes'
fo'mite'
Fong lesion
Fon·se'ca disease
Fon·se·cae'a
Fon·tan'a
—spaces
—stain
fon'ta·nel' or fon·ta·nelle'
Fon·tan' operation
fon·tic'u·li' cra'ni·i'
fon·tic'u·lus pl. -li'
—anterior
—fron·ta'lis
—mas·toi'de·us
—oc·cip'i·ta'lis
—posterior
—sphe·noi'da'lis
foot
foot'-can·dle
foot'plate'
foot'-pound'
for'age, -aged, -ag·ing
fo·ra'men pl. -mens or
fo·ram'i·na
—a'pi·cis den'tis
—cae'cum lin'guae'
—caecum me·dul'lae'
ob'lon·ga'tae'
—caecum os'sis fron·ta'lis

—ca·rot'i·cum ex·ter'num
—caroticum in·ter'num
—ce'cum
—cecum lin'guae'
—cecum os'sis fron·ta'lis
—cos'to·trans'ver·sar'i·um
—di'a·phrag'ma·tis sel'lae'
—ep'i·plo'i·cum
—eth'moi·da'le' an·te'ri·us
—ethmoidale pos·te'ri·us
—fron·ta'le'
—in·ci'si'vum
—in'fra·or'bi·ta'le'
—in'fra·pir'i·for'me'
—in·nom'i·na'tum
—in·ter·ven·tric'u·lar'e'
—in·ter·ver'te·bra'le
—is·chi·ad'i·cum ma'jus
—ischiadicum mi'nus
—jug'u·lar'e'
—lac'er·um
—mag'num
—man·dib'u·lae'
—man·dib'u·lar'e'
—mas·toi'de·um
—men·ta'le'
—nu·tri'ci·um
—ob'tu·ra'tum
—oc·cip'i·ta'le' mag'num
—of Boch'da·lek'
—of Husch'ke
—of Key
—of Lusch'ka
—of Ma·gen'die
—of Mon·ro'
—of Mor'ga'gni
—of Ret'zi·us
—of Scar'pa
—of Sten'sen
—of Ve·sa'li·us
—of Wins'low'
—op'ti·cum
—o·va'le'
—ovale cor'dis
—ovale os'sis sphe·noi·
da'lis
—ovale pri'mum
—pal'a·ti'num ma'jus
—pa·ri'e·ta'le'
—pri'mum
—ro·tun'dum
—rotundum os'sis
sphe'noi·da'lis

—se·cun'dum
—sin'gu·lar'e'
—sphe'no·pal'a·ti'num
—spi·no'sum
—sty'lo·mas·toi'de·um
—su'pra·or·bi·ta'lis
—su'pra·pir'i·for'me'
—thy're·oi'de·um
—thy·roi'de·um
—trans·ver·sar'i·um
—ve'nae' ca'vae'
—ve·no'sum
—ver'te·bra'le'
—zy'go·mat'i·co·fa·ci·a'le'
—zy'go·mat'i·co·or·bi·ta'le'
—zy'go·mat'i·co·tem·po·ra'le'
fo·ra'mens
—of Scar'pa
—of Sten'sen
fo·ram'i·na
—al've·o·lar'i·a max·il'lae'
—eth'moi·da'li·a
—in·ci·si'va
—in·ter·ver'te·bra'li·a os'sis
    sa'cri'
—na·sa'li·a
—ner·vo'sa lam'i·nae'
    spi·ra'lis
—nervosa lim'bus lam'i·
    nae' spi·ra'lis
—pal'a·ti'na mi·no'ra
—pap'il·lar'i·a re'nis
—sa·cra'li·a an·te'ri·o'ra
—sacralia dor·sa'li·a
—sacralia pel·vi'na
—sacralia pos·te'ri·o'ra
—ve·nar'um min'i·mar'um
    cor'dis
fo·ram'i·nal
fo·ram'i·nif'er·ous
fo·ram'i·not'o·my
fo'ra·min·u'late'
fo'ra·min·u'lum pl. -la
Forbes'-Al'bright
    syndrome
Forbes disease
force
for'ceps
Forch'hei'mer sign
for'ci·pate'
for'cip'i·tal
for'ci·pres'sure
fore'arm'

fore'brain'
fore'con'scious
fore'fin'ger
fore'foot'
fore'gut'
fore'head'
for'eign
fore'kid'ney
Fo·rel'
—bundle
—decussation
fore'leg'
fore'milk'
fo·ren'sic
fore'play'
fore'pleas'ure
fore'skin'
fore'stom'ach
fore'wa'ters
form
for·mal'de·hyde'
for'ma·lin
for'ma·lin·ize'
form·am'ide'
for'mate'
for·ma'ti·o' pl. -ma·ti·o'nes'
—re·tic'u·lar'is
—reticularis me·dul'lae'
    ob'lon·ga'tae'
—reticularis medullae
    spi·na'lis
—reticularis mes'en·ceph'-
    a·li'
—reticularis pe·dun'cu·li'
    cer'e·bri'
—reticularis pon'tis
for·ma'tion
for'ma·tive
for'ma·zan
forme fruste pl. formes
    frustes
for'mic
for'mi·cant
for'mi·ca'tion
for'mi·ci·a·sis
for·mim'i·no·glu·tam'ic
for·mim'i·no·trans'fer·ase'
for'mo·cre'sol'
for'mol'
for'mu·la pl. -las or -lae'
for'mu·lar'y
for'myl
for'myl·am'ide'

for'myl·ase'
for'ni·cal
for'ni·cate', -cat'ed, -cat'ing
for'ni·ca'tion
for'nix pl. -ni·ces'
—cer'e·bri'
—con'junc·ti'vae' inferior
—conjunctivae superior
—pha·ryn'gis
—sac'ci' lac'ri·ma'lis
—va·gi'nae'
Fors'gren method
for'sko·lin
Forss'man antigens
Fort Bragg fever
for'ti·fi·ca'tion
fos·car'net
Fo·shay' test (tularemia)
    ♦ Fouchet test
fo·sin'o·pril
fos'pi·rate'
fos'sa pl. -sae'
—ac'e·tab'u·li'
—ant·hel'i·cis
—ax·il·lar'is
—cae·ca'lis
—ca·ni'na
—ca·rot'i·ca
—cer'e·bri' lat'er·a'lis
    (Syl'vi·i')
—con'dy·lar'is
—con'dy·loi'de·a
—cor'o·noi'de·a
—cra'ni·i' anterior
—cranii me'di·a
—cranii posterior
—cu·bi·ta'lis
—di·gas'tri·ca
—duc'tus ve·no'si'
—ep'i·gas'tri·ca
—glan'du·lae' lac'ri·ma'lis
—hy'a·loi'de·a
—hy'po·phys'e·os'
—hy'po·phys'i·a'lis
—i·li'a·ca
—i·li'a·co·sub·fas'ci·a'lis
—il'i·o·pec·tin'e·a
—in·ci·si'va
—in·cu'dis
—in'fra·spi·na'ta
—in'fra·tem'po·ra'lis
—in'gui·na'lis lat'er·a'lis
—inguinalis me'di·a'lis

—in·nom′i·na′ta
—in′ter·con′dy·lar′is
  fem·or·is
—in′ter·con′dy·loi′de·a
  anterior tib′i·ae′
—intercondyloidea fem′o·ris
—intercondyloidea posterior
  tib′i·ae′
—in′ter·pe·dun′cu·lar′is
—is·chi·o·rec′ta′lis
—jug′u·lar′is
—jugularis os′sis tem′po·
  ra′lis
—la·ter·a′lis cer′e·bri′
—mal·le′o·li′ lat′er·a′lis
—man·dib′u·lar′is
—na·vic′u·lar′is u·re′thrae′
—navicularis ves·tib′u·li′
  va·gi′nae′
—oc·cip′i·ta′lis
—o′le·cra′ni′
—o·va′lis
—ovalis cor′dis
—ovalis fas′ci·ae′ la′tae′
—ovalis fem′o·ris
—pop·lit′e·a
—prae′na·sa′lis
—pter′y·goi′de·a
—pter′y·go·pal′a·ti′na
—ra′di·a′lis
—ret′ro·man·dib′u·lar′is
—rhom·boi′de·a
—sac′ci′ lac′ri·ma′lis
—sag′it·ta′lis si·nis′tra
  hep′a·tis
—sca·phoi′de·a
—scar′pae′ major
—sem′i·lu·nar′is
—sub·ar′cu·a′ta
—sub·in′gui·na′lis
—sub·scap′u·lar′is
—su′pra·cla·vic′u·lar′is
  major
—supraclavicularis minor
—su′pra·spi·na′ta
—su′pra·ton′sil·lar′is
—su′pra·ves′i·ca′lis
—tem′po·ra′lis
—ton′sil·lar′is
—tri·an′gu·lar′is au·ric′u·lar′e′
—tro′chan·ter′i·ca
—ve′nae′ ca′vae′
—venae um·bil′i·ca′lis

—ve·si′cae′ fel′le·ae′
—ves·tib′u·li′ va·gi′nae′
fos′sae sag′it·ta′les′
  dex′trae′ hep′a·tis
fos·sette′
fos′su·la *pl.* -lae′
  —fe·nes′trae′ coch′le·ae′
  —fenestrae ves·tib′u·li′
  —pe·tro′sa
  —post fe·nes′tram
fos′su·lae′
  —ton·sil·lar′es′ ton·sil′lae′
    pal′a·ti′nae′
  —tonsillares tonsillae
    pha·ryn′ge·ae′ee
fos′su·late′
Fos′ter Ken′ne·dy
  syndrome
Fos′ter rule
Foth′er·gill disease
Fou·chet′ reagent
Fou·chet′ test *(bilirubin)*
  ◆ *Foshay test*
fou·droy′ant
foul
fou·lage′
four·chette′
Fou·rier′
  —analysis
  —transform
fo′ve·a *pl.* -ae′
  —ar·tic′u·lar′is inferior
    at·lan′tis
  —articularis superior
    atlantis
  —cap′i·tis fem′o·ris
  —ca·pit′u·li′ ra′di·i′
  —cen·tra′lis
  —cos·ta′lis inferior
  —costalis superior
  —costalis trans′ver·sa′lis
  —den′tis at·lan′tis
  —hem′i·el·lip′ti·ca
  —hem′i·sphe′ri·ca
  —inferior fos′sae′ rhom·
    boi′de·ae′
  —in′gui·na′lis lat′er·a′lis
  —inguinalis me′di·a′lis
  —nu′chae′
  —ob·lon′ga car′ti·lag′i·nis
    ar′y·tae·noi′de·ae′
  —oblonga cartilaginis
    ar′y·te·noi′de·ae′

—pal′a·ti′na
—pter′y·goi′de·a man·dib′-
  u·lae′
—pterygoidea pro·ces′sus
  con′dy·loi′de·i′
—sa′cro·coc·cyg′e·a
—sub·lin·gua′lis
—sub′man·dib′u·lar′is
—sub·max′il·lar′is
—superior fos′sae′ rhom·
  boi′de·ae′
—su′pra·ves′i·ca′lis per′i·
  to·nae′i′
—tri·an′gu·lar′is car′ti·lag′-
  i·nis
—triangularis cartilaginis
  ar′y·te·noi′de·ae′
—troch′le·ar′is
fo′ve·ae′ ar·tic′u·lar′es′
  in·fe′ri·o′res′ at·lan′tis
fo′ve·al
fo′ve·ate′
fo′ve·a′tion
fo·ve·o′la *pl.* -lae′ *or* -las
  —coc·cyg′e·a
  —pal′a·ti′na
fo·ve·o′lae′
  —gas′tri·cae′
  —gran′u·lar′es′
fo·ve·o′lar
fo·ve·o′late′
Fo′ville paralysis
Fow′ler
  —incision
  —position
  —solution
fox′glove′
frac′tion
frac′tion·al
frac′tion·ate′, -at·ed, -at·ing
frac′tion·a′tion
frac′ture, -tured, -tur·ing
frac′ture
–en coin
–en rave
frad′i·cin
Fraenk′el
  —glands
  —nodule
Fraentz′el murmur
frag′ile
fra·gil′i·tas
  —cri′ni·um

—os'si·um
fra·gil'i·ty
fra·gil'o·cyte'
fra·gil'o·cy·to'sis *pl.* -ses'
frag'ment
frag'men·tar'y
frag'men·ta'tion
fraise
fram·be'si·a
frame
Frame, Rus'sell, and
  Wil'hel'mi method
frame'shift'
frame'work'
Fran'ce·schet'ti syndrome
Fran'ci·sel'la
—tu'la·ren'sis
Fran'cis test
fran'ci·um
Fran·çois' syndrome
frang'u·lin
frank
Frank
—capillary toxicosis
—operation
Frän'kel sign
Franke method
Frank'en·häu'ser ganglion
Frank'fort horizontal plane
frank'in·cense'
frank'lin·ic
Frank'-Star'ling law
frap·page'
fra·ter'nal
frat'ri·cide'
Fraun'ho'fer lines
fray
frax'in
freck'le
Fre·det'-Ram'stedt
  operation
Free'man rule
freeze, froze, fro'zen,
  freez'ing
Frei
—disease
—test
Frei'berg' disease
frem'i·tus
fre'nal
French scale
fre·nec'to·my
fre·net'ic *var. of* phrenetic

fre'no·plas'ty
fre·not'o·my
fren'u·lec'to·my
fren'u·lum *pl.* -la
—cli·to'ri·dis
—la'bi·i' in·fe'ri·o'ris
—labii su·pe'ri·o'ris
—la'bi·o'rum pu·den'di'
—lin'guae'
—of Gia'co·mi'ni
—pre·pu'ti·i' pe'nis
—val'vae' il'e·o·ce·ca'lis
—val'vu·lae' co'li'
—ve'li' med'ul·lar'is
  an·te'ri·o'ris
—veli medullaris
  su·pe'ri·o'ris
fre'num *pl.* -nums *or* -na
Fren'zel maneuver
fren'zy
fre'quen·cy
Frer'ich theory
fre'tum
—hal'ler·i'
freud'i·an
Freund adjuvant
Freund'lich adsorption
  equation
Frey syndrome
fri'a·bil'i·ty
fri'a·ble
fric'tion
fric'tion·al
Frid'er·ich·sen
—syndrome
—test
Frie'de·mann and Grae'ser
  method
Frie'den·wald' nomogram
Fried'län'der
—bacillus
—cells
—pneumonia
Fried'mann vasomotor
  symptom complex
Fried'man test
Fried'reich'
—ataxia
—disease
—sign
Fried'rich-Bau'er operation
Fried rule
frig'id

fri·gid'i·ty
frig'o·la'bile'
frig'o·rif'ic
frig'o·sta'ble
fringe
Frisch bacillus
frit
frog'leg'
Froh'de reagent
Fröh'lich
—dystrophy
—syndrome
Froin syndrome
frole·ment'
Fro'ment sign
From'mann line
From'mel
—disease
—operation
frond
frons
fron'tad'
fron'tal
fron·ta'lis
fron·tip'e·tal
fron'to·eth'moid'
fron'to·lac'ri·mal
fron'to·ma'lar
fron'to·max'il·lar'y
fron'to·men'tal
fron'to·na'sal
fron'to·oc·cip'i·tal
fron'to·pa·ri'e·tal
fron'to·pon'tine'
fron'to·pon'to·cer'e·bel'lar
fron'to·sphe'noid'
fron'to·tem'por·al
fron'to·tem'po·ra'le'
  pl. -ra'li·a
fron'to·zy'go·mat'ic
Fro'riep'
—ganglion
—induration
frost
frost'bite'
froth
froth'y
frot·tage'
frot·teur'
fruc·tiv'o·rous
fruc'to·fu·ran'o·san'
fruc'to·fu'ra·nose'
fruc'to·fu·ran'o·side'

fruc'to·ki'nase'
fruc'to·py'ra·nose'
fruc'to·san'
fruc'tose'
fruc'to·se'mi·a
fruc'to·side'
fruc'to·su'ri·a
fru·giv'o·rous
fru'men·ta'ceous
fru·men'tum
frus'trate', -trat'ed, -trat'ing
frus·tra'tion
Fryk'man
 —fracture
 —classification
Fuchs
 —dystrophy
 —iridocyclitis
 —phenomenon
fuch'sin
fuch·sin'o·phil'
fuch·sin·o·phil'i·a
fuch·sin·o·phil'ic
fu'cose'
fu·co'si·dase'
fu·co·si·do'sis pl. -ses'
Fuer'bring'er
 —law
 —sign
fu·ga'cious
fu'gi·tive
fugue
ful'gu·rant
ful'gu·rate', -rat'ed, -rat'ing
ful'gu·ra'tion
fu·lig'i·nous
Ful'ler Al'bright'
 syndrome
Ful'ler operation
full'ness
ful'mi·nant
ful'mi·nat'ing
fu'ma·gil'lin
fu'ma·rase'
fu'ma·rate'
Fu·mar'i·a·ce·ae'
fu·mar'ic
fu·mig'a·cin
fu'mi·gant
fu'mi·gate', -gat'ed, -gat'ing
fu'mi·ga'tion
fum'ing

func'ti·o'
 —lae'sa
func'tion
func'tion·al
func'tion·al·ly
fun'dal
fun'da·ment
fun'da·men'tal
fun·dec'to·my
fun'dic
fun'di·form'
fun'do·plas'ty
fun'do·pli·ca'tion
fun'do·scop'ic
fun·dos'co·py
fun'dus pl. -di'
 —fla'vi·mac'u·la'tus
 —fol·lic'u·li' pi'li'
 —me·a'tus a·cu'sti·ci'
  in·ter'ni'
 —oc'u·li'
 —u'ter·i'
 —ven·tric'u·li'
 —ve·si'cae' fel'le·ae'
 —vesicae u'ri·nar'i·ae'
fun'du·scope'
fun'du·scop'ic
fun·dus'co·py
fun'du·sec'to·my
fun'gal
fun'gate', -gat'ed, -gat'ing
fun·ge'mi·a
fun'gi·cid'al
fun'gi·cide'
fun'gi·form'
fun'gi·sta'sis
fun'gi·stat'
fun'gi·stat'ic
fun'gi·tox'ic
fun'gi·tox·ic'i·ty
fun'goid'
fun·gos'i·ty
fun'gous (of a fungus)
 ◆fungus
fun'gus (plant), pl. -gi' or
 -gus·es
 ◆fungous
fu'nic
fu'ni·cle
fu·nic'u·lar
fu·nic'u·li' me·dul'lae'
 spi·na'lis
fu·nic'u·li'tis

fu·nic'u·lus pl. -li'
 —anterior me·dul'lae'
  spi·na'lis
 —cu·ne·a'tus me·dul'lae'
  ob'lon·ga'tae'
 —grac'i·lis me·dul'lae'
  ob'lon·ga'tae'
 —lat·er·a'lis me·dul'lae'
  ob'lon·ga'tae'
 —lateralis medullae
  spi·na'lis
 —posterior medullae
  spinalis
 —sep'a·rans'
 —sper·mat'i·cus
 —um·bil'i·ca'lis
fu'ni·form'
fu'nis
fu'nis·i'tis
fun'nel
fu'ra·nose'
fu'ra·zol'i·done'
fu'ra·zo'li·um
fur·az'o·sin
fur'ca pl. -cae'
 —or'bi·ta'lis
fur'cal
fur·ca'lis
fur'cate'
fur·ca'tion
fur·cu'la pl. -lae'
fur'fur pl. -fu'res'
fur·fu·ra'ceous
fur'fur·al
fu'ri·bund'
Fur'ness anastomosis
fu'ror'
 —am'a·to'ri·us
 —ep'i·lep'ti·cus
 —gen'i·ta'lis
fu'ro·sem'ide
fur'row
fur'sa·lan'
fu'run·cle
fu·run'cu·lar
fu·run'cu·loid'
fu·run'cu·lo'sis pl. -ses'
 —o'ri·en·ta'lis
fu·run'cu·lus pl. -li'
Fu·sar'i·um
fus'cin
fuse, fused, fus'ing
fu·seau' pl. -seaux'

fu′sel
fu′si·ble
fu′si·form′
Fu′si·for′mis
fu′si·mo′tor
fu′sion
fu′so·bac·te′ri·um *pl.* -ri·a
Fu′so·bac·te′ri·um
— fu′si·for′me′
— plau′ti-vin·cen′ti′
fu′so·cel′lu·lar
fu′so·spi′ro·che′tal
fu′so·spi′ro·che·to′sis
  pl. -ses′
fus′ti·ga′tion

G

G′-ac′tin
gad′fly′
gad′o·lin′i·um
gad′o·pen′te·tate′
Gaert′ner tonometer
Gaff′ky·a
— te·trag′e·na
gag, gagged, gag′ging
gain
Gais′böck′
— disease
— syndrome
gait
ga·lac′ta·cra′si·a
ga·lac′ta·gog′in
ga·lac′ta·gogue′
ga·lac′tan′
ga·lac′tase′
gal·ac·te′mi·a
ga·lact′hi·dro′sis
ga·lac′tic
ga·lac′tin
gal·ac·tis′chi·a
ga·lac′to·blast′
ga·lac′to·bol′ic
ga·lac′to·cele′
ga·lac′to·fla′vin
ga·lac′toid′
ga·lac′to·ki′nase′
ga·lac′to·lip′id
ga·lac′to·lip′in
gal·ac′to·ma *pl.* -mas *or*
  -ma·ta
gal·ac·ton′ic
ga·lac′to·pex′ic

ga·lac′to·pex′y
gal·ac·toph′a·gous
  (subsisting on milk)
  ♦galactophygous
gal·ac·toph′ly·sis *pl.* -ses′
ga·lac′to·phore′
gal·ac·toph′o·ri′tis
gal′ac·toph′o·rous
gal·ac·toph′y·gous
  (arresting the secretion of milk)
  ♦galactophagous
ga·lac′to·pla′ni·a
ga·lac′to·poi·e′sis *pl.* -ses′
ga·lac′to·poi·et′ic
ga·lac′to·py′ra
ga·lac′to·py′ra·nose′
ga·lac′to·py·ret′ic
ga·lac′tor·rhe′a
ga·lac′tos·am′ine′
gal·ac·tos′che·sis
ga·lac′to·scope′
ga·lac′tose′
ga·lac′to·se′mi·a
ga·lac′to·sid′ase′
ga·lac′to·side′
gal′ac·to′sis *pl.* -ses′
gal′ac·tos′ta·sis *pl.* -ses′
ga·lac′to·su′ri·a
ga·lac′to·tox′i·con′
ga·lac′to·tox′in
ga·lac′to·tox′ism
gal′ac·tot′ro·phy
ga·lac′to·zy′mase′
gal′ac·tu′ri·a
ga·lac′tu·ron′ic
gal′a·nin
Gal′ant
— reflex
— response
ga·le′a *pl.* -as *or* -ae′
— ap′o·neu·rot′i·ca
— cap′i·tis
Ga′le·az′zi
— fracture
— sign
gal′e·ro′pi·a
gall
gal′la·mine′ tri·eth·i′o·
  dide′
Gal′la·var′din phenome-
  non
gall′blad′der
gal′ler·y

Gal′lie-Le Me·su′ri·er
  operation
Gal′lie operation
gal′li·um
gal′lop
gal′lon
gall′stone′
Gal′ton
— bar
— law
— system
— whistle
gal·van′ic
gal′va·nism
gal′va·ni·za′tion
gal′va·nize′, -nized′, -niz′ing
gal′va·no·cau′ter·y
gal′va·no·con′trac·til′i·ty
gal′va·nom′e·ter
gal′va·no·mus′cu·lar
gal′va·no·punc′ture
gal′va·no·sur′ger·y
gal′va·no·tax′is *pl.* -es
gal′va·no·ther′a·py
gal′va·no·ther′my
gal′va·not′o·nus
gal′va·not′ro·pism
gam′a·soi·do′sis *pl.* -ses′
gam′bir
gam·boge′
Gam·bu′si·a
gam′e·tan′gi·um *pl.* -gi·a
gam′ete′
ga·met′ic
ga·me′to·cide′
ga·me′to·cyte′
gam′e·to·gen′e·sis
gam′e·to·gen′ic
gam′e·tog′o·ny
gam′e·toid′
gam′e·to·ki·net′ic
gam′e·tox′ine′
gam′ic
gam′ma
— globulin
gam′ma·cism
gam′ma·glob′u·lin·op′-
  a·thy
Gam′mel syndrome
gam·mop′a·thy
Gam′na
— disease
— nodules

—spleen
Gam'na-Fa'vre bodies
Gam'na-Gan'dy
—bodies
—nodules
gam'o·gen'e·sis *pl.* -ses'
gam'o·ge·net'ic
gam'o·pho'bi·a
gam'o·sep'al·ous
Gam'per bowing reflex
Gam'storp' disease
gan·ci'clo·vir'
Gan'dy-Gam'na
—nodules
—spleen
Gan'dy-Nan'ta disease
gan'gli·a
—a·or'ti·co·re·na'li·a
—car·di'a·ca
—ce·li'a·ca
—coe·li'a·ca
—in'ter·me'di·a
—lum·ba'li·a
—pel·vi'na
—phren'i·ca
—plex'u·um au'to·nom'i·
　co'rum
—plexuum sym·path'i·
　co'rum
—re·na'li·a
—sa·cra'li·a
—tho'ra·ca'li·a
—tho·ra'ci·ca
—trun'ci' sym·path'i·ci'
gan'gli·al
gan'gli·ar
gan'gli·at'ed
gan'gli·ec'to·my
gan'gli·form'
gan'gli·i'tis
gan'gli·o·blast'
gan'gli·o·cyte'
gan'gli·o·cy·to'ma *pl.* -mas
　or -ma·ta
gan'gli·o·gli·o'ma *pl.* -mas
　or -ma·ta
gan'gli·oid'
gan'gli·o'ma *pl.* -mas *or*
　-ma·ta
gan'gli·on *pl.* -gli·a *or*
　-gli·ons
—car·di'a·cum
　(Wris'ber·gi')

—cer'vi·ca'le' in·fe'ri·us
—cervicale medium
—cervicale su·pe'ri·us
—cer'vi·co·tho·ra'ci·cum
—cil'i·ar'e'
—ge·nic'u·li'
—ha·ben'u·lae'
—im'par'
—in·fe'ri·us
—inferius ner'vi' glos'so·
　pha·ryn'ge·i'
—inferius nervi va'gi'
—jug'u·lar'e' ner'vi' va'gi'
—mes'en·ter'i·cum
　in·fe'ri·us
—mesentericum su·pe'ri·us
—mol'le'
—no·do'sum
—o'ti·cum
—pe·tro'sum
—pter'y·go·pal'a·ti'num
—re·na'le'
—sphe'no·pa·lat'i·num
—spi·na'le'
—spi·ra'le' coch'le·ae'
—splanch'ni·cum
—stel·la'tum
—sub'man·dib'u·lar'e'
—sub'max'il·lar'e'
—su·pe'ri·us
—superius ner'vi'
　glos'so·pha·ryn'ge·i'
—superius nervi va'gi'
—ter'mi·na'le'
—tri'gem'i·na'le'
—tym·pan'i·cum
—ver'te·bra'le'
—ves·tib'u·lar'e'
gan'gli·o·nat'ed
gan'gli·on·ec'to·my
Gan'gli·o·ne'ma
gan'gli·o·neu'ro·blas·to'ma
　pl. -mas *or* -ma·ta
—sim'plex'
—sym·path'i·cum
gan'gli·o·neu'ro·cy·to'ma
　pl. -mas *or* -ma·ta
gan'gli·o·neu·ro'ma
　pl. -mas *or* -ma·ta
—te·lan'gi·ec·ta'tum cys'ti·
　cum
gan'gli·on'ic
gan'gli·on·i'tis

gan'gli·o·ple'gic
gan'gli·o·side'
gan'gli·o·si·do'sis'
gan'gli·o·sym·path'i·co·
　blas·to'ma *pl.* -mas *or*
　-ma·ta
gan·go'sa
gan'grene'
gan'gre·no'sis *pl.* -ses'
gan'gre·nous
gan'o·blast'
Gan'ser
—commissure
—ganglion
—syndrome
Gant operation
gan'try
Gant'zer muscle
gap, gapped, gap'ping
Gar'den fracture
Gard'ner syndrome
gar'gle, -gled, -gling
gar'goyl·ism
Gar'land triangle
Gar·ré'
—disease
—osteomyelitis
Gar'rod test
Gart'ner
—cyst
—duct
gas, gassed, gas'sing
gas'e·ous
gas·om'e·ter
gas'o·met'ric
gasp
gas·se'ri·an
gas'si·ness
gas'sy
Gas·taut' disease
gas'ter
Gas'ter·oph'i·lus
—hem'or·rhoi·da'lis
—in·tes'ti·na'lis
—na·sa'lis
gas·trad'e·ni'tis
gas'tral
gas·tral'gi·a
gas·tral'go·ke·no'sis
gas·tras·the'ni·a
gas'tra·tro'phi·a
gas'trec·ta'si·a
gas·trec'to·my

gas'tric
gas'trin
gas'tri·no'ma *pl.* -mas *or*
  -ma·ta
gas·trit'ic
gas·tri'tis
gas'tro·a·ceph'a·lus *pl.* -li'
gas'tro·a·mor'phus *pl.* -phi'
gas'tro·a·nas'to·mo'sis
gas'tro·a·to'ni·a
gas'tro·cam'er·a
gas'tro·car'di·ac'
Gas'troc·cult' test
gas'tro·cele' *(hernia of the*
  stomach)
  ♦ *gastrocoel*
gas'tro·cne·mi·us *pl.* -mi·i'
gas'tro·coel' *(archenteron)*
  ♦ *gastrocele*
gas'tro·col'ic
gas'tro·co·li'tis
gas'tro·co·los'to·my
gas'tro·co·lot'o·my
gas'tro·col·pot'o·my
gas'tro·cu·ta'ne·ous
gas'tro·did'y·mus *pl.* -mi'
gas'tro·dis·ci'a·sis *pl.* -ses'
Gas'tro·dis·coi'des'
  —hom'i·nis
gas'tro·disk'
gas'tro·du'o·de'nal
gas'tro·du'o·de·nec'to·my
gas'tro·du'o·de·ni'tis
gas'tro·du'o·de·nos'co·py
gas'tro·du'o·de·nos'to·my
gas'tro·dyn'i·a
gas'tro·en'ter·al'gi·a
gas'tro·en·ter'ic
gas'tro·en'ter·it'ic
gas'tro·en'ter·i'tis
gas'tro·en'ter·o·a·nas'to·
  mo'sis
gas'tro·en'ter·o·co·li'tis
gas'tro·en'ter·ol'o·gist
gas'tro·en'ter·ol'o·gy
gas'tro·en'ter·op'a·thy
gas'tro·en'ter·op·to'sis
gas'tro·en'ter·os'to·my
gas'tro·en'ter·ot'o·my
gas'tro·ep'i·plo'ic
gas'tro·e·soph'a·ge'al
gas'tro·e·soph'a·gi'tis
gas'tro·e·soph'a·go·plas'ty

gas'tro·e·soph'a·gos'to·my
gas'tro·fi'ber·scope'
gas'tro·gas·tros'to·my
gas'tro·ga·vage'
gas'tro·gen'ic
gas'tro·graph'
gas'tro·he·pat'ic
gas'tro·hep'a·ti'tis
  pl. -tis·es *or* -tit'i·des'
gas'tro·hy'per·ton'ic
gas'tro·il'e·ac'
gas'tro·il'e·i'tis
gas'tro·il'e·os'to·my
gas'tro·in·tes'ti·nal
gas'tro·je·ju'nal
gas'tro·je·ju·ni'tis
gas'tro·je·ju·no·col'ic
gas'tro·je·ju·nos'to·my
gas'tro·la·vage'
gas'tro·li'e·nal
gas'tro·lith'
gas'tro·li·thi'a·sis *pl.* -ses'
gas·trol'o·gist
gas·trol'o·gy
gas·trol'y·sis *pl.* -ses'
gas'tro·ma·la'ci·a
gas'tro·meg'a·ly
gas·trom'e·lus
gas'tro·mes'en·ter'ic
gas'tro·my·co'sis *pl.* -ses'
gas'tro·my·ot'o·my
gas'tro·myx'or·rhe'a
gas'tro·pan'cre·at'ic
gas'tro·pan'cre·a·ti'tis
gas'tro·par'a·si'tus
gas'tro·pa·re'sis di'a·bet'i·
  co'rum
gas'tro·path'ic
gas·trop'a·thy
gas'tro·per'i·to·ni'tis
gas'tro·pex'y
gas'tro·phren'ic
gas'tro·phthi'sis *pl.* -ses'
gas'tro·plas'ty
gas'tro·ple'gi·a
gas'tro·pli·ca'tion
Gas·trop'o·da
gas'tro·pore'
gas'tro·pto'sis
gas'tro·pul'mo·nar'y
gas'tro·py'lo·rec'to·my
gas'tro·py·lor'ic
gas'tro·ra·dic'u·li'tis

gas'tror·rha'gi·a
gas·tror'rha·phy
gas'tror·rhe'a
gas'tror·rhex'is
gas'tro·sal'i·var'y
gas·tros'chi·sis
gas'tro·scope'
gas'tro·scop'ic
gas·tros'co·py
gas·tro'sis *pl.* -ses'
gas'tro·spasm
gas'tro·splen'ic
gas'tro·stax'is
gas'tro·ste·no'sis *pl.* -ses'
gas·tros'to·ga·vage'
gas·tros'to·la·vage'
gas·tros'to·ma *pl.* -mas *or*
  -ma·ta
gas·tros'to·my
gas'tro·suc'cor·rhe'a
gas'tro·tho'ra·cop'a·gus
  pl. -gi'
gas'tro·tome'
gas·trot'o·my
gas'tro·to·nom'e·ter
gas'tro·tox'ic
gas'tro·tox'in
gas'tro·trop'ic
gas'tro·tym'pa·ni'tes'
gas·tru'la *pl.* -las *or* -lae'
gas·tru·la'tion
Gatch bed
gatched
gate, gat'ed, gat'ing
gat'o·phil'i·a
gat'o·pho'bi·a
Gau·cher'
  —cells
  —disease
  —lipid
gauge
gaul·the'ri·a
gaul'the·rin
Gault reflex
gaunt'let
gauss
Gaus·sel' sign
Gauss'i·an
  —distribution
  —points
gauze
ga·vage'
Gay'nor-Hart' position

gaze, gazed, gaz'ing
g'-com·po'nent
Gee'-Her'ter disease
Gee'-Her'ter-Heub'ner
—disease
—syndrome
Gee'-Thay'sen disease
Ge'gen·baur' muscle
ge'gen·hal'ten
Gei'gel reflex
Gei'ger
—counter
—region
—threshold
—tube
Gei'ger-Mül'ler
—counter
—counting circuit
—tube
gel
ge·las'mus
ge·las'tic
gel'ate'
ge·lat'i·fi·ca'tion
gel'a·tin
ge·lat'i·nase'
ge·lat'i·nif'er·ous
ge·lat'i·ni·za'tion
ge·lat'i·nize', -nized', -niz'ing
ge·lat'i·noid'
ge·lat'i·no·lyt'ic
ge·lat'i·no'sa
ge·lat'i·nous
ge·la'tion
gel'a·tose'
Gé'li·neau'-Red'lich
  syndrome
Gé'li·neau' syndrome
Gel·lé' test
gel'o·ple'gi·a
gel'ose'
ge·lo'sis pl. -ses'
gel'se·mine'
gem·fib'ro·zil
gem'i·nate', -nat'ed, -nat'ing
gem'i·na'tion
gem'i·nous
ge·mis'to·cyte'
ge·mis'to·cyt'ic
gem'ma pl. -mae'
gem·ma'tion
gem'mule'
gem·py'lid poisoning

ge'na pl. -nae'
ge'nal
gen'der
Gen'dre fixing fluid
gene
gen'er·al·i·za'tion
gen'er·al·ize', -ized', -iz'ing
gen'er·a'tor
ge·ner'ic
ge·ne'si·al
ge·nes'ic
ge·ne'si·ol'o·gy
gen'e·sis pl. -ses'
ge·net'ic
ge·net'i·cist
ge·net'ics
ge·net'o·troph'ic
gen'e·tous
ge'ni·al
gen'ic
ge·nic'u·lar
ge·nic'u·late'
ge·nic'u·lo·cal'ca·rine'
ge·nic'u·lo·tem'po·ral
ge·nic'u·lum pl. -la
  —ca'na'lis fa·ci·a'lis
  —ner'vi' fa·ci·a'lis
ge'ni·o·glos'sus pl. -si'
ge'ni·o·hy'o·glos'sus pl. -si'
ge'ni·o·hy'oid'
ge·ni'on'
ge'ni·o·pha·ryn'ge·us
ge'ni·o·plas'ty
gen'i·tal
gen'i·ta'li·a
gen'i·tal'i·ty
gen'i·tal·oid'
gen'i·to·cru'ral
gen'i·to·der'ma·to'sis
  pl. -ses'
gen'i·to·fem'o·ral
gen'i·to·plas'ty
gen'i·to·u'ri·nar'y
gen'i·to·ves'i·cal
gen'ius
  —ep'i·dem'i·cus
  —mor'bi'
gen'o·blast'
gen'o·cide'
gen'o·der'ma·to'sis pl. -ses'
ge'nome'
gen'o·pho'bi·a
gen'o·type'

gen'o·typ'ic or
  gen'o·typ'i·cal
gen'ta·mi'cin
gen'tian
ge'nu pl. gen'u·a
  —cap'su·lae' in·ter'nae'
  —cor'po·ris cal·lo'si'
  —ex·tror'sum
  —fa·ci·a'lis
  —im·pres'sum
  —in·tror'sum
  —ner'vi' fa·ci·a'lis
  —rad'i·cis ner'vi' fa·ci·a'lis
  —re'cur·va'tum
  —val'gum
  —var'um
gen'u·al
gen'u·cu'bi·tal
gen'u·fa'cial
gen'u·pec'to·ral
ge'nus pl. gen'er·a
gen'y·an'trum
gen'y·plas'ty
ge'o·graph'ic
ge'o·med'i·cine
ge'o·pha'gi·a
ge·oph'a·gism
ge·oph'a·gist
ge·oph'a·gous
ge·oph'a·gy
Geor'gi-Sachs' test
ge'o·tax'is
ge·ot'ri·cho'sis pl. -ses'
Ge·ot'ri·chum
Ger'agh·ty operation
ge·rat'ic
ger'a·tol'o·gy
Ger'dy tubercle
Ger'hardt'
—disease
—sign
ger'i·at'ric
ger'i·at'rics
ger'i·o·psy·cho'sis pl. -ses'
Ger'lach' tubal tonsil
Ger'li·er
—disease
—syndrome
germ
germ'-free'
ger'mi·cid'al
ger'mi·cide'
ger'mi·nal

ger'mi·nate', -nat'ed, -nat'ing
ger'mi·na'tion
ger'mi·na·tive
ger'mi·no'ma *pl.* -mas *or*
   -ma·ta
Ger'mis·ton fever
ger'o·co'mi·a
ger'o·com'i·cal
ge·roc'o·my
ger'o·der'ma
ger'o·don'ti·a
ger'o·don'tic
ger'o·don'tics
ger'o·don·tol'o·gy
ger'o·ma·ras'mus
ger'o·mor'phism
ge·ron'tal
ge·ron'tic
ger'on·tol'o·gy
ge·ron'to·phil'i·a
ge·ron'to·pho'bi·a
ge·ron'to·ther'a·peu'tics
ge·ron'to·ther'a·py
ger'on·tox'on'
Ge·ro'ta fascia
Gersh'-Ma·cal'lum method
Gerst'mann syndrome
Ge·sell'
  —developmental schedule
  —scale
ges'ta·gen
ge·stalt'
ge·stalt'ism
ge·stalt'ist
ges'tate', -tat'ed, -tat'ing
ges·ta'tion
ges·ta'tion·al
ges·to'sis *pl.* -ses'
Get'so·wa adenoma
Ghon
  —complex
  —lesion
  —tubercle
ghost
Gia·co·mi'ni
  —band
  —frenulum
Gian·nuz'zi
  —cells
  —crescent
Gia·not'ti-Cro'sti
  syndrome
gi'ant

gi'ant·ism
Gi·ar'di·a
  —intestinalis
  —lam'bli·a
gi'ar·di'a·sis *pl.* -ses'
gib'ber·el'lic
gib'ber·el'lin
Gib'bon-Lan'dis test
gib·bos'i·ty
gib'bous *(swollen, convex, or
  protuberant)*
  ♦*gibbus*
Gibbs adsorption law
Gibbs'-Don'nan
  equilibrium
Gibbs'-Helm'holtz'
  equation
gib'bus *(a hump)*
  ♦*gibbous*
Gi·bral'tar fever
Gib'son rule
Giem'sa stain
Giem'sa-Wright' stain
Gier'ke
  —corpuscles
  —disease
  —respiratory bundle
Gif'ford
  —operation
  —reflex
  —sign
gig'a·hertz'
gi·gan'tism
gi·gan'to·blast'
gi·gan'to·chro'mo·blast'
gi·gan'to·cyte'
gi·gan'to·mas'ti·a
Gi'gli operation
Gil·bert'
  —disease
  —sign
  —syndrome
Gil'christ disease
gild'ing
Gil'e·ad balm
Gil'ford-Hutch'in·son
  disease
gill
Gilles de la Tou·rette'
  —disease
  —syndrome
Gil'lies operation
Gill'-Stein' operation

Gim'ber·nat' ligament
gin'ger
gin'gi·va *pl.* -vae'
gin'gi·val
gin'gi·val·ly
gin'gi·vec'to·my
gin'gi·vi'tis
gin'gi·vo·ax'i·al
gin'gi·vo·buc'cal
gin'gi·vo·glos'sal
gin'gi·vo·glos·si'tis
gin'gi·vo·la'bi·al
gin'gi·vo·plas'ty
gin'gi·vo'sis *pl.* -ses'
gin'gi·vo·sto'ma·ti'tis
gin'gly·form'
gin'gly·mo·ar·thro'di·al
gin'gly·moid'
gin'gly·mus *pl.* -mi'
Gi·ral'dés organ
gir'dle
Gir'dle·stone' operation
Gir'dle·stone'-Tay'lor
  operation
girth
git'a·lin
Git'lin syndrome
git·og'e·nin
git'o·nin
gi·tox'i·gen'in
gi·tox'in
Gjes'sing syndrome
gla·bel'la *pl.* -lae'
gla·bel'lar
gla'brate'
gla'brous
gla'cial
gla'di·ate'
glad'i·o'lic
glad'i·o'lus *pl.* -li'
glair'in
glair'y
gland
  —of Bar'tho·lin
  —of Vir'chow-Troi'si·er
glan'ders
glands
  —of Lie'ber·kühn
  —of Sham'baugh'
  —of Zeis
glan'du·la *pl.* -lae'
  —bul'bo·u're·thra'lis
  —lac'ri·ma'lis

—lacrimalis inferior
—lacrimalis superior
—lin·gua′lis anterior
—mam·mar′i·a
—mu·co′sa
—par′a·thy·roi′de·a inferior
—parathyroidea superior
—pa·ro′tis
—parotis ac′ces·so′ri·a
—pi·tu′i·tar′i·a
—se·ro·mu·co′sa
—se·ro′sa
—sub′lin·gua′lis
—sub′man·dib′u·lar′is
—sub′max′il·lar′is
—su′pra·re·na′lis
—thy′re·oi′de·a
—thyreoidea ac′ces·so′ri·a
  su′pra·hy·oi′de·a
—thy·roi′de·a
—tym·pan′i·ca
—ves·tib′u·lar′is major
glan′du·lae′
—ar′e·o·lar′es′
—bron′chi·a′les′
—buc·ca′les′
—ce·ru′mi·no′sae′
—cer·vi·ca′les′ u′ter·i′
—cil′i·ar′es′
—cir′cum·a·na′les′
—con·junc′ti·va′les′
—cu′tis
—du·o·de·na′les′
—e′so·pha′ge·ae′
—gas′tri·cae′
—glom′i·for′mes′
—in·tes′ti·na′les′ in′tes·ti′ni′
  cras′si′
—intestinales intestini
  ten′u·is
—intestinales rec′ti′
—la·bi·a′les′
—lac′ri·ma′les′ ac′ces·so′-
  ri·ae′
—la·ryn′ge·ae′
—laryngeae an·te′ri·o′res′
—laryngeae me′di·ae′
—laryngeae pos·te′ri·o′res′
—lin·gua′les′
—mo·lar′es′
—mu·co′sae′ bil′i·o′sae′
—mucosae tu′ni·cae′ con′-
  junc·ti′vae′

—mucosae u′re·te′ris
—na·sa′les′
—ol′fac·to′ri·ae′
—o′ris
—pal′a·ti′nae′
—pel′vis re·na′lis
—pha·ryn′ge·ae′
—prae·pu′ti·a′les′
—pre·pu′ti·a′les′
—pro′pri·ae′
—py·lo′ri·cae′
—se·ba′ce·ae′
—sebaceae a·re′o·lae′
  mam′mae′
—sebaceae
  con·junc′ti·va′les′
—sebaceae la′bi·o′rum
  pu·den′di′
—si′ne′ duc′ti·bus
—su′do·rif′er·ae′
—su′pra·re·na′les′
  ac′ces·so′ri·ae′
—tar·sa′les′
—thy′re·oi′de·ae′
  ac′ces·so′ri·ae′
—thy·roi′de·ae′
  ac′ces·so′ri·ae′
—tra′che·a′les′
—tu·bar′i·ae′
—u′re·thra′les′
—urethrales u·re′thrae′
  mu′li·e′bris
—u′ter·i′nae′
—ves·i·ca′les′
—ves·tib′u·lar′es′ mi·no′res′
glan′du·lar
glans pl. glan′des′
—cli·to′ri·dis
—pe′nis
Glanz′mann disease
Gla·se′ri·an fissure
glass′es
Glau′ber salt
glau·co′ma
glau·co′ma·to·cy·clit′ic
glau·co′ma·tous
Glea′son score
gleet
gleet′y
Glé·nard′ disease
Glenn anastomosis
glen′o·hu′mer·al
gle′noid′

gle′no·plas′ty
Gley
—cells
—glands
gli′a
gli′a·cyte′
gli′a·din
gli′al
gli′o·bac·te′ri·a
gli′o·blast′
gli′o·blas·to′ma pl. -mas or
  -ma·ta
—i′so·mor′phe′
—mul′ti·for′me′
gli′o·car′ci·no′ma pl. -mas
  or -ma·ta
gli′o·coc′cus pl. -ci′
gli′o·fi′bro·sar·co′ma
  pl. -mas or -ma·ta
gli·og′e·nous
gli·o′ma pl. -mas or -ma·ta
gli′o·ma·to′sis pl. -ses′
—cer′e·bri′
gli·om′a·tous
gli′o·neu′ro·blas·to′ma
  pl. -mas or -ma·ta
gli′o·neu·ro′ma pl. -mas or
  -ma·ta
gli′o·sar·co′ma pl. -mas or
  -ma·ta
gli·o′sis pl. -ses′
gli′o·some′
gli′o·tox′in
Glis′son
—capsule
—disease
glis·so′ni′tis
glis′ten·ing
glob′al
globe
Glo·bid′i·um
glo′bin
glo′boid′
glo′bose′
glo′bo·side′
glob′u·lar
glob′ule′
glob′u·lin
a-globulin
b-globulin
g-globulin
glob′u·lin·e′mi·a
glob′u·li·nu′ri·a

glob′u·lo·max′il·lar′y
glo′bus *pl.* -bi′
—hys·ter′i·cus
—major ep′i·di·dym′i·dis
—minor epididymidis
—pal′li·dus
glo′man·gi·o′ma *pl.* -mas *or*
-ma·ta
glome
glo·mec′to·my
glom′er·a a·or′ti·ca
glom′er·ate
glo·mer′u·lar
glom′er·ule′
glo·mer′u·li′
—ar·te′ri·o′si′ coch′le·ae′
—re′nis
glo·mer′u·li′tis
glo·mer′u·lo·ne·phri′tis
glo·mer′u·lop′a·thy
glo·mer′u·lo·scle·ro′sis
pl. -ses′
glo·mer′u·lose′
glo·mer′u·lo·tro′pin
glo·mer′u·lus *pl.* -li′
glo′mic
glo′mus *pl.* glom′er·a
—a·or′ti·cum
—ca·rot′i·cum
—cho′ri·oi′de·um
—cho·roi′de·um
—coc·cyg′e·um
—jug′u·lar′e′
glon′o·in
glos′sa *pl.* -sae′
glos′sal
glos·sal′gi·a
glos·san′thrax′
glos·sec′to·my
Glos·si′na
glos·sit′ic
glos·si′tis
—ar′e·a′ta ex·fo′li·a·ti′va
glos′so·cele′
glos′so·dy′na·mom′e·ter
glos′so·dyn′i·a
—ex·fo′li·a·ti′va
glos′so·ep′i·glot′tic
glos′so·ep′i·glot·tid′e·an
glos′so·graph′
glos′so·hy′al
glos′so·hy′oid′
glos′so·kin′es·thet′ic

glos′so·la′bi·al
glos′so·la′bi·o·la·ryn′ge·al
glos′so·la′bi·o·pha·ryn′-
ge·al
glos′so·la′li·a
glos·sol′o·gy
glos′so·man′ti·a
glos′so·pal′a·tine′
glos′so·pal′a·ti′nus
glos′so·pal′a·to·la′bi·al
glos·sop′a·thy
glos′so·pha·ryn′ge·al
glos′so·pha·ryn′ge·o·la′-
bi·al
glos′so·pha·ryn′ge·us
glos′so·plas′ty
glos′so·ple′gi·a
glos·sop·to′sis *pl.* -ses′
glos′so·py·ro′sis
glos·sor′rha·phy
glos·sos′co·py
glos′so·spasm
glos·sot′o·my
glos′so·trich′i·a
glot′tal
glot′tic
glot·tid′e·an
glot′tis *pl.* -tis·es *or* -ti·des′
glu′ca·gon′
glu′ca·go·no′ma *pl.* -mas *or*
-ma·ta
glu′can
glu′ca·to′ni·a
glu·cep′tate′
glu′cide′
glu·cid′ic
glu′co·a·scor′bic
glu′co·cor′ti·coid′
glu′co·fu′ra·nose′
glu′co·gen′ic
glu′co·he′mi·a
glu′co·ki′nase′
glu′co·ki·net′ic
glu′co·kin′in
glu′co·lip′ids
glu·col′y·sis *pl.* -ses′
glu′co·nate′
glu′co·ne·o′gen′e·sis
glu·con′ic
glu′co·pro′tein′
glu′co·pyr′a·nose′
glu′co·sa·mine′
glu′co·sans′

glu′cose′
glu·co′si·dase′
glu′co·side′
glu′co·sin
glu·co′sone′
glu′co·sul′fone′
glu·co·su′ri·a
glu·cu·ron′i·dase′
glu·cu′ro·nide′
glu′ta·mate′
glu·tam′ic
glu·tam′i·nase′
glu′ta·mine′
glu′ta·min′ic
glu′ta·myl
glu′ta·ral′de·hyde′
glu·tar′ic
glu′ta·thi′one′
glu′ta·thi′o·nu′ri·a
glu′te·al
glu′te·lin
glu′ten *(a mixture of proteins found in cereal seeds)*
♦*glutin*
glu′te·nin
glu′te·o·fas′ci·al
glu′te·o·fem′o·ral
glu′te·o·in′gui·nal
glu′te·o·tro′chan·ter′ic
glu·teth′i·mide′
glu′te·us *pl.* -te′i′
—max′i·mus
—me′di·us
—min′i·mus
glu′tin *(a protein obtained from gelatin)*
♦*gluten*
glu′ti·nous
gly·bu′ride′
gly′can
gly′case′
gly·ce′mi·a
gly·ce′mic
glyc·er′al′de·hyde′
gly·cer′ic
glyc′er·i·dase′
glyc′er·ide′
glyc′er·in
glyc′er·in·at′ed
glyc′er·ite′
glyc′er·o·gel′a·tin
glyc′er·ol′
glyc′er·o·phos′phate′

glyc′er·o·phos·phor′ic
glyc′er·ose′
glyc′er·yl
gly′ci·nate′
gly′cine′
gly′ci·nin
gly′ci·nu′ri·a
gly′co·bi·ar′sol′
gly′co·ca′lyx
gly′co·ca′li·cin
gly′co·cho′late′
gly′co·cho′lic
gly′co·con′ju·gate
gly′co·cy·am′i·nase′
gly′co·cy′a·mine′
gly′co·gen
gly′co·ge·nase′
gly′co·gen′e·sis *(process of formation of glycogen)*
   ♦*glycogenosis*
gly′co·ge·net′ic
gly′co·gen′ic
gly′co·ge·nol′y·sis *pl.* -ses′
gly′co·gen′o·lyt′ic
gly′co·gen·o′sis *(one of several inborn errors in the metabolism of glycogen), pl.* -ses′
   ♦*glycogenesis*
gly·cog′e·nous
gly′co·geu′si·a
gly′co·he′mi·a
gly′co·his·tech′i·a
gly′col′
gly′col·al′de·hyde′
gly′col·ic
gly′co·lip′id
gly′co·lyl
gly·col′y·sis *pl.* -ses′
gly′co·lyt′ic
gly′co·met′a·bol′ic
gly′co·me·tab′o·lism
gly′co·ne′o·gen′e·sis *pl.* -ses′
gly′co·pe′ni·a
gly′co·pep′tide′
gly′co·pex′is
gly′co·phil′i·a
gly′co·pro′tein′
gly′co·pty′a·lism
gly′co·pyr′ro·late′
gly′cor·rha′chi·a
gly′cor·rhe′a
gly·co′sa·mine′

gly′cos·a·mi′no·gly′can
gly′co·se·cre′to·ry
gly′co·se′mi·a
gly′co·si·al′i·a
gly′co·sid′al
gly′co·si·dase′
gly′co·side′
gly′co·sid′ic
gly′co·som′e·ter
gly′co·sphin′go·lip′id
gly′co·sphin′go·side′
gly′co·stat′ic
gly′co·su′ri·a
gly′co·su′ric
gly·cos′y·lat′ed
gly·cos′y·la′tion
gly′co·troph′ic
glyc·u·re′sis *pl.* -ses′
gly′cu·ron′ic
gly′cu·ron′i·dase′
gly′cu′ro·nide′
gly′cu·ro·nu′ri·a
glyc′yl
glyc′yr·rhi′za
glyc′yr·rhi′zic
glyc′yr·rhi′zin
gly·hex′a·mide′
gly·oc′ta·mide′
gly′ox′al
gly·ox′a·lase′
gly·ox′a·line′
gly′ox·yl′ic
gly·par′a·mide′
Gmel′in test
gnat
gna·thal′gi·a
gnath′ic
gna′thi·on′
gna·thi′tis
gnath′o·ceph′a·lus *pl.* -li′
gnath′o·dy′na·mom′e·ter
gnath′o·dyn′i·a
gnath′o·pal′a·tos′chi·sis
   pl. -ses′
gna′tho·plas′ty
gna·thos′chi·sis *pl.* -ses′
Gna·thos′to·ma
  —his′pi·dum
  —spi·nig′er·um
gna·thos′to·mi′a·sis
gnaw′ing
gno′si·a
gno′sis *pl.* -ses′

gnos′tic
gno′to·bi·ol′o·gy
gno′to·bi·o′ta
gno′to·bi·ote′
gno′to·bi·ot′ic
gno′to·bi·ot′ics
gob′let
go·det′
Godt′fred′sen syndrome
Goetsch test
Gof′man test
goi′ter
goi′trin
goi′tro·gen
goi′tro·gen′ic
goi′tro·ge·nic′i·ty
goi′trous
Gold′ber′ger limb lead
Gold′blatt′
  —hypertension
  —kidney
  —phenomenon
Gol′den·har′ syndrome
gold′en·rod′
Gold′flam′
  —disease
  —symptom complex
Gold′schei′der disease
Gold′stein′
  —cannula
  —reaction
  —retractor
Gold′stein′-Schee′rer tests
Gold′thwait′ operation
Gol′gi
  —apparatus
  —body
  —bottle neuron
  —cells
  —cisternae
  —complex
  —corpuscle
  —element
  —law
  —material
  —membranes
  —method
  —network
  —remnant
  —substance
  —tendon organ
  —zone
Gol′gi-Maz·zo′ni corpuscle

Gol'gi-Rez·zon'i·co spirals
Goll
—column
—nucleus
—tract
Goltz syndrome
Gom·bault'
—degeneration
—demyelination
—neuritis
Gom·bault'-Phi·lippe'
triangle
go·mit'o·li'
Go·mo'ri stain
gom·pho'sis *pl.* -ses'
gon'a·cra'ti·a
go'nad'
go·nad'al
go·na·dec'to·mize', -mized',
-miz'ing
go'nad·ec'to·my
go·nad'o·blas·to'ma
pl. -mas *or* -ma·ta
go·nad'o·cen'tric
go·nad'o·in·hib'i·to'ry
go·nad'o·ki·net'ic
go·nad'o·lib'er·in
go·na·dop'a·thy
go·nad'o·ther'a·py
go·nad'o·trop'ic
go·nad'o·tro'pin
gon'a·duct'
go·nag'ra
go·nal'gi·a
gon·an'gi·ec'to·my
gon'ar·thri'tis
gon'ar·thro'sis *pl.* -ses'
gon'ar·throt'o·my
go·nat'o·cele'
Gon'da reflex
gon'e·cys·ti'tis
gon'e·cys'to·lith
gon'e·cys'to·py·o'sis
gon'e·i'tis
Gon'gy·lo·ne'ma
—pul'chrum
gon'gy·lo'ne·mi'a·sis
pl. -ses'
go'ni·al
gon'ic
go·nid'i·al
go·nid'i·um *pl.* -i·a
go'ni·o·chei·los'chi·sis

go'ni·o·cra'ni·om'e·try
go'ni·om'e·ter
go'ni·on'
go'ni·o·punc'ture
go'ni·o·scope'
go'ni·o·scop'ic
go'ni·os'co·py
go'ni·ot'o·my
go·ni'tis
gon'o·blast'
gon'o·blen'nor·rhe'a
gon'o·camp'sis
gon'o·cele'
gon'o·coc'cal
gon'o·coc·ce'mi·a
gon'o·coc'cic
gon'o·coc'cide'
gon'o·coc'cus *pl.* -ci'
gon'o·cyte'
gon'o·cy·to'ma *pl.* -mas *or*
-ma·ta
gon·nom'er·y
gon'or·rhe'a
gon'or·rhe'al
Gon'y·au'lax
gon'y·camp'sis
gon'y·o·cele'
gon'y·on'cus
Gon·za'les blood group
Goo·dell' sign
Good'e·nough' test
Good'pas'ture
—stain
—syndrome
Good'sall rule
Good syndrome
goose'neck' deformity
Gop'a·lan' syndrome
Gor'di·a'ce·a
Gor'don
—reflex
—test
Gor'don-Tay'lor operation
gorge
gor'get
Gor'lin
—formula
—syndrome
Gos'se·lin fracture
Gos·syp'i·um
gos'sy·pol
Gott'lieb' cuticle
Gott'schaldt' figures

gouge
Gou'ger·ot'-Blum' disease
Gou'ger·ot'-Hou'wer-
Sjö'gren syndrome
Gou·lard' extract
goun'dou'
gout
gout'y
Gow'er-Hen'ry reflex
Gow'ers
—column
—fasciculus
—myopathy
—phenomenon
—sign
—solution
—syndrome
—tract
graaf'i·an
grab'ber
grac'ile
grac'i·lis
gra·da'tim
Gra'de·ni'go
—sign
—syndrome
gra'di·ent
grad'u·ate
grad'u·at'ed
Grae'fe sign
Grae'ser method
Graff method
graft
Gra'ham
—law
—operation
Gra'ham-Cole' test
Gra'ham Steell' murmur
grain
grain'age
gram
Gram
—iodine
—method
—stain
Gram'-Clau'di·us stain
gram'i·ci'din
Gram'-neg'a'tive
Gram'-pos'i·tive
gra'na
gra·na'tum
Gran·cher'
—pneumonia

—system
grand
　—hys·té·rie'
　—mal
Gran'dry-Mer'kel
　corpuscle
Gran'ger line
gran'u·la
gran'u·lar
gran'u·lar'i·ty
gran'u·late'
gra'nu·la'ti·o' pl. -la'ti·o'nes'
gran'u·la'tion
gran'u·la'ti·o'nes'
　a·rach'noi·de·a'les'
gran'ule'
gran'u·li·form'
gran'u·lo·blast'
gran'u·lo·blas'to·sis pl. -ses'
gran'u·lo·cyte'
gran'u·lo·cyt'ic
gran'u·lo·cy'to·pe'ni·a
gran'u·lo·cy'to·poi·e'sis
　pl. -ses'
gran'u·lo·cy'to·poi·et'ic
gran'u·lo·cy'to·sis pl. -ses'
gran'u·lo'ma pl. -mas or
　-ma·ta
　—an'nu·lar'e'
　—con·ta'gi·o'sa
　—fa'ci·a'le'
　—faciale e'o·sin'o·phil'i·cum
　—fis'su·ra'tum
　—fun·goi'des'
　—gen'i·to·in'gui·na'le'
　—in'gui·na'le'
　—pen'du·lum
　—py'o·gen'i·cum
　—tel·an'gi·ec'ti·cum
　—trop'i·cum
　—ve·ne're·um
gran'u·lo·ma·to'sis pl. -ses'
　—dis'ci·for'mis chron'i·ca
　　pro'gres·si'va
　—in·fan'ti·sep'ti·ca
gran'u·lom'a·tous
gran'u·lo·mere'
gran'u·lo·pe'ni·a
gran'u·lo·plasm
gran'u·lo·plas'tic
gran'u·lo·poi·e'sis pl. -ses'
gran'u·lo·poi·et'ic

gran'u·lo'sa
gran'u·lo'sis pl. -ses'
　—ru'bra na'si'
gra'num pl. -na
graph
graph'an·es·the'si·a
graph'es·the'si·a
graph'ic
graph'ite'
gra·phol'o·gy
graph'o·ma'ni·a
graph'o·mo'tor
graph'o·pho'bi·a
graph'or·rhe'a
graph'o·spasm
Gra'ser diverticulum
grasp
grasp'ers
Gras·set'-Gaus·sel'
　—phenomenon
　—sign
Gras·set' law
grate
Gra'tio·let' optic radiation
grat·tage'
grave
grav'el
Graves disease
grav'id
grav'i·da pl. -das or -dae'
gra·vid'ic
grav'id·ism
gra·vid'i·tas
　—ex·am'i·na'lis
　—ex'o·cho'ri·a'li·a
gra·vid'i·ty
grav'i·do·car'di·ac'
gra·vim'e·ter
grav'i·met'ric
gra·vim'e·try
grav'is ne'o·na·to'rum
　jaundice
grav'i·stat'ic
grav'i·tate', -tat'ed, -tat'ing
grav'i·ta'tion
grav'i·ta'tion·al
grav'i·ty
Gra'witz tumor
gray
gray'-out'
Gray'son ligament
Gray stain
Green'berg' method

Green'field' disease
green'stick' fracture
gref'fo·tome'
greg'a·loid'
Greg'a·ri'na
greg'a·rine'
Greg'er·sen test
Greg'o·ry powder
Greig hypertelorism
grenz
Greu'lich and Pyle bone
　age
Grey Tur'ner sign
grid
Grieg disease
Grie'sin'ger
　—disease
　—sign
Grif'fith method
grind, ground, grind'ing
grind'er
grip
grippe
gris'e·o·ful'vin
gris'e·o·my'cin
Gri·solle' sign
gris'tle
Grit'ti-Stokes' amputation
Groc'co
　—sign
　—triangle
Gro'cott-Go·mo'ri stain
Groen'blad-Strand'berg'
　syndrome
Groe'nouw corneal
　dystrophy
groin
grom'met
groove
gross
Gross disease
gross'ly
growth
Gru'ber
　—fossa
　—ligament
　—muscle
　—syndrome
　—test
gru'mose'
gru'mous
grunt'ing
Grün'wald' stain

Gryn'feltt' triangle
gry'o·chrome'
gry·po'sis *pl.* -ses'
G'-stro·phan'thin
G'-suit'
gua'co
guai'ac'
guai'a·col'
guai·fen'e·sin
Gua·ma fever
gua'na·cline'
gua'na·drel'
gua'nase'
guan·cy'dine'
guan·eth'i·dine'
gua'ni·dine'
gua·ni·di·no·a·ce'tic
gua'nine'
guan·i'so·quin
gua'no·clor'
guan·oc'tine'
gua'no·sine'
guan·ox'an'
guan·ox'y·fen'
gua·nyl'ic
gua·ra'na
guard
Guar·ni·e'ri bodies
Gua·ro'a fever
gua'za
gu'ber·nac'u·lar
gu'ber·nac'u·lum *pl.* -la
  —den'tis
  —tes'tis
Gu'bler paralysis
Gud'den
  —atrophy
  —commissure
Gu'der·natsch' test
Gué·neau' de Mus·sy' point
Gué·rin'
  —fold
  —fracture
  —sinus
  —valve
guide
Guil·lain'-Bar·ré'
  —disease
  —syndrome
Guil·lain' sign
guil'lo·tine'
guin'ea pig

Guld'berg-Waa'ge law
Gu'le·ke-Stoo'key operation
Gull
  —and Sut'ton disease
  —disease
gul'let
gu'lose'
gum
gum'boil'
gum'ma *pl.* -mas *or* -ma·ta
gum'ma·tous
gum'my
Gum'precht' shadows
Gun'ning
  —point
  —test
Gün'ther disease
gur'gle
gur'ney
Gur'vich radiation
gus·ta'tion
gus·ta·to'ry
gus·to·lac'ri·mal
gut
Guth'rie test
Gut'stein' stain
gut'ta *pl.* -tae'
gut'ta-per'cha
gut'tate'
gut'ta'tim
gut'ter
gut'ti·form'
Gutt'mann sign
gut'tur·al
gut'tur·oph'o·ny
gut'tur·o·tet'a·ny
Gut'zeit' test
Gu·yon'
  —amputation
  —canal
  —isthmus
  —sign
Gwath'mey method
gym·ne'mic
gym'no·cyte'
gym'no·pho'bi·a
gym'no·spore'
gym·no·tho'rax' poisoning
gynaec-. See words spelled *gynec-.*
gynaeco-. See words spelled *gyneco-.*

gy·nan'der
gy·nan'dri·a
gy·nan'drism
gy·nan'dro·blas·to'ma *pl.* -mas *or* -ma·ta
gy·nan'droid'
gy·nan'dro·morph'
gy·nan'dro·mor'phic
gy·nan'dro·mor'phism
gy·nan'dro·mor'phous
gy·nan'drous
gy·nan'dry
gyn·a'tre'si·a
gy·ne'cic
gyn·e'co·gen
gy·ne·co·gen'ic
gy·ne·cog'ra·phy
gy·ne·coid'
gy·ne·co·log'ic *or* gy·ne·co·log'i·cal
gy·ne·col'o·gist
gy·ne·col'o·gy
gy·ne·co·ma'ni·a
gy·ne·co·mas'ti·a
gy·ne·co·mas'ty
gy·ne·co·ma·zi·a
gy·ne·co·cop'a·thy
gy·ne·pho'bi·a
gy·ne·phor'ic
gy·ni·at'rics
gy·no·gam'one'
gy·no·gen'e·sis
gyn·o·mer'o·gon
gyn·o·me·rog'o·ny
gyn·o·path'ic
gy'no·plas'tic
gy'no·plas'ty
gyp'sum
gy'ral
gy'rate'
gy·ra'tion
Gy·rau'lus
  —sai'go·nen'sis
gy·rec'to·my
gyr'en·ceph'a·late'
gyr'en·ce·phal'ic
gyr'en·ceph'a·lous
gy'ri'
  —An'dre·ae' Ret'zi·i'
  —an'nec'ten'tes'
  —brev'es' in'su·lae'
  —cer'e·bel'li'
  —cer'e·bri'

—in′su·lae′
—oc·cip′i·ta′les′ lat′er·a′les′
—occipitales su·pe′ri·o′res′
—o·per′ti′
—or′bi·ta′les′
—pro·fun′di′ cer′e·bri′
—tem′po·ra′les′ trans·ver′si′
—tran′si·ti′vi′ cer′e·bri′
gy′ro·mag·net′ic
gy′rose′
gy′ro·spasm
gy′rus *pl.* -ri′
—am′bi·ens
—an′gu·lar′is
—cal·lo′sus
—cen·tra′lis anterior
—centralis posterior
—cin′gu·li′
—cu′ne·us
—den·ta′tus
—ep′i·cal·lo′sus
—fas·ci·o·lar′is
—for′ni·ca′tus
—fron·ta′lis inferior
—frontalis me′di·us
—frontalis superior
—fu′si·for′mis
—hip′po·cam′pi′
—in′fra·cal·ca·ri′nus
—in′tra·lim′bi·cus
—lim′bi·cus
—lin·gua′lis
—lon′gus in′su·lae′
—mar′gi·na′lis
—oc·cip′i·to·tem′po·ra′lis lat′er·a′lis
—occipitotemporalis me′di·a′lis
—of Bro′ca
—ol′fac·to′ri·us
—par′a·hip′po·cam·pa′-lis
—par′a·ter′mi·na′lis
—post′cen·tra′lis
—pre′cen·tra′lis
—rec′tus
—ro·lan′di·cus
—sem′i·lu·nar′is
—sub′cal·lo′sus
—su′pra·cal·lo′sus
—su′pra·mar′gi·na′lis
—tem′po·ra′lis inferior

—temporalis me′di·us
—temporalis superior
—un′ci·na′tus

H

Haab reflex
Haa′se rule
ha·be′na
ha·be′nar
ha·ben′u·la *pl.* -lae′
—per′fo·ra′ta
ha·ben′u·lar
ha·ben′u·lo·pe·dun′cu·lar
ha·bil′i·ta′tion
hab′it
hab′i·tat′
ha·bit′u·al
ha·bit′u·a′tion
hab′i·tus
—ap′o·plec′ti·cus
—phthis′i·cus
Hab′ro·ne′ma
hab′ro·ne·mi′a·sis *pl.* -ses′
hache·ment′
hack′ing
Had′e·field′-Clarke′ syndrome
Ha′den-Haus′ser method
haem-. See words spelled *hem-.*
haema-. See words spelled *hema-.*
Hae′ma·dip′sa
Hae′ma·gog′us
Haem′a·phys′a·lis
haemat-. See words spelled *hemat-.*
haemato-. See words spelled *hemato-.*
haemo-. See words spelled *hemo-.*
Hae′nel
—sign
—variant
Hae′ser
—coefficient
—formula
Haff disease
Haff′kine vaccine
Haf′ni·a al′ve·i′
haf′ni·um
Hag′e·dorn′ and Jen′sen method

Ha′ge·man
—factor
—trait
Hag′lund
—deformity
—disease
Hag′ner
—bag
—disease
Hahn′e·mann·ism
Hai′din·ger brushes
Hai′ley-Hai′ley disease
Haines test
hair′ball′
hair′line′
Ha′jek operation
ha·la′tion
hal′a·zone′
Hal′ber·staedt′er bodies
hal·be′ta·sol′
hal·cin′o·nide′
Hal′dane′
—chamber
—scale
half′-life′
half′-val′ue
hal′ide′
hal′i·ste·re′sis *pl.* -ses′
hal′i·ste·ret′ic
hal′i·to′sis *pl.* -ses′
hal′i·tus
Hall
—muscle
—sign
hal′la·chrome′
Hal′lé point
Hal′ler
—habenula
—isthmus
Hal′ler·mann-Streiff′-Fran·çois′ syndrome
Hal′ler·vor′den-Spatz′
—disease
—syndrome
Hal′lion law
Hal′lo·peau′ disease
hal′lu·cal
hal·lu′ci·nate′, -nat′ed, -nat′ing
hal·lu′ci·na′tion
hal·lu′ci·na·tive
hal·lu′ci·na·to′ry
hal·lu′ci·no·gen

hal·lu′ci·no·gen′e·sis
hal·lu′ci·no·gen′ic
hal·lu′ci·no′sis *pl.* -ses′
hal·lu′ci·not′ic
hal′lux *pl.* -lu·ces′
—flex′us
—mal′le·us
—rig′i·dus
—val′gus
—var′us
hal′ma·to·gen′e·sis *pl.* -ses′
ha′lo′
hal′o·gen
hal′o·gen·ate′, -at′ed, -at′ing
hal′oid′
ha·lom′e·ter
hal′o·per′i·dol′
hal′o·phile′
hal′o·phil′ic
hal′o·pro·ges′ter·one′
hal′o·pro′gin
hal′o·thane′
hal′qui·nols′
Hal′stead tests
Hal′sted
—herniorrhaphy
—mastectomy
—technique
hal·ter
ham′a·me′lis
ha·mar′ti·a
ha·mar′to·blas·to′ma
pl. -mas *or* -ma·ta
ham′ar·to′ma *pl.* -mas *or*
-ma·ta
ham′ar·to′ma·tous
ham′ar·to·pho′bi·a
ha′mate′
ha·ma′tum *pl.* -ta
Ham′bur′ger rule
Ham′il·ton sign
Ham′man
—disease
—murmur
—sign
Ham′man-Rich′ syndrome
Ham′mar·sten test
ham′mer
Ham′mer·schlag′ method
ham′mer·toe′
ham′mock
Ham′mond disease
Hamp′ton

—hump
—line
—maneuver
—technique
ham′string′
ham′u·lar
ham′u·late′
ham′u·lus *pl.* -li′
—lac′ri·ma′lis
—lam′i·nae′ spi·ra′lis
—os′sis ha·ma′ti′
—pter′y·goi′de·us
ha·my′cin
hand
—sign of Brun
hand′breadth′
hand′ed·ness
hand′grip′
hand′i·cap′
han′dle
Hand′ley method
hand′piece′
hand′print′
Hand′-Schül′ler-Chris′tian
disease
hang
Hang′er test
hang′man′s fracture
hang′nail′
hang′o′ver
Ha·not′
—cirrhosis
—disease
Ha·not′-Chauf·fard′
syndrome
Han′sen
—bacillus
—disease
han′se·nid
H antigen
hap′a·lo·nych′i·a
haph′al·ge′si·a
haph′e·pho′bi·a
hap′lo·dont′
hap′loid′
hap′loi·dy
hap·lol′o·gy
hap′lo·my·co′sis
hap·lo′pi·a
hap′lo·scope′
hap′lo·scop′ic
hap′lo·type′
hap′ten

hap·ten′ic
hap′te·pho′bi·a
hap′tic
hap′tics
hap′to·dys·pho′ri·a
hap′to·glo′bin
hap′tom′e·ter
hap′to·phore′
Ha·ra′da syndrome
hard′en
Har′den-Young′ ester
Har·de′ri·an gland
Har′ding-Pas′sey
melanoma
hard′ness
hard′-of-hear′ing
Har′dy-Wein′berg′
equilibrium
hare′lip′
Hare syndrome
Har′kins method
Har′ley disease
har·mo′ni·a
har·mon′ic
har′mo·ny
har′ness
har′pax·o·pho′bi·a
har·poon′
Har′ring·ton operation
Har′ris
—hematoxylin
—syndrome
Har′ris and Ben′e·dict
standards
Har′ri·son
—curve
—groove
—speculum
—sulcus
—test
Har′row·er-Er′ick·son test
Hart′ley-Krause′ operation
Hart′mann
—point
—pouch
Hart′man·nel′la
—cas′tel·lan′i·i′
—hy′a·li′na
Hart′nup disease
harts′horn′
har′vest
Hash′i·mo′to
—disease

—struma
—thyroiditis
hash'ish'
Has'kins test
Has'ner valve
Has'sall
—body
—corpuscle
Has'sall-Hen'le warts
Hau'dek' niche
haunch
Hau'ser procedure
haus·to'ri·um *pl.* -ri·a
haus'tra co'li'
haus'tral
haus·tra'tion
haus'trum *pl.* -tra
haut mal
haus'tus *pl.* haus'tus
Ha'ver·hill fever
Ha'ver·hil'li·a
mul'ti·for'mis
Ha'vers glands
ha·ver'sian
Haxt'hau'sen disease
Hay'em
—corpuscle
—solution
Hay'em-Wi·dal' syndrome
Hay'garth' nodes
Haynes operation
head
Head
—areas
—zones
head'ache'
head'cap'
head'hunt'er catheter
head'lock'
head'rest'
heal
health
health'y
hear, heard, hear'ing
heart
heart'beat'
heart'burn'
heat'stroke'
heave
heaves
heav'i·ness
heav'y
he'be·phre'ni·a

he'be·phren'ic
Heb'er·den
—arthritis
—disease
—node
Heb'er·den-Ro'sen·bach'
node
he·bet'ic
heb'e·tude'
heb'e·tu'di·nous
he'bi·at'rics
he·bos'te·ot'o·my
he·bot'o·my
Heb'ra pityriasis
hec'a·ter·o·mer'ic *or*
hec'a·to·mer'ic
Hecht'-Schla'er adapt-
ometer
hec'tic
hec'to·gram'
hec'to·li'ter
Hed'blom' syndrome
he'de·o'ma
he·do'ni·a
he·don'ic
he·don·ism
he'don·is'tic
he'don·o·pho'bi·a
heel
heel'stick'
Heer'fordt' disease
Hef'ke-Tur'ner sign
Hegg'lin anomaly
Hei'den·hain'
—cells
—iron hematoxylin
—pouch
Hei'den·heim' disease
height
Heim'-Krey'sig sign
Heim'lich maneuver
Hei'ne·ke-Mik'u·licz
—operation
—pyloroplasty
Hei'ne-Med'in disease
Hei'ner syndrome
Heinz bodies
Heinz'-Ehr'lich bodies
Heis'ter valve
Hek'toen' phenomenon
hel'coid'
hel·co'ma *pl.* -mas *or* -ma·ta
hel·co'sis

hel·cot'ic
Held
—spaces
—stria
he'li·an'thine'
hel'i·cal
he·lic'i·form'
hel'i·cine'
hel'i·coid'
hel'i·co·pod'
hel'i·co·po'di·a
hel'i·co·tre'ma
he'li·en·ceph'a·li'tis
he'li·o·pho'bi·a
he'li·o'sis *pl.* -ses'
he'li·o·tax'is
he'li·o·ther'a·py
he'li·o·trop'ic
he'li·o·tro'pin
he'li·ot'ro·pism
he'li·ox'
he'li·um
he'lix *pl.* -lix·es *or* hel'i·ces'
Hel'ke·si·mas'tix
—fae·cic'o·la
hel'le·bore'
Hel'ler-Döh'le disease
Hel'ler test
Hel'li·ge method
Hel'lin law
Hel'ly fixing fluid
Helm'holtz'
—coil
—theory
hel'minth'
hel·min'tha·gogue'
hel'min·them'e·sis
hel'min·thi'a·sis *pl.* -ses'
—e·las'ti·ca
hel·min'thic
hel'minth·ism
hel'min'thoid'
hel'min·thol'o·gist
hel'min·thol'o·gy
hel'min·tho'ma *pl.* -mas *or*
-ma·ta
hel·min'thous
He'lo·der'ma
—hor'ri·dum
—sus·pec'tum
he·lo'ma *pl.* -mas *or* -ma·ta
he·lot'o·my
help'er cell

Hel'weg'
—bundle
—tract
he'ma·chro'ma·to'sis
he'ma·chrome'
he'ma·chro'sis
he'ma·cy·tom'e·ter
he'ma·cy'to·zo'on
hem'a·den
he'ma·do·ste·no'sis pl. -ses'
he'ma·dro'mo·graph'
he'ma·dro·mom'e·ter
hem'ad·sorp'tion
he'ma·dy'na·mom'e·try
he'ma·fa'cient
he'mag·glu'ti·na'tion
he'mag·glu'ti·nin
he'mal
he·mal'um
hem'a·nal'y·sis pl. -ses'
he·man'gi·ec·ta'si·a
he·man'gi·ec'ta·sis pl. -ses'
he·man'gi·ec·tat'ic
he·man'gi·o·am'e·lo·blas·
    to'ma pl. -mas or -ma·ta
he·man'gi·o·blast'
he·man'gi·o·blas·to'ma
    pl. -mas or -ma·ta
he·man'gi·o·blas'to·ma·to'-
    sis
he·man'gi·o·cy·to'ma
    pl. -mas or -ma·ta
he·man'gi·o·e·las'to·
    myx·o'ma pl. -mas or
    -ma·ta
he·man'gi·o·en'do·the'li·
    o·blas·to'ma pl. -mas or
    -ma·ta
he·man'gi·o·en'do·the'li·
    o'ma pl. -mas or -ma·ta
he·man'gi·o·en'do·the'li·
    o·sar·co'ma pl. -mas or
    -ma·ta
he·man'gi·o·fi·bro'ma
    pl. -mas or -ma·ta
he·man'gi·o·li·po'ma
    pl. -mas or -ma·ta
he·man'gi·o'ma pl. -mas or
    -ma·ta
he·man'gi·o·ma·to'sis
    pl. -ses'
—ret'i·nae'
he·man'gi·om'a·tous

he·man'gi·o·my'o·li·po'ma
    pl. -mas or -ma·ta
he·man'gi·o·per'i·cy·to'ma
    pl. -mas or -ma·ta
he·man'gi·o·sar·co'ma
    pl. -mas or -ma·ta
he'ma·phe'ic
he'ma·phe'in
hem'a·poph'y·sis pl. -ses'
hem'ar·thro'sis pl. -ses'
he'ma·te'in
he'ma·tem'e·sis
he'mat·en·ceph'a·lon
he'ma·therm'
he'ma·ther'mal
he'ma·ther'mous
he'mat·hi·dro'sis
he·mat'ic
he'ma·ti·dro'sis
he'ma·tim'e·ter
he'ma·tim'e·try
he'ma·tin
he'ma·tin·e'mi·a
he'ma·tin'ic
he'ma·ti·nom'e·ter
he'ma·ti·nu'ri·a
he'ma·tite'
he'ma·to·bil'i·a
he'ma·to·blast'
he'ma·to·cele'
he'ma·to·che'zi·a
he'ma·to·chro·ma·to'sis
    pl. -ses'
he'ma·to·chro'mi·a
he'ma·to·chy'lo·cele'
he'ma·to·chy'lu·ri·a
he'ma·to·coe'li·a
he'ma·to·col'po·me'tra
he'ma·to·col'pos
he·mat'o·crit'
he'ma·toc'ry·al
he'ma·to·crys'tal·lin
he'ma·to·cyst'
he'ma·to·cys'tic
he'ma·to·cyte'
he'ma·to·cy·tol'y·sis
    pl. -ses'
he'ma·to·cy·tom'e·ter
he'ma·to·cy·to'sis pl. -ses'
he'ma·to·cy'to·zo'on
he'ma·to·cy·tu'ri·a
he'ma·to·dys·cra'si·a
he'ma·to·en'ce·phal'ic

he'mat'o·gen'
he'ma·to·gen'e·sis pl. -ses'
he'ma·to·gen'ic
he'ma·tog'e·nous
he'ma·to·glo'bin
he·mat'o·gone'
he'ma·to·hi·dro'sis
he'ma·toid'
he'ma·toi'din
he'ma·to·log'ic
he'ma·to·log'i·cal
he'ma·tol'o·gist
he'ma·tol'o·gy
he'ma·to·lym'phan'-
    gi·o'ma pl. -mas or -ma·ta
he'ma·to·lym·phu'ri·a
he'ma·tol'y·sis pl. -ses'
he'ma·to·lyt'ic
he'ma·to·lyt'o·poi·et'ic
he'ma·to'ma pl. -mas or
    -ma·ta
he'ma·to·me'di·as·ti'num
he'ma·tom'e·ter
he'ma·tom'e·tra
he'ma·tom'e·try
he·mat'o·mole'
he'ma·tom·phal'o·cele'
he'ma·to·my'e·li·a
he'ma·to·my'e·li'tis
he'ma·to·my'e·lo·pore'
he'ma·ton'ic
he'ma·to·pa·thol'o·gy
he'ma·top'a·thy
he'ma·to·pe'ni·a
he'ma·to·per'i·car'di·um
he'ma·to·per'i·to·ne'um
he'ma·to·phage'
he'ma·to·pha'gi·a
he'ma·toph'a·gous
he'ma·to·phil'i·a
he'ma·to·pho'bi·a
he'ma·to·phyte'
he'ma·to·plas'tic
he'ma·to·poi·e'sis pl. -ses'
he'ma·to·poi·et'ic
he'ma·to·por·phyr'i·a
he'ma·to·por'phy·rin
he'ma·to·por'phy·rin·e'-
    mi·a
he'ma·to·por'phy·ri·nu'ri·a
he'ma·to·pre·cip'i·tin
he'ma·tor'rha·chis
he'ma·tor·rhe'a

he′ma·to·sal′pinx
he′ma·to·scope′
he′ma·tose′
he′ma·to′sis *pl.* -ses′
he′ma·to·spec′tro·scope′
he′ma·to·spec·tros′co·py
he′ma·to·sper′ma·to·cele′
he′ma·to·sper′mi·a
he′ma·to·stat′ic
he′ma·tos′te·on′
he′ma·to·ther′a·py
he′ma·to·ther′mal
he′ma·to·ther′mous
he′ma·to·tho′rax′
he′ma·to·tox′ic
he′ma·to·tox·ic′i·ty
he′ma·to·tox′i·co′sis
he′ma·to·trop′ic
he′ma·to·tym′pa·num
he′ma·tox′y·lin
he′ma·tox′y·lin·o·phil′ic
he′ma·to·zo′ic
he′ma·to·zo′on *pl.* -zo′a
he′ma·tu′ri·a
he′ma·tu′ric
heme
hem′er·a·lo′pi·a
hem′i·a·blep′si·a
hem′i·a·car′di·us
hem′i·a·ceph′a·lus *pl.* -li′
hem′i·ac′e·tal
hem′i·a·chro′ma·top′si·a
hem′i·a·gen′e·sis
hem′i·a·geu′si·a
hem′i·al′bu·mose′
hem′i·al′bu·mo·su′ri·a
hem′i·al′gi·a
hem′i·am′bly·o′pi·a
hem′i·a·my′os·the′ni·a
hem′i·an′a·cu′si·a
hem′i·an·al·ge′si·a
hem′i·an·en·ceph′a·ly
hem′i·an·es·the′si·a
hem′i·a·no′pi·a
hem′i·a·no′pic
hem′i·a·nop′si·a
hem′i·an·os′mi·a
hem′i·a·prax′i·a
hem′i·ar′thro·plas′ty
hem′i·ar·thro′sis *pl.* -ses′
hem′i·a·tax′i·a
hem′i·ath′e·to′sis *pl.* -ses′
hem′i·at′ro·phy

hem′i·az′y·gos′
hem′i·bal′lism
hem′i·bal·lis′mus
he′mic
hem′i·car′di·a
hem′i·cel′lu·lose′
hem′i·cen′trum
hem′i·ce·pha′li·a
hem′i·ceph′a·lus *pl.* -li′
hem′i·ceph′a·ly
hem′i·cer′e·bral
hem′i·cer′e·brum *pl.*
 -brums *or* -bra
hem′i·cho·re′a
hem′i·chro′ma·top′si·a
hem′i·co·lec′to·my
hem′i·con·vul′sion
hem′i·cra′ni·a
hem′i·cra′ni·ec′to·my
hem′i·cra′ni·o′sis
hem′i·cra′ni·ot′o·my
hem′i·cys·tec′to·my
hem′i·de·cor′ti·ca′tion
hem′i·di′a·pho·re′sis
hem′i·di′a·phragm′
hem′i·dro′sis
hem′i·dys·es·the′si·a
hem′i·dys′tro·phy
hem′i·ec′tro·me′li·a
hem′i·el·lip′tic
hem′i·ep′i·lep′sy
hem′i·fa′cial
hem′i·gas·trec′to·my
hem′i·geu′si·a
hem′i·glos′sal
hem′i·glos·sec′to·my
hem′i·glos·si′tis
hem′i·glos·so·ple′gic
hem′i·gna′thi·a
hem′i·gnath′us
hem′i·hi·dro′sis *pl.* -ses′
hem′i·hyp′al·ge′si·a
hem′i·hy′per·es·the′si·a
hem′i·hy′per·hi·dro′sis
hem′i·hy′per·pla′si·a
hem′i·hy′per·to′ni·a
hem′i·hy′per·tro·phy
hem′i·hyp·es·the′si·a
hem′i·hy′po·to′ni·a
hem′i·kar′y·on
hem′i·lam′i·nec′to·my
hem′i·lar′yn·gec′to·my
hem′i·lar′ynx

hem′i·lat′er·al
hem′i·mac′ro·ceph′a·ly
hem′i·man·dib′u·lec′-
 to·my
hem′i·man·dib′u·lo·glos·
 sec′to·my
hem′i·max′il·lec′to·my
hem′i·me′li·a
hem′i·me′lus *pl.* -li′
hem′i·me·tab′o·lous
he′min
hem′i·ne·phrec′to·my
hem′i·o′pi·a
hem′i·op′ic
he·mip′a·gus *pl.* -gi′
hem′i·pal′a·tec′to·my
hem′i·pal′pa·to·la·ryn′go·
 ple′gi·a
hem′i·pa·ral′y·sis
hem′i·par·an·es·the′si·a
hem′i·par′a·ple′gi·a
hem′i·pa·re′sis *pl.* -ses′
hem′i·par·es·the′si·a
hem′i·pa·ret′ic
hem′i·par′kin·son·ism
hem′i·pel·vec′to·my
hem′i·pel′vis
hem′i·ple′gi·a
 —al′ter·nans′
 —cru′ci·a′ta
hem′i·ple′gic
hem′i·pros′ta·tec′to·my
He·mip′ter·a
he·mip′ter·ous
hem′i·ra·chis′chi·sis *pl.*
 -ses′
hem′i·sco·to′sis *pl.* -ses′
hem′i·sect′
hem′i·sec′tion
hem′i·sep′tum *pl.* -tums *or*
 -ta
hem′i·so′mus
hem′i·spasm
hem′i·sphae′ri·a bul′bi·
 u·re′thrae′
hem′i·sphae′ri·um
 —cer′e·bel′li′
 —tel′en·ceph′a·li′
hem′i·sphere′
hem′i·spher·ec′to·my
hem′i·spher′ic
hem′i·spher′i·cal
hem′i·sphe′ri·um

—cer′e·bel′li′
—cer′e·bri′
hem′i·spo·ro′sis *pl.* -ses′
hem′i·sys′to·le
hem′i·ter′a·ta
hem′i·te·rat′ic
hem′i·tho′rax′
hem′i·thy′roi·dec′to·my
hem′i·ver′te·bra
hem′i·zy·gos′i·ty
hem′i·zy′gote′
hem′i·zy′gous
hem′lock′
Hem′me·ler thrombopathy
he′mo·ag·glu′ti·nin
he′mo·al′ka·lim′e·ter
he′mo·bil′i·a
he′mo·bil′i·ru′bin
he′mo·blast′
he′mo·blas′tic
he′mo·blas·to′sis *pl.* -ses′
he′mo·ca·ther′e·sis
he′mo·cath′er·et′ic
He′moc·cult′ test
he′mo·che′zi·a
he′mo·cho′le·cys·ti′tis
he′mo·cho′ri·al
he′mo·chro′ma·to′sis
 pl. -ses′
he′mo·chro′ma·tot′ic
he′mo·chrome′
he′mo·chro′mo·gen
he′mo·chro·mom′e·ter
he′mo·cid′al
he′mo·cla′si·a
he·moc′la·sis *pl.* -ses′
he′mo·clas′tic
he′mo·clip′
he′mo·co·ag′u·la′tion
he′mo·co·ag′u·lin
he′mo·coe′lom
he′mo·con′cen·tra′tion
he′mo·co′ni·a
he′mo·co·ni·o′sis *pl.* -ses′
he′mo·crine
he′mo·crin′i·a
he′mo·cry·os′co·py
he′mo·cul′ture
he′mo·cu′pre·in
he′mo·cy′a·nin
he′mo·cyte′
he′mo·cy′to·blast′
he′mo·cy′to·blas′tic

he′mo·cy′to·blas·to′ma
 pl. -mas *or* -ma·ta
he′mo·cy′to·ca·ther′e·sis
he′mo·cy′to·gen′e·sis
 pl. -ses′
he′mo·cy·tol′o·gy
he′mo·cy·tol′y·sis *pl.* -ses′
he′mo·cy′to·lyt′ic
he′mo·cy·to′ma *pl.* -mas *or*
 -ma·ta
he′mo·cy′tom′e·ter
he′mo·cy′tom′e·try
he′mo·cy′to·poi·e′sis
 pl. -ses′
hem′o·cy′to·trip′sis
he′mo·di′ag·no′sis *pl.* -ses′
he′mo·di·al′y·sis *pl.* -ses′
hem′o·di′a·lyz′er
he′mo·di′a·stase′
he′mo·di·lu′tion
he′mo·drom′o·graph′
he′mo·dy·nam′ic
he′mo·dy·nam′i·cal·ly
he′mo·dy·nam′ics
he′mo·dy′na·mom′e·ter
he′mo·dy′na·mom′e·try
he′mo·en′do·the′li·al
he′mo·e·ryth′rin
he′mo·fil·tra′tion
he′mo·flag′el·late′
he′mo·fus′cin
he′mo·gen′e·sis *pl.* -ses′
he′mo·gen′ic
he·mog′e·nous
he′mo·glo′bin
he′mo·glo′bin·e′mi·a
he′mo·glo′bi·nif′er·ous
he′mo·glo′bi·nol′y·sis
he′mo·glo′bi·nom′e·ter
he′mo·glo′bi·nom′e·try
he′mo·glo′bi·nop′a·thy
he′mo·glo′bi·no·phil′ic
he′mo·glo′bin·ous
he′mo·glo′bi·nu′ri·a
he′mo·glo′bi·nu′ric
he′mo·gram′
he′mo·his′ti·o·blast′
he′mo·hy′dro·sal′pinx
he′mo·ki·ne′sis *pl.* -ses′
he′mo·ki·net′ic
he′mo·lymph′
he′mo·lym·phat′ic
he′mo·lym·phan′gi·o·ma

 pl. -mas *or* -ma·ta
he·mol′y·sate′
he·mol′y·sin
he·mol′y·sis *pl.* -ses′
he′mo·lyt′ic
he′mo·lyt′o·poi·et′ic
he′mo·ly·za′tion
he′mo·lyze′, -lyzed′, -lyz′ing
he′mo·ma·nom′e·ter
he′mo·me′di·as·ti′num
he·mom′e·ter
he′mo·me′tra
he·mom′e·try
he′mo·my′e·lo·gram′
he′mo·ne·phro′sis
he′mo·path′ic
he′mo·pa·thol′o·gy
he·mop′a·thy
he′mo·per·fu′sion
he′mo·per′i·car′di·um
he′mo·per′i·to·ne′um
he′mo·pex′in
he′mo·phage′
he′mo·pha′gi·a
he′mo·pha′gic
he′mo·phag′o·cyte′
he′mo·phag′o·cyt′ic
he·moph′a·gous
he′mo·phil′
he′mo·phil′i·a
he′mo·phil′i·ac′
he′mo·phil′ic
he′mo·phil′i·oid′
He·moph′i·lus
 —ae·gyp′ti·us
 —bron′chi·sep′ti·ca
 —con·junc′ti·vi′ti·dis
 —du·crey′i′
 —gal′li·nar′um
 —in′flu·en′zae′
 —par′a·per′tus′sis
 —per·tus′sis
 —su′is
he′mo·pho′bi·a
he′mo·pho′bic
he′moph·thal′mi·a
he′moph·thal′mos
he′moph′thi·sis *pl.* -ses′
he′mo·plas′tic
he′mo·pleu′ra
he′mo·pneu′mo·per′i·car′-
di·um
he′mo·pneu′mo·tho′rax′

he′mo·poi·e′sis *pl.* -ses′
he′mo·poi·et′ic
he′mo·poi′e·tin
he′mo·por′phy·rin
he′mo·po′si·a
he′mo·pre·cip′i·tin
he′mo·pro′tein′
he′mo·pro′to·zo′a
he·mop′tic
he·mop′ty·sis *pl.* -ses′
hem′or·rhage
hem′or·rhag′ic
hem′or·rha′gin
hem′or·rhe′a
he′mor·rhe·ol′o·gy
hem′or·rhoid′
hem′or·rhoi′dal
hem′or·rhoi·dec′to·my
he′mo·sal′pinx
he′mo·sid′er·in
he′mo·sid′er·i·nu′ri·a
he′mo·sid′er·o′sis *pl.* -ses′
he′mo·sper′mi·a
he′mo·sta′si·a
he′mo·sta′sis *pl.* -ses′
he′mo·stat′
he′mo·stat′ic
he′mo·styp′tic
he′mo·ta·chom′e·ter
he′mo·ther′a·py
he′mo·tho′rax′
he′mo·tox′ic
he′mo·tox·ic′i·ty
he′mo·tox′in
he′mo·troph′ic
he′mo·tym′pa·num
he′mo·zo′on
hen′bane′
Hench and Al′drich test
Hen′der·son-Jones′ disease
Hen′der·son operation
Hen′le
—ampulla
—layer
—ligament
—loop
—muscle
—sheath
—spine
—warts
Hen′le-Coe′nen test
Hen′ne·berg′
—disease

—reflex
Hen′och-Schön′lein′
   purpura
hen·pu′ye
Hen·ri′ques-Sor′en·sen
   method
hen′ry *pl.* -rys *or* -ries
Hen′ry
—law
—melanoflocculation test
Hen′sen
—canal
—disk
—duct
—knot
—node
he′par′
—lo·ba′tum
—sul′fu·ris
hep′a·rin
hep′a·rin·e′mi·a
hep′a·rin·i·za′tion
hep′a·rin·ize′, -ized′, -iz′ing
hep′a·rin·oid′
hep′a·tal′gi·a
hep′a·tec′to·mize′
hep′a·tec′to·my
he·pat′ic
he·pat′i·co·du′o·de·nos′-
   to·my
he·pat′i·co·en′ter·os′to·my
he·pat′i·co·gas·tros′to·my
he·pat′i·co·je′ju·nos′to·my
He·pat′i·co′la he·pat′i·ca
he·pat′i·co·li·thot′o·my
he·pat′i·co·lith′o·trip′sy
he·pat′i·co·pan′cre·at′ic
he·pat′i·co·pul′mo·nar′y
he·pat′i·co·re′nal
he·pat′i·cos′to·my
he·pat′i·cot′o·my
hep′a·ti′tis *pl.* -tis·es *or*
   -tit′i·des′
hep′a·ti·za′tion
hep′a·tized′
hep′a·to·bil′i·ar′y
hep′a·to·blas·to′ma *pl.*
   -mas *or* -ma·ta
hep′a·to·bron′chi·al
hep′a·to·car′ci·no′ma
   pl. -mas *or* -ma·ta
he·pat′o·cele′
hep′a·to·cel′lu·lar

hep′a·to·chol·an′gi·o·du′-
   o·de·nos′to·my
hep′a·to·chol·an′gi·o·en′-
   ter·os′to·my
hep′a·to·chol·an′gi·o·gas·
   tros′to·my
hep′a·to·chol·an′gi·o·je′ju·
   nos′to·my
hep′a·to·chol·an·gi′tis
hep′a·to′cir·rho′sis *pl.* -ses′
hep′a·to·col′ic
hep′a·to·cu′pre·in
hep′a·to·cys′tic
hep′a·to·cyte′
hep′a·to·du′o·de′nal
hep′a·to·du′o·de·nos′-
   to·my
hep′a·to·dyn′i·a
hep′a·to·dys′tro·phy
hep′a·to·en·ter′ic
hep′a·to·en′ter·os′to·my
hep′a·to·fla′vin
hep′a·to·gas′tric
hep′a·to·gen′ic
hep′a·tog·e′nous
hep′a·to·gram′
hep′a·tog′ra·phy
hep′a·toid′
hep′a·to·je·ju′nal
hep′a·to·jug′u·lar
hep′a·to·len·tic′u·lar
hep′a·to·li·e′nal
hep′a·to·li·e·nog′ra·phy
hep′a·to·lith′
hep′a·to·li·thec′to·my
hep′a·to·li·thi′a·sis *pl.* -ses′
hep′a·tol′o·gist
hep′a·tol′o·gy
hep′a·tol′y·sin
hep′a·to·lyt′ic
hep′a·to′ma *pl.* -mas *or*
   -ma·ta
hep′a·to·ma·la′ci·a
hep′a·to·me·ga′li·a
hep′a·to·meg′a·ly
hep′a·to·mel′a·no′sis
   pl. -ses′
hep′a·tom·phal′o·cele′
hep′a·to·neph′ric
hep′a·to·ne·phri′tis
hep′a·to·pan′cre·at′ic
hep′a·top′a·thy
hep′a·to·pex′y

hep'a·to·pleu'ral
hep'a·to·pneu·mon'ic
hep'a·to·por'tal
hep'a·top·to'sis
hep'a·to·pul'mo·nar'y
hep'a·to·re'nal
hep'a·tor'rha·phy
hep'a·tor·rhex'is *pl.* -es'
hep'a·to·scan'
hep'a·tos'co·py
hep'a·to'sis *pl.* -ses'
hep'a·to·sple·ni'tis
hep'a·to·sple·nog'ra·phy
hep'a·to·sple·no·meg'a·ly
hep'a·to·sple·nop'a·thy
hep'a·to·ther'a·py
hep'a·tot'o·my
hep'a·to·tox'ic
hep'a·to·tox·ic'i·ty
hep'a·to·tox'in
hep'a·to·trop'ic
hep'a·to·u'ro·log'ic
hep'ta·bar'bi·tal'
hep'ta·chro'mic
hep'tad
hep'to·glo'bin
hep'tose'
hep'tu·lose'
her'ald
herb
her·ba'ceous
herb'al
herb'al·ist
her'bi·cid'al
her'bi·cide'
her'bi·vore'
her·biv'o·rous
Herbst
—bodies
—corpuscles
he·red'i·tar'y
he·red'i·ty
her'e·do·de·gen'er·a'tion
her'e·do·de·gen'er·a'tive
her'e·do·fa·mil'i·al
her'e·do·mac'u·lar
Her'ing
—canal
—theory
Her'ing-Breu'er reflex
her'i·ta·bil'i·ty
her'i·ta·ble
her'i·tage

Her·man'sky-Pud'lak'
   syndrome
her·maph'ro·dism
her·maph'ro·dite'
her·maph'ro·dit'ic
her·maph'ro·dit·ism
her·maph'ro·di·tis'mus
Her·me'ti·a
her·met'ic
her·met'i·cal·ly
her'ni·a *pl.* -as *or* -ae'
her'ni·al
her'ni·ate', -at'ed, at'ing
her'ni·a'tion
her'ni·oid'
her'ni·o·plas'ty
her'ni·or'rha·phy
her'ni·o·tome'
her'ni·ot'o·my
her'o·in
her'o·in·ism
her'pan·gi'na
her'pes'
—cir'ci·na'tus
—des·qua'mans'
—fa'ci·a'lis
—fe·bri'lis
—gen'i·ta'lis
—ges·ta·ti'o'nis
—hom'i·nis
—i'ris
—la'bi·a'lis
—oph·thal'mi·cus
—pro·gen'i·ta'lis
—re·cur'rens
—sim'i·ae'
—sim'plex'
—ton·su'rans'
—tonsurans mac·u'lo·sus
—zos'ter
—zoster au·ric'u·lar'is
—zoster oph·thal'mi·cus
—zoster o'ti·cus her'pes·vi'-
   rus
—zos'ter var'i·cel·lo'sus
Her'pes·vi'rus
—su'is
—var'i·cel'lae
her·pet'ic
her·pet'i·form'
Her'pe·tom'o·nas
Her'rick anemia
Her'ring bodies

Hers disease
Her'ter-Fos'ter method
Her'ter-Heub'ner disease
Her'ter infantilism
Hert'wig root sheath
hertz
Her'yng
—benign ulcer
—sign
herz'stoss
Heschl gyri
hes·per'i·din
Hes'sel·bach'
—ligament
—triangle
het'a·cil'lin
het'a·starch'
het'er·a·del'phus
het'er·a·de'ni·a
het'er·a·den'ic
Het'er·a'kis
het'er·a'li·us
het'er·aux·e'sis
het'er·ax'i·al
het'er·e'cious
het'er·er'gic
het'er·es·the'si·a
het'er·o·ag·glu'ti·nin
het'er·o·al'bu·mose'
het'er·o·al'bu·mo·su'ri·a
het'er·o·al·lele'
het'er·o·an'ti·bod'y
het'er·o·at'om
het'er·o·aux'in
het'er·o·blas'tic
het'er·o·cel'lu·lar
het'er·o·ceph'a·lus
het'er·o·chro·mat'ic
het'er·o·chro'ma·tin
het'er·o·chro'mi·a
het'er·o·chro'mic
het'er·o·chro'mo·some'
het'er·o·chro'mous
het'er·o·chro'ni·a
het'er·o·chron'ic
het'er·och'ro·nous
het'er·och'ro·ny
het'er·och'tho·nous
het'er·o·crine
het'er·o·cy'cle
het'er·o·cy'clic
het'er·o·cyst'
het'er·o·cy'to·trop'ic

Het′er·od′er·a
—rad′i·cic′o·la
het′er·o·dont′
het′er·od′ro·mous
het′er·o·e·rot′ic
het′er·o·e·rot′i·cism
het′er·o·er′o·tism
het′er·o·fer·men′ta·tive
het′er·o·gam′ete′
het′er·o·ga·met′ic
het′er·o·gam′e·try
het′er·og′a·mous
het′er·og′a·my
het′er·o·ge·ne′i·ty
het′er·o·ge′ne·ous
het′er·o·gen′e·sis
het′er·o·ge·net′ic
het′er·o·gen′ic
het′er·og′e·nous
het′er·o·geu′si·a
het′er·og′o·ny
het′er·o·graft′
het′er·o·he′mag·glu′ti·nin
het′er·o·he·mol′y·sin
het′er·o·hyp·no′sis
het′er·o·im·mu′ni·ty
het′er·o·in·tox′i·ca′tion
het′er·o·kar′y·on
het′er·o·kar′y·ot′ic
het′er·o·ker′a·to·plas′ty
het′er·o·ki·ne′si·a
het′er·o·ki·ne′sis pl. -ses′
het′er·o·lac′tic
het′er·o·la′li·a
het′er·o·lat′er·al
het′er·ol′o·gous
het′er·ol′o·gy
het′er·ol′y·sin
het′er·ol′y·sis
het′er·o·lyt′ic
het′er·o·mas′ti·gote′
het′er·o·mer′ic
het′er·om′er·ous
het′er·o·met′a·pla′si·a
het′er·o·met′ric
het′er·o·me·tro′pi·a
het′er·o·mor′phic
het′er·o·mor′phism
het′er·o·mor·pho′sis
    pl. -ses′
het′er·o·mor′phous
het′er·on′o·mous
het′er·on′o·my

het′er·o·os′te·o·plas′ty
het′er·op′a·gus pl. -gi′
het′er·o·path′ic
het′er·op′a·thy
het′er·o·pha′si·a
het′er·o·phe′mi·a
het′er·oph′e·my
het′er·o·phil′
het′er·o·phil′ic
het′er·o·pho·ni·a
het′er·o·pho·ral′gi·a
het′er·o·pho·ri·a
het′er·o·phor′ic
Het′er·oph′y·es′
het′er·o·phy·i′a·sis
het′er·o·phy′id
het′er·o·phy′i·di·a·sis
het′er·o·pla′si·a
het′er·o·plasm
het′er·o·plas′tic
het′er·o·plas′ty
het′er·o·ploid′
het′er·o·ploi′dy
het′er·o·pol′y·sac′cha·ride′
het′er·o·pro′so·pus
het′er·op′si·a
Het′er·op′ter·a
het′er·op′tics
het′er·o·pyk·no′sis
het′er·o·pyk·not′ic
het′er·o·sac′cha·ride′
het′er·o·scope′
het′er·o·scop′ic
het′er·os′co·py
het′er·o·sex′u·al
het′er·o·sex′u·al′i·ty
het′er·o·sex′u·al·ly
het′er·os′mi·a
het′er·o·some′
het′er·os′po·rous
het′er·o·sug·ges′ti·bil′i·ty
het′er·o·sug·ges′tion
het′er·o·tax′i·a
het′er·o·tax′ic
het′er·o·tax′is pl. -tax′es′
het′er·o·tax′y
het′er·o·therm′
het′er·o·ther′my
het′er·o·to′ni·a
het′er·o·ton′ic
het′er·o·to′pi·a
het′er·o·top′ic
het′er·ot′o·pous

het′er·ot′o·py
het′er·o·tox′in
het′er·o·trans′plant′
het′er·o·trans′plan·ta′tion
het′er·o·tri·cho′sis pl. -ses′
het′er·o·troph′
het′er·o·troph′ic
het′er·o·tro′pi·a
het′er·ot′ro·py
het′er·o·typ′ic or het′er·o·
    typ′i·cal
het′er·o·xan′thine′
het′er·ox′e·nous
het′er·ox′e·ny
het′er·o·zy′go·sis pl. -ses′
het′er·o·zy′gos′i·ty
het′er·o·zy′gote′
het′er·o·zy′gous
Heth′er·ing·ton stain
Heub′ner
—disease
—endarteritis
Heub′ner-Her′ter disease
heu·ris′tic
Heu′ser membrane
hex′a·canth′
hex′a·chlo′ro·cy′clo·hex′-
    ane′
hex′a·chlo′ro·phene′
hex′a·chro′mic
hex′ad′
hex′a·dac′tyl·ism
hex′a·dac′ty·ly
hex′a·dec′a·no′ic
hex′a·dec′yl
hex′a·di·meth′rine′
hex′a·eth′yl tet′ra·phos′-
    phate′
hex′a·fluo·re′ni·um
hex·al′de·hyde′
hex′a·me·tho′ni·um
hex′a·mine′
hex′ane′
hex′a·no′ic
hex′a·ploid′
hex′a·ploi′dy
hex′a·va′lent
hex′a·vi′ta·min
hex·ax′i·al
hex′es·trol′
hex·e′thal′
hex·et′i·dine′
hex·o·bar′bi·tal′

hex′o·bar′bi·tone′
hex′o·cy′cli·um
hex′o·ki′nase′
hex′one′
hex′os·am′ine′
hex′os·a·min′i·dase′
hex′o·san′
hex′ose′
hex′u·lose′
hex′u·ron′ic
hex′yl
hex′yl·caine′
hex′yl·re·sor′ci·nol′
Hey amputation
hi·a′tal
hi·a′tus
—ad′duc·to′ri·us
—a·or′ti·cus
—ca·na′lis fa·ci·a′lis
—canalis ner′vi′ pe·tro′si′
  ma·jo′ris
—canalis nervi petrosi
  mi·no′ris
—e′so·phag′e·us
—eth′moi·da′lis
—max′il·lar′is
—oe′so·phag′e·us
—of Fal·lo′pi·us
—of Schwal′be
—pleu′ro·per′i·to′ne·a′lis
—sa·cra′lis
—sa·phe′nus
—sem′i·lu·nar′is
—ten·din′e·us
Hibbs operation
hi′ber·nate′, -nat′ed, -nat′ing
hi′ber·na′tion
hi′ber·no′ma pl. -mas or
  -ma·ta
Hib′i·clens′ solution
hic′cup
hick′o·ry-stick′ fracture
Hicks
—sign
—version
hi·drad′e·ni′tis
—ax′il·lar′is
—sup′pu·ra·ti′va
hi′drad·e·no·car′ci·no′ma
  pl. -mas or -ma·ta
hi·drad′e·noid′
hi·drad′e·no′ma pl. -mas or
  -ma·ta

—pap′il·lif′e·rum
hid′ro·cyst·ad′e·no′ma
  pl. -mas or -ma·ta
hid′ro·cys·to′ma pl. -mas or
  -ma·ta
hid′ro·poi·e′sis pl. -ses′
hid′ro·poi·et′ic
hid′ror·rhe′a
hi′dros·ad′e·ni′tis
hi·dros′che·sis pl. -ses′
hi′drose′
hi·dro′sis pl. -ses′
hi·drot′ic
hi′er·al′gi·a
hi′er·et′ic
hi′er·o·lis′the·sis
hi′er·o·pho′bi·a
high′-risk′
hi′lar
Hill
—reaction
—sign
Hill′-Flack′ sign
Hil′liard lupus
hill′ock
Hil′ton law
hi′lum pl. -la
hi′lus pl. -li′
—glan′du·lae′ su′pra·re·
  na′lis
—li·e′nis
—lym′pho·glan′du·lae′
—no′di′ lym·phat′i·ci′
—nu′cle·i′ den·ta′ti′
—nuclei ol′i·var′is
—o·var′i·i′
—pul·mo′nis
—re′na′lis
hind′brain′
hind′foot′
hind′gut′
Hines and Brown test
hinge
Hin′kle pill
Hin′ton test
hip
Hip′pe·la′tes′
—fla′vi·pes′
—pu′si·o′
Hip′pel-Lin′dau′ disease
Hip′po·bos′ca
Hip′po·bos′ci·dae′
hip′po·cam′pal

hip′po·cam′pus pl. -pi′
Hip·poc′ra·tes′ maneuver
hip′po·crat′ic
hip′po·lith′
hip′pu·ran′
hip′pu·rase′
hip′pu·rate′
hip·pu′ri·a
hip·pu′ric
hip·pu′ri·case′
hip′pus
hir′ci′ sing. -cus
hir·cis′mus
Hirsch′berg′
—reflex
—sign
—test
Hirsch′feld′
—nerve
—point
Hirsch′sprung′ disease
hir′sute′
hir′sut·ism
hir′tel·lous
Hirtz rale
hi·ru′di·cide′
hir′u·din
Hir′u·din′e·a
hir′u·din′e·an
hir′u·di·ni′a·sis pl. -ses′
His
—band
—bundle
—canal
—perivascular space
—spindle
—tubercle
His′-Held′ space
His′-Pur·kin′je system
His spaces
Hiss serum water
his·tam′i·nase′
his′ta·mine′
his′ta·mi·ne′mi·a
his′ta·min·ic
His′-Ta·wa′ra
—node
—system
his′ti·dase′
his′ti·dine′
his′ti·di·ne′mi·a
his′ti·di·nu′ri·a
his′ti·dyl

his'ti·o·cyte'
his'ti·o·cyt'ic
his'ti·o·cy'toid
his'ti·o·cy·to'ma *pl.* -mas *or*
 -ma·ta
his'ti·o·cy·to'ma·to'sis
 pl. -ses'
his'ti·o·cy'to·sar·co'ma
 pl. -mas *or* -ma·ta
his'ti·o·cy·to'sis *pl.* -ses'
his'ti·o·gen'ic
his'ti·oid'
his'ti·o'ma *pl.* -mas *or* -ma·ta
his'ti·o·troph'ic
his'to·blast'
his'to·chem'i·cal
his'to·chem'is·try
his'to·com·pat'i·bil'i·ty
his'to·com·pat'i·ble
his'to·cyte'
his'to·di·al'y·sis *pl.* -ses'
his'to·dif·fer·en'ti·a'tion
his'to·fluo·res'cence
his'to·gen'e·sis
his'to·ge·net'ic
his·tog'e·nous
his·tog'e·ny
his'to·gram'
his'to·he'ma·tin
his'toid'
his'to·in'com·pat'i·bil'i·ty
his'to·in'com·pat'i·ble
his'to·ki·ne'sis
his'to·log'ic *or* his'to·log'i·cal
his'to·log'i·cal·ly
his·tol'o·gist
his·tol'o·gy
his·tol'y·sis
his'to·lyt'ic
his·to'ma *pl.* -mas *or* -ma·ta
his'to·mor·phol'o·gy
his'to·my·co'sis *pl.* -ses'
his'tone'
his'to·neu·rol'o·gy
his·ton'o·my
his'to·nu'ri·a
his'to·path'o·log'ic
his'to·path'o·log'i·cal
his'to·pa·thol'o·gist
his'to·pa·thol'o·gy
his'to·phys'i·ol'o·gy
His'to·plas'ma
 —cap'su·la'tum

his'to·plas'min
his'to·plas·mo'ma *pl.* -mas
 or -ma·ta
his'to·plas·mo'sis *pl.* -ses'
his'to·ra'di·og'ra·phy
his'to·ry
his·to·spec·tros'co·py
his'to·ther'a·py
his'to·throm'bin
his'to·tome'
his·tot'o·my
his·to·tox'ic
his·to·troph'ic
his·to·trop'ic
his'to·zo'ic
his'to·zyme'
his'tri·on'ic
his'tri·o·nism
His'-Wer'ner disease
hitch
Hitch'cock' reagent
Hit'zig center
HIV (human
 immunodeficiency virus)
hives
Hjär're disease
hoarse
hoarse'ness
hoar'y
hob'ble, -bled, -bling
Hoch'sin'ger sign
Hodg'kin
 —disease
 —granuloma
 —lymphoreticuloma
 —sarcoma
Hodg'kin-Key' murmur
Hodg'son disease
ho'do·neu'ro·mere'
ho'do·pho'bi·a
hoe
Hoeh'ne sign
hof
Hof'bau'er cell
Hof'fa
 —disease
 —operation
Hoff'mann
 —anodyne
 —atrophy
 —drops
 —duct
 —finger reflex

 —phenomenon
 —sign
 —syndrome
Hoff'mann-Werd'nig
 —disease
 —syndrome
Hof'meis'ter
 —gastroenterostomy
 —operation
 —series
Hö'gyes treatment
Hoke operation
hol·an'dric
hol'ar·thri'tis
hold'er
hole
Hol'ger Niel'sen method
ho'lism
ho·lis'tic
Hol'la disease
Hol·lande' solution
Hol'lan·der test
Hol'len·horst'
 —bodies
 —plaque
hol'low
Holmes
 —phenomenon
 —sign
Holm'gren-Gol'gi canals
Holm'gren test
hol'mi·um
hol'o·a·car'di·us
 —a·ceph'a·lus
 —a·cor'mus
 —a·mor'phus
hol'o·a·cra'ni·a
hol'o·blas'tic
hol'o·ce·phal'ic
hol'o·crine
ho·loc'ri·nous
hol'o·di·as·tol'ic
hol'o·en·dem'ic
hol'o·en'zyme'
ho·log'a·my
hol'o·gas·tros'chi·sis
 pl. -ses'
hol'o·gram'
hol'o·graph'ic
ho·log'ra·phy
hol'o·gyn'ic
hol'o·mas'ti·gote'
hol'o·me·tab'o·lous

hol'o·mi·crog'ra·phy
hol'o·mor·pho'sis *pl.* ses'
hol'o·phyt'ic
hol'o·pros'en·ceph'a·ly
hol'o·ra·chis'chi·sis *pl.* -ses'
hol'o·sys·tol'ic
hol'o·zo'ic
Hol'ter-Doyle' method
Hol'ter monitor
Holt'-O'ram syndrome
hom'a·lo·ceph'a·lus *pl.* -li'
hom'a·lu'ri·a
Ho'mans sign
ho·mat'ro·pine'
hom·ax'i·al
Home
 —gland
 —lobe
ho'me·o·chrome'
ho'me·o·ki·ne'sis *pl.* -ses'
ho'me·o·met'ric
ho'me·o·mor'phous
ho'me·o·path'
ho'me·o·path'ic
ho'me·op'a·thist
ho'me·op'a·thy
ho'me·o·pla'si·a
ho'me·o·plas'tic
ho'me·o'sis *pl.* -ses'
ho'me·o·sta'sis *pl.* -ses'
ho'me·o·stat'ic
ho'me·o·ther'a·py
ho'me·o·ther'mal
ho'me·o·ther'mic
ho'me·ot'ic
ho'me·o·trans'plant'
ho'me·o·typ'ic
ho·mer'gic
Ho'mer-Wright' rosette
hom'i·cid'al
hom'i·cide'
hom'i·nid
Ho·min'i·dae'
Hom'i·noi'de·a
Ho'mo
 —sa'pi·ens
ho'mo·al·lele'
ho'mo·bi'o·tin
ho'mo·blas'tic
ho'mo·cen'tric *or*
 ho'mo·cen'tri·cal
ho·moch'ro·nous
ho'mo·clad'ic

ho'mo·cys'tine'
ho'mo·cys'ti·ne'mi·a
ho'mo·cys'ti·nu'ri·a
ho'mo·cys'to·trop'ic
ho·mod'ro·mous
ho'mo·dy·nam'ic
ho'mo·dy'na·my
ho'mo·e·rot'ic
ho'mo·er'o·tism
ho'mo·ga·met'ic
ho'mo·fer·men'ta·tive
ho·mog'a·my
ho'mog'e·nate'
ho'mo·ge·ne'i·ty
ho'mo·ge'ne·ous
ho'mo·gen'e·sis *pl.* -ses'
ho'mo·ge·net'ic
ho'mo·gen'ic
ho'mog'e·ni·za'tion
ho'mog'e·nize', -nized',
 -niz'ing
ho'mog'e·nous
ho'mo·gen·tis'ic
ho'mog'e·ny
ho'mo·glan'du·lar
ho'mo·graft'
ho'mo·lac'tic
ho'mo·lat'er·al
ho'mo·log'ic
ho·mol'o·gous
ho'mo·logue'
ho·mol'o·gy
ho·mol'y·sin
ho·mol'y·sis *pl.* -ses'
ho'mo·mor'phic
ho·mon'y·mous
ho'mo·phil
ho'mo·phil'ic
ho'mo·pho'bi·a
ho'mo·pho'bic
ho'mo·plast'
ho'mo·plas'tic
ho'mo·plas'ty
ho'mo·pol'y·mer
hom·or'gan·ic
ho'mo·ser'ine'
ho'mo·sex'u·al
ho'mo·sex'u·al'i·ty
ho'mo·ther'mal
ho'mo·top'ic
ho'mo·trans'plant'
ho'mo·trans'plan·ta'tion
ho'mo·type'

ho'mo·typ'ic
ho'mo·zy·gos'i·ty
ho'mo·zy'gote'
ho'mo·zy'gous
hon'ey·comb'
honk
hood
hood'ed
hook
Hooke law
Hook'er method
hook'let
hook'worm'
Hoo'ver sign
Hope murmur
Hopf disease
Hop'kins-Cole' reaction
Hop'mann polyp
Hop'pe-Gold'flam'
 —disease
 —symptom complex
ho'qui·zil
ho'ra
 —de·cu'bi·tus
 —som'ni'
hor·de'o·lum *pl.* -la
ho·ri'zon
hor'i·zon'tal
hor'i·zon·ta'lis
hor·me'sis
hor'mi·on'
Hor'mo·den'drum
hor·mo'nal
hor'mone'
hor·mon'ic
hor·mo'no·poi·e'sis *pl.* -ses'
hor·mo'no·poi·et'ic
horn
Hor'ner
 —law
 —muscle
 —syndrome
horn'i·fi·ca'tion
horn'y
ho·rop'ter
hor·op'ter·ic
hor·rip'i·la'tion
horse'shoe'
Hors'ley
 —operation
 —sign
Hor·te'ga
 —cell

—silver stain
Hor'ton
—disease
—headache
—syndrome
hos'pi·tal
hos'pi·tal·ism
hos'pi·tal·i·za'tion
hos'pi·tal·ize', -ized', -iz'ing
host
hos'tile
hos·til'i·ty
Hotch'kiss
—method
—operation
Hot'ten·tot'
—apron
—bustle
hot'ten·tot·ism
Houns'field' unit
hour'glass'
house'fly'
Hous·say'
—animal
—phenomenon
Hous'ton
—muscle
—valves
ho'ven
How'ard-Dol'man test
How'ard method
How'ell-Jol'ly bodies
How'ship lacunas
How'ship-Rom'berg'
—sign
—syndrome
Hub'bard tank
Hu·chard'
—disease
—sign
Hud'dle·son test
Hud'son line
Hud'son-Stäh'li line
hue
Hug'gins-Mil'ler-Jen'sen test
Hug'gins test
Hughes reflex
Hugh'ston view
Hu·guier'
—canal
—disease
Huh'ner test

hum
hu'man
hu'man·is'tic
hu·man'o·scope'
hu·mec'tant
hu·mec·ta'tion
hu'mer·al
hu'mer·o·ra'di·al
hu'mer·o·scap'u·lar
hu'mer·o·ul'nar
hu'mer·us pl. -mer·i'
hu'mic
hu·mic'o·lin
hu'mid
hu·mid'i·fi·ca'tion
hu·mid'i·fi'er
hu·mid'i·fy
hu·mid'i·ty
hu'min
hu'mor
—a·quo'sus
—vit're·us
hu'mor·al
hump
hump'back'
Hum'phry operation
hu'mu·lene'
hu'mu·lus
hunch'back'
hun'ger
Hun'ner ulcer
Hunt
—atrophy
—neuralgia
—syndrome
—tremor
Hun'ter
—canal
—glossitis
—line
—operation
—syndrome
Hun'ter·i·an chancre
Hun'ter-Schre'ger bands
Hun'ting·ton
—chorea
—disease
—sign
Hup'pert test
Hur'ler syndrome
Hürth'le cells
Husch'ke
—cartilage

—foramen
—ligaments
—papilla
—teeth
Hutch'in·son
—disease
—freckle
—prurigo
—pupil
—teeth
—triad
Hutch'in·son-Boeck' disease
Hutch'in·son-Gil'ford syndrome
hutch'in·so'ni·an
Hutch'i·son type
hy'a·lin
hy'a·line'
hy'a·lin·i·za'tion
hy'a·lin·ize', -ized', -iz'ing
hy'·li·no'sis pl. -ses'
hy'a·li·nu'ri·a
hy'a·li'tis
hy·al'o·gen
hy'a·loid'
hy'a·loi'de·o·cap'su·lar
hy'a·loid·i'tis
hy'a·lo·mere'
hy'a·lo·mu'coid'
hy'a·lo·nyx'is
hy'a·lo·pha'gi·a
hy'a·lo·plasm
hy'a·lo·se'ro·si'tis
hy·al'o·some'
hy'a·lu'ro·nate'
hy'a·lu·ron'ic
hy'a·lu·ron'i·dase'
hy·ben'zate'
hy'brid
hy'brid·ism
hy·brid'i·ty
hy'brid·i·za'tion
hy'brid·ize'
hy·can'thone'
hy'clate'
hy·dan'to·ic
hy·dan'to·in
hy·dan·to'in·ate'
hy·dat'ic
hy·dat'id
—of Mor·ga'gni
hy'da·tid'i·form'

hy′da·tid′o·cele′
hy′da·ti·do′sis *pl.* -ses′
hy′da·ti·dos′to·my
Hyde disease
hyd′no·car′pus
hy·drac′e·tin
hy·drac′id
hy·dra′er·o·per′i·to·
  ne′um
hy′dra·gogue′
hy·dral′a·zine′
hy·dram′ni·on′
hy·dram′ni·os′
hy·dran·en·ceph′a·ly
hy·drar·gyr′i·a
hy·drar′gy·ri′a·sis
hy·drar′gyr·oph·thal′mi·a
hy·drar′gy·rum
hy′drar·thro′sis *pl.* -ses′
hy′drase′
hy·dras′tis
hy′drate′
hy′drat′ed
hy·dra′tion
hy·drau′lics
hy′dra·zide′
hy′dra·zine′
hy′dra·zone′
hy·dre′mi·a
hy·dre′mic
hy′dren·ceph′a·lo·cele′
hy′dren·ceph′a·lo·me·nin′-
  go·cele′
hy′drep′i·gas′tri·um
hy′dric
hy′dride′
hy′dri·od′ic
hy·dri′o·dide′
hy·dro′a
  —her·pet′i·for′me′
  —vac·cin′i·for′me′
hy′dro·ap·pen′dix
  pl. -dix·es *or* -di·ces′
hy′dro·bil′i·ru′bin
hy′dro·bleph′a·ron′
hy′dro·bro′mate′
hy′dro·bro′mic
hy′dro·bro′mide′
hy′dro·cal′y·co′sis *pl.* -ses′
hy′dro·ca′lyx
hy′dro·car′bon
hy′dro·cele′
  —her′ni·a′lis

hy′dro·ce·lec′to·my
hy′dro·ce·phal′ic
hy′dro·ceph′a·lo·cele′
hy′dro·ceph′a·loid′
hy′dro·ceph′a·lus
hy′dro·ceph′a·ly
  —ex vac′u·o
hy′dro·chlo·ret′ic
hy′dro·chlo′ric
hy′dro·chlo′ride′
hy′dro·chlo·ro·thi′a·zide′
hy′dro·cho·le·cys′tis
hy′dro·chol′er·e′sis *pl.* -ses′
hy′dro·chol′er·et′ic
hy′dro·cho·les′ter·ol′
hy′dro·cir′so·cele′
hy′dro·co′done′
hy′dro·col′loid′
hy′dro·col′pos
hy′dro·co′ni·on′
hy′dro·con′qui·nine′
hy′dro·cor′ta·mate′
hy′dro·cor′ti·sone′
hy′dro·co·tar′nine′
hy′dro·cy·an′ic
hy′dro·cyst′ad·e·no′ma
  pl. -mas *or* -ma·ta
hy′dro·dip′si·a
hy′dro·dip′so·ma′ni·a
hy′dro·di′u·re′sis *pl.* -ses′
hy′dro·dy·nam′ic
hy′dro·dy·nam′ics
hy′dro·en·ceph′a·lo·cele′
hy′dro·er·got′i·nine′
hy′dro·flu′me·thi′a·zide′
hy′dro·fluor′ic
hy′dro·gel
hy′dro·gen
hy·drog′e·nase′
hy′dro·gen·at′ed
hy′dro·gen·a′tion
hy′dro·gen·ly′ase′
hy′dro·gym·nas′tics
hy′dro·he′ma·to·ne·phro′-
  sis
hy′dro·he′ma·to·sal′pinx
hy′dro·hep′a·to′sis *pl.* -ses′
hy′dro·ki·net′ic
hy′dro·ki·net′ics
hy′drol′
hy′dro·la′bile
hy′dro·la·bil′i·ty
hy′dro·lase′

hy·drol′o·gy
hy′dro·ly′ase′
hy·drol′y·sate′
hy·drol′y·sis *pl.* -ses′
hy′dro·lyt′ic
hy′dro·lyze′, -lyzed′, -lyz′ing
hy·dro′ma
hy′dro·mas·sage′
hy′dro·men·in′gi′tis
hy′dro·me·nin′go·cele′
hy·drom′e·ter
hy′dro·me′tra
hy′dro·met′ric
hy′dro·me·tro·col′pos
hy·drom′e·try
hy′dro·mi′cro·ceph′a·ly
hy′dro·mor′phone′
hy·drom′pha·lus
hy′dro·my·e′li·a
hy′dro·my′e·lo·cele′
hy′dro·my′e·lo·me·nin′go·
  cele′
hy′dro·my·o′ma *pl.* -mas *or*
  -ma·ta
hy′dro·ne·phro′sis *pl.* -ses′
hy′dro·ne·phrot′ic
hy·dro·path′ic
hy·drop′a·thy
hy′dro·pel′vis
hy′dro·pe′ni·a
hy′dro·pe′nic
hy′dro·per′i·car·di′tis
hy′dro·per′i·car′di·um
hy′dro·per′i·ne·phro′sis
  pl. -ses′
hy′dro·per′i·on′
hy′dro·per′i·to·ne′um
hy′dro·pex′ic
hy′dro·phag′o·cy·to′sis
  pl. -ses′
hy′dro·phil′
hy′dro·phil′i·a
hy′dro·phil′ic
hy′droph′i·lism
hy′droph′i·lous
hy′dro·pho′bi·a
hy′dro·pho′bic
hy′dro·phone′
hy′droph·thal′mos
hy·drop′ic
hy·dro·pleu′ra
hy′dro·pneu′ma·to′sis
  pl. -ses′

hy′dro·pneu′mo·per′i·car′-
di·um
hy′dro·pneu′mo·per′i·to·
ne′um
hy′dro·pneu′mo·tho′rax′
hy′drops′
—an′tri′
—ar·tic′u·lo′rum
—fe·ta′lis
—grav′i·dar′um
hy′dro·py′o·ne·phro′sis
   pl. -ses′
hy′dro·quin′i·dine′
hy′dro·quin′ine′
hy′dro·quin′ol′
hy·dro·qui·none′
hy·dror′a·chis
hy·dro·ra·chi′tis
hy·dror·rhe′a
—grav′i·dar′um
hy′dro·sal′pinx
hy′dro·sar′co·cele′
hy′dro·sol′
hy′dro·sol′u·ble
hy′dro·sper′ma·to·cele′
hy′dro·sper′ma·to·cyst′
hy′dro·spi·rom′e·ter
hy′dro·stat′
hy′dro·stat′ic
hy′dro·sul·fu′ric
hy′dro·sy·rin′go·my·e′li·a
hy′dro·tax′is   *pl.* -es
hy′dro·ther′a·peu′tic
hy′dro·ther′a·peu′tics
hy′dro·ther′a·py
hy′dro·ther′mal
hy′dro·thi·o′ne·mi·a
hy′dro·thi·o′nu·ri·a
hy′dro·tho·rac′ic
hy′dro·tho′rax′
hy′dro′tis
hy·drot′ro·pism
hy·dro·tym′pa·num
hy′dro·u·re′ter
hy′dro·u·re′ter·o·ne·phro′-
sis   *pl.* -ses′
hy′dro·u·re′ter·o′sis
   pl. -ses′
hy′dro·u′ri·a
hy′drous
hy′dro·var′i·um
hy·drox′ide′
hy·drox′o·co·bal′a·min

hy·drox′y·a·ce′tic
hy·drox′y·am·phet′a·mine
hy·drox′y·ap′a·tite′
hy·drox′y·ben′zene′
hy·drox′y·ben·zo′ic
hy·drox′y·chlo′ro·quine′
hy·drox′y·cor′ti·cos′ter·
   one′
hy·drox′y·di′one′
hy·drox′yl
hy·drox′yl·am′ine′
hy·drox′yl·ase′
hy·drox′yl·at′ed
hy·drox′yl·a′tion
hy·drox′y·pro·ges′ter·one′
hy·drox′y·pro′line′
hy·drox′y·pro′li·ne·mi·a
hy·drox′y·quin′o·line′
hy·drox′y·ste′a·rin
hy·drox′y·stil·bam′i·dine′
hy·drox′y·u·re′a
hy·drox′y·zine′
Hy′dro·zo′a
hy′dro·zo′an
hy·dru′ri·a
hy·dru′ric
hy′giene′
hy·gien′ic
hy·gien′ist
hy′gre·che′ma
hy′gric
hy′gro·ble·phar′ic
hy′gro·ma   *pl.* -mas *or* -ma·ta
—cys′ti·cum col′li′
hy·gro′ma·tous
hy·grom′e·ter
hy′gro·met′ric *or* hy′gro·
   met′ri·cal
hy·grom′e·try
hy′gro·pho′bi·a
hy′gro·scop′ic
hy′lic
hy′lo·pho′bi·a
hy′men
hy′men·al
hy′men·ec′to·my
hy′men·i′tis
hy′me·no·le·pi′a·sis   *pl.* -ses′
Hy′me·no·le·pid′i·dae′
Hy′me·nol′e·pis
—dim′i·nu′ta
—na′na
hy′men·ol′o·gy

Hy′me·nop′ter·a
hy′me·nop′ter·an
hy′me·nop′ter·ism
hy′me·nop′ter·ous
hy′men·or·rha′phy
hy·men′o·tome′
hy′men·ot′o·my
hy′o·de·ox′y·cho′lic
hy′o·ep′i·glot′tic
hy′o·ep′i·glot·tid′e·an
hy′o·glos′sal
hy′o·glos′sus   *pl.* -si′
hy′oid′
hy′o·man·dib′u·lar
hy′o·scine′
hy′o·scy′a·mine′
hy′o·scy′a·mus
hy′o·sta·pe′di·al
hy′o·thy′roid′
hyp′a·cu′si·a
hyp′a·cu′sis
hyp′al·bu′min·e′mi·a
hyp′al·bu′mi·no′sis
hyp′al·ge′si·a
hyp′al·ge′sic
hyp·al′gi·a
hy′pam·ni′on
hy′pam·ni′os
hy·pan′a·ki·ne′sis
hyp′a·ni·sog′na·thism
hy′paph·o′rine
hyp′ar·te′ri·al
hyp′as·the′ni·a
hyp·ax′i·al
hy·paz′o·tu′ri·a
hy·pen′gy·o·pho′bi·a
hyp′e·o·sin′o·phil
hy′per·ab·duc′tion
hy′per·ac′id
hy′per·ac′id·am′i·nu′ri·a
hy′per·a·cid′i·ty
hy′per·ac′tive
hy′per·ac·tiv′i·ty
hy′per·a·cu′i·ty
hy′per·a·cu′si·a
hy′per·a·cu′sis
hy′per·a·cute′
hy′per·ad′e·no′sis   *pl.* -ses′
hy′per·ad′i·po′sis   *pl.* -ses′
hy′per·a·dre′nal
hy′per·a·dre′nal·cor′ti·cal·
ism
hy′per·a·dre′nal·ism

hy'per·a·dre'ni·a
hy'per·a·dre'no·cor'ti·cism
hy'per·af·fec'tive
hy'per·af·fec·tiv'i·ty
hy'per·a·geu'si·a
hy'per·al·bu'min·e'mi·a
hy'per·al·bu'mi·no'sis
   pl. -ses'
hy'per·al'do·ster·o·ne'mi·a
hy'per·al'do·ster'o·nism
hy'per·al'do·ster·o·nu'ri·a
hy'per·al·ge'si·a
hy'per·al·ge'sic
hy'per·al'i·men·ta'tion
hy'per·al'i·men·to'sis
   pl. -ses'
hy'per·al·ka·lin'i·ty
hy'per·am'i·no·ac'i·du'ri·a
hy'per·am·mo·ne'mi·a
hy'per·am·ne'si·a
hy'per·am'y·las·e'mi·a
hy'per·an·a'ki·ne'si·a
   —ven·tric'u·li'
hy'per·a'phi·a
hy'per·aph'ic
hy'per·az'o·te'mi·a
hy'per·az'o·tu'ri·a
hy'per·bar'ic
hy'per·bar'ism
hy'per·be'ta·lip'o·pro'-
   tein·e'mi·a
hy'per·bil'i·ru'bin·e'mi·a
hy'per·blas·to'sis *pl.* -ses'
hy'per·brach'y·ce·phal'ic
hy'per·brach'y·ceph'a·ly
hy'per·brach'y·cra'ni·al
hy'per·bu'li·a
hy'per·cal·ce'mi·a
hy'per·cal·ce'mic
hy'per·cal·ci·nu'ri·a
hy'per·ca·lor'ic
hy'per·cap'ni·a
hy'per·cap'nic
hy'per·car'bi·a
hy'per·car'o·te·ne'mi·a
hy'per·cat'a·bol'ic
hy'per·ca·thar'sis *pl.* -ses'
hy'per·ca·thar'tic
hy'per·ca·thex'is
hy'per·cel'lu·lar
hy'per·cel'lu·lar'i·ty
hy'per·ce'men·to'sis
   pl. -ses'

hy'per·ce'nes·the'si·a
hy'per·chlo·re'mi·a
hy'per·chlo·re'mic
hy'per·chlor·hy'dri·a
hy'per·cho·les'ter·e'mi·a
hy'per·cho·les'ter·ol·e'mi·a
hy'per·cho·les'ter·ol·e'mic
hy'per·cho'li·a
hy'per·chon'dro·pla'si·a
hy'per·chro'maf·fin·ism
hy'per·chro·ma'si·a
hy'per·chro·mat'ic
hy'per·chro·ma·tism
hy'per·chro·ma·to'sis
   pl. -ses'
hy'per·chro'mi·a
hy'per·chro'mic
hy'per·chy'li·a
hy'per·chy'lo·mi'cron·e'-
   mi·a
hy'per·co·ag'u·la·bil'i·ty
hy'per·con'cen·tra'tion
hy'per·cor'ti·cism
hy'per·cre'a·ti·ne'mi·a
hy'per·cri'nism
hy'per·cry'al·ge'si·a
hy'per·cry'es·the'si·a
hy'per·cu·pre'mi·a
hy'per·cu'pri·u'ri·a
hy'per·cy'a·not'ic
hy'per·cy·the'mi·a
hy'per·cy·to'sis *pl.* -ses'
hy'per·dac·tyl'i·a
hy'per·dac'ty·ly
hy'per·di·crot'ic
hy'per·di·cro'tism
hy'per·dip'loid'
hy'per·dip'loi·dy
hy'per·dip'si·a
hy'per·dis·ten'tion
hy'per·di·u·re'sis *pl.* -ses'
hy'per·dol'i·cho·cra'ni·al
hy'per·dy·na'mi·a
hy'per·dy·nam'ic
hy'per·e·che'ma
hy'per·e·cho'ic
hy'per·e·las'tic
hy'per·e·las·tic'i·ty
hy'per·em'e·sis *pl.* -ses'
   —grav'i·dar'um
   —lac'ten'ti·um
hy'per·e·met'ic
hy'per·e'mi·a

hy'per·e'mic
hy'per·en·dem'ic
hy'per·en·de·mic'i·ty
hy'per·en·do·crin·ism
hy'per·e·o·sin'o·phil'i·a
hy'per·ep'i·thy'mi·a
hy'per·e'qui·lib'ri·um
hy'per·er'gi·a
hy'per·er'gic
hy'per·er'gy
hy'per·e·ryth'ro·cy·the'-
   mi·a
hy'per·es·o·pho'ri·a
hy'per·es·the'si·a
   —un'gui·um
hy'per·es·thet'ic
hy'per·es'trin·ism
hy'per·es'tro·gen·e'mi·a
hy'per·es'tro·gen·ism
hy'per·ex·cit'a·bil'i·ty
hy'per·ex'o·pho'ri·a
hy'per·ex·ten'si·ble
hy'per·ex·ten'sion
hy'per·fer·re'mi·a
hy'per·fi·brin'o·gen·e'mi·a
hy'per·fi'brin·ol'y·sis
hy'per·flex'ion
hy'per·fo'cal
hy'per·func'tion
hy'per·ga·lac'ti·a
hy'per·ga·lac·to'sis
hy'per·ga·lac'tous
hy'per·gam'ma·glob'u·lin·
   e'mi·a
hy'per·gen·e·sis *pl.* -ses'
hy'per·ge·net'ic
hy'per·gen'i·tal·ism
hy'per·geu'ses·the'si·a
hy'per·geu'si·a
hy'per·glan'du·lar
hy'per·glob·u'li·a
hy'per·glob'u·lin·e'mi·a
hy'per·gly·ce'mi·a
hy'per·gly·ce'mic
hy'per·gly·ci·ne'mi·a
hy'per·gly'co·ge·nol'y·sis
   pl. -ses'
hy'per·gly'cor·rha'chi·a
hy'per·gly'co·su'ri·a
hy'per·gly·ox'a·la·tu'ri·a
hy'per·go'nad·ism
hy'per·go'ni·a
hy'per·he·do'ni·a

hy′per·he′don·ism
hy′per·he′mo·glo′bin·e′-
mi·a
hy′per·he′mo·lyt′ic
hy′per·hep′a·rin·e′mi·a
hy′per·hi·dro′sis *pl.* -ses′
hy′per·his′ta·mi·ne′mi·a
hy′per·hor·mon′al
hy′per·hy·dra′tion
hy·per′i·cin
hy′per·im·mune′
hy′per·im′mu·no·glob′u·
lin·e′mi·a
hy′per·in·fla′tion
hy′per·in·o·se′mi·a
hy′per·in′su·lin·ism
hy′per·in·vo·lu′tion
hy′per·ir′ri·ta·bil′i·ty
hy′per·i′so·ton′ic
hy′per·ka·le′mi·a
hy′per·ka·le′mic
hy′per·ker′a·tin·i·za′tion
hy′per·ker′a·to′sis *pl.* -ses′
—ex·cen′tri·ca
—fol·lic′u·lar′is par′a·fol·
lic′u·lar′is
—lac′u·nar′is pha·ryn′gis
—lin′guae′
—sub′un·gua′lis
hy′per·ker′a·tot′ic
hy′per·ke′to·ne′mi·a
hy′per·ke′to·nu′ri·a
hy′per·ki·ne′mi·a
hy′per·ki·ne′si·a
hy′per·ki·ne′sis
hy′per·ki·net′ic
hy′per·lac·ta′tion
hy′per·leu′ko·cy·to′sis
pl. -ses′
hy′per·li·pe′mi·a
hy′per·li·pe′mic
hy′per·lip′i·de′mi·a
hy′per·lip′i·dem′ic
hy′per·lip′o·pro′tein·e′-
mi·a
hy′per·li·po′sis
hy′per·lith′ic
hy′per·li·thu′ri·a
hy′per·lor·do′sis
hy′per·lu′cen·cy
hy′per·mag·ne′se·mi·a
hy′per·ma′ni·a
hy′per·man′ic

hy′per·mas′ti·a
hy′per·ma·ture′
hy′per·mel′a·no′sis *pl.* -ses′
hy′per·mel′a·not′ic
hy′per·men′or·rhe′a
hy′per·met′a·bol′ic
hy′per·me·tab′o·lism
hy′per·met′a·mor′pho·sis
pl. -ses′
—of Wer′nick·e
hy′per·met′a·pla′si·a
hy′per·met′rope′
hy′per·me·tro′pi·a
hy′per·me·tro′pic
hy′per·mi′cro·so′ma
hy′per·mim′i·a
hy′per·min′er·al·o·cor′ti·
coid·ism
hy′perm·ne′si·a
hy′perm·ne′sic
hy′per·morph′
hy′per·mo·til′i·ty
hy′per·my′o·to′ni·a
hy′per·my·ot′ro·phy
hy′per·na·tre′mi·a
hy′per·na·tre′mic
hy·per′ne′a
hy′per·ne·o′cy·to′sis
hy′per·ne·phri′tis
hy′per·neph′roid′
hy′per·ne·phro′ma *pl.* -mas
or -ma·ta
hy′per·noi′a
hy′per·nor′mal
hy′per·nu·tri′tion
hy′per·on′to·morph′
hy′per·o·nych′i·a
hy′per·ope′
hy′per·o′pi·a
hy′per·op′ic
hy′per·or′chi·dism
hy′per·o·rex′i·a
hy′per·or′tho·cy·to′sis
hy′per·os′mi·a
hy′per·os·mo·lar′i·ty
hy′per·os·mot′ic
hy′per·os·te·og′e·ny
hy′per·os·to′sis *pl.* -ses′
hy′per·os·tot′ic
hy′per·ox′a·lu′ri·a
hy′per·ox·e′mi·a
hy′per·ox′i·a
hy′per·ox′ic

hy′per·par′a·site′
hy′per·par′a·sit′ic
hy′per·par′a·thy′roid·ism
hy′per·path′i·a
hy′per·path′ic
hy′per·pep′sin′i·a
hy′per·per′i·stal′sis *pl.* -ses′
hy′per·per′me·a·bil′i·ty
hy′per·pex′i·a
hy′per·pha′gi·a
hy′per·pha′gic
hy′per·pha·lan′gi·a
hy′per·pha·lan′gism
hy′per·pha·lan′gy
hy′per·phen′yl·al′a·ni·ne′-
mi·a
hy′per·pho·ne′sis
hy′per·pho′ni·a
hy′per·pho′ri·a
hy′per·phos′pha·te′mi·a
hy′per·phos′pha·tu′ri·a
hy′per·phos′pho·re′mi·a
hy′per·phre′ni·a
hy′per·pi·e′si·a
hy′per·pi·e′sis
hy′per·pi·et′ic
hy′per·pig′men·ta′tion
hy′per·pi·tu′i·ta·rism
hy′per·pi·tu′i·tar′y
hy′per·pla′si·a
hy′per·plas′mi·a
hy′per·plas′tic
hy′per·plat′y·mer′ic
hy′per·ploid′
hy′per·ploi′dy
hy′perp·ne′a
hy′perp·ne′ic
hy′per·po·lar′i·za′tion
hy′per·po·ne′sis
hy′per·po·ro′sis *pl.* -ses′
hy′per·po·si′a
hy′per·po·tas′se′mi·a
hy′per·pra′gi·a
hy′per·prag′ic
hy′per·prax′i·a
hy′per·pre·be′ta·lip′o·pro′-
tein·e′mi·a
hy′per·pres′by·o′pi·a
hy′per·pro·lac′tin·e′mi·a
hy′per·pro·li·ne′mi·a
hy′per·pro·sex′i·a
hy′per·pro′tein·e′mi·a
hy′per·pro·te·o′sis

hy′per·psy·cho′sis
hy′per·py·re′mi·a
hy′per·py·ret′ic
hy′per·py·rex′i·a
hy′per·re·ac′tive
hy′per·re·flex′i·a
hy′per·re·flex′ic
hy′per·ren·in·e′mi·a
hy′per·res′o·nance
hy′per·res′o·nant
hy′per·sa·le′mi·a
hy′per·sal′i·va′tion
hy′per·se·cre′tion
hy′per·se·cre′to·ry
hy′per·seg′men·ta′tion
hy′per·sen′si·tive
hy′per·sen′si·tiv′i·ty
hy′per·sen′si·ti·za′tion
hy′per·ser′o·to·nin·e′mi·a
hy′per·sex′u·al′i·ty
hy′per·som′ni·a
hy′per·son′ic
hy′per·splen′ic
hy′per·sple·nism
hy′per·sthe′ni·a
hy′per·sthe′nic
hy′per·sus·cep′ti·bil′i·ty
hy′per·syn′chro·nism
hy′per·syn′chro·ny
hy′per·tel′o·rism
hy′per·ten·sin·o·gen
hy′per·ten′sion
hy′per·ten′sive
hy′per·ten′sor
hy′per·the·co′sis *pl.* -ses′
hy′per·the′li·a
hy′per·ther′mal
hy′per·ther·mal·ge′si·a
hy′per·ther·mes·the′si·a
hy′per·ther′mi·a
hy′per·ther′mic
hy′per·ther·mo·es·the′si·a
hy′per·ther′my
hy′per·throm′bin·e′mi·a
hy′per·thy′mi·a
hy′per·thy′mic
hy′per·thy′mism
hy′per·thy′mi·za′tion
hy′per·thy′roid′
hy′per·thy′roid·ism
hy′per·thy·roi·do′sis
hy′per·thy·rox·i′ne′mi·a
hy′per·to′ni·a

hy′per·ton′ic
hy′per·to·nic′i·ty
hy′per·to′nus
hy′per·tri·cho′sis *pl.* -ses′
hy′per·tri·glyc′er·i·de′mi·a
hy′per·tro′phic
hy·per′tro·phy
hy′per·tro′pi·a
hy′per·ty′ro·si·ne′mi·a
hy′per·u·re′sis *pl.* -ses′
hy′per·u·ri·ce′mi·a
hy′per·u·ri·ce′mic
hy′per·u·ri·co·su′ri·a
hy′per·val′i·ne′mi·a
hy′per·vas′cu·lar
hy′per·veg′e·ta′tive
hy′per·ven′ti·la′tion
hy′per·vis·cos′i·ty
hy′per·vis′cous
hy′per·vi′ta·min·o′sis
  pl. -ses′
hy′per·vo·le′mi·a
hy′per·vo·le′mic
hy′per·vo·lu′mic
hy′pes·the′si·a
hy′pes·the′sic
hy′pes·thet′ic
hy′pha *pl.* -phae′
hy′phal
hyp′he·do′ni·a
hy·phe′ma
hy·phe′mi·a
hyp′hi·dro′sis
hy′pho·my·co′sis
hyp′na·gog′ic
hyp′na·gogue′
hyp·nal′gi·a
hyp′nic
hyp′no·a·nal′y·sis *pl.* -ses′
hyp′no·an·es·the′si·a
hyp′no·ca·thar′sis
hyp′no·don′ti·a
hyp′no·don′tics
hyp′no·gen′e·sis
hyp′no·gen′ic
hyp·nog′e·nous
hyp′noid′
hyp′noi′dal
hyp′no·lep′sy
hyp·nol′o·gy
hyp′no·nar·co′sis *pl.* -ses′
hyp′no·pho′bi·a
hyp′no·pom′pic

hyp·no′sis *pl.* -ses′
hyp′no·ther′a·py
hyp·not′ic
hyp′no·tism
hyp′no·tist
hyp′no·tize′, -tized′, -tiz′ing
hyp′no·toid′
hyp′no·tox′in
hy′po
hy′po·a·cid′i·ty
hy′po·ac′tive
hy′po·ac·tiv′i·ty
hy′po·a·cu′si·a
hy′po·a·cu′sis
hy′po·a·dre′nal
hy′po·a·dren·a·li·ne′mi·a
hy′po·a·dre′nal·ism
hy′po·a·dre′ni·a
hy′po·a·dre·no·cor′ti·cism
hy′po·aer·a′tion
hy′po·af·fec′tive
hy′po·af·fec·tiv′i·ty .
hy′po·ag′na·thus
hy′po·al·bu′min·e′mi·a
hy′po·al·bu′mi·no′sis
hy′po·al·dos′ter·on·ism
hy′po·al′i·men·ta′tion
hy′po·al′ka·line
hy′po·al′ler·gen′ic
hy′po·az′o·tu′ri·a
hy′po·bar′ic
hy′po·bar′ism
hy′po·ba·rop′a·thy
hy′po·be′ta·lip′o·pro′-
  tein·e′mi·a
hy′po·bil′i·ru′bin·e′mi·a
hy′po·blast′
hy′po·blas′tic
hy′po·bran′chi·al
hy′po·bro′mite′
hy′po·bro′mous
hy′po·bu′li·a
hy′po·cal·ce′mi·a
hy′po·cal·ce′mic
hy′po·cal·cif′ic
hy′po·cal·ci·fi·ca′tion
hy′po·cal′ci·fy′, -fied′, -fy′ing
hy′po·cal·ci·u′ri·a
hy′po·cap′ni·a
hy′po·car′bi·a
hy′po·ca·thex′is
hy′po·cel′lu·lar
hy′po·cel′lu·lar′i·ty

hy′po·ce′lom
hy′po·ce·ru′lo·plas′min·e′-
mi·a
hy′po·chlo·re′mi·a
hy′po·chlo·re′mic
hy′po·chlor·hy′dri·a
hy′po·chlo′rite′
hy′po·chlo′ri·za′tion
hy′po·chlo′rous
hy′po·chlor·u′ri·a
hy′po·cho·les′ter·ol·e′mi·a
hy′po·chon′dri·a
hy′po·chon′dri·ac′
hy′po·chon·dri′a·cal
hy′po·chon′dri·al
hy′po·chon·dri′a·sis
　　pl. -ses′
hy′po·chon′dri·um
　　pl. -dri·a
hy′po·chord′al
hy′po·chro·ma′si·a
hy′po·chro·mat′ic
hy′po·chro′ma·tism
hy′po·chro·ma·to′sis
hy′po·chro·me′mi·a
hy′po·chro·mi·a
hy′po·chro′mic
hy′po·chy′li·a
hy′po·ci·ne′si·a
hy′po·coe′lom
hy′po·com′ple·ment·e′mi·a
hy′po·con′dy·lar
hy′po·cone′
hy′po·con′id
hy′po·con′ule′
hy′po·con′u·lid
hy′po·crine
hy′po·crin′i·a
hy′po·cri′nism
hy′po·cu·pre′mi·a
hy′po·cy·clo′sis *pl.* -ses′
hy′po·cys·tot′o·my
hy′po·cy·the′mi·a
hy′po·cy·to′sis *pl.* -ses′
hy′po·dac′ty·ly
hy′po·de·pres′sion
hy′po·derm′
Hy′po·der′ma
hy′po·der·mat′ic
hy′po·der·mat′o·my
hy′po·der·mi′a·sis *pl.* -ses′
hy′po·der′mic
hy′po·der′mis

hy′po·der·moc′ly·sis
　　pl. -ses′
hy′po·der′mo·li·thi′a·sis
　　pl. -ses′
hy′po·di′a·phrag·mat′ic
hy′po·dip′loid′
hy′po·dip′loi·dy
hy′po·dip′si·a
hy′po·don′ti·a
hy′po·dy·na′mi·a
hy′po·dy·nam′ic
hy′po·ec·cris′i·a
hy′po·e·cho′ic
hy′po·en′do·crin·ism
hy′po·e·o′sin·o·phil′i·a
hy′po·er′gi·a
hy′po·er′gic
hy′po·er′gy
hy′po·es′o·pho′ri·a
hy′po·es·the′si·a
hy′po·es′trin·ism
hy′po·es·tro·gen·e′mi·a
hy′po·ex′o·pho′ri·a
hy′po·fer·re′mi·a
hy′po·fer′rism
hy′po·fi′bri·no·gen·e′mi·a
hy′po·func′tion
hy′po·func′tion·al
hy′po·ga·lac′ti·a
hy′po·gam′ma·glob′u·
lin·e′mi·a
hy′po·gas′tric
hy′po·gas′tri·um *pl.* -tri·a
hy′po·gas·trop′a·gus
hy′po·gas·tros′chi·sis
　　pl. -ses′
hy′po·gen′e·sis
hy′po·ge·net′ic
hy′po·gen′i·tal·ism
hy′po·geu′si·a
hy′po·glan′du·lar
hy′po·glos′sal
hy′po·glos′sus *pl.* -si′
hy′po·glot′tis
hy′po·gly·ce′mi·a
hy′po·gly·ce′mic
hy′po·gly′ce·mo′sis *pl.* -ses′
hy′po·gly′cin
hy′po·gly′co·ge·nol′y·sis
　　pl. -ses′
hy′po·gly′cor·rha′chi·a
hy′pog′na·thous
hy′po·go′nad·ism

hy′po·gon′a·do·trop′ic
hy′po·gran′u·lo·cy·to′sis
　　pl. -ses′
hy′po·hi·dro′sis *pl.* -ses′
hy′po·in′su·lin·ism
hy′po·ka·le′mi·a
hy′po·ka·le′mic
hy′po·ker′a·to′sis *pl.* -ses′
hy′po·ki·ne′si·a
hy′po·ki·ne′sis *pl.* -ses′
hy′po·ki·net′ic
hy′po·lar′ynx *pl.* -ynx·es *or*
-la·ryn′ges′
hy′po·lem′mal
hy′po·leu′ko·cyt′ic
hy′po·ley′dig·ism
hy′po·li·pe′mi·a
hy′po·li·pe′mic
hy′po·lip′o·pro′tein·e′mi·a
hy′po·li·po′sis *pl.* -ses′
hy′po·lo′gi·a
hy′po·lu·te′mi·a
hy′po·mag′ne·se′mi·a
hy′po·ma′ni·a
hy′po·man′ic
hy′po·mas′ti·a
hy′po·ma′zi·a
hy′po·mel′a·nism
hy′po·mel′a·no′sis *pl.* -ses′
hy′po·mel′a·not′ic
hy′po·men′or·rhe′a
hy′po·mere′
hy′po·me·tab′o·lism
hy′po·me′tri·a
hy′po·me·tro′pi·a
hy′po·mi′cron′
hy′po·mi′cro·so′ma
hy′pom·ne′si·a
hy′po·morph′
hy′po·mo·til′i·ty
hy′po·myx′i·a
hy′po·na·tre′mi·a
hy′po·ne·o′cy·to′sis
hy′po·ni′trous
hy′po·noi′a
hy′po·nych′i·al
hy′po·nych′i·um
hy′po·or′chi·dism
hy′po·os·to′sis *pl.* -ses′
hy′po·o·var′i·an·ism
hy′po·pan′cre·a·tism
hy′po·par′a·thy′roid′
hy′po·par′a·thy′roid·ism

hy′po·per·fu′sion
hy′po·per′i·stal′sis *pl.* -ses′
hy′po·per′me·a·bil′i·ty
hy′po·pha·lan′gism
hy′po·pha·ryn′ge·al
hy′po·phar′yn·gi′tis
hy′po·phar′yn·gos′co·py
hy′po·phar′ynx
hy′po·pho·ne′sis
hy′po·pho′ni·a
hy′po·pho′ri·a
hy′po·phos′pha·ta′si·a
hy′po·phos′pha·te′mi·a
hy′po·phos′pha·tu′ri·a
hy′po·phos′phite′
hy′po·phra′si·a
hy′po·phre′ni·a
hy′po·phren′ic
hy′poph′y·se′al
hy·poph′y·sec′to·mize′,
   -mized′, -miz′ing
hy·poph′y·sec′to·my
hy·poph′y·se′o·por′tal
hy′po·phys′i·o·priv′ic
hy·poph′y·sis *pl.* -ses′
   —cer′e·bri′
hy·poph′y·si′tis
hy′po·pi·e′si·a
hy′po·pi·e′sis *pl.* -ses′
hy′po·pi·et′ic
hy′po·pig′men·ta′tion
hy′po·pin′e·al·ism
hy′po·pi·tu′i·ta·rism
hy′po·pi·tu′i·tar′y
hy′po·pla′si·a
   —cu′tis con·gen′i·ta
hy′po·plas′tic
hy′po·plas′ty
hy′po·ploid′
hy′po·ploi′dy
hy′po·pne′a
hy′po·po·ro′sis *pl.* -ses′
hy′po·po′si·a
hy′po·po′tas·se′mi·a
hy′po·po′tas·se′mic
hy′po·prax′i·a
hy′po·pro·sex′ia
hy′po·pros′o·dy
hy′po·pro′tein·e′mi·a
hy′po·pro·tein′ic
hy′po·pro·throm′bin·e′-
   mi·a
hy′po·psel′a·phe′si·a

hy′po·psy·cho′sis *pl.* -ses′
hy·po′py·on′
hy′po·re·ac′tive
hy′po·re·flex′i·a
hy′po·re·flex′ic
hy′po·ren′in·e′mi·a
hy′po·ri′bo·fla′vi·no′sis
   pl. -ses′
hy′po·sal′i·va′tion
hy′po·scle′ral
hy′po·se·cre′tion
hy′po·sen′si·tive
hy′po·sen′si·tiv′i·ty
hy′po·sen′si·ti·za′tion
hy′po·sen′si·tize′
hy′po·sex′u·al′i·ty
hy·pos′mi·a
hy′po·so′mi·a
hy′po·som′ni·a
hy′po·spa′di·ac′
hy′po·spa′di·as
hy′po·sper′ma·to·gen′e·sis
   pl. -ses′
hy·pos′ta·sis *pl.* -ses′
hy′po·stat′ic
hy′po·sthe′ni·a
hy′po·sthe′ni·ant
hy′po·sthen′ic
hy·po′sthe·nu′ri·a
hy′po·sto′mi·a
hy′po·styp′sis
hy′po·styp′tic
hy′po·syn·er′gi·a
hy′po·sys′to·le
hy′po·tax′i·a
hy′po·tax′is
hy′po·tel′o·rism
hy′po·ten′sion
hy′po·ten′sive
hy′po·ten′sor
hy′po·tha·lam′ic
hy′po·thal′a·mo·hy′po·
   phys′e·al
hy′po·thal′a·mus
hy′po·the′nar
hy′po·ther′mal
hy′po·ther′mes·the′si·a
hy′po·ther′mi·a
hy′po·ther′mic
hy′po·ther′my
hy·poth′e·sis *pl.* -ses′
hy′po·throm′bin·e′mi·a
hy′po·thy′mi·a

hy′po·thy′mism
hy′po·thy′roid′
hy′po·thy′roid′ism
hy′po·thy·ro′sis
hy′po·to′ni·a
hy′po·ton′ic
hy′po·to·nic′i·ty
hy′po·to′nus
hy·pot′o·ny
hy′po·tox·ic′i·ty
hy′po·trans·fer′rin·e′mi·a
hy′po·tri·cho′sis
hy·pot′ro·phy
hy′po·tro′pi·a
hy′po·tym·pan′ic
hy′po·tym′pa·num
hy′po·u·re′mi·a
hy′po·var′i·a
hy′po·va·so·pres′sin·e′mi·a
hy′po·veg′e·ta′tive
hy′po·ve·nos′i·ty
hy′po·ven′ti·la′tion
hy′po·vir·gil′i·ty
hy′po·vi′ta·min·o′sis
   pl. -ses′
hy′po·vo·le′mi·a
hy′po·vo·le′mic
hy′po·vo′li·a
hy′po·vo·lu′mic
hy′po·xan′thine′
hy·pox·e′mi·a
hy·pox·e′mic
hy·pox′i·a
hy·pox′ic
hy′po·zinc·e′mi·a
hyp′sar·rhyth′mi·a
hyp′sar·rhyth′moid′
hyp′si·brach′y·ce·phal′ic
hyp′si·ce·phal′ic
hyp′si·ceph′a·lous
hyp′si·ceph′a·ly
hyp′si·conch′
hyp′si·con′chous
hyp′si·loid′
hyp′si·sta·phyl′i·a
hyp′si·sta·phyl′ic
hyp′si·staph′y·line′
hyp′so·ceph′a·lous
hyp′so·chro′mic
hyp′so·dont′
hyp·so·ki·ne′sis *pl.* -ses′
Hyrtl loop
hys′ter·al′gi·a

hys'ter·al'gic
hys'ter·a·tre'si·a
hys'ter·ec'to·my
hys'ter·e'sis *pl.* -ses'
hys'ter·eu·ryn'ter
hys'ter·eu'ry·sis
hys·te'ri·a
hys·ter'ic *or* hys·ter'i·cal
hys·ter'i·cal·ly
hys·ter'i·cism
hys·ter'ics
hys·ter'i·form'
hys·ter·i'tis
hys'ter·o·bu·bon'o·cele'
hys'ter·o·car'ci·no'ma
 pl. -mas *or* -ma·ta
hys'ter·o·cele'
hys'ter·o·clei'sis *pl.* -ses'
hys'ter·o·col·pec'to·my
hys'ter·o·cys'tic
hys'ter·o·cys'to·clei'sis
 pl. -ses'
hys'ter·o·cys'to·pex'y
hys'ter·o·dyn'i·a
hys'ter·o·ep'i·lep'tic
hys'ter·o·ep'i·lep'sy
hys'ter·o·gen'ic
hys'ter·og'e·nous
hys'ter·o·gram'
hys'ter·o·graph'
hys'ter·og'ra·phy
hys'ter·oid'
hys'ter·oi'dal
hys'ter·o·lap'a·rot'o·my
hys'ter·o·lith'
hys'ter·o·li·thi'a·sis *pl.* -ses'
hys'ter·ol'o·gy
hys'ter·ol'y·sis *pl.* -ses'
hys'ter·o·ma'ni·a
hys'ter·om'e·ter
hys'ter·om'e·try
hys'ter·o·my·o'ma *pl.* -mas
 or -ma·ta
hys'ter·o·my'o·mec'to·my
hys'ter·o·my·ot'o·my
hys'ter·o·neu'ras·the'ni·a
hys'ter·o-o'o·pho·rec'-
 to·my
hys'ter·o·path'ic
hys'ter·op'a·thy
hys'ter·o·pex'y
hys'ter·o'pi·a
hys'ter·o·plas'ty

hys'ter·op·to'sis
hys'ter·or'rha·phy
hys'ter·or·rhex'is
 pl. -rhex'es'
hys'ter·o·sal'pin·gec'to·my
hys'ter·o·sal'pin·go·gram'
hys'ter·o·sal'pin·gog'ra·
 phy
hys'ter·o·sal'pin·go-
 o'o·pho·rec'to·my
hys'ter·o·sal'pin·gos'to·my
hys'ter·o·scope'
hys'ter·o·scop'ic
hys'ter·os'co·py
hys'ter·o·sys·ton'ic
hys'ter·o·tome'
hys'ter·ot'o·my
hys'ter·o·tra'che·lec'to·my
hys'ter·o·tra'che·lo·plas'ty
hys'ter·o·tra'che·lor'rha·
 phy
hys'ter·o·tra'che·lot'o·my
hys'ter·o·trau·mat'ic
hys'ter·o·trau'ma·tism
hys'ter·o·tu·bog'ra·phy

I

i'am·a·tol'o·gy
i·at'ric
i·at'ro·chem'i·cal
i·at'ro·chem'is·try
i·at'ro·gen'e·sis
i·at'ro·gen'ic
i·at'ro·tech'ni·cal
i·at'ro·tech'nics
i·at'ro·tech'nique'
i'bo·ga'ine'
i·bu'fe·nac'
i·bu·pro'fen
Ice'land
 —disease
 —moss
 —spar
ich'no·gram'
i'chor'
i'chor·e'mi·a
i'chor·oid'
i'chor·ous
i'chor·rhe'a
i'chor·rhe'mi·a
ich'tham·mol'
ich'thy·ism

ich'thy·o·col'la
ich'thy·oid'
ich'thy·oph'a·gous
ich'thy·o·pho'bi·a
ich'thy·o·sar'co·tox'in
ich'thy·o·sar'co·tox'ism
ich'thy·o'si·form'
ich'thy·o'sis *pl.* -ses'
 —con·gen'i·ta
 —fe·ta'lis
 —fol·lic'u·lar'is
 —hys'trix
 —le·tha'lis
 —sim'plex'
 —vul·gar'is
ich'thy·ot'ic
ich'thy·o·tox'in
ich'thy·o·tox'ism
ich'thy·o·tox·is'mus
i'con·o·ma'ni·a
ic'tal
Ic'ta·lu'ri·dae'
ic·ter'ic
ic'ter·o·a·ne'mi·a
ic'ter·o·gen'ic
ic'ter·og'e·nous
ic'ter·o·he'ma·tu'ri·a
ic'ter·o·he'ma·tu'ric
ic'ter·o·he'mo·lyt'ic
ic'ter·o·hem'or·rhag'ic
ic'ter·o·hep'a·ti'tis *pl.* -tis·es
 or -tit'i·des'
ic'ter·oid'
ic'ter·us
 —grav'is
 —ne'o·na·to'rum
ic'tus
id
i'da·ru'bi·cin
i·de'al·i·za'tion
i·de·a'tion
i·de·a'tion·al
i·dée' fixe'
i·den'ti·cal
i·den'ti·fi·ca'tion
i·den'ti·fy
i·den'ti·ty
i'de·o·ge·net'ic
i'de·og'e·nous
i'de·o·glan'du·lar
i'de·o·ki·net'ic
i'de·ol'o·gy
i'de·o·met'a·bol'ic

i'de·o·me·tab'o·lism
i'de·o·mo'tion
i'de·o·mo'tor
i'de·o·mus·cu·lar
i'de·o·pho'bi·a
i'de·o·phre'ni·a
i'de·o·plas'ty
i'de·o·vas·cu·lar
id'i·o·blast'
id'i·o·chro'mo·some'
id'i·o·cra'si·a
id'i·oc'ra·sis *pl.* -ses'
id'i·oc'ra·sy
id'i·o·crat'ic
id'i·o·cy
id'i·o·dy·nam'ics
id'i·og'a·mist
id'i·o·gen'e·sis
id'i·o·glos'si·a
id'i·o·glot'tic
id'i·o·gram'
id'i·o·het'er·ol'y·sin
id'i·o·hyp'no·tism
id'i·ol'o·gism
id'i·o·me·tri'tis
id'i·o·mus·cu·lar
id'i·o·neu·ro'sis *pl.* -ses'
id'i·o·pa·thet'ic
id'i·o·path'ic
id'i·op'a·thy
id'i·o·phren'ic
id'i·o·plasm
id'i·o·re'flex'
id'i·o·ret'i·nal
id'i·o·some'
id'i·o·spasm
id'i·o·spas'tic
id'i·o·syn'cra·sy
id'i·o·syn·crat'ic
id'i·ot
  —sa·vant'
id'i·o·tope'
id'i·o·tox'in
id'i·o·trop'ic
id'i·o·var'i·a'tion
id'i·o·ven·tric'u·lar
i'do·lo·ma'ni·a
i'dox·u'ri·dine'
ig·na'ti·a
ig'ni·punc'ture
ig·ni'tion
il'e·ac' *(pertaining to the ileum)*
  ♦*iliac*

il'e·al
il'e·ec'to·my
il'e·i'tis
il'e·o·ap'pen·dic'u·lar
il'e·o·ce'cal
il'e·o·ce·cos'to·my
il'e·o·ce'cum
il'e·o·col'ic
il'e·o·co·li'tis
il'e·o·co·lon'ic
il'e·o·co·los'to·my
il'e·o·co·lot'o·my
il'e·o·cu·ta'ne·ous
il'e·o·cys'to·plas'ty
il'e·o·cys·tos'to·my
il'e·o·il'e·al
il'e·o·il'e·os'to·my
il'e·o·proc·tos'to·my
il'e·o·rec'tal
il'e·o·rec·tos'to·my
il'e·or'rha·phy
il'e·o·sig'moid'
il'e·o·sig'moid·os'to·my
il'e·os'to·my
il'e·ot'o·my
il'e·o·trans·verse'
il'e·o·trans·ver'sos·to·my
il'e·o·typh·li'tis
il'e·o·ves'i·cal
I·le'sha fever
il'e·tin
il'e·um *(lower portion of the small intestine)*, *pl.* -e·a
  ♦*ilium*
il'e·us
il'i·ac' *(pertaining to the ilium)*
  ♦*ileac*
i·li'a·cus *pl.* -ci'
il'i·a·del'phus
il'i·o·cap'su·lar'is
il'i·o·coc·cyg'e·al
il'i·o·coc·cyg'e·us
il'i·o·co·lot'o·my
il'i·o·cos'tal
il'i·o·cos·ta'lis
  —cer'vi·cis
  —dor'si'
  —lum·bo'rum
  —tho·ra'cis
il'i·o·cos·to·cer'vi·ca'lis
il'i·o·fem'o·ral
il'i·o·hy'po·gas'tric
il'i·o·in'gui·nal

il'i·o·lum'bar
il'i·op'a·gus
il'i·o·pec·tin'e·al
il'i·o·pel'vic
il'i·o·pop·lit'e·al
il'i·o·pso'as
il'i·o·pu'bic
il'i·o·sa'cral
il'i·o·tho'ra·cop'a·gus
il'i·o·tib'i·al
il'i·o·tro'chan·ter'ic
il'i·o·xi·phop'a·gus
il'i·um *(the flank)*, *pl.* -i·a
  ♦*ileum*
I·li'za·rov procedure
ill
il·laq'ue·ate', -at'ed, -at'ing
il·laq'ue·a'tion
il'le·git'i·ma·cy
il'le·git'i·mate
il·lic'it
il·li'ci·um
il'li·ni'tion
il·lin'i·um
ill'ness
il·lu'mi·nance
il·lu'mi·nate', -nat'ed, -nat'ing
il·lu'mi·na'tion
il·lu'mi·na'tor
il·lu'mi·nism
il·lu'sion
il·lu'sion·al
il·lu'sion·ar'y
il·lu'so·ry
i'ma
im'age
im'age·ry
i·mag'i·nal
i·mag'i·nar'y
i·mag'i·na'tion
i·mag'ine
i·ma'go *pl.* -goes *or* i·mag'i·nes'
im·bal'ance
im·be·cile
im·be·cil'i·ty
im·bed', -bed'ded, -bed'ding, *var. of* embed
im·bibe', -bibed', -bib'ing
im·bi·bi'tion
im'bri·cate', -cat'ed, -cat'ing
im'bri·ca'tion

im′i·daz′ole′
im′i·daz′o·lyl
im′ide′
i·mid′o·line′
i·mi′no
im′i·no·gly′ci·nu′ri·a
im′i·no·u·re′a
im′i·pen′em
i·mip′ra·mine′
im′i·tate′, -tat′ed, -tat′ing
im′i·ta′tion
im′i·ta′tive
im·ma·ture′
im·ma·tu′ri·ty
im·me′di·ate
im·med′i·ca·ble
im·merse′, -mersed′,
    -mers′ing
im·mer′sion
im·mis′ci·ble
im′mo·bil′i·ty
im·mo′bi·li·za′tion
im·mo′bi·lize′, -lized′,
    -liz′ing
im·mo′bi·liz′er
im·mor·tal′i·ty
im·mune′
im·mu′ni·fa′cient
im·mu′ni·ty
im′mu·ni·za′tion
im′mu·nize′, -nized′, -niz′ing
im·mu·no·ad·he′sion
im′mu·no·as′say′
im′mu·no·bi·ol′o·gy
im′mu·no·blast′
im′mu·no·blas′tic
im′mu·no·chem′is·try
im′mu·no·com′pe·tence
im′mu·no·com′pe·ten·cy
im′mu·no·com′pe·tent
im′mu·no·con·glu′ti·nin
im′mu·no·cyte′
im′mu·no·cy′to·chem′is·
    try
im′mu·no·de·fi′cien·cy
im′mu·no·de·pres′sive
im′mu·no·di·ag·no′sis
    pl. -ses′
im′mu·no·dif·fu′sion
im′mu·no·e·lec′tro·pho·
    re′sis *pl.* -ses′
im′mu·no·e·lec′tro·pho·
    ret′ic

im′mu·no·fer′ri·tin
im′mu·no·fil·tra′tion
im′mu·no·fluo·res′cence
im′mu·no·fluo·res′cent
im′mu·no·gen
im′mu·no·ge·net′ic
im′mu·no·ge·net′ics
im′mu·no·gen′ic
im′mu·no·ge·nic′i·ty
im′mu·no·glob′u·lin
im′mu·no·glob′u·lin·op′a·
    thy
im′mu·no·he′ma·tol′o·gy
im′mu·no·he′mo·lyt′ic
im′mu·no·his′to·chem′is·
    try
im′mu·no·log′ic
im′mu·no·log′i·cal
im′mu·nol′o·gist
im′mu·nol′o·gy
im′mu·no·path′o·log′ic *or*
    im′mu·no·path′o·log′i·cal
im′mu·no·pa·thol′o·gist
im′mu·no·pa·thol′o·gy
im′mu·no·pho·re′sis
    pl. -ses′
im′mu·no·pre·cip′i·ta′tion
im′mu·no·pro·lif′er·a·tive
im′mu·no·pro′tein′
im′mu·no·re·ac′tion
im′mu·no·re·ac′tive
im′mu·no·re·ac·tiv′i·ty
im′mu·no·sor′bent
im′mu·no·sup·pres′sant
im′mu·no·sup·pres′sion
im′mu·no·sup·pres′sive
im′mu·no·ther′a·py
im′mu·no·tox′in
im′mu·no·trans·fu′sion
im·pact′ed
im·pac′tion
im·pac′tor
im·pal′pa·ble
im·pair′
im·pair′ment
im′par′
im·par′i·dig′i·tate′
im′passe′
im·pa′ten·cy
im·pa′tent
im·ped′ance
im·per′a·tive
im′per·cep′ti·ble

im′per·cep′tion
im·per′fo·rate
im·per′fo·ra′tion
im·per′me·a·ble
im·per′me·a·bil′i·ty
im·per′son·al·i·za′tion
im·per′vi·ous
im′pe·tig′i·ni·za′tion
im′pe·tig′i·noid′
im′pe·tig′i·nous
im·pe·ti′go
    —cir′ci·na′ta
    —cir′cum·pi·lar′is
    —con·ta·gi·o′sa
    —fol·lic′u·lar′is
    —her·pet′i·for′mis
    —ne·o·na′to′rum
    —vul·gar′is
im′pe·tus
im′pinge′
im·pinge′ment
im·ping′er
im·plant′
im·plant′a·ble
im·plan·ta′tion
im·plan·tol′o·gist
im·plan·tol′o·gy
im·plic′it
im′po·tence
im′po·ten·cy
im′po·tent
im·po·ten′ti·a
    —co′e·un·di′
    —er′i·gen·di′
im·preg′nate′, -nat′ed,
    -nat′ing
im·preg′na′tion
im·pres′si·o′ *pl.* im·pres′si·
    o′nes′
    —car·di′a·ca hep′a·tis
    —cardiaca pul·mo′nis
    —co′li·ca
    —du·o′de·na′lis hep′a·tis
    —e·so·pha′ge·a hep′a·tis
    —gas′tri·ca hep′a·tis
    —gastrica re′nis
    —he·pat′i·ca re′nis
    —lig·a·men′ti′ cos′to·cla·
        vic′u·lar′is
    —mus·cu·lar′is re′nis
    —oe·so·pha′ge·a hep′a·tis
    —pe·tro′sa cer′e·bri′
    —re·na′lis hep′a·tis

—su′pra·re′na′lis hep′a·tis
—tri·gem′i·ni′ os′sis
tem′po·ra′lis
im·pres′sion
im·pres′si·o′nes′ dig′i·ta′-
tae′
im·print′
im·print′ing
im·pro′cre·ance
im·pro′cre·ant
im·prove′
im·prove′ment
im·pu′ber·al
im·pu′ber·ism
im·pu′bic
im′pulse
im·pul′sion
im·pul′sive
im·pul′sive·ness
im·pu′ni·tive
im·pu′ta·bil′i·ty
im′vic
in′a·cid′i·ty
in·ac′tion
in·ac′ti·vate′, -vat′ed,
-vat′ing
in·ac′ti·va′tion
in·ac′tive
in·ac·tiv′i·ty
in·ad′e·qua·cy
in·ad′e·quate
in·ad′e·quate·ly
in·al′i·men′tal
in·an′i·mate
in′a·ni′tion
in·ap′par′ent
in·ap′pe·tence
in·ar·tic′u·late
in ar·tic·u·lo′ mor′tis
in·as·sim′i·la·ble
in′born′
in′bred′
in′breed′ing
In′ca bone
in·ca·nous
in·ca·pac′i·tate′
in·ca·pac′i·ta′tion
in·car′cer·ate′, -at′ed, -at′ing
in·car′cer·a′tion
in·car′i·al
in·car′nant
in·car·na′ti·o′ un′guis
in·car′na·tive

in·case′ment
in·cen′di·a·rism
in·cen′di·ar′y
in·cen′tive
in·cep′tion
in·cep′tus
in′cest′
in·ces′tu·ous
in′ci·dence
in′ci·dent
in′ci·den′tal
in·cin′er·ate′, -at′ed, -at′ing
in·cin′er·a′tion
in·cin′er·a′tor
in·cip′i·ence
in·cip′i·en·cy
in·cip′i·ent
in·ci′sal
in·cise′, -cised′, -cis′ing
in·ci′sion
in·ci′sion·al
in·ci′sive
in′ci·si′vus
—la′bi·i′ in·fe′ri·o′ris
—labii su·pe′ri·o′ris
in·ci′so·la′bi·al
in·ci′so·lin′gual
in·ci′so·prox′i·mal
in·ci′sor
in′ci·su′ra *pl.* -rae′
—ac′e·tab′u·li′
—an′gu·lar′is
—anterior au′ris
—ap′i·cis cor′dis
—car·di′a·ca
—cardiaca pul·mo′nis
si′nis·tri′
—cardiaca ven·tric′u·li′
—cer′e·bel′li′ anterior
—cerebelli posterior
—cla·vic′u·lar′is
—cos·ta′lis
—eth′moi·da′lis
—fib′u·lar′is
—fron·ta′lis
—in′ter·ar′y·tae·noi′de·a
—in′ter·ar′y·te·noi′de·a
—in′ter·lo·bar′is pul·mo′nis
—in′ter·trag′i·ca
—is′chi·ad′i·ca major
—ischiadica minor
—jug′u·lar′is os′sis oc·cip′i·
ta′lis

—jugularis ossis tem′po·
ra′lis
—jugularis ster′ni′
—lac′ri·ma′lis
—lig′a·men′ti′ te′re·tis
—man·dib′u·lae′
—mas·toi′de·a
—na·sa′lis
—pan·cre′a·tis
—pa·ri′e·ta′lis
—pre′oc·cip′i·ta′lis
—pter′y·goi′de·a
—ra′di·a′lis
—scap′u·lae′
—sem′i·lu·nar′is
—sphe′no·pal′a·ti′na
—su′pra·or′bi·ta′lis
—ten·to′ri·i′
—ter′mi·na′lis au′ris
—thy′re·oi′de·a inferior
—thyreoidea superior
—thy·roi′de·a inferior
—thyroidea superior
—troch′le·ar′is
—tym·pan′i·ca
—ul·nar′is
—um·bil′i·ca′lis
—ver′te·bra′lis inferior
—vertebralis superior
in′ci·su·rae′
—car′ti·lag′i·nis me·a′tus
a·cu′sti·ci′
—cartilaginis meatus
acustici ex·ter′ni′
(San·to·ri′ni)
—cos·ta′les′
—hel′i·cis
in·ci′su·ral
in·ci′sure
—of Ri·vi′nus
—of Schmidt′-Lan′ter·mann
in·ci′tant
in·cli·na′ti·o′ *pl.* -na′ti·o′nes′
in·cli·na′tion
in·cline′, -clined′, -clin′ing
in·cli·nom′e·ter
in·clu′sion
in·co·ag′u·la·bil′i·ty
in·co·ag′u·la·ble
in·co·her′ence
in·co·her′ent
in·com·pat′i·bil′i·ty
in·com·pat′i·ble

in·com'pe·tence
in·com'pe·ten·cy
in·com'pe·tent
in'com·plete'
in·con'gru·ence
in·con'gru·ent
in·con·gru'i·ty
in·con'stant
in·con'ti·nence
in·con'ti·nent
in·con'ti·nen'ti·a
—al'vi'
—pig'men'ti'
—u·ri'nae'
—vul'vae'
in·co·or'di·nate
in·co·or'di·na'tion
in·cor'po·rate', -rat'ed,
-rat'ing
in·cor'po·ra'tion
in·co·sta·pe'di·al
in'crease'
in'cre·ment
in·cre·men'tal
in·cre'to·ry
in'cross'
in·crust'
in·crus·ta'tion
in'cu·bate', -bat'ed, -bat'ing
in·cu·ba'tion
in'cu·ba'tor
in'cu·bus *pl.* -bi' *or* -bus·es
in'cu·dal
in·cu·dec'to·my
in·cu'di·form'
in·cu·do·mal'le·al
in·cu·do·sta·pe'di·al
in·cur'a·ble
in·cur'vate', -vat'ed, -vat'ing
in·cur·va'tion
in'cus *pl.* in·cu'des'
in·cy'clo·pho'ri·a
in·cy'co·tro'pi·a
in·dent'
in·den·ta'tion
in·de·ter'mi·nate
in'dex' *pl.* -dex'es *or* -di·ces'
—of Flow'er
In'dex' Med'i·cus
In'di·a ink
—method
—nucleus
—stain

in'di·can'
in'di·cant
in'di·ca·nu'ri·a
in'di·ca'ti·o'
—cau·sa'lis
—cu·ra·ti'va
—symp'to·mat'i·ca
in'di·ca'tion
in'di·ca'tor
in'di·co·phose'
in di'es
in·dif'fer·ent
in·dig'e·nous
in'di·gest'i·ble
in'di·gest'i·bil'i·ty
in'di·ges'tion
in·dig'i·ta'tion
in'di·go
in·dig'o·tin
in'di·go·u'ri·a
in'di·rect'
in·di·ru'bin
in·dis'crete'
in·dis·crim'i·nate
in·dis·posed'
in·dis·po·si'tion
in·dis'tinct'
in'di·um
in·di·vid'u·al·i·za'tion
in·di·vid'u·al·ize', -ized',
-iz'ing
in·di·vid'u·a'tion
in·do·cy'a·nine'
in·dol·ac'e·tu'ri·a
in'dole'
in'dole·a·ce'tic
in'do·lent
in'dole·pro'pi·on'ic
in'dole·py·ru'vic
in·do·log'e·nous
in·do·lu'ri·a
in·do·lyl·a·cryl'o·yl·gly'-
cine
in·do·lyl·a·cryl'o·yl·gly'ci·
nu'ri·a
in·do·meth'a·cin
in·do·phe'nol'
in·dox'ole'
in·dox'yl
in·dox'yl·e'mi·a
in·dox'y·log'e·nous
in·dox'yl·sul'fate'
in·dox'yl·sul·fu'ric

in·dox'yl·u'ri·a
in'dri·line'
in·duce', -duced', -duc'ing
in·duc'er
in·duc'i·ble
in·duc'tance
in·duc'tion
in·duc'tive
in·duc'to·py·rex'i·a
in·duc'to·ri·um
in·duc'to·ther'my
in'du·lin
in'du·rate', -rat'ed, -rat'ing
in'du·ra'tion
in'du·ra'tive
in·du'si·um *pl.* -si·a
—gris'e·um
in'dwell'ing
in·e'bri·ant
in·e'bri·ate', -at'ed, -at'ing
in·e'bri·a'tion
in·e'bri'e·ty
in·ef·fi·ca'cious
in·ef·fi·ca·cy
in·e·las'tic
in·ert'
in·er'tia
in ex·tre'mis
in'fan·cy
in'fant
in·fan'ti·cide'
in·fan'tile'
in·fan'ti·lism
in'farct'
in·farc·tec'to·my
in·farc'tion
in·fect'
in·fec'tion
in·fec'tious
in·fec'tive
in·fec·tiv'i·ty
in·fe·cun'di·ty
in·fe'ri·or
in·fe'ri·or'i·ty
in·fer·o·lat'er·al
in·fer·o·me'di·al
in·fer·o·pa·ri'e·tal
in·fer·o·pos·te'ri·or
in·fer'tile
in·fer·til'i·ty
in·fest'
in'fes·ta'tion
in·fes'tive

in·fib′u·la′tion
in′fil·trate′, -trat′ed, -trat′ing
in′fil·tra′tion
in·fin′i·ty
in·firm′
in·fir′ma·ry
in·fir′mi·ty
in·flame′, -flamed′,
  -flam′ing
in·flam′ma·ble
in·flam·ma′tion
in·flam′ma·to′ry
in·flate′, -flat′ed, -flat′ing
in·fla′tion
in·fla′tor
in·flec′tion
in·flo·res′cence
in′flow′
in·flu·en′za
in·flu·en′zal
in′fold′
in′foot′ed
in′fra·al′ve·o′lar
in′fra·au·ric′u·lar
in′fra·ax′il·lar′y
in′fra·bo′ny
in′fra·bulge′
in′fra·car′di·ac′
in′fra·cla·vic′u·lar
in′fra·cla·vic′u·lar′is
in′fra·cli′noid′
in′fra·clu′sion
in′fra·con′dy·lism
in′fra·cor′ti·cal
in′fra·cos′tal
in·frac′tion
in′fra·den·ta′le′
in′fra·di·a·phrag·mat′ic
in′fra·gle′noid′
in′fra·glot′tic
in′fra·gran′u·lar
in′fra·hy′oid′
in′fra·mam′ma·ry
in′fra·man·dib′u·lar
in′fra·mar′gin·al
in′fra·max′il·lar′y
in′fra·na′sal
in′fra·na′tant
in′fra·nu′cle·ar
in′fra·oc·clu′sion
in′fra·or′bi·tal
in′fra·pa·tel′lar
in′fra·phys′i·o·log′ic

in′fra·place′ment
in′fra·red′
in′fra·scap′u·lar
in′fra·son′ic
in′fra·spi·na′tus
in′fra·spi′nous
in′fra·ster′nal
in′fra·struc′ture
in′fra·tem′po·ral
in′fra·tem′po·ra′le′
in′fra·ten·to′ri·al
in′fra·tra′che·al
in′fra·troch′le·ar
in′fra·tur′bin·al
in′fra·um·bil′i·cal
in′fra·vag′i·nal
in′fra·ver′sion
in′fra·ves′i·cal
in′fra·zy′go·mat′ic
in·fric′tion
in·fun·dib′u·lar
in·fun·dib′u·lec′to·my
in·fun·dib′u·li·form′
in·fun·dib′u·lo′ma pl. -mas
  or -ma·ta
in·fun·dib′u·lo·pel′vic
in·fun·dib′u·lo·ven·tric′u·
  lar
in·fun·dib′u·lum pl. -la
  —eth′moi·da′le′
  —hy′po·thal′a·mi′
  —tu′bae′ u′te·ri′nae′
in·fuse′
in·fus′i·ble
in·fu′sion
in·gest′
in·ges′ta
in·ges′tant
in·gest′i·ble
in·ges′tion
in·ges′tive
In·gras′si·a wings
in′gra·ves′cent
in·gre′di·ent
in′grow′ing
in′grown′
in′growth′
in′guen pl. -gui·na
in′gui·nal
in′gui·no·ab·dom′i·nal
in′gui·no·cru′ral
in′gui·no·dyn′i·a
in′gui·no·la′bi·al

in′gui·no·scro′tal
in·hal′ant
in·ha·la′tion
in·ha·la′tor
in·hale′, -haled′, -hal′ing
in·hal′er
in·her′ent
in·her′ent·ly
in·her′it
in·her′it·a·ble
in·her′i·tance
in·hib′in
in·hib′it
in·hi·bi′tion
in·hib′i·tive
in·hib′i·tor
in·hib′i·to′ry
in·ho·mo·ge·ne′i·ty
in·ho·mo·ge′ne·ous
in′i·al
in′i·en·ceph′a·lus
in′i·en·ceph′a·ly
in′i·od′y·mus
in′i·on′
in′i·op′a·gus
in′i·ops′
i·ni′tial
i·ni′ti·a′tor
in·i′tis
in·ject′
in·ject′a·ble
in·jec′ti·o′ pl. in·jec′ti·o′nes′
in·jec′tion
in·jec′tor
in·ju′ri·ous
in′ju·ry
ink′blot′
in′lay′
in′let′
in′ly′ing
in′nate′
in′ner
in′ner·vate′ (to supply with
  nerves), -vat′ed, -vat′ing
  ♦enervate
in′ner·va′tion
in·nid′i·a′tion
in·no′cent
in·noc′u·ous
in·nom′i·na′tal
in·nom′i·nate
in·nox′ious
in′nu·tri′tion

in'o·blast'
in'oc·ci·pit'i·a
in'o·chon·dri'tis
in·oc'u·la·bil'i·ty
in·oc'u·la·ble
in·oc'u·late', -lat'ed, -lat'ing
in·oc'u·la'tion
in·oc'u·la'tive
in·oc'u·la'tor
in·oc'u·lum pl. -la
in'o·cyte'
in'o·gen
in'o·gen'e·sis
in·og'e·nous
in·og'li·a
in'o·lith'
in·op'er·a·ble
in'or·gan'ic
in·os'co·py
in·os'cu·late', -lat'ed, -lat'ing
in·os'cu·la'tion
in·ose'
in'o·se'mi·a
in'o·sine'
in'o·sin'ic
in·o'si·tol'
in'o·si·tu'ri·a
in'o·su'ri·a
in'o·trope'
in'o·trop'ic
in'pa'tient
in'put'
in'quest'
in'qui·line'
in'ruc·ta'tion
in·sal'i·vate', -vat'ed, -vat'ing
in·sal'i·va'tion
in·sa·lu'bri·ous
in·sa·lu'bri·ty
in·sane'
in·san'i·tar'y
in·san'i·ty
in·scrip'ti·o'
   pl. in·scrip'ti·o'nes'
in·scrip'tion
in'sect'
In·sec'ta
in·sec'ti·cid'al
in·sec'ti·cide'
in·sec'ti·fuge'
in·se·cure'
in·se·cure'ly
in·se·cur'i·ty

in·sem'i·nate'
in·sem'i·na'tion
in·se·nes'cence
in·sen'si·bil'i·ty
in·sen'si·ble
in·sen'si·bly
in·sert' v.
in'sert' n.
in·sert'er
in·ser'tion
in·sid'i·ous
in'sight'
in·sip'id
in si'tu
in·so·la'tion
in·sol'u·bil'i·ty
in·sol'u·ble
in·som'ni·a
in·som'ni·ac'
in·sorp'tion
in·spec'tion
in·sper'sion
in·spi·ra'tion
in·spi·ra'tor
in·spi'ra·to'ry
in·spire'
in·spi·rom'e·ter
in·spis'sate', -sat'ed, -sat'ing
in·spis·sa'tion
in·spis'sa·tor
in·sta·bil'i·ty
in'stance
in·stan·ta'ne·ous
in'star'
in'step'
in·still'
in·stil·la'tion
in·stil·la'tor
in'stinct
in·stinc'tive
in·stinc'tive·ly
in·stinc'tu·al
in'sti·tute'
in·sti·tu'tion·al
in'stru·ment
in'stru·men'tal
in'stru·men·tar'i·um pl. -i·a
in'stru·men·ta'tion
in'su·date'
in'suf·fi'cien·cy
in'suf·fi'cient
in'suf·fi'cient·ly
in'suf·flate'

in'suf·fla'tion
in'suf·fla'tor
in'su·la pl. -lae'
in'su·lar
in'su·late'
in'su·la'tion
in'su·la'tor
in'su·lin
in'su·lin·ase'
in'su·lin·e'mi·a
in'su·lin·o'gen·e'sis pl. -ses'
in'su·lin·o'gen'ic
in'su·li·no'ma pl. -mas or
  -ma·ta
in'su·lo'ma pl. -mas or -ma·ta
in'sult'
in'sus·cep'ti·bil'i·ty
in·tact'
in'take'
in'te·gral
in'te·grate'
in'te·gra'tion
in·teg'ri·ty
in·teg'u·ment
in·teg'u·men'tal
in·teg'u·men'ta·ry
in·teg'u·men'tum
  —com·mu'ne'
in'tel·lect'
in'tel·lec'tu·al
in'tel·lec'tu·al·i·za'tion
in'tel·lec'tu·al·ize', -ized',
  -iz'ing
in·tel'li·gence
in·tel'li·gent
in·tem'per·ance
in·tem'per·ate
in·tem'per·ate·ly
in·tense'
in·ten·si·fi·ca'tion
in·ten'si·fy', -fied', -fy'ing
in·ten·sim'e·ter
in·ten'si·ty
in·ten'sive
in·ten'tion
in·ten'tion·al
in·ter·ac·ces'so·ry
in·ter·ac'i·nar
in·ter·ac'i·nous
in'ter·al·ve'o·lar
in'ter·an'nu·lar
in'ter·ar·tic'u·lar
in'ter·ar'y·te'noid'

in'ter·ar'y·te·noi'de·us
in'ter·a'tri·al
in'ter·ax'o·nal
in'ter·bod'y
in'ter·brain'
in'ter·ca·lar'y
in'ter·ca·late', -lat'ed, -lat'ing
in'ter·ca·la'tion
in'ter·can'a·lic'u·lar
in'ter·cap'il·lar'y
in'ter·ca·rot'id
in'ter·car'pal
in'ter·car'ti·lag'i·nous
in'ter·cav'er·nous
in'ter·cel'lu·lar
in'ter·cen'tral
in'ter·cer'e·bral
in'ter·chon'dral
in'ter·cil'i·um
in'ter·clav'i·cle
in'ter·cla·vic'u·lar
in'ter·cli'noid'
in'ter·coc·cyg'e·al
in'ter·co·lum'nar
in'ter·con'dy·lar
in'ter·con'dy·loid'
in'ter·cor'o·nar'y
in'ter·cos'tal
in'ter·cos'to·bra'chi·al
in'ter·cos'to·hu'mer·al
in'ter·cou'pler
in'ter·course'
in'ter·cri'co·thy·rot'o·my
in'ter·cris'tal
in'ter·cross'
in'ter·cru'ral
in'ter·cur'rent
in'ter·cus·pa'tion
in'ter·cusp'ing
in'ter·den'tal
in'ter·den'ti·um
in'ter·dic'tion
in'ter·dig'it
in'ter·dig'i·tal
in'ter·dig'i·tate', -tat'ed,
   -tat'ing
in'ter·dig'i·ta'tion
in'ter·dis'ci·pli·nar'y
in'ter·duc'tal
in'ter·face' *(a surface forming*
   the boundary between two
   phases)
   ♦*interphase*

in'ter·fa'cial
in'ter·fas·cic'u·lar
in'ter·fem'o·ral
in'ter·fere', -fered', -fer'ing
in'ter·fer'ence
in'ter·fe·rom'e·ter
in'ter·fer'o·met'ric
in'ter·fe·rom'e·try
in'ter·fer'on'
in'ter·fer·on'o·gen
in'ter·fi'bril·lar
in'ter·fi'bril·lar'y
in'ter·fi'brous
in'ter·fil'a·men'tous
in'ter·fi'lar
in'ter·fol·lic'u·lar
in'ter·fo·ve'o·lar
in'ter·fron'tal
in'ter·fur'ca *pl.* -cae'
in'ter·gem'mal
in'ter·glob'u·lar
in'ter·glu'te·al
in'ter·go'ni·al
in'ter·grade'
in'ter·gran'u·lar
in'ter·gy'ral
in'ter·he'mal
in'ter·hem'i·cer'e·bral
in'ter·hem'i·spher'ic
in'ter·ic'tal
in·te'ri·or
in'ter·ja'cent
in'ter·ki·ne'sis *pl.* -ses'
in'ter·la'bi·al
in'ter·lace'
in'ter·la·mel'lar
in'ter·lam'i·nar
in'ter·leu'kin
in'ter·lig'a·men'ta·ry
in'ter·lig'a·men'tous
in'ter·lo'bar
in'ter·lob'u·lar
in'ter·mal·le'o·lar
in'ter·mam'ma·ry
in'ter·mar'riage
in'ter·max·il'la *pl.* -lae' *or*
   -las
in'ter·max'il·lar'y
in'ter·me'di·ar'y
in'ter·me'di·ate
in'ter·me'din
in'ter·me'di·o·lat'er·al
in'ter·me'di·o·me'di·al

in'ter·me'di·us
in'ter·mem'bra·nous
in'ter·me·nin'ge·al
in'ter·men'stru·al
in·ter'ment
in'ter·mes'en·ter'ic
in'ter·mes'o·blas'tic
in'ter·met'a·car'pal
in'ter·met'a·mer'ic
in'ter·met'a·tar'sal
in'ter·mis'sion
in'ter·mi·tot'ic
in'ter·mit'tence
in'ter·mit'ten·cy
in'ter·mit'tent
in'ter·mix'
in'ter·mu'ral
in'ter·mus'cu·lar
in'tern'
in·ter'nal
in·ter'nal·i·za'tion
in·ter'nal·ize'
in'ter·nar'i·al
in'ter·na'sal
in'ter·na'tal
in'ter·neu'ral
in'ter·neu'ron'
in'ter·neu'ro·nal
in·tern'ist
in'ter·nod'al
in'ter·node'
in'tern·ship'
in'ter·nu'cle·ar
in'ter·nun'ci·al
in·ter'nus
in'ter·oc·clu'sal
in'ter·o·cep'tive
in'ter·o·cep'tor
in'ter·o·fec'tion
in'ter·o·fec'tive
in'ter·o·ges'tate'
in'ter·ol'i·var'y
in'ter·or'bi·tal
in'ter·os'se·al
in'ter·os'se·i' *sing.* -se·us
in'ter·os'se·ous
in'ter·pal'a·tine'
in'ter·pal'pe·bral
in'ter·pap'il·lar'y
in'ter·pa·ri'e·tal
in'ter·par'ox·ys'mal
in'ter·pe·dic'u·late'
in'ter·pe·dun'cu·lar

in′ter·pel′vi·o·ab·dom′i·nal
in′ter·per′son·al
in′ter·pha·lan′ge·al
in′ter·phase′ *(a period in the life of a cell during which there is no mitotic division)*
 ♦interface
in′ter·pha′sic
in′ter·plant′
in′ter·pleu′ral
in·ter′po·late′, -lat′ed, -lat′ing
in·ter′po·la′tion
in·ter′pose′, -posed′, -pos′ing
in·ter′po·si′tion
in·ter·pre·ta′tion
in·ter·pris·mat′ic
in·ter·prox′i·mal
in·ter·prox′i·mate
in·ter·pu′bic
in·ter·pulse′
in·ter·pu′pil·lar′y
in·ter·py·ram′i·dal
in·ter·ra′di·al
in·ter·ra·dic′u·lar
in·ter·re′nal
in·ter·re·tic′u·lar
in·ter·rupt′ed
in·ter·scap′u·lar
in·ter·scap′u·lo·tho·rac′ic
in·ter·sect′
in·ter·sec′ti·o′ *pl.* -sec′ti·o′- nes′
in·ter·sec′tion
in·ter·sec′ti·o′nes′ ten·din′- e·ae′
in·ter·seg·men′tal
in·ter·sen′so·ry
in·ter·sep′tal
in·ter·sep′to·val′vu·lar
in·ter·sep′tum *pl.* -tums *or* -ta
in·ter·sex′
in·ter·sex′u·al
in·ter·sex′u·al′i·ty
in·ter·sig′moid′
in·ter·space′
in·ter·sphe′noid′
in·ter·spi′nal
in·ter·spi·na′les′ *sing.* -na′lis
in·ter·spi′nous
in·ter·stic·es *sing.* -stice
in·ter·sti′tial

in·ter·sti′ti·o′ma *pl.* -mas *or* -ma·ta
in·ter·sti′ti·um
in·ter·sys·tol′ic
in·ter·tar′sal
in·ter·ter′ri·to′ri·al
in·ter·tho·rac′i·co·scap′u· lar
in·ter·trans′ver·sa′les′
in·ter·trans′ver·sa′lis
in·ter·trans·verse′
in·ter·tri·gem′i·nal
in·ter·trig′i·nous
in·ter·tri′go
in·ter·tro′chan·ter′ic
in·ter·tu′ber·al
in·ter·tu·ber′cu·lar
in·ter·tu′bu·lar
in·ter·u′re·ter·al
in·ter·u′re·ter′ic
in·ter·vag′i·nal
in·ter·val
in·ter·val′vu·lar
in·ter·vas′cu·lar
in·ter·ve′nous *(between veins)*
 ♦intravenous
in′ter·ven′tion
in′ter·ven′tion·al
in′ter·ven·tric′u·lar *(situated between ventricles)*
 ♦intraventricular
in′ter·ver′te·bral
in′ter·vil′lous
in′ter·zo′nal
in·tes′ti·nal
in·tes′tine
in·tes·ti′num *pl.* -na
 —cae′cum
 —cras′sum
 —il′e·um
 —je·ju′num
 —rec′tum
 —ten′u·e′
 —tenue mes·en·ter′i·a′le′
in′ti·ma
in′ti·mal
in′ti·mec′to·my
in′ti·mi′tis
in′tine′
in′toe′
in·tol′er·ance
in·tor′sion
in·tort′

in·tort′er
in·tox′i·cant
in·tox′i·cate′
in·tox′i·ca′tion
in′tra·ab·dom′i·nal
in′tra·ac′i·nar
in′tra·al·ve′o·lar
in′tra·a·or′tic
in′tra·ar·te′ri·al
in′tra·ar·te′ri·al·ly
in′tra·ar·tic′u·lar
in′tra·a′tri·al
in′tra·au′ral
in′tra·au·ric′u·lar
in′tra·bron′chi·al
in′tra·bron·chi′o·lar
in′tra·buc′cal
in′tra·cal′y·ce′al
in′tra·can·a·lic′u·lar
in′tra·cap′su·lar
in′tra·car′di·ac′
in′tra·car′pal
in′tra·car′ti·lag′i·nous
in′tra·cav′er·nous
in′tra·cav′i·tar′y
in′tra·cel′lu·lar
in′tra·ce·phal′ic
in′tra·cer′e·bel′lar
in′tra·cer′e·bral
in′tra·cer′vi·cal
in′tra·chon′dri·al
in′tra·cho′ri·on′ic
in′tra·cho·roi′dal
in′tra·cis·ter′nal
in′tra·col′ic
in′tra·cor′ne·al
in′tra·co·ro′nal
in′tra·cor·po′re·al
in′tra·cor·pus′cu·lar
in′tra·cor′ti·cal
in′tra·cos′tal
in′tra·cra′ni·al
in·trac′ta·ble
in′tra·cu·ta′ne·ous
in′tra·cu·tic′u·lar
in′tra·cys′tic
in′tra·cy′to·plas′mic
in′tra·der′mal
in′tra·der′mic
in·tra·duc′tal
in·tra·du′ral
in′tra·em′bry·on′ic
in′tra·ep′i·der′mal

in′tra·ep′i·the′li·al
in′tra·e·ryth′ro·cyt′ic
in′tra·e·soph′a·ge′al
in′tra·fa′cial
in′tra·fal·lo′pi·an
in′tra·fas·cic′u·lar
in′tra·fi′lar
in′tra·fis′su·ral
in′tra·fis′tu·lar
in′tra·fol·lic′u·lar
in′tra·fu′sal
in′tra·gas′tric
in′tra·gem′mal
in′tra·gen′ic
in′tra·glan′du·lar
in′tra·glob′u·lar
in′tra·glu′te·al
in′tra·gy′ral
in′tra·he·pat′ic
in′tra·hy′oid′
in′tra·ic′tal
in′tra·in·tes′ti·nal
in′tra·jug′u·lar
in′tra·lam′i·nar
in′tra·la·ryn′ge·al
in′tra·le′sion·al
in′tra·leu′ko·cyt′ic
in′tra·lig′a·men′tous
in′tra·lo′bar
in′tra·lob′u·lar
in′tra·loc′u·lar
in′tra·lu′mi·nal
in′tra·mam′ma·ry
in′tra·mar′gin·al
in′tra·med′ul·lar′y
in′tra·mem′bra·nous
in′tra·me·nin′ge·al
in′tra·men′stru·al
in′tra·mo·lec′u·lar
in′tra·mu·co′sal
in′tra·mu′ral
in′tra·mus′cu·lar
in′tra·my′o·car′di·al
in′tra·my′o·me′tri·al
in′tra·nar′i·al
in′tra·na′sal
in′tra·na′tal
in′tra·neu′ral
in′tra·nu′cle·ar
in′tra·oc′u·lar
in′tra·op′er·a·tive
in′tra·op′er·a·tive·ly
in′tra·op′tic

in′tra·o′ral
in′tra·or′bi·tal
in′tra·os′se·ous
in′tra·os′te·al
in′tra·pan′cre·at′ic
in′tra·pa·ren′chy·mal
in′tra·pa·ri′e·tal
in′tra·par′tum
in′tra·pel′vic
in′tra·per′i·car′di·ac′
in′tra·per′i·car′di·al
in′tra·per′i·ne′al
in′tra·per′i·to·ne′al
in′tra·pha·lan′ge·al
in′tra·pi′al
in′tra·pla·cen′tal
in′tra·pleu′ral
in′tra·pros·tat′ic
in′tra·psy′chic
in′tra·pul′mo·nar′y
in′tra·py·ret′ic
in′tra·rec′tal
in′tra·re′nal
in′tra·ret′i·nal
in′tra·scap′u·lar
in′tra·scle′ral
in′tra·scro′tal
in′tra·seg·men′tal
in′tra·sel′lar
in′tra·se′rous
in′tra·spi′nal
in′tra·spi′nous
in′tra·sple′nic
in′tra·ster′nal
in′tra·sti′tial
in′tra·stro′mal
in′tra·syn·o′vi·al
in′tra·tar′sal
in′tra·tes·tic′u·lar
in′tra·the′cal
in′tra·tho·rac′ic
in′tra·ton′sil·lar
in′tra·tra·bec′u·lar
in′tra·tra′che·al
in′tra·tro·chan·ter′ic
in′tra·tu′bal
in′tra·tu′bu·lar
in′tra·tym·pan′ic
in′tra·um·bil′i·cal
in′tra·u·re′ter·al
in′tra·u·re′thral
in′tra·u′ter·ine
in′tra·vag′i·nal

in·trav′a·sate′
in·trav′a·sa′tion
in′tra·vas′cu·lar
in′tra·vas′cu·lar·ly
in′tra·ve·na′tion
in′tra·ve′nous *(within the veins)*
   ♦ *intervenous*
in′tra·ven·tric′u·lar *(located within a ventricle)*
   ♦ *interventricular*
in′tra·ver′te·bral
in′tra·ves′i·cal
in′tra·vi′tal
in′tra·vi·tel′line′
in′tra·vit′re·ous
in·trin′sic
in·tro·ces′sion
in·tro·duc′er
in·tro·flex′ion
in·troi′tal
in·troi′tus *pl.* in·troi′tus
in·tro·jec′tion
in·tro·mis′sion
in·tro·mit′tent
in·tro·pu′ni·tive
in·tro·spec′tion
in·tro·spec′tive
in·tro·sus·cep′tion
in·tro·ver′sion
in′tro·vert′
in·trude′, -trud′ed, -trud′ing
in′tu·bate′, -bat′ed, -bat′ing
in′tu·ba′tion
in′tu·ba′tor
in·tu·i′tion
in·tu′i·tive
in′tu·mesce′
in′tu·mes′cence
in′tu·mes′cent
in·tu′mes·cen′ti·a *pl.* -ae′
   —cer′vi·ca′lis
   —lum·ba′lis
   —tym·pan′i·ca
in′tus·sus·cep′tion
in′tus·sus·cep′tum
in′tus·sus·cip′i·ens
in·u′lase′
in·u′lin
in·unc′tion
in u′ter·o′
in vac′u·o′
in·vade′, -vad′ed, -vad′ing

in·vad'er
in·vag'i·nate', -nat'ed,
  -nat'ing
in·vag'i·na'tion
in'va·lid
in'va·lid·ism
in·va'sin
in·va'sion
in·va'sive
in·va'sive·ness
in'ven·to'ry
in·verse'
in·ver'sion
in·ver'sive
in·ver'sus
in·vert' v.
in·vert' n.
in·ver'tase'
in·ver'te·bral
in·ver'te·brate'
in·vert'ed
in·ver'tin
in·ver'tor
in·ver'tose'
in·vest'
in·vest'ment
in·vet'er·ate
in'vi·ril'i·ty
in'vis·ca'tion
in vi'tro'
in vi'vo'
in'vo·lu'cre
in'vo·lu'crum pl. -cra
in·vol'un·tar'y
in'vo·lute'
in'vo·lu'tion
in'vo·lu'tion·al
i'o·ben·zam'ic
i·o'ce·tam'ic
i·o'da·mide'
I·o'da·moe'ba
  —bütsch'li·i'
  —wil·liam'si'
i'o·date'
i'od'ic
i'o·dide'
i'o·dim'e·try
i·o'di·nate'
i·o'di·na'tion
i'o·dine'
i·od'i·nin
i'o·din'o·phil'
i'o·din'o·phil'i·a

i'o·din'o·phil'ic
i'o·dip'a·mide'
i'o·dism
i'o·dize', -dized', -diz'ing
i·o'do·a·ce'tic
i·o'do·al·phi·on'ic
i·o'do·ca'sein'
i·o'do·chlor'hy·drox'y·
  quin
i·o'do·de·ox'y·u'ri·dine'
i·o'do·der'ma
i·o'do·form'
i·o'do·glob'u·lin
i·o'do·gor·go'ic
i·o'do·met'ric
i'o·dom'e·try
i·o'do·nat'ed
i·o'do·pa·no'ic
i·o'do·phe'nol'
i·o'do·phil'
i·o'do·phil'i·a
i·o'do·phor'
i·o'do·phthal'ein'
i·o'do·pro'tein'
i'o·dop'sin
i·o'do·pyr'a·cet
i·o'do·ther'a·py
i·o'do·thy'ro·glob'u·lin
i'o·dox'yl
i'o·gly·cam'ic
i'o·hex'ol
i'on'
I'o·nes'cu method
i·on'ic
i·o'ni·um
i'on·i·za'tion
i'on·ize', -ized', -iz'ing
i'on·om'e·ter
i·on'to·pho·re'sis pl. -ses'
i·on'to·pho·ret'ic
i'o·no'phose'
i'o·pam'i·dol'
i'o·pan·o'ic
i'o·pen'tol'
i'o·phen'dy·late'
i'o·phen·ox'ic
i'o·pho'bi·a
i'o·py'dol'
i'o·py'done'
i'o·thal'a·mate'
i'o·tha·lam'ic
i'o·thi'o·u'ra·cil
i·o'ver·sol'

i·ox'a·glate'
ip'e·cac'
i'po·date'
ip'o·me'a
i·prin'dole'
i'pro·ni'a·zid
i'pro·nid'a·zole'
ip·sa'tion
ip'sa·tive
ip'si·lat'er·al
ip'si·lat'er·al·ly
ip'si·ver'sive
i·ras'ci·bil'i·ty
i'ri·dal
i'ri·dal'gi·a
ir'id·aux'e·sis pl. -ses'
ir'i·dec'ta·sis
ir'i·dec'tome'
ir'i·dec'to·mize', -mized',
  -miz'ing
ir'i·dec'to·my
ir'i·dec·tro'pi·um
ir'i·de'mi·a
ir'i·den·clei'sis pl. -ses'
ir'i·den·tro'pi·um
ir'i·de·re'mi·a
ir'i·des'cence
ir'i·des'cent
i·rid'e·sis pl. -ses'
i·rid'i·al
i·rid'i·an
i·rid'ic
ir'i·din
i·rid'i·um
ir'i·di·za'tion
ir'i·do·a·vul'sion
ir'i·do·cap'su·li'tis
ir'i·do·cap'su·lot'o·my
i·rid'o·cele'
ir'i·do·cho'roi·di'tis
ir'i·do·col'o·bo'ma
ir'i·do·con·stric'tor
ir'i·do·cor'ne·al
ir'i·do·cy·clec'to·my
ir'i·do·cy·cli'tis
ir'i·do·cy'clo·cho'roi·di'tis
ir'i·do·cys·tec'to·my
ir'i·dod'e·sis pl. -ses'
ir'i·do·di·ag·no'sis pl. -ses'
ir'i·do·di·al'y·sis pl. -ses'
ir'i·do·di·as'ta·sis pl. -ses'
ir'i·do·di·la'tor
ir'i·do·do·ne'sis pl. -ses'

ir'i·do·ker'a·ti'tis
ir'i·do·ki·ne'si·a
ir'i·do·ki·ne'sis *pl.* -ses'
ir'i·do·ki·net'ic
ir'i·do·lep·tyn'sis
ir'i·dol'o·gy
ir'i·dol'y·sis *pl.* -ses'
ir'i·do·ma·la'ci·a
ir'i·do·mes'o·di·al'y·sis
ir'i·do·mo'tor
ir'id·on·co'sis
ir'i·don'cus
ir'i·do·pa·ral'y·sis *pl.* -ses'
ir'i·do·pa·re'sis *pl.* -ses'
ir'i·dop'a·thy
ir'i·do·ple'gi·a
ir'i·dop·to'sis *pl.* -ses'
ir'i·do·pu'pil·lar'y
ir'i·do·rhex'is *pl.* -rhex'es'
ir'i·dos'chi·sis *pl.* -ses'
ir'i·do·schis'ma
ir'i·do·scle·rot'o·my
ir'i·do·ste·re'sis *pl.* -ses'
ir'i·dot'a·sis *pl.* -ses'
ir'i·do·tome'
ir'i·dot'o·my
i'ris *pl.* i'ri·des'
—bom·bé'
i'ri·sin
i·ri'tis
ir'i·to·ec'to·my
i·rit'o·my
ir'i·um
i'ron
i·rot'o·my
ir·ra'di·ate', -at'ed, -at'ing
ir·ra'di·a'tion
ir·ra'tion·al
ir·ra'tion·al'i·ty
ir·ra'tion·al·ly
ir·re·duc'i·ble
ir·reg'u·lar
ir·reg'u·lar'i·ty
ir·re'me·a·ble
ir·re'me·di·a·ble
ir·res·pi'ra·ble
ir·re·sus'ci·ta·ble
ir·re·ver'si·bil'i·ty
ir·re·ver'si·ble
ir'ri·gate', -gat'ed, -gat'ing
ir'ri·ga'tion
ir'ri·ga'tor
ir'ri·ta·bil'i·ty

ir'ri·ta·ble
ir'ri·tant
ir'ri·tate'
ir'ri·ta'tion
ir'ri·ta'tive
ir'ru·ma'tion
I'saac' granules
I·sam'bert' disease
i'sa·tin
is·aux·e'sis *pl.* -ses'
is·che'mi·a
is·che'mic
is·che'sis
is'chi·ad'ic
is'chi·al
is'chi·al'gi·a
is'chi·al'gic
is'chi·at'ic
is'chi·a·ti'tis
is'chi·dro'sis *pl.* -ses'
is'chi·drot'ic
is'chi·ec'to·my
is·chi·o·a'nal
is'chi·o·bul'bar
is'chi·o·cap'su·lar
is'chi·o·cav'er·no'sus
is'chi·o·cav'er·nous
is'chi·o·cele'
is'chi·o·coc·cyg·e'al
is'chi·o·coc·cyg'e·us
is'chi·o·did'y·mus
is'chi·o·dyn'i·a
is'chi·o·fem'o·ral
is'chi·o·fem'o·ra'lis
is'chi·o·fib'u·lar
is'chi·om'e·lus
is'chi·o·my'e·li'tis
is'chi·o·neu·ral'gi·a
is'chi·o·ni'tis
is'chi·op'a·gus
—tet'ra·pus
—tri'pus
is'chi·op'a·gy
is'chi·o·pu'bic
is'chi·o·pu'bi·cus
is'chi·o·pu'bis
is'chi·o·rec'tal
is'chi·o·sa'cral
is'chi·o·vag'i·nal
is'chi·um *pl.* -chi·a
is'cho·ga·lac'tic
is'cho·gy'ri·a
is'cho·me'ni·a

is'cho·pho'ni·a
is·chu'ri·a
is·ei·kon'ic
i'se·thi'o·nate'
i'se·thi·on'ic
Ish'i·ha'ra test
is'land
—of Lang'er·hans'
—of Reil
is'let
i'so·a·dre'no·cor'ti·cism
i'so·ag·glu'ti·na'tion
i'so·ag·glu'ti·nin
i'so·ag·glu'ti·no·gen
i'so·al·lox'a·zine'
i'so·am'yl
i'so·an·dros'ter·one'
i'so·an'ti·bod'ies
i'so·an'ti·bod'y
i'so·an'ti·gen
i'so·bar'
i'so·bar'ic
i'so·bor'nyl thi'o·cy·a·no·ac'e·tate'
i'so·bu'caine'
i'so·bu'tyl
i'so·bu·tyr'ic
i'so·ca·lor'ic
i'so·car·box'a·zid
i'so·cel'lo·bi'ose'
i'so·cel'lu·lar
i'so·cho·les'ter·ol'
i'so·chor'ic
i'so·chro·mat'ic
i'so·chro·mat'o·phil'
i'so·chro'mo·some'
i·soch'ro·nal
i'so·chro'ni·a
i·soch'ro·nic
i·soch'ro·nism
i·soch'ro·nous
i'so·cit'ric
i'so·com'ple·ment
i'so·co'ri·a
i'so·cor'tex'
i'so·cy'a·nide'
i'so·cy'tol'y·sin
i'so·cy·to'sis
i'so·dac'tyl·ism
i'so·dac'ty·lous
i'so·di·a·met'ric
i'so·dont'
i'so·dose'

i′so·dy·nam′ic
i′so·e·lec′tric
i′so·en′er·get′ic
i′so·en′zyme′
i′so·eth′a·rine′
i′so·feb′ri·fu′gine′
i′so·flu′ro·phate′
i′so·gam′ete′
i′so·ga·met′ic
i′so·gam′e·ty
i·sog′a·mous
i·sog′a·my
i′so·gen′e·sis *pl.* -ses′
i′so·gen′ic
i·sog′e·nous
i′so·ger′mine′
i·sog′na·thous
i′so·graft′
i′so·he′mag·glu′ti·na′tion
i′so·he′mag·glu′ti·nin
i′so·he·mol′y·sin
i′so·he·mol′y·sis *pl.* -ses′
i′so·he·mo·lyt′ic
i′so·hy′dric
i′so·hy′per·cy·to′sis
i′so·hy′po·cy·to′sis
i′so·i·co′ni·a
i′so·i·con′ic
i′so·im·mune′
i′so·im′mu·ni·ty
i′so·im′mu·ni·za′tion
i′so·im′mu·nize′
i′so·i·on′ic
i′so·lac′tose′
i′so·late′, -lat′ed, -lat′ing
i′so·lat′er·al
i′so·la′tion
i′so·la′tor
i′so·lec′i·thal
i′so·leu′cine′
i′so·leu′cyl
i·sol′o·gous
i·sol′y·sin
i·sol′y·sis
i′so·mal′tose′
i′so·mer
i·som′er·ase′
i·som′er·ic
i·som′er·ide′
i·som′er·ism
i·som′er·i·za′tion
i·som′er·ize′, -ized′, -iz′ing
i·som′er·ous

i′so·meth′a·done′
i′so·me·thep′tene′
i′so·met′ric
i′so·met′rics
i′so·me·tro′pi·a
i·som′e·try
i′so·morph′
i′so·mor′phic
i′so·mor′phism
i′so·mor′phous
i′so·ni′a·zid
i′so·nic′o·tin′ic
i′so·nic′o·tin′o·yl·hy′dra·
zine′
i′so·nip′e·caine′
i′so·ni′trile
i′so·os·mot′ic
i′so·path′ic
i·sop′a·thy
i′so·phane′
i′so·pho′ri·a
i·so′pi·a
i′so·plas′tic
i′so·pre·cip′i·tin
i′so·pren′a·line′
i′so·prene′
i′so·pren′oid′
i′so·prin′o·sine′
i′so·pro′pa·mide′
i′so·pro′pa·nol′
i′so·pro′pyl
i′so·pro′pyl·ar·te′re·nol′
i′so·pro·te′re·nol′
i·sop′ter
i′so·pyk·no′sis
i′so·quin′o·line′·
i′so·rau·wol′fine′
i′so·rhyth′mic
i′so·ri′bo·fla′vin
i·sor′rhe′a
i′so·scope′
i′so·ser′ine′
i·sos′mot′ic
i′so·sor′bide′
I·sos′po·ra
—bel′li
—hom′i·nis
i′so·spo·ro′sis *pl.* -ses′
i′so·stere′
i′so·ster′ic
i·sos′ter·ism
i·sos′the·nu′ri·a
i′so·therm′

i′so·ther′mal
i′so·ther′mic
i′so·thi′o·cy′a·nate′
i′so·tone′
i′so·to′ni·a
i′so·ton′ic
i′so·to·nic′i·ty
i′so·tope′
i′so·top′ic
i′so·trop′ic
i·sot′ro·pous
i·sot′ro·py
i′so·typ′i·cal
i′so·va·ler′ic
i′so·va·ler′ic·ac′i·de′mi·a
i′so·vol′u·met′ric
i′so·vol′u′mic
i′sox·su′prine′
i′so·zyme′
is′sue
isth·mec′to·my
isth′mi·an
isth′mic
isth′mo·pa·ral′y·sis
isth′mo·ple′gi·a
isth′mus
—a·or′tae′
—car′ti·lag′i·nis au′ris
—fau′ci·um
—glan′du·lae′ thy′re·oi′-
de·ae′
—glandulae thy·roi′de·ae′
—gy′ri′ cin′gu·li′
—gyri for′ni·ca′ti′
—hip′po·cam′pi′
—pros′ta·tae′
—rhom′ben·ceph′a·li′
—tu′bae′ au′di·ti′vae′
—tubae u′ter·i′nae′
—u′ter·i′
i·su′ri·a
it′a·con′ic
I·ta′qui fever
itch
itch′i·ness
itch′y
i′ter
—ad in′fun·dib′u·lum
—chor′dae′ an·te′ri·us
—chordae pos·te′ri·us
—den′ti·um
i′ter·al
it′er·a′tion

it′er·o·par′i·ty
ith′y·lor·do′sis *pl.* -ses′
ith′y·o·ky·pho′sis *pl.* -ses′
I′to-Reen·stier′na
—reaction
—test
Ive′mark′ syndrome
i′ver·mec′tin
I′vy
—bleeding time
—method
—test
I′wa·noff′ cysts
Ix·o′des′
—dam′mi·ni
—pa·cif′i·cus
—scap′u·la′ris
ix′o·di′a·sis
ix·od′ic
ix·od′id
Ix·od′i·dae′
Ix′o·doi′de·a
ix′y·o·my′e·li′tis

J

jab′o·ran′di
Ja·bou·lay′
—amputation
—button
—method
—operation
—pyloroplasty
Jac·coud′
—arthritis
—fever
—sign
jack′et
jack′knife′
jack′screw′
Jack′son
—membrane
—re-evolution
—sign
—syndrome
—veil
Jack′son-Bab′cock′
operation
Jack·so′ni·an
—convulsion
—epilepsy
—march
Ja′cob·sohn reflex

Ja′cob·son
—cartilage
—nerve
—plexus
Ja′cob ulcer
Ja·cod′
—syndrome
—triad
Jacque′mi·er′ sign
Jac·quet′ erythema
jac·ta′tion
jac′ti·ta′tion
jac′u·lif′er·ous
Jad′as·sohn
—disease
—nevus
Jad′as·sohn-
Lew′an·dow′sky law
Jad′as·sohn-Ti·èche′ nevus
Jae′ger test
Jaf·fé′
—reaction
—test
Jaf′fe disease
Jaf·fé′-Lich′ten·stein′
—disease
—syndrome
Ja′kob-Creutz′feldt′
—disease
—syndrome
ja′mais vu′
jam′bul
James fiber
James′-Lang′e theory
Ja·net′
—disease
—test
Jane′way′ lesions
jan′i·ceps′
—a·sym′me·tros′
—a·te′le·us
Jan′sen
—operation
—syndrome
—test
Jan′sky
—classification
—groups
ja′nus
—a·sym′me·tros′
Ja′nus green
Ja·nu′si·an
ja′ra·rac′a

Jar′isch-Herx′hei′mer
reaction
Jat′ro·pha
jaun′dice
jaw
jaw′bone′
Ja·wor′ski
—corpuscles
—test
jec′o·rize′
Jed′dah ulcer
Jef′fer·son fracture
Jegh′ers-Peutz′ syndrome
je·ju′nal
je′ju·nec′to·my
je′ju·ni′tis
je·ju′no·ce·cos′to·my
je·ju′no·co·los′to·my
je·ju′no·gas′tric
je·ju′no·il′e·al
je·ju′no·il′e·i′tis
je·ju′no·il′e·os′to·my
je·ju′no·il′e·um
je·ju′no·je′ju·nos′to·my
je′ju·nor′rha·phy
je·ju′nos′to·my
je·ju′not′o·my
je·ju′num *pl.* -na
Jel′li·nek′ sign
jel′ly
—of Whar′ton
jel′ly·fish′
Je′na Nom′i·na An′a·tom′-
i·ca
Jenck′el cholecystoduode-
nostomy
Jen′dra·sic test
Jen′dras·sik maneuver
Jen·ne′ri·an
—vaccination
—vaccine
Jen′ner stain
Jen′sen
—method
—retinopathy
—sarcoma
jerk
jerk′y
Jew′ett nail
Jez′ler-Ta·ka′ta test
jig
jig′ger
Jirgl reaction

jit'ter·y
Jo·bert' fossa
Jobst stockings
Job syndrome
Jof'froy
—reflex
—sign
Joh'ne bacillus
John'son operation
joint
Jol'ly
—bodies
—reaction
—sign
Jo'nas modification
Jones
—criteria
—hammer toe operation
—position
—test
Jor'ge Lo'bo blastomycosis
Jo'seph syndrome
joule
Joule equivalent
juc·cu'ya
Judd operation
Ju·det' operation
Jud'kins
—coronary arteriography
—technique
ju'ga
—al·ve'o·lar'i·a man·dib'u·
lae'
—alveolaria max·il'lae'
—cer'e·bra'li·a os'si·um
cra'ni·i'
ju'ga al·ve·o·lar'i·a
max·il'lae'
ju'gal
ju·ga'le
jug'u·lar
jug'u·la'tion
jug'u·lo·di·gas'tric
jug'u·lo·ve'nous
jug'u·lum _pl._ -la
ju'gum _pl._ -ga
—sphe'noi·da'le'
juice
Jukes unit
jump'ers
jump'ing French'men of
Maine disease
junc'tion

junc'tion·al
junc·tu'ra _pl._ -rae'
—car'ti·la·gin'e·a
—fi·bro'sa
—lum'bo·sa·cra'lis
—os'si·um
—sac'ro·coc·cyg'e·a
—sy'no·vi·a'lis
junc·tu'rae'
—cin'gu·li' mem'bri'
in·fe'ri·o'ris
—cinguli membri
su·pe'ri·o'ris
—co·lum'nae' ver'te·bra'lis,
tho·ra'cis, et cra'ni·i'
—mem'bri' in·fe'ri·o'ris
lib'er·i'
—membri su·pe'ri·o'ris
lib'er·i'
—os'si·um
—ten'di·num
junc'ture
—zyg'a·poph'y·se·a'les'
Jung'i·an
Jüng'ling disease
Jung muscle
ju'ni·per
Ju'ni·us-Kuhnt' disease
ju'ris·pru'dence
Jus'ter reflex
jus'to
—major
—minor
ju·van'ti·a
ju've·nile'
jux'ta-ar·tic'u·lar
jux'ta-ar·tic'u·la'tion
jux'ta·cor'ti·cal
jux'ta·e·piph'y·se'al
jux'ta·glo·mer'u·lar
jux·tal'lo·cor'tex
jux'ta·pap'il·lar'y
jux'ta·pose', -posed', -pos'ing
jux'ta·po·si'tion
jux'ta·py·lor'ic
jux'ta·res'ti·form'
jux'ta·spi'nal

K

Ka'der operation
Ka'der-Senn' operation
Kaes'-Bekh'ter·ev layer

Kaes line
Kaf'fir pox
Kahl'den tumor
Kah'ler disease
Kahn
—method
—test
kai'nate'
kai'nic
Kai'ser·ling method
kak'er·ga'si·a
ka'la a·zar'
ka'la·fun'gin
ka·le'mi·a
ka·lim'e·ter
ka'li·o·pe'nic
Kal'i·scher disease
ka'li·um
kal'i·u·re'sis
kal'i·u·ret'ic
kal'lak
kal'li·din
kal'li·kre'in
kal'li·krei'no·gen
kam'a·la
Kam'mer·er-Bat'tle
incision
Kan'a·ga'wa phenomenon
kan'a·my'cin
Kan'a·vel
—operation
—sign
Kan'da·har' sore
Kan·din'sky complex
Kan'ner syndrome
ka'o·lin
ka·o·li·no'sis _pl._ -ses'
Ka·po'si
—disease
—sarcoma
—syndrome
—varicelliform eruption
ka·ra'ya
Kar'men unit
Karr method
Kar'ta·gen'er syndrome
kar'y·en'chy·ma
kar'y·o·blast'
kar'y·o·chrome'
kar'y·oc'la·sis _pl._ -ses'
kar'y·o·clas'tic
kar'y·o·cyte'
kar'y·o·gam'ic

kar'y·og'a·my
kar'y·o·gen'
kar'y·o·gen'e·sis
kar'y·o·gen'ic
kar'y·o·ki·ne'sis *pl.* -ses'
kar'y·o·ki·net'ic
kar'y·o·lo'bic
kar'y·ol'o·gy
kar'y·o·lymph'
kar'y·ol'y·sis
kar'y·o·lyt'ic
kar'y·o·meg'a·ly
kar'y·o·mere'
kar'y·om'e·try
kar'y·o·mi'cro·so'ma
kar'y·o·mi'cro·some'
kar'y·o·mi'tome'
kar'y·o·mi·to'sis *pl.* -ses'
kar'y·o·mi·tot'ic
kar'y·o·mor'phism
kar'y·on'
kar'y·o·phage'
kar'y·o·plasm
kar'y·o·plas'mic
kar'y·o·pyk·no'sis
kar'y·o·pyk·not'ic
kar'y·or·rhec'tic
kar'y·or·rhex'is *pl.* -rhex'es'
kar'y·o·some'
kar'y·os'ta·sis *pl.* -ses'
kar'y·o·the'ca
kar'y·o·type'
kar'y·o·typ'ic
Kas'a·bach-Mer'ritt
  syndrome
ka·sai'
Ka·shi'da thermic sign
Kash'in-Beck' disease
Kast syndrome
kat'a·chro'ma·sis *pl.* -ses'
kat'a·did'y·mus
kat'a·ther·mom'e·ter
Kat'a·ya'ma
  —for'mo·sa'na
  —no·soph'o·ra
Ka'to test
katz'en·jam'mer
Katz'-Wach'tel sign
Kauff'mann medium
ka'va
Ka'wa·sa'ki
  —disease
  —syndrome

Kay'-Gra'ham
  pasteurization test
Kay'ser-Flei'scher ring
Ka·zan'ji·an operation
Kearns'-Say'er syndrome
ked
Ke·da'ni fever
keel
Keen
  —point
  —sign
Kehr
  —operation
  —sign
Kehr'er reflex
Keith
  —bundle
  —node
Keith'-Wag'e·ner-Bar'ker
  classification
Kell blood group system
Kel'ler
  —micromethod
  —operation
Kel'ling test
Kel'ly-Pat'er·son
  syndrome
Kel'ly sign
ke'loid'
ke·loi'dal
ke·lo'ma *pl.* -mas *or* -ma·ta
kelp
kel'vin
Kel'vin scale
Kemp'ner rice diet
Ken'ne·dy
  —classification
  —syndrome
Ken'ny treatment
ken'o·pho'bi·a
ken'o·tox'in
Kent
  —bundle
  —mental test
Kent'-His' bundle
Ker'an·del' sign
ker'a·phyl'lo·cele'
ker'a·sin
ker'a·tal'gi·a
ker'a·tec·ta'si·a
ker'a·tec'to·my
ke·rat'ic
ker'a·tin

ker'a·tin·ase'
ker'a·tin·i·za'tion
ker'a·tin·ize'
ke·rat'i·no·cyte'
ker'a·tin·oid'
ke·rat'i·nous
ker'a·tit'ic
ker'a·ti'tis
  —ar'bo·res'cens
  —bul·lo'sa
  —dis'ci·for'mis
  —neu'ro·par'a·lyt'i·ca
  —pa·ren'chy·ma·to'sa
    an'a·phy'lac'ti·ca
  —punc·ta'ta
  —punctata le·pro'sa
  —punctata pro·fun'da
  —pu'ru·len'ta
  —pus'tu·li·for'mis
    pro·fun'da
  —ro·sa'ce·a
  —sic'ca
ker'a·to·ac'an·tho'ma
  pl. -mas *or* -ma·ta
ker'a·to·cele'
ker'a·to·cen·te'sis *pl.* -ses'
ker'a·to·chro'ma·to'sis
  pl. -ses'
ker'a·to·con·junc'ti·vi'tis
  —sic'ca
ker'a·to·co'nus
ker'a·to·cyte'
ker'a·to·der'ma
  —blen'nor·rhag'i·cum
  —cli'mac·ter'i·cum
  —punc·ta'tum
ker'a·to·der·mat'o·cele'
ker'a·to·der'mi·a
ker'a·to·ec·ta'si·a
ker'a·tog'e·nous
ker'a·to·gen'e·sis *pl.* -ses'
ker'a·to·glo'bus
ker'a·to·hel'co·sis
ker'a·to·he'mi·a
ker'a·to·hy'a·lin
ker'a·toid'
ker'a·to·i·rid'o·scope'
ker'a·to·i·ri'tis
ker'a·to·lep·tyn'sis
ker'a·to·leu·ko'ma *pl.* -mas
  or -ma·ta
ker'a·tol'y·sis
ker'a·to·lyt'ic

ker'a·to'ma
—sul·ca'tum plan·tar'um
ker'a·to·ma·la'ci·a
ker'a·tome'
ker'a·to·meg'a·ly
ker'a·tom'e·ter
ker'a·tom'e·try
ker'a·to·my'co'sis *pl.* -ses'
ker'a·ton'o·sus
ker'a·to·nyx'is *pl.* -es'
ker'a·top'a'thy
ker'a·to·plas'tic
ker'a·to·plas'ty
ker'a·to·pre·cip'i·tate
ker'a·to·pros·the'sis
ker'a·tor·rhex'is *pl.* -rhex'es'
ker'a·to·scle·ri'tis
ker'a·to·scope'
ker'a·tos'co·py
ker'a·tose'
ker'a·to'sis *pl.* -ses'
—blen'nor·rhag'i·ca
—fol·lic'u·lar'is
—ni'gri·cans'
—pal·mar'is et plan·tar'is
—pha·ryn'ge·us
—pi·lar'is
—punc·ta'ta
—seb'or·rhe'i·ca
—se·ni'lis
—u'ni·ver·sa'lis
con·gen'i·ta
ker'a·to·sul'fate'
ker'a·to·sul'fa·tu'ri·a
ker'a·tot'ic
ker'a·tot'o·my
ker'a·to·to'rus
Kerck'ring
—folds
—ossicle
ker'i·on' cel'si'
Ker'ley lines
ker·nic'ter·us
Ker'nig sign
Ker'no·han' syndrome
Ker'no·han'-Wolt'man
syndrome
ker'o·sene'
ke'ta·mine'
ke'tene'
ke·tip'ra·mine'
ke'to
ke'to·ac'i·do'sis *pl.* -ses'

ke'to·ac'i·du'ri·a
ke'to·a·dip'ic
ke'to·bem'i·done'
ke'to·con'a·zole'
ke'to·gen'e·sis
ke'to·gen'ic
ke'to·glu·tar'ic
ke'to·hep'tose'
ke'to·hex'ose'
ke'to·hy·drox'y·es'trin
ke'tol'
ke·tol'y·sis
ke'to·lyt'ic
ke'tone'
ke'to·ne'mi·a
ke'to·ne'mic
ke·ton'ic
ke'to·nu'ri·a
ke'tose'
ke'to·side'
ke·to'sis *pl.* -ses'
ke'to·ste'roid'
ke'to·su'ri·a
ke·tot'ic
ke·tox'ime'
key'ridge'
key'way'
khel'lin
khel'li·nin
kick
Kidd blood group system
Kid'ner operation
kid'ney
Kien'böck'
—atrophy
—disease
—dislocation
Kier'nan spaces
Kies'sel·bach'
—area
—triangle
Kil'i·an line
Kil'li·an operation
kil'o·cal'o·rie
kil'o·cy'cle
kil'o·gram'
kil'o·hertz'
kil'o·joule'
kil'o·li'ter
kil'o·me'ter
kil'o·nem'
kil'o·pas·cal'
kil'o·u'nit

kil'o·volt'
kil'o·watt'
Kim'mel·stiel-Wil'son
disease
ki'nase'
kin'e·mat'o·graph'
ki·ne'mi·a
ki·ne'mic
kin'e·plas'tic
kin'e·plas'ty
kin'es·al'gi·a
kin'e·scope'
ki·ne'si·a
ki·ne'si·at'rics
ki·ne'sic
ki·ne'si·es·the'si·om'e·ter
kin'e·sim'e·ter
ki·ne'si·ol'o·gy
ki·ne'sis *pl.* -ses'
—par'a·dox'a
ki·ne'si·ther'a·py
ki·ne'so·pho'bi·a
kin'es·the'si·a
kin'es·the·si·om'e·ter
kin'es·the'sis *pl.* -ses'
kin'es·thet'ic
ki·net'ic
ki·net'i·cist
ki·net'ics
ki·ne'tin
ki·ne'tism
ki·ne'to·car'di·o·gram'
ki·ne'to·chore'
ki·ne'to·gen'ic
ki·ne'to·graph'ic
ki·ne'to·nu'cle·us
ki·ne'to·plasm
ki·ne'to·plast'
kin'e·to'sis *pl.* -ses'
ki·ne'to·some'
ki·ne'to·ther'a·py
King'-Arm'strong unit
King operation
Kings'bur·y test
ki'nin
ki·nin'o·gen
kink
Kin'ney law
Kin'ni·er Wil'son sign
ki'no·cen'trum
ki'no·cil'i·um
ki'no·plasm
ki'no·plas'mic

kin'ship'
Kin'youn stain
Kirch'ner diverticulum
Kirk'-Bent'ley method
Kir·mis'sion operation
Kirsch'ner
—operation
—traction
Kisch reflex
ki·ta'sa·my'cin
Kjel'dahl' method
Klatsch preparation
Klebs disease
Kleb'si·el'la
—gran'u·lo'ma·tis
—ox'y·to'ca
—o·zae'nae'
—pneu'mo'ni·ae'
—rhi'no·scle·ro'ma·tis
Klebs'-Loef'fler bacillus
klee'blatt·schä'del
    deformity syndrome
Kleine'-Lev'in syndrome
Klein'ert
—flap
—operation
Klein muscle
Klem'per·er
—disease
—tuberculin
klep'to·lag'ni·a
klep'to·ma'ni·a
klep'to·ma'ni·ac'
klep'to·pho'bi·a
Kline'fel'ter-Ref'fen·stein-
    Al'bright' syndrome
Kline'fel'ter syndrome
Kline test
Klip'pel disease
Klip'pel-Feil syndrome
Klip'pel-Tré'nau·nay'-
    We'ber syndrome
Klip'pel-Weil' sign
Klump'ke paralysis
knee
knee'cap'
Knies sign
knife pl. knives
knob
knob'by
knock
knock'-knee'
Knoop theory

Knopf treatment
Knop test
knot
knuck'le
Ko'belt' cyst
Ko'bert test
Koch
—law
—node
—phenomenon
Koch'er
—maneuver
—operation
—reflex
Koch'er-De·bré'-
    Sé·mé·laigne' syndrome
koch'er·i·za'tion
Koch'-Mc·Mee'kin
    method
Koch'-Weeks'
—bacillus
—conjunctivitis
Koeb'ner phenomenon
Koep'pe nodules
Koer'ber-Sa'lus-Elsch'nig
    syndrome
Köh'ler
—disease
—method
—tarsal scaphoiditis
Köhl'mei'er-De·gos'
    disease
Kohn'stamm
—maneuver
—phenomenon
Kohs test
koi'lo·cy·to'sis
koi'lo·cy·tot'ic
koi'lo·nych'i·a
koi'lor·rhach'ic
koi'lo·ster'ni·a
koi'no·trop'ic
koi'not'ro·py
ko'jic
ko'la
Kol'mer test
Kom'mer·ell diverticulum
Kon·do'lé·on operation
Kö'nig disease
ko'ni·o·cor'tex'
ko·phe'mi·a
Kop'lik spots
kop'ro·ste'a·rin

Korff fibers
Kor'ner-Shil'ling·ford
    method
ko'ro
ko'ro·cyte'
ko·ros'co·py
Ko·rot'kov'
—method
—sounds
—test
Kor'sa·koff' syndrome
Kos'sel test
Koss koilocytotic atypia
kou'miss
Ko·zhev'ni·kov' epilepsy
Krab'be disease
Krae'pe·lin classification
Krae'pe·lin-Mo'rel' disease
krait
Kra'mer-Tis'dall method
Kras'ke
—operation
—position
kra·tom'e·ter
krau·ro'sis pl. -ses'
Krause
—corpuscle
—glands
—membrane
Krause'-Wolfe' graft
Kraus fetal cells
kre'a·tin
kre·at'i·nine'
Krebs
—cycle
—tumor
Krebs'-Hen'se·leit' cycle
kre'o·tox'in
kre'o·tox'ism
Kretsch'mer type
Kreu'scher bunionectomy
Krey'sig sign
Krom'pech'er tumor
Krö'nig
—fields
—isthmus
Kru'ken·berg'
—operation
—spindle
—tumor
kryp'ton
ku·bis'a·ga'ri
Ku'der Preference Record

Kufs disease
Ku'gel artery
Ku'gel·berg'-Wel'an·der
  syndrome
Kuhnt'-Ju'ni·us disease
Kul·chit'sky
  —carcinoma
  —cell
  —hematoxylin
Kum'lin·ge disease
Küm'mell disease
Kun'drat' lymphosarcoma
Kun'kel
  —syndrome
  —test
Kupf'fer cells
kur'chi
Kur'lov'
  —bodies
  —cell
ku'ru
Kus·kok'wim disease
Küss'-Ghon' focus
Kuss'maul'
  —disease
  —respiration
  —sign
Kuss'maul-Mai'er
  disease
Kut'ter flap
Kveim
  —antigen
  —test
kwa'shi·or'kor'
Kwi·leck'i method
ky'a·nop'si·a
Kya·sa'nur forest disease
kyl·lo'sis
ky'ma·tism
ky'mo·gram'
ky'mo·graph'
ky'mo·graph'ic
ky·mog'ra·phy
ky·nu're·nine'
ky'pho·ra·chit'ic
ky'pho·ra·chi'tis
ky'phos'
ky'pho·sco'li·o'sis *pl.* -ses'
ky'pho·sco'li·ot'ic
ky·pho'sis *pl.* -ses'
ky·phot'ic
Kyrle disease
kyr'tor·rhach'ic

L

Lab'ar·raque' solution
la'bel
la·bet'a·lol'
la'bi·a
  —ma·jo'ra
  —mi·no'ra
  —o'ris
  —pu·den'di'
la'bi·al
la'bi·al·ism
La'bi·a'tae'
la'bile'
la·bil'i·ty
la'bi·o·al·ve'o·lar
la'bi·o·cer'vi·cal
la'bi·o·cho·re'a
la'bi·o·cli·na'tion
la'bi·o·den'tal
la'bi·o·gin'gi·val
la'bi·o·glos'so·la·ryn'ge·al
la'bi·o·glos'so·pha·ryn'-
  ge·al
la'bi·o·graph'
la'bi·o·in·ci'sal
la'bi·o·lin'gual
la'bi·o·men'tal
la'bi·o·my·co'sis *pl.* -ses'
la'bi·o·na'sal
la'bi·o·pal'a·tine'
la'bi·o·plas'ty
la'bi·o·scro'tal
la'bi·o·ver'sion
la'bi·um *pl.* -bi·a
  —an·te'ri·us os'ti·i' u'ter·i'
  —anterius por'ti·o'nis
    vag'i·na'lis u'ter·i'
  —anterius tu'bae'
    au'di·ti'vae'
  —ex·ter'num cris'tae'
    i·li'a·cae'
  —in·fe'ri·us o'ris
  —inferius val'vu·lae' co'li'
  —in·ter'num cris'tae'
    i·li'a·cae'
  —lat'er·a'le' lin'e·ae'
    as'per·ae' fem'o·ris
  —lep'o·ri'num
  —lim'bi' tym·pan'i·cum
  —limbi ves·tib'u·lar'e'
  —ma'jus
  —majus pu·den'di'

  —me'di·a'le' lin'e·ae'
    as'per·ae' fem'o·ris
  —mi'nus
  —minus pu·den'di'
  —pos·te'ri·us os'ti·i' u'-
    ter·i'
  —posterius por'ti·o'nis
    vag'i·na'lis u'ter·i'
  —posterius tu'bae'
    au'di·ti'vae'
  —su·pe'ri·us o'ris
  —superius val'vu·lae' co'li'
  —tym·pan'i·cum
  —ves·tib'u·lar'e'
  —vo·ca'le'
la'bor
lab'o·ra·to'ry
La·borde' method
lab·ra'le
  —in·fe'ri·us
  —su·pe'ri·us
lab'ro·cyte'
la'brum
  —ac'e·tab'u·lar'e'
  —glen'oi·da'le'
  —glenoidale ar·tic'u·la'ti·o'-
    nis cox'ae'
  —glenoidale articulationis
    hu'mer·i'
lab'y·rinth'
lab'y·rin·thec'to·my
lab'y·rin'thine'
lab'y·rin·thi'tis
lab'y·rin·thot'o·my
lab'y·rin'thus *pl.* -thi'
  —eth'moi·da'lis
  —mem'bra·na'ce·us
  —os'se·us
lac *pl.* lac'ta
  —fem'i·ni'num
  —sul·fu'ris
lac'case'
lace'like'
lac'er·ate', -at'ed, -at'ing
lac'er·a'tion
lac'er·o·con'dy·lar
la·cer'tus
  —fi·bro'sus
  —mus'cu·li' rec'ti'
    lat'er·a'lis
Lach'e·sis mu'tus
la·cin'i·ate'
la·con'ic

lac'ri·ma *pl.* -mae'
lac'ri·mal *(pertaining to tears)*
  ♦*lacrimale*
lac'ri·ma'le' *(a point in the skull)*
  ♦*lacrimal*
lac'ri·ma'tion
lac'ri·ma'tor
lac'ri·ma·to'ry
lac'ri·mo·max'il·lar'y
lac'ri·mo·na'sal
lac'ri·mot'o·my
lac·tac'i·de'mi·a
lac·tac'i·du'ri·a
lac'ta·gogue'
lac'tal·bu'min
lac'tam'
lac·tam'ic
lac·tam'ide'
lac'ta·ro·vi'o·lin
lac'tase'
lac'tate', -tat'ed, -tat'ing
lac·ta'tion
lac·ta'tion·al
lac'te·al
lac·tes'cence
lac·tes'cent
lac'tic
lac·ti·ce'mi·a
lac·tif'er·ous
lac'ti·fuge'
lac·tig'e·nous
lac·tig'er·ous
lac'tim
lac'tin
lac'ti·su'gi·um
lac·tiv'o·rous
Lac'to·bac'il·la'ce·ae'
lac'to·ba·cil'lic
lac'to·ba·cil'lin
Lac'to·ba·cil'lus
  —ac'i·doph'i·lus
  —bi'fi·dus
  —bul·gar'i·cus
  —ca'se·i' factor
  —gas·troph'i·lus
  —lac'tis Dor'ner
  —of Bo'as-Op'pler
lac'to·cele'
lac'to·crit
lac'to·fer'rin
lac'to·fla'vin
lac'to·gen

lac'to·gen'e·sis *pl.* -ses'
lac'to·gen'ic
lac'to·glob'u·lin
lac·tom'e·ter
lac'tone'
lac·ton'ic
lac'to·per·ox'i·dase'
lac'to·phos'phate'
lac'to·pro'tein'
lac'tor·rhe'a
lac'tose'
lac'to·su'ri·a
lac'to·ther'a·py
lac'to·tox'in
lac'to·veg'e·tar'i·an
lac'tu·car'i·um
lac'tu·lose'
la·cu'na *pl.* -nas *or* -nae'
  —mag'na
  —mus'cu·lo'rum
  —va·so'rum
  —ve·no'sa du'rae' ma'tris
la·cu'nae'
  —lat'er·a'les'
  —u're·thra'les'
la·cu'nar
la·cu'nas of Mor·ga'gni
la·cu'nule'
la'cus
  —lac'ri·ma'lis
Ladd
  —band
  —operation
  —procedure
Ladd'-Frank'lin theory
Lad'e·wig stain
Laehr'-Hen'ne·berg' hard palate reflex
Laen·nec'
  —cirrhosis
  —pearl
  —thrombus
lae've
La·fo'ra
  —body
  —disease
lag
la·ge'na *pl.* -nas *or* -nae'
la·ge'ni·form'
lag'oph·thal'mi·a
lag'oph·thal'·mic
lag'oph·thal'mos
La·grange' operation

la grippe'
Laid'law' stain
Laid'low' method
lake
lak'y
l-al'a·nine'
la·li'a·try
lal'i·o·pho'bi·a
lal·la'tion
lal'ling
lal'og·no'sis
la·lop'a·thy
lal'o·pho'bi·a
lal'o·ple'gi·a
lal'or·rhe'a
La·maze' method
lamb'da
lamb'da·cism
lamb'doid'
lam'bert
Lam'bert law
Lambl excrescences
Lam'bli·a
lam·bli'a·sis *pl.* -ses'
lame
la·mel'la *pl.* -las *or* -lae'
la·mel'lar
lam'el·lat'ed
lam'i·na *pl.* -nas *or* -nae'
  —af·fix'a
  —a'lar'is
  —anterior va·gi'nae' mus'-cu·li' rec'ti' ab·dom'i·nis
  —ar'cus ver'te·brae'
  —ba·sa'lis
  —basalis cho'ri·oi'de·ae'
  —basalis cho'roi'de·ae'
  —basalis cor'po·ris cil'i·ar'is
  —bas'i·lar'is
  —car'ti·lag'i·nis cri·coi'-de·ae'
  —cartilaginis lat'er·a'lis tu'bae' au'di·ti'vae'
  —cartilaginis me'di·a'lis tu'bae' au'di·ti'vae'
  —cho'ri·o·cap'il·lar'is
  —cho'ri·oi'de·a ep'i·the'li·a'lis ven·tric'u·li' lat'er·a'-lis
  —chorioidea epithelialis ventriculi quar'ti'
  —cho'roi'do·cap'il·lar'is
  —ci·ne're·a

—cri·bro′sa
—cribrosa os′sis
eth′moi·da′lis
—cribrosa scle′rae′
—dex′tra car′ti·lag′i·nis
thy·roi′de·ae′
—du′ra
—e·las′ti·ca
—elastica anterior
—elastica posterior
—ep′i·scle·ra′lis
—ep′i·the′li·a′lis
—ex·ter′na os′si·um cra′ni·i′
—fi′bro·car′ti·la·gin′e·a
in′ter·pu′bi·ca
—for′ni·cis
—fus′ca scle′rae′
—ho′ri·zon·ta′lis os′sis
pal′a·ti′ni′
—in·ter′na os′si·um cra′ni·i′
—lat′er·a′lis pro·ces′sus
pter′y·goi′de·i′
—lim′i·tans′ anterior
cor′ne·ae′
—limitans posterior corneae
—me′di·a′lis pro·ces′sus
pter′y·goi′de·i′
—med′ul·lar′is lat′er·a′lis
cor′po·ris stri·a′ti′
—medullaris me′di·a′lis
cor′po·ris stri·a′ti′
—mem′bra·na′ce·a tu′bae′
au′di·ti′vae′
—mo·di′o·li′
—mus′cu·lar′is mu·co′sae′
—muscularis mucosae co′li′
—muscularis mucosae
e·soph′a·gi′
—muscularis mucosae
in′tes·ti′ni′ cras′si′
—muscularis mucosae
intestini ten′u·is
—muscularis mucosae
oe·soph′a·gi′
—muscularis mucosae
rec′ti′
—muscularis mucosae
ven·tric′u·li′
—or′bi·ta′lis
—pap′y·ra′ce·a
—pa·ri′e·ta′lis per′i·car′di·i′
—parietalis tu′ni·cae′ vag′-
i·na′lis pro·pri·ae′ tes′tis

—parietalis tunicae vaginalis
tes′tis
—per′pen·dic′u·lar′is os′sis
eth′moi·da′lis
—perpendicularis ossis
pal′a·ti′ni′
—posterior va·gi′nae′ mus′-
cu·li′ rec′ti′ ab·dom′i·nis
—pre·tra′che·a′lis fas′ci·ae′
cer′vi·ca′lis
—pre·ver′te·bra′lis
fas′ci·ae′ cer′vi·ca′lis
—pro·fun′da fas′ci·ae′
tem′po·ra′lis
—profunda mus′cu·li′
lev′a·to′ris pal·pe′brae′
su·pe′ri·o′ris
—pro·pri·a mem·bra′nae′
tym′pa·ni′
—propria mu·co′sae′
—qua′dri·gem′i·na
—ros·tra′lis
—sep′ti′ pel·lu′ci·di′
—si·nis′tra car′ti·lag′i·nis
thy·roi′de·ae′
—spi·ra′lis os′se·a
—spiralis sec′un·dar′i·a
—su′per·fi′ci·a′lis fas′ci·ae′
cer′vi·ca′lis
—superficialis fasciae
tem′po·ra′lis
—superficialis mus′cu·li′
lev′a·to′ris pal·pe′brae′
su·pe′ri·o′ris
—su′pra·cho′ri·oi′de·a
—su′pra·cho·roi′de·a
—tec′ti′
—ter′mi·na′lis
—tra′gi′
—vas′cu·lo′sa cho′ri·oi′-
de·ae′
—vasculosa cho·roi′de·ae′
—vasculosa tes′tis
—vis′ce·ra′lis per′i·car′di·i′
—visceralis tu′ni·cae′ vag′-
i·na′lis pro·pri·ae′ tes′tis
—visceralis tunicae vaginalis
tes′tis
—vit′re·a
lam′i·nae′
—al′bae′ cer′e·bel′li′
—car′ti·lag′i·nis thy·roi′-
de·ae′

—me′di·as′ti·na′les′
—med′ul·lar′es′ cer′e·bel′li′
—medullares thal′a·mi′
lam′i·na·gram′
lam′i·na·graph′
lam′i·nag′ra·phy
lam′i·nar
Lam′i·nar′i·a
lam′i·nate′, -nat′ed, -nat′ing
lam′i·na′tion
lam′i·nec′to·my
lam′i·nog′ra·phy
lam′i·not′o·my
lam′pro·phon′ic
lam·proph′o·ny
La′mus me·gis′tus
la·nat′o·side′
Lan′cas′ter advancement
lance, lanced, lanc′ing
Lance′field′ groups
Lan′ce·reaux′
—diabetes
—law
lan′cet
lan′ci·nate′, -nat′ed, -nat′ing
Lan·ci′si
—sign
—striae
Lan′dau′ position
Lan′dis-Gib′bon test
land′mark′
Lan′dolt′
—broken C test
—ring
Lan·dou′zy
—disease
—purpura
—sciatica
Lan·dou′zy-Dé′je·rine′
dystrophy
Lan·dou′zy-Gras·set′ law
Lan·dry′-Guil·lain′-Bar·ré′
syndrome
Lan·dry′ paralysis
Land′stei′ner classification
Land′ström muscle
Lane
—band
—disease
—kink
—method
—operation
—plates

Lang'don Down anomaly
Lang'e
—method
—repair
—test
Lang'en·beck' operation
Lang'en·dorf' preparation
Lang'er·hans'
—adenoma
—cell granule
—layer
Lang'er·hans'i·an
adenoma
Lang'er lines
Lang'hans'
—cell
—layer
—stria
lan'guor
Lan'ne·longue' operation
lan'o·lin
la·nos'ter·ol'
Lan'sing virus
Lan'ter·mann incisure
lan'tha·nic
lan'tha·nides'
lan'tha·num
la·nu'gi·nous
la·nu'go
lan'u·lous
la·pac'tic
lap'a·rec'to·my
lap'a·ro·cele'
lap'a·ro·co·lec'to·my
lap'a·ro·cys·tec'to·my
lap'a·ro·cys·tot'o·my
lap'a·ro·en'ter·os'to·my
lap'a·ro·en'ter·ot'o·my
lap'a·ro·gas·tros'co·py
lap'a·ro·gas·tros'to·my
lap'a·ro·gas·trot'o·my
lap'a·ro·hep'a·tot'o·my
lap'a·ro·hys'ter·ec'to·my
lap'a·ro·hys'ter·ot'o·my
lap'a·ro·il'e·ot'o·my
lap'a·ro·my·i'tis
lap'a·ro·my'o·mec'to·my
lap'a·ro·ne·phrec'to·my
lap'a·ror'rha·phy
lap'a·ro·sal'pin·gec'to·my
lap'a·ro·sal'pin·go-
o·oph'o·rec'to·my
lap'a·ro·sal'pin·got'o·my

lap'a·ro·scope'
lap'a·ros'co·py
lap'a·ro·sple·nec'to·my
lap'a·ro·sple·not'o·my
lap'a·ro·tome'
lap'a·rot'o·my
lap'a·ro·trach'e·lot'o·my
lap'is
—cal'a·mi·nar'is
—im·pe'ri·a'lis
—in'fer·na'lis
La·place' law
lap'sus *pl.* lap'sus
—cal'a·mi'
—lin'guae'
—me·mo'ri·ae'
—pal·pe'brae' su·pe'ri·o'ris
—pi·lo'rum
—un'gui·um
lar·da'ceous
lark'spur'
Lar'mor
—equation
—frequency
La·ron' dwarfism
La Roque' sign
La'roy·enne' operation
Lar·rey' sign
Lar'sen
—disease
—syndrome
Lar'sen-Jo·han'sson
disease
lar'va *pl.* -vae'
—mi'grans'
lar'val
lar'vate'
lar'vi·cide'
lar'yn·gal'gi·a
la·ryn'ge·al
lar'yn·gec'to·my
lar'yn·gem·phrax'is
lar'yn·gis'mal
lar'yn·gis'mus *pl.* -mi'
—stri'du·lus
lar'yn·git'ic
lar'yn·gi'tis
—sic'ca
la·ryn'go·cele'
la·ryn'go·cen·te'sis
la·ryn'go·fis'sure
la·ryn'go·gram'
la·ryn'go·graph'

lar'yn·gog'ra·phy
lar'yn·go·log'ic
lar'yn·gol'o·gist
lar'yn·gol'o·gy
lar'yn·gom'e·try
la·ryn'go·pa·ral'y·sis
  pl. -ses'
lar'yn·gop'a·thy
la·ryn'go·phan'tom
la·ryn'go·pha·ryn'ge·al
la·ryn'go·phar'yn·gec'-
  to·my
la·ryn'go·pha·ryn'ge·us
la·ryn'go·phar'yn·gi'tis
la·ryn'go·phar'ynx
lar'yn·goph'o·ny
lar'yn·goph'thi·sis
la·ryn'go·plas'ty
la·ryn'go·ple'gi·a
la·ryn'go·pto'sis
la·ryn'go·rhi·nol'o·gy
la·ryn'gor·rha'gi·a
lar'yn·gor'rha·phy
la·ryn'gor·rhe'a
la·ryn'go·scle·ro'ma
la·ryn'go·scope'
la·ryn'go·scop'ic
la·ryn'gos'co·py
la·ryn'go·spasm
lar'yn·gos'ta·sis
la·ryn'go·stat'
la·ryn'go·ste·no'sis *pl.* -ses'
lar'yn·gos'to·my
la·ryn'go·stro'bo·scope'
la·ryn'go·stro·bos'co·py
la·ryn'go·tome'
lar'yn·got'o·my
la·ryn'go·tra'che·al
la·ryn'go·tra'che·i'tis
la·ryn'go·tra'che·o·bron·
  chi'tis
la·ryn'go·tra'che·os'co·py
la·ryn'go·tra'che·ot'o·my
la·ryn'go·ves·tib'u·li'tis
la·ryn'go·xe·ro'sis
lar'ynx *pl.* -ynx·es *or*
  la·ryn'ges'
La·sègue'
—disease
—law
—sign
—test
la'ser

Lash′met and New′burgh′
test
Las·kow′ski method
Las′sa
—fever
—virus
Las·saigne′ test
las′si·tude′
la′ta
la′ten·cy
la′tent
la·ten′ti·a′tion
lat′er·ad′
lat′er·al
lat′er·al′is
lat′er·al′i·ty
lat′er·al·i·za′tion
lat′er·al·ize′, -ized′, -iz′ing
lat′er·o·ab·dom′i·nal
lat′er·o·duc′tion
lat′er·o·flex′ion
lat′er·o·mar′gin·al
lat′er·o·pul′sion
lat′er·o·tor′sion
lat′er·o·ver′sion
la′tex′ *pl.* -ti·ces′ *or* -tex′es
lath′y·rism
lath′y·rit′ic
lath′y·ro·gen′ic
la·tis′si·mus
—dor′si′
—tho·ra′cis
lat′ro·dec′tism
Lat′ro·dec′tus
lat′tice (*a network*)
  ♦*latus*
la′tus (*the flank*)
  ♦*lattice*
laud′a·ble
lau′da·no·sine′
lau′da·num
Laugh′len test
Lau′gi·er′ sign
Lau′rence-Moon′-Bie′dl
syndrome
lau′ric
Lauth violet
la·vage′
la·va′tion
La′ve·ran′ bodies
la·veur′
Lav·ren′ti·ev phenomenon
law

—of A′vo·ga′dro
—of Bun′sen-Ros′coe
—of Du·long′ and Pe·tit′
—of Lam′bert
—of Wal·ler′i·an
degeneration
Law
—projection
—view
lax·a′tion
lax′a·tive
lax′a·tor
lax′i·ty
lay′er
—of Hen′le
—of Lang′hans′
laz′a·ret′to
Laz·a·row′ method
la′zy
l-do′pa
leach (*to percolate away*)
  ♦*leech*
lead
Lead′bet′ter
—maneuver
—procedure
leaf′let
leak
leak′age
Leake and Guy method
leak′y
Le′ber disease
Le·cat′ gulf
lech′o·py′ra
lec′i·thal
lec′i·thal·bu′min
lec′i·thin
lec′i·tho·blast′
lec′i·tho·pro′tein′
lec′i·tho·vi·tel′lin
lec′tin
Led′der·hose′ disease
Led′er·er acute anemia
Le·Duc′-Ca′mey
ileocystoplasty
Le·duc′ current
leech (*parasitic annelid*)
  ♦*leach*
Lee test
Lee′-White′ method
Le Fort′
—amputation
—fracture

—operation
—repair
left′-eyed′
left′-foot′ed
left′-hand′ed
leg
Le′gal
—disease
—test
Legg′-Cal·vé′-Per′thes
disease
Legg′-Cal·ve′-
Wal′den·ström′ disease
Legg disease
Legg′-Per′thes disease
Le′gion·el′la
—mic·da′de·i′
—pneu′mo·phil′i·a
le′gion·el·lo′sis *pl.* -ses′
leg′ume
le·gu′min
Lei′boff′ and Kahn method
Leich′ten·stern′
—encephalitis
—phenomenon
—sign
Leif′son method
Leigh syndrome
Lei′ner disease
lei′o·der′ma·tous
lei′o·der′mi·a
lei′o·dys·to′ni·a
lei′o·my′o·blas·to′ma
  pl. -mas *or* -ma·ta
lei′o·my′o·fi·bro′ma
  pl. -mas *or* -ma·ta
lei′o·my′o·ma *pl.* -mas *or*
  -ma·ta
lei′o·my′o·ma·to′sis
lei′o·my′o·sar·co′ma
  pl. -mas *or* -ma·ta
lei·ot′ri·chous
Leish′man-Don′o·van
—bodies
—parasite
Leish·ma′ni·a
—bra·sil′i·en′sis
—don′o·va′ni′
—in·fan′tum
—pe·ru′vi·a′na
—trop′i·ca
leish·ma′ni·al
leish′ma·ni·a·sis *pl.* -ses′

—a·mer'i·ca'na
Leish'man stain
le'ma
Lem'bert suture
le'mic
lem'mo·blast'
lem'mo·blas'tic
lem'mo·blas·to'ma pl. -mas or -ma·ta
lem'mo·cyte'
lem'mo·cy·to'ma pl. -mas or -ma·ta
lem·nis'cal
lem·nis'cus pl. -ci'
—a·cus'ti·cus
—lat'er·a'lis
—me'di·a'lis
—op'ti·cus
—sen'si·ti'vus
—spi·na'lis
—tri·gem'i·na'lis
le'mo·pa·ral'y·sis pl. -ses'
le'mo·ste·no'sis pl. -ses'
Lem'pert operation
Len'drum stain
length'wise'
Len'hartz' diet
len'i·ceps'
len'i·quin'sin
len'i·tive
Lenn'hoff
—index
—sign
Len'nox-Gas'taut' syndrome
Len'nox syndrome
lens
—crys'tal·li'na
lens·om'e·ter
len·tec'to·mize', -mized', -miz'ing
len·tec'to·my
len'ti·co'nus
len·tic'u·la
len·tic'u·lar
len·tic'u·late'
len·tic'u·lo·stri·ate'
len·tic'u·lo·tha·lam'ic
len'ti·form'
len·tig'i·nes' le·pro'sae'
len·tig'i·no'sis
len·tig'i·nous
len'ti·glo'bus

len·ti'go pl. -tig'i·nes'
—ma·lig'na
len'ti·vi'rus
len'tu·la
lep'er
lep'i·do'ma pl. -mas or -ma·ta
Lep'i·dop'ter·a
L'E·pis'co·po operation
lep'o·thrix'
lep'ra
lep're·chaun·ism
lep'rid
lep·rol'o·gist
lep·rol'o·gy
lep·ro'ma pl. -mas or -ma·ta
lep·ro'ma·tous
lep'ro·min
lep·ro·pho'bi·a
lep·ro·sar'i·um pl. -i·ums or -i·a
lep'ro·stat'ic
lep'ro·sy
lep·rot'ic
lep'rous
lep·tan'dra
lep'ta·zol'
lep'to·ce·pha'li·a
lep'to·ceph'a·lous
lep'to·ceph'a·lus pl. -li'
lep'to·chro·mat'ic
lep'to·cyte'
lep'to·cyt'ic
lep'to·cy·to'sis pl. -ses'
lep'to·dac'ty·lous
lep'to·don'tous
lep'to·me·nin'ge·al
lep'to·me·nin'ges'
lep'to·me·nin·gi·o'ma pl. -mas or -ma·ta
lep'to·men·in·gi'tis
lep'to·men·in·gop'a·thy
lep'to·me'ninx pl. -me·nin'ges'
lep'to·mo'nad
Lep'to·mo'nas
lep'to·pel'lic
lep'to·pho'ni·a
lep'to·phon'ic
lep'to·pro·so'pi·a
lep'to·pro·so'pic
lep'tor·rhine'
lep'to·scope'

Lep'to·sphaer'i·a sen'e·gal·en'sis
lep'to·spi'ra pl. -ras or -rae'
Lep'to·spi'ra
—au'tum·na'lis
—ca·nic'o·la
—grip·po·ty·pho'sa
—heb·dom'a·dis
—ic'ter·o·haem'or·rha'gi·ae'
lep'to·spi'ral
lep'to·spire'
lep'to·spi·ro'sis pl. -ses'
—ic'ter·o·hem'or·rhag'i·ca
lep'to·tene'
Lep'to·trich'i·a buc·ca'lis
lep'to·tri·cho'sis pl. -ses'
—con'junc·ti'vae'
le·re'sis
Lé·ri'
—disease
—sign
Le·riche'
—operation
—syndrome
Ler'man-Means' scratch
Ler'mo·yez' syndrome
les'bi·an
les'bi·an·ism
Lesch'ke method
Lesch'-Ny'han' disease
Le'ser-Tré'lat sign
le'sion
Les'ter Mar'tin modification
le'thal
le·thal'i·ty
le·thar'gic
leth·ar'gy
le'the
leth'o·log'i·ca
Let'o·noff' and Rein'hold' method
Let'ter·er-Si'we disease
leuc-. See words spelled leuk-.
leu'cine'
leu·ci·nu'ri·a
leuco-. See words spelled leuko-.
Leu'co·nos'toc'
leu'co·sin
leu'co·vor'in
leu'cyl

Leu·det′ sign
leu′ka·ne′mi·a
leu·kas′mus
leu·ke′mi·a
leu·ke′mic
leu·ke′mid
leu·ke′mo·gen
leu·ke′mo·gen′esis *pl.* -ses′
leu·ke′mo·gen′ic
leu·ke′moid′
leu′kin
leu′ko·blast′
leu′ko·blas·to′sis *pl.* -ses′
leu·ko·ci′din
leu·ko·co′ri·a
leu′ko·cyte′
leu′ko·cy·the′mi·a
leu′ko·cyt′ic
leu′ko·cy′to·blast′
leu′ko·cy′to·gen′e·sis
  pl. -ses′
leu′ko·cy·tol′o·gy
leu′ko·cy·tol′y·sin
leu′ko·cy·tol′y·sis *pl.* -ses′
leu′ko·cy′to·lyt′ic
leu′ko·cy′to·ma *pl.* -mas *or*
  -ma·ta
leu′ko·cy′tom′e·ter
leu′ko·cy′to·pe′ni·a
leu′ko·cy′to·pla′ni·a
leu′ko·cy′to·poi·e′sis
  pl. -ses′
leu′ko·cy′to·poi·et′ic
leu′ko·cy′to·sis *pl.* -ses′
leu′ko·cy′to·tax′is
leu′ko·cy′tot′ic
leu′ko·cy′to·tox′in
leu′ko·cy·tu′ri·a
leu′ko·der′ma
  —ac′qui·si′tum cen·trif′u·
   gum
  —col′li′
  —pso′ri·at′i·cum
  —punc·ta′tum
leu′ko·der′mic
leu′ko·dys′tro·phy
leu′ko·e·de′ma *pl.* -mas *or*
  -ma·ta
leu′ko·en·ceph′a·li′tis
leu′ko·en·ceph′a·lop′a·thy
leu′ko·en·ceph′a·ly
leu′ko·e·ryth′ro·blas′tic
leu′ko·e·ryth′ro·blas·to′sis

leu′ko·ker′a·to′sis *pl.* -ses′
leu′ko·ki·ne′sis *pl.* -ses′
leu′ko·ki′net′ic
leu′ko·ko′ri·a
leu′ko·krau·ro′sis
leu′ko·lym′pho·sar·co′ma
  pl. -mas *or* -ma·ta
leu·kol′y·sin
leu·kol′y·sis *pl.* -ses′
leu′ko·lyt′ic
leu·ko′ma *pl.* -mas *or* -ma·ta
leu·ko′ma·tous
leu′ko·my′e·li′tis
leu′ko·my′e·lop′a·thy
leu′ko·my·o′ma *pl.* -mas *or*
  -ma·ta
leu′ko·ne·cro′sis
leu′ko·nych′i·a
  —par′ti·a′lis
  —stri·a′ta
  —striata lon′gi·tu′di·na′lis
  —to·ta′lis
leu′ko·path′i·a
leu·kop′a·thy
leu′ko·pe·de′sis *pl.* -ses′
leu′ko·pe′ni·a
leu′ko·pe′nic
leu′ko·phe·re′sis *pl.* -ses′
leu′ko·phleg·ma′si·a
leu′ko·phyll
leu′ko·pla′ki·a
  —buc·ca′lis
  —o′ris
  —vul′vae′
leu′ko·pla′ki·al
leu′ko·pla′si·a
leu′ko·plas′tid
leu′ko·poi·e′sis *pl.* -ses′
leu′ko·poi·et′ic
leu′ko·pro′te·ase′
leu′kop′sin
leu′kor·rha′gi·a
leu′kor·rhe′a
leu′kor·rhe′al
leu′ko·sar·co′ma *pl.* -mas *or*
  -ma·ta
leu′ko·sar·co′ma·to′sis
  pl. -ses′
leu·ko′sis *pl.* -ses′
leu′ko·tac′tic
leu′ko·tax′ine′
leu′ko·tax′is
leu·ko·throm′bo·pe′ni·a

leu′ko·tome′
leu·kot′o·my
leu′ko·tox′ic
leu′ko·tox′in
leu′ko·trich′i·a
leu·kot′ri·chous
leu′ko·u·ro·bil′in
leu′kous
Lev′a·di′ti
  —method
  —spirochete stain
lev′al·lor′phan
lev′am·fet′a·mine′
le·vam′i·sole′
lev′ar·te′re′nol′
le·va′tor *pl.* lev′a·to′res′
  —an′gu·li′ o′ris
  —anguli scap′u·lae′
  —a′ni′
  —cla·vic′u·lae′
  —ep′i·glot′ti·dis
  —glan′du·lae′ thy·roi′de·ae′
  —la′bi·i′ su·pe′ri·o′ris
  —labii superioris a·lae′que′
   na′si′
  —men′ti′
  —pa·la′ti′
  —pal·pe′brae′ su·pe′ri·o′ris
  —pros′ta·tae′
  —scap′u·lae′
  —ve′li′ pal·a·ti′ni′
lev′a·to′res′ cos·tar′um
lev′el
le·vid′u·lin·ose′
lev′i·gate′, -gat′ed, -gat′ing
lev′i·ga′tion
Lé·vi′-Lo·rain′ disease
Le·vine′ clenched′-fist′ sign
Lev′in·son test
Lé·vi′ syndrome
lev′i·ta′tion
le′vo·car′di·a
le′vo·car′di·o·gram′
le′vo·cli·na′tion
le′vo·con′dy·lism
le′vo·cy′clo·ver′sion
le′vo·do′pa
le′vo·duc′tion
le′vo·gram′
le′vo·gy′ral
le′vo·gy′rate′
le′vo·nor·de′frin
le′vo·nor·ges′trel

le'vo·pho'bi·a
le'vo·pro·pox'y·phene'
le'vo·ro·ta'tion
le'vo·ro'ta·to·ry
lev·or'pha·nol
le'vo·sco'li·o'sis
le'vo·thy·rox'ine'
le'vo·tor'sion
le'vo·ver'sion
lev'u·lin
lev'u·lin'ic
lev'u·lo·san'
lev'u·lose'
lev'u·lo·se'mi·a
lev'u·lo·su'ri·a
lev'u·rid
Le'vy-Pal'mer method
Lé·vy'-Rous·sy' syndrome
Le'vy test
Lew'is
—blood group system
—disease
lew'is·ite'
Lew'y body
Ley'den
—ataxia
—crystals
—disease
—jar
—neuritis
Ley'den-Mö'bi·us dystrophy
Ley'dig
—cell
—pause
ley'dig·ar'che
Ley'dig-cell' tumor
Lher·mitte' sign
li'a·bil'i·ty
li'ai·son'
li·bid'i·nal
li·bid'i·ni·za'tion
li·bid'i·nous
li·bi'do
Lib'man-Sacks'
—disease
—endocarditis
—syndrome
li'bra *pl.* -brae'
li'cense
li·cen'ti·ate
li'chen
—chron'i·cus sim'plex'

—cor'ne·us hy'per·troph'-i·cus
—myx'e·de'ma·to'sus
—nit'i·dus
—ob'tu'sus cor'ne·us
—pi·lar'is
—pla'nus
—ru'ber a·cu'mi·na'tus
—ruber mo·nil'i·for'mis
—scle·ro'sus et a·troph'i·cus
—scrof'u·lo'sus
—spi'nu·lo'sus
—stri·a'tus
—trop'i·cus
—ur'ti·ca'tus
li·chen·i·fi·ca'tion
li·chen'i·for'min
li'chen·in
li'chen·i·za'tion
li'chen·oid'
li'chen·ous
Licht'heim'
—aphasia
—syndrome
lid
li'do·caine'
li'do·fla'zine'
Lie'ben test
Lie'ber·kühn'
—crypts
—follicles
—glands
Lie'ber·mann-Bur'chard reaction
Lie'ber·mann reaction
Lie'big test
li'en
—ac'ces·so'ri·us
li·e'nal
li·en'cu·lus *pl.* -li'
li·e'ni·tis
li·e'no·cele'
li·e'nog'ra·phy
li·e'no·ma·la'ci·a
li·e'no·med'ul·lar'y
li·e'no·my'e·log'e·nous
li·e'no·my'e·lo·ma·la'ci·a
li·e'no·pan'cre·at'ic
li'e·nop'a·thy
li·e'no·re'nal
li·e'no·tox'in
li'en·ter'ic
li'en·ter'y

li·e'nun'cu·lus *pl.* -li'
Liep'mann apraxia
Lie'se·gang' phenomenon
life *pl.* lives
life'style'
lift
lig'a·ment
—of Coo'per
—of Treitz
—of Zinn
lig'a·men'ta
—ac'ces·so'ri·a plan·tar'i·a
—accessoria vo·lar'i·a
—a·lar'i·a ar·tic'u·la'ti·o'nis at·lan'to·ax'i·a'lis me·di·a'nae'
—an'nu·lar'i·a dig'i·to'rum ma'nus
—annularia digitorum pe'dis
—annularia tra'che·a'li·a
—an'u·lar'i·a tra'che·a'li·a
—au·ric'u·lar'i·a
—ba'si·um os'si·um met'a·car·pa'li·um dor·sa'li·a
—basium ossium metacarpalium in'ter·os'se·a
—basium ossium metacarpalium vo·lar'i·a
—basium ossium met'a·tar·sa'li·um dor·sa'li·a
—basium ossium metatarsalium in'ter·os'se·a
—basium ossium metatarsalium plan·tar'i·a
—ca·pit'u·li' fib'u·lae'
—ca·pit'u·lo'rum os'si·um met'a·car·pa'li·um trans·ver'sa
—capitulorum ossium met'a·tar·sa'li·um trans·ver'sa
—car·po·met'a·car'pe·a dor·sa'li·a
—carpometacarpea pal·mar'i·a
—carpometacarpea vo·lar'i·a

—cer′a·to·cri·coi′de·a
lat′er·a′li·a
—ceratocricoidea
pos·te′ri·o′ra
—cin′gu·li′ ex·trem′i·ta′tis
in·fe′ri·o′ris
—cinguli extremitatis
su·pe′ri·o′ris
—col·lat′er·a′li·a
ar·tic′u·la′ti·o′num
dig′i·to′rum ma′nus
—collateralia articula-
tionum digitorum pe′dis
—collateralia articulationum in′ter·pha·lan′ge·ar′-
um ma′nus
—collateralia articulationum interphalangearum
pe′dis
—collateralia articulationum met′a·car′po·pha·
lan′ge·ar′um
—collateralia articulationum met′a·tar′so·pha·lan′-
ge·ar′um
—co·lum′·nae′
ver′te·bra′lis et cra′ni·i′
—cos′to·xi·phoi′de·a
—cru′ci·a′ta dig′i·to′rum
ma′nus
—cruciata digitorum pe′dis
—cruciata ge′nu′
—cruciata ge′nus
—cu′ne·o·met′a·tar′se·a
in′ter·os′se·a
—cu′ne·o·na·vic′u·lar′i·a
dor·sa′li·a
—cuneonavicularia
plan·tar′i·a
—ex′tra·cap′su·lar′i·a
—fla′va
—glen′o·hu·mer·a′li·a
—in′ter·car′pe·a dor·sa′li·a
—intercarpea in′ter·os′se·a
—intercarpea pal·mar′i·a
—intercarpea vo·lar′i·a
—in′ter·cos·ta′li·a
—intercostalia ex·ter′na
—intercostalia in·ter′na
—in′ter·cu′ne·i·for′mi·a
dor·sa′li·a
—intercuneiformia
in′ter·os′se·a

—intercuneiformia
plan·tar′i·a
—in′ter·spi·na′li·a
—in′ter·trans·ver′sar′i·a
—in′tra·cap′su·lar′i·a
—met′a·car′pe·a dor·sa′-
li·a
—metacarpea in′ter·os′se·a
—metacarpea pal·mar′i·a
—met′a·tar′se·a dor·sa′li·a
—metatarsea in′ter·os′se·a
—metatarsea plan·tar′i·a
—os′sic′u·lo′rum au·di′tus
—pal·mar′i·a ar·tic′u·la′ti·
o′num in′ter·pha·lan′-
ge·ar′um ma′nus
—palmaria articulationum
met′a·car′po·pha·lan′ge·
ar′um
—plan·tar′i·a ar·tic′u·la′ti·
o′num in′ter·pha·lan′-
ge·ar′um pe′dis
—plantaria articulationum
met′a·tar′so·pha·lan′ge·
ar′um
—py′lo′ri′
—sac′ro·i·li′a·ca
an·te′ri·o′ra
—sacroiliaca dor·sa′li·a
—sacroiliaca in′ter·os′se·a
—sacroiliaca ven·tra′li·a
—ster′no·cos·ta′li·a
ra·di·a′ta
—ster′no·per′i·car·di′a·ca
—sus′pen′so′ri·a mam′mae′
—tar′si′ dor·sa′li·a
—tarsi in′ter·os′se·a
—tarsi plan·tar′i·a
—tarsi pro·fun′da
—tar′so·met′a·tar′se·a
dor·sa′li·a
—tarsometatarsea
in′ter·os′se·a
—tarsometatarsea
plan·tar′i·a
—vag′i·na′li·a dig′i·to′rum
ma′nus
—vaginalia digitorum pe′dis
lig′a·men′tal
lig′a·men′to·pex′y
lig′a·men′tous
lig′a·men′tum pl. -ta
—a·cro′mi·o·cla·vic′u·lar′e′

—an′nu·lar′e′ ba′se·os′
sta·pe′dis
—annulare ra′di·i′
—a′no·coc·cyg′e·um
—an′u·lar′e′ ra′di·i′
—anulare sta·pe′dis
—a′pi·cis den′tis
—ar′cu·a′tum lat′er·a′le′
—arcuatum me′di·a′le′
—arcuatum me′di·a′num
—arcuatum pu′bis
—ar·te′ri·o′sum
—au·ric′u·lar′e′ an·te′ri·us
—auriculare pos·te′ri·us
—auriculare su·pe′ri·us
—bi′fur·ca′tum
—cal·ca′ne·o·cu·boi′de·um
—calcaneocuboideum
plan·tar′e′
—cal·ca′ne·o·fib′u·lar′e′
—cal·ca′ne·o·na·vic′u·lar′e′
—calcaneonaviculare
dor·sa′le′
—calcaneonaviculare
plan·tar′e′
—cal·ca′ne·o·tib′i·a′le′
—cap′i·tis cos′tae′
in′tra·ar·tic′u·lar′e′
—capitis costae ra′di·a′tum
—capitis fem′o·ris
—capitis fib′u·lae′ an·te′-
ri·us
—capitis fibulae pos·te′ri·us
—ca·pit′u·li′ cos′tae′
in′ter·ar·tic′u·lar′e′
—capituli costae ra′di·a′tum
—car′pi′ dor·sa′le′
—carpi ra′di·a′tum
—carpi trans·ver′sum
—carpi vo·lar′e′
—cau′da′le′
—cer′a·to·cri·coi′de·um
an·te′ri·us
—col·lat′er·a′le′ car′pi′
ra·di·a′le′
—collaterale carpi ul·nar′e′
—collaterale fib′u·lar′e′
—collaterale ra′di·a′le′
—collaterale tib′i·a′le′
—collaterale ul·nar′e′
—col′li′ cos′tae′
—co·noi′de·um
—co·ra′co·a·cro′mi·a′le′

—co′ra·co·cla′vic′u·lar′e′
—co′ra·co·hu′mer·a′le′
—co′ro·nar′i·um hep′a·tis
—cos′to·cla·vic′u·lar′e′
—cos′to·trans·ver·sar′i·um
—costotransversarium
an·te′ri·us
—costotransversarium
lat′er·a′le′
—costotransversarium
pos·te′ri·us
—costotransversarium
su·pe′ri·us
—cri′co·ar′y·tae·noi′de·um
pos·te′ri·us
—cri′co·ar′y·te·noi′de·um
pos·te′ri·us
—cri′co·pha·ryn′ge·um
—cri′co·thy′re·oi′de·um
—cri′co·thy′roi′de·um
—cri′co·tra′che·a′le′
—cru·ci·a′tum an·te′ri·us
—cruciatum at·lan′tis
—cruciatum cru′ris
—cruciatum pos·te′ri·us
—cru′ci·for′me′ at·lan′tis
—cu·boi′de·o′na·vic′u·lar′e′
dor·sa′le′
—cuboideonaviculare
plan·tar′e′
—cu′ne·o·cu·boi′de·um
dor·sa′le′
—cuneocuboideum
in′ter·os′se·um
—cuneocuboideum
plan·tar′e′
—del·toi′de·um
—den·tic′u·la′tum
—du′o·de′no·re′na′le′
—ep′i·di·dym′i·dis
in·fe′ri·us
—epididymidis su·pe′ri·us
—fal′ci·for′me′ hep′a·tis
—fla′vum
—fun′di·for′me′ pe′nis
—gas′tro·co′li·cum
—gas′tro·li′e·na′le′
—gas′tro·phren′i·cum
—gen′i·to·in′gui·na′le′
—hep′a·to·co′li·cum
—hep′a·to·du′o·de·na′le′
—hep′a·to·gas′tri·cum
—hep′a·to·re′na′le′

—hy′o·ep′i·glot′ti·cum
—hy′o·thy′re·oi′de·um
lat′er·a′le′
—hyothyreoideum
me′di·um
—il′i·o·fem′o·ra′le′
—il′i·o·lum·ba′le′
—in·cu′dis pos·te′ri·us
—incudis su·pe′ri·us
—in′gui·na′le′
—in′ter·cla·vic′u·lar′e′
—in′ter·fo′ve·o′lar′e′
—in′ter·spi·na′le′
—in′ter·trans·ver·sar′i·um
—is′chi·o·cap′su·lar′e′
—is′chi·o·fem′o·ra′le′
—la·cin′i·a′tum
—lac′u·nar′e′
—lat′er·a′le′
—la′tum u′ter·i′
—li′e·no·re·na′le′
—lon′gi·tu·di·na′le′
an·te′ri·us
—longitudinale pos·te′ri·us
—mal′le·i′ an·te′ri·us
—mallei lat′er·a′le′
—mallei su·pe′ri·us
—mal′le·o·li′ lat′er·a′lis
an·te′ri·us
—malleoli lateralis
pos·te′ri·us
—me′di·a′le′
—me·nis′co·fem′o·ra′le′
an·te′ri·us
—meniscofemorale
pos·te′ri·us
—met′a·car′pe·um trans·
ver′sum pro·fun′dum
—metacarpeum trans-
versum su′per·fi′ci·a′le′
—met′a·tar′se·um trans·
ver′sum pro·fun′dum
—metatarseum transversum
su′per·fi′ci·a′le′
—nu′chae′
—o·var′i·i′ pro′pri·um
—pal′pe·bra′le′ lat′er·a′le′
—palpebrale me′di·a′le′
—pa·tel′lae′
—pec′ti·na′tum an′gu·li′
i′ri·do·cor′ne·a′lis
—pectinatum i′ri·dis
—pec·tin′e·a′le′

—phren′i·co·co′li·cum
—phren′i·co·li′e·na′le′
—pi′so·ha·ma′tum
—pi′so·met′a·car′pe·um
—plan·tar′e′ lon′gum
—pop′lit′e·um ar·cu′a′-
tum
—popliteum o·bli′quum
—pter′y·go·spi·na′le′
—pter′y·go·spi·no′sum
—pu′bi·cum su·pe′ri·us
—pu′bo·cap′su·lar′e′
—pu′bo·fem′o·ra′le′
—pu′bo·pros·tat′i·cum
—puboprostaticum
lat′er·a′le′
—puboprostaticum
me′di·um
—pu′bo·ves′i·ca′le′
—pubovesicale lat′er·a′le′
—pubovesicale me′di·um
—pul′mo·na′le′
—pul′mo·nis
—qua·dra′tum
—ra·di·o·car′pe·um
dor·sa′le′
—radiocarpeum pal·mar′e′
—radiocarpeum vo·lar′e′
—re·flex′um
—sac′ro·coc′cyg′e·um
an·te′ri·us
—sacrococcygeum dor·sa′-
le′ pro·fun′dum
—sacrococcygeum dorsale
su′per·fi′ci·a′le′
—sacrococcygeum
lat′er·a′le′
—sacrococcygeum pos·te′-
ri·us pro·fun′dum
—sacrococcygeum posterius
su′per·fi′ci·a′lis
—sacrococcygeum
ven·tra′le′
—sac′ro·i·li′a·cum
pos·te′ri·us brev′e′
—sacroiliacum posterius
long′um
—sac′ro·spi·na′le′
—sac′ro·spi·no′sum
—sac′ro·tu′ber·a′le′
—sac′ro·tu′ber·o′sum
—se·ro′sum
—sphe′no·man·dib′u·lar′e′

—spi·ra'le' coch'le·ae'
—ster'no·cla·vic'u·lar'e'
—sternoclaviculare
 an·te'ri·us
—sternoclaviculare
 pos·te'ri·us
—ster'no·cos·ta'le'
 in'ter·ar·tic'u·lar'e'
—sternocostale
 in'tra·ar·tic'u·lar'e'
—sty'lo·hy·oi'de·um
—sty'lo·man·dib'u·lar'e'
—su'pra·spi·na'le'
—sus·pen·so'ri·um
 cli·to'ri·dis
—suspensorium o·var'i·i'
—suspensorium pe'nis
—ta'lo·cal·ca'ne·um
 an·te'ri·us
—talocalcaneum
 in'ter·os'se·um
—talocalcaneum lat'er·a'le'
—talocalcaneum me'di·a'le'
—talocalcaneum pos·te'-
 ri·us
—ta'lo·fib'u·lar'e' an·te'-
 ri·us
—talofibulare pos·te'ri·us
—ta'lo·na·vic'u·lar'e'
—ta'lo·tib'i·a'le' an·te'ri·us
—talotibiale pos·te'ri·us
—tem'po·ro·man'dib'u·lar'e'
—te'res' fem'o·ris
—teres hep'a·tis
—teres u'ter·i'
—tes'tis
—thy're·o·ep'i·glot'ti·cum
—thy'ro·ep'i·glot'ti·cum
—thy'ro·hy·oi'de·um
—thyrohyoideum me'di·a'-
 num
—tib'i·o·fib'u·lar'e'
 an·te'ri·us
—tibiofibulare pos·te'ri·us
—tib'i·o·na·vic'u·lar'e'
—trans·ver'sum
 ac'e·tab'u·li'
—transversum at·lan'tis
—transversum cru'ris
—transversum gen'u'
—transversum ge'nus
—transversum pel'vis
—transversum per'i·ne'i'

—transversum scap'u·lae'
 in·fe'ri·us
—transversum scapulae
 su·pe'ri·us
—trap'e·zoi'de·um
—tri·an'gu·lar'e' dex'trum
—triangulare si·nis'trum
—tu·ber'cu·li' cos'tae'
—ul'no·car'pe·um pal·
 mar'e'
—um·bil'i·ca'le' lat'er·a'le'
—umbilicale me'di·a'le'
—umbilicale me'di·a'num
—umbilicale me'di·um
—vag'i·na'le'
—ve'nae' ca'vae' si·nis'trae'
—ve·no'sum
—ven·tric'u·lar'e'
—ves·tib'u·lar'e'
—vo·ca'le'
lig'and'
li'gase'
li'gate', -gat'ed, -gat'ing
li·ga'tion
li'ga·tor
lig'a·ture
Lig'et sign
light
light'-head'ed
Li·gnac'-de To'ni-Fan·co'ni
 syndrome
Li·gnac'-Fan·co'ni
 syndrome
lig'ne·ous
lig'nin
lig'no·caine'
lig'no·cer'ic
lig'num
lig'ro·in
lig'u·la *pl.* -las *or* -lae
lig'ule
Lil'i·en·thal' operation
limb
lim'bal
lim'ber·neck'
lim'bi'
 —pal'pe·bra'les'
  an·te'ri·o'res'
 —palpebrales pos·te'ri·o'res'
lim'bic
lim'bus *pl.* -bus·es *or* -bi'
 —al've·o·lar'is man·dib'-
  u·lae'

—alveolaris max·il'lae'
—cor'ne·ae'
—fos'sae' o·va'lis
—lam'i·nae' spi·ra'lis
 os'se·ae'
—mem·bra'nae' tym'pa·ni'
—pal'pe·bra'lis anterior
—palpebralis posterior
—sphe'noi·da'lis
—spi·ra'lis
li'men *pl.* lim'i·na
—in'su·lae'
—na'si'
lim'i·nal
lim'i·nom'e·ter
lim'it
lim'i·tans'
lim'i·ta'tion
lim'i·troph'ic
Lim·na'tis
—ni·lot'i·ca
lim'o·nene'
li·moph'thi·sis
li·mo'sis
limp
lin'co·my'cin
linc'tus
lin'dane'
Lin'dau' disease
Lind'bergh' flask
Lin'der·strom-Lang'-
 Dus·pi'va method
Lin'der·strom-Lang'-
 En'gel method
Lin'der·strom-Lang'-
 Glick' method
Lin'der·strom-Lang'-
 Hol'ter method
Lin'der·strom-Lang'-Lanz'
 method
Lin'der·strom-Lang'
 method
Lin'der·strom-Lang'-Weil'-
 Hol'ter methods
line
—of Gen'na'ri
—of Zahn
lin'e·a *pl.* -ae'
—al'ba
—ar·cu·a'ta os'sis il'i·i'
—arcuata ossis il'i·um
—arcuata va·gi'nae' mus'-
 cu·li' rec'ti' ab·dom'i·nis

—as′per·a
—ax′il·lar′is
—ep′i·phy′si·a′lis
—glu′tae·a anterior
—glutaea inferior
—glutaea posterior
—glu′te·a anterior
—glutea inferior
—glutea posterior
—in′ter·con′dy·lar′is
—in′ter·con′dy·loi′de·a
—in′ter·me′di·a
—in′ter·tro′chan·ter′i·ca
—mam′mil·lar′is
—me′di·a′na anterior
—mediana posterior
—me′di·o·cla·vic′u·lar′is
—men·sa′lis
—mus′cu·li′ so′le·i′
—my′lo·hy·oi′de·a
—ni′gra
—nu′chae′ inferior
—nuchae superior
—nuchae su·pre′ma
—o·bli′qua car′ti·lag′i·nis
   thy·roi′de·ae′
—obliqua man·dib′u·lae′
—par′a·ster·na′lis
—pec·tin′e·a
—pop·lit′e·a
—scap′u·lar′is
—sem′i·cir′cu·lar′is
   (Doug′la·si′)
—sem′i·lu·nar′is
—sin′u·o′sa a·na′lis
—splen′dens
—ster·na′lis
—tem′po·ra′lis inferior
   os′sis pa·ri·e·ta′lis
—temporalis ossis fron·
   ta′lis
—temporalis superior ossis
   pa·ri·e·ta′lis
—ter′mi·na′lis
—trap′e·zoi′de·a
lin′e·ae′
—al′bi·can′tes′
—grav′i·dar′um
—mus′cu·lar′es′ scap′u·lae′
—trans·ver′sae′ os′sis sa′cri′
lin′e·al
lin′e·ar
lines

—of Bail·lar·ger′
—of O′wen
—of Ret′zi·us
—of Sal′ter
—of Schre′ger
lin′gua pl. -guae′
—ni′gra
—pli·ca′ta
lin′gual
lin·gua′le
lin·gua′lis
lin′gual·ly
Lin·gua′tu·la
—ser·ra′ta
lin′gui·form′
lin′gu·la pl. -lae′
—cer′e·bel′li′
—man·dib′u·lae′
—pul·mo′nis si·nis′tri′
—sphe′noi·da′lis
lin′gu·lar
lin′gu·lec′to·my
lin′guo·ax′i·al
lin′guo·ax′i·o·gin′gi·val
lin′guo·cer′vi·cal
lin′guo·den′tal
lin′guo·dis′tal
lin′guo·gin′gi·val
lin′guo·in·ci′sal
lin′guo·me′si·al
lin′guo·oc·clu′sal
lin′guo·pap′il·li·ti′tis
lin′guo·pul′pal
lin′guo·ver′sion
lin′i·ment
li′nin
li·ni′tis
—plas′ti·ca
link′age
lin′o·le′ic
lin′seed
lin′tin
Linz′en·mei′er test
li·o·thy′ro·nine′
li·o′trix′
lip
lip·ac·i·de′mi·a
lip·ac·i·du′ri·a
li·par′o·cele′
lip′a·roid′
lip′a·ro·trich′i·a
lip′a·rous
li′pase′

lip′a·su′ri·a
li·pec′to·my
lip′e·de′ma pl. -mas or
   -ma·ta
li·pe′mi·a
—ret′i·na′lis
lip′id
lip′i·dase′
lip′i·de′mi·a
li·pid′ic
lip′i·dol′y·sis pl. -ses′
lip′i·do′sis pl. -ses′
lip′i·du′ri·a
lip′o·ad′e·no′ma pl. -mas or
   -ma·ta
lip′o·ar·thri′tis
lip′o·at′ro·phy
lip′o·blast′
lip′o·blas′tic
lip′o·blas·to′ma pl. -mas or
   -ma·ta
lip′o·blas·to′ma·to′sis
   pl. -ses′
lip′o·blas·to′sis
lip′o·ca′ic
lip′o·car′di·ac′
lip′o·cat′a·bol′ic
lip′o·cele′
lip′o·cere′
lip′o·chon′dro·dys′tro·phy
lip′o·chon·dro′ma pl. -mas
   or -ma·ta
lip′o·chrome′
lip′o·chro·me′mi·a
lip′o·cor′ti·coid′
lip′o·cyte′
lip′o·di·er′e·sis pl. -ses′
lip′o·dys·tro′phi·a
—pro·gres·si′va
lip′o·dys·tro·phy
lip′o·fi·bro′ma pl. -mas or
   -ma·ta
lip′o·fi′bro·myx·o′ma
   pl. -mas or -ma·ta
lip′o·fi′bro·sar·co′ma
   pl. -mas or -ma·ta
lip′o·fus′cin
lip′o·gen·e′sis pl. -ses′
lip′o·gen′ic
li·pog′e·nous
lip′o·gran′u·lo′ma pl. -mas
   or -ma·ta
lip′o·gran′u·lo·ma·to′sis

lip'o·he'mar·thro'sis
   pl. -ses'
li·po'ic
lip'oid'
lip·oi'dal
lip·oi·de·mi·a
li·poi'dic
lip'oi·do'sis *pl.* -ses'
   —cor'ne·ae'
   —cu'tis et mu·co'sae'
li·pol'y·sis *pl.* -ses'
lip'o·lyt'ic
li·po'ma *pl.* -mas *or* -ma·ta
   —foe·ta'lo'cel'lu·lar'e'
li·po'ma·toid'
lip'o·ma·to'sis *pl.* -ses'
li·po'ma·tous
lip'o·mel'a·not'ic
lip'o·me·nin'go·cele'
lip'o·me·ri·a
lip'o·met'a·bol'ic
lip'o·me·tab'o·lism
lip'o·my'e·lo·me·nin'go·
   cele'
lip'o·my'o·he·man'gi·o'ma
   pl. -mas *or* -ma·ta
lip'o·my'o·ma *pl.* -mas *or*
   -ma·ta
lip'o·my'o·sar·co'ma
   pl. -mas *or* -ma·ta
lip'o·myx·o'ma *pl.* -mas *or*
   -ma·ta
lip'o·myx'o·sar·co'ma
   pl. -mas *or* -ma·ta
lip'o·ne·phro'sis
Lip'o·nys'sus
   —ba·co'ti
lip'o·pe·ni·a
lip'o·pe'nic
lip'o·pep'tide'
lip'o·pex'i·a
lip'o·phage'
lip'o·pha'gi·a
lip'o·pha'gic
lip'o·pha'gy
lip'o·phan'e·ro'sis *pl.* -ses'
lip'o·phil'
lip'o·phil'i·a
lip'o·phil'ic
lip'o·phore'
lip'o·phren'ic
lip'o·plas'tic
lip'o·pol'y·sac'cha·ride'

lip'o·pro'tein'
lip'o·rho'din
lip'o·sar·co'ma *pl.* -mas *or*
   -ma·ta
lip'o·sar·co'ma·tous
li·po'sis *pl.* -ses'
li·pos'i·tol'
lip'o·sol'u·ble
lip'o·some'
li·pos'to·my
lip'o·suc'tion
li'po·thy'mi·a
lip'o·tro'pi·a
lip'o·troph'ic
li·pot'ro·phy
lip'o·trop'ic
li·pot'ro·py
lip'o·vac'cine
lip'o·vi·tel'lin
li·pox'e·nous
li·pox'e·ny
li·pox'i·dase'
li·pox'y·ge·nase'
lip'pa
lip'ping
lip'pi·tude'
lip'pi·tu'do
Lip'schütz'
   —body
   —cell
li·pu'ri·a
li·pu'ric
liq'ue·fa'cient
liq'ue·fac'tion
liq'ue·fac'tive
liq'ue·fy', -fied', -fy'ing
li·ques'cent
liq'uid
liq'uo·gel'
liq'uor
   —am'ni·i'
   —amnii spu'ri·us
   —cer'e·bro·spi'na'lis
   —fol·lic'u·li'
   —per'i·car'di·i'
   —san'gui·nis
   —se'mi·nis
li·quo'res'
Lis'franc'
   —amputation
   —tubercle
li·sin'o·pril
lisp

Lis'sau'er
   —column
   —paralysis
Lis'sen·ceph'a·la
lis'sen·ce·pha'li·a
lis'sen·ce·phal'ic
lis'sen·ceph'a·ly
lis'sive
list
lis'ter·el·lo'sis *pl.* -ses'
Lis·te'ri·a
   —mon'o·cy·tog'e·nes'
lis·te'ri·al
lis·te'ri·o'sis *pl.* -ses'
lis'ter·ism
Lis'ting law
li'ter *also* litre
lith'a·gogue'
li·thec'ta·sy
li·thec'to·my
li·the'mi·a
li·the'mic
lith'i·a
li·thi'a·sic
li·thi'a·sis *pl.* -ses'
lith'ic
lith'i·co'sis *pl.* -ses'
lith'i·um
lith'o·cho'lic
lith'o·clast'
lith'o·cys·tot'o·my
lith'o·di·al'y·sis
lith'o·gen'e·sis
lith'o·ge·net'ic
li·thog'e·nous
li·thog'e·ny
lith'oid'
lith'o·kel'y·pho·pe'di·on'
lith'o·kel'y·phos'
lith'o·labe'
li·thol'a·pax'y
li·thol'o·gy
li·thol'y·sis
lith'o·lyte'
lith'o·ne·phri'tis
lith'o·ne·phrot'o·my
lith'o·pe'di·on'
lith'o·scope'
lith'o·tome'
li·thot'o·mist
li·thot'o·my
lith'o·trip'sy
lith'o·trip'tic

lith′o·trip′tor
lith′o·trip′to·scope′
lith′o·trip·tos′co·py
lith′o·trite′
lith′o·trit′ic
li·thot′ri·ty
lith′o·troph′
lith′o·troph′ic
lith′ous
lith′u·re′sis
li·thu′ri·a
lit′mus
li′tre *var. of* liter
Lit′ten sign
lit′ter
Lit′tle disease
Lit′tle League elbow
Lit′tler operation
Litt′man ox′-gall′ medium
Lit·tré′
　—crypts
　—glands
　—hernia
　—operation
　—space
lit·tri′tis
Litz′mann ob·liq′ui·ty
live′-born′
li·ve′do
　—re·tic′u·lar′is
li·ve′doid′
liv′er
liv′er·wort′
liv′e·tin
liv′id
li·vid′i·ty
Li·vi·e′ra′to sign
li′vor′
　—mor′tis
lix·iv′i·a′tion
Li′zars operation
Lju·bin′sky stain
load
Lo′a lo′a
lo′bar
lo′bate′
lo′bat′ed
lobe
lo·bec′to·my
lo·be′li·a
lo·be·line′
lo′bi′
　—cer′e·bri′

—glan′du·lae′ mam·mar′-
　i·ae′
—mam′mae′
—re·na′les′
lo·bi′tis
lo′bo·cyte′
lo′bo·po′di·um *pl.* -di·a
Lo′bo′s disease
lo·bot′o·my
Lob′stein′ disease
lob′u·lar
lob′u·lat′ed
lob′u·la′tion
lob′ule′
lob′u·li′
　—cor′ti·ca′les′ re′nis
　—ep′i·di·dym′i·dis
　—glan′du·lae′ mam·mar′-
　i·ae′
　—glandulae thy′re·oi′de·ae′
　—glandulae thy·roi′de·ae′
　—hep′a·tis
　—mam′mae′
　—pul·mo′num
　—tes′tis
　—thy′mi′
lob′u·lose′
lob′u·lus *pl.* -li′
　—au·ric′u·lae′
　—bi·ven′ter
　—cen′tra′lis
　—me′di·us me·di·a′nus
　—par′a·cen·tra′lis
　—pa·ri′e·ta′lis inferior
　—parietalis superior
　—qua·dran′gu·lar′is
　—sem′i·lu·nar′is inferior
　—semilunaris superior
　—sim′plex′
lo′bus *pl.* -bi′
　—anterior hy′po·phys′e·os′
　—cau·da′tus
　—fron·ta′lis
　—glan′du·lae′ thy′re·oi′-
　de·ae′
　—glandulae thy·roi′de·ae′
　—hep′a·tis dex′ter
　—hepatis si·nis′ter
　—inferior pul·mo′nis
　—inferior pulmonis dex′tri′
　—inferior pulmonis
　si·nis′tri′
　—me′di·us pros·ta′tae′

—medius pul·mo′nis
　dex′trae′
—medius pulmonis dex′tri′
—oc·cip′i·ta′lis
—ol′fac′to′ri·us
—pa·ri′e·ta′lis
—posterior hy′po·phy′-
　se·os′
—pros′ta·tae′
—py·ram′i·da′lis
—qua′dra′tus
—superior pul·mo′nis
—superior pulmonis dex′tri′
—superior pulmonis
　si·nis′tri′
—tem′po·ra′lis
—thy′mi′
lo′cal
lo′cal·i·za′tion
lo′cal·ize′, -ized′, -iz′ing
lo′cal·iz′er
lo′cal·ly
lo′ca′tor
lo′chi·a
　—al′ba
　—cru·en′ta
　—ru′bra
　—se·ro′sa
lo′chi·al
lo′chi·o·col′pos′
lo′chi·o·cyte′
lo′chi·o·me′tra
lo′chi·o·me·tri′tis
lo′chi·or·rha′gi·a
lo′chi·or·rhe′a
lo′chi·os′che·sis
lo′cho·me·tri′tis
lo′cho·per′i·to·ni′tis
Locke′-Rin′ger solution
lock′jaw′
Lock′wood′ sign
lo′co·mo′tion
lo′co·mo′tive
lo′co·mo′tor
loc′u·lar
loc′u·late′
loc′u·lat′ed
loc′u·la′tion
loc′u·lus *pl.* -li′
lo′cum ten′ens
lo′cus *pl.* -ci′
　—cae·ru′le·us
　—ce·ru′le·us

—mi·no'ris res'is·ten'ti·ae'
—per'fo·ra'tus
Loeb decidual reaction
Loef'fler
—stain
Loele method
Loe'wen·thal' tract
Loe'wi sign
Löff'ler
—disease
—endocarditis
—eosinophilia
—pneumonia
—syndrome
log'a·dec'to·my
log'ag·no'si·a
log'a·graph'i·a
log'am·ne'si·a
log'a·pha'si·a
log'o·clo'ni·a
log'o·ko·pho'sis *pl.* -ses'
log'o·ma'ni·a
log'o·neu·ro'sis *pl.* -ses'
lo·gop'a·thy
log'o·pe'di·a
log'o·pe'dics
log'o·pha'si·a
log'o·ple'gi·a
log'or·rhe'a
log'o·spasm
log'o·ther'a·py
Loh'mann reaction
lo·i'a·sis *pl.* -ses'
loin
lol'i·ism
Lol'i·um tem'u·len'tum
lo'mo·fun'gin
Londe atrophy
Long coefficient
lon·gev'i·ty
lon'gi·lin'e·al
lon'gi·ma'nous
lon'gi·ped'ate'
lon·gis'si·mus
lon'gi·tu'di·nal
lon'gi·tu'di·na'lis
lon'gi·typ'i·cal
long'stand'ing
lon'gus
—cap'i·tis
—cer'vi·cis
—col'li
Loo'ney and Dy'er method

loop (*a bend in a cordlike*
structure)
♦*loupe*
—of Hen'le
Loo'ser-Milk'man
syndrome
Loo'ser zones
lo·per'a·mine'
loph'o·dont'
Lo·phoph'o·ra
lo·phoph'o·rine'
lo·phot'ri·cate'
lo·phot'ri·chous
lo·quac'i·ty
Lo·rain'-Lé·vi' syndrome
lo·raz'e·pam'
lor'do·sco'li·o'sis *pl.* -ses'
lor·do'sis *pl.* -ses'
lor·dot'ic
Lo'renz
—method
—osteotomy
—procedure
—sign
Lo·ri'ga disease
Lor·rain' Smith stain
loss
Los'sen operation
Lo'theis'sen operation
lo'ti·o'
lo'tion
Lou Geh'rig disease
Lou·is'
—angle
—law
Lou·is'-Bar' syndrome
loupe (*a magnifying lens*)
♦*loop*
loup'ing ill
louse *pl.* lice
lous'y
lov'age
lo'va·stat'in
Lo'vén reflex
Love'set maneuver
Lo'vi·bond' unit
Low'-Beers' projection
Lö'wen·stein'-Jen'sen
medium
Low'er tubercle
Lowe syndrome
Lowe'-Ter'ry-
Mc·Clach'lan syndrome

Lown'-Gan'ong-Le·vine'
syndrome
Low'ry-Lo'pez-Bes'sey
method
Low'sley operation
lox'i·a
Lox·os'ce·les
lox·os'ce·lism
loz'enge
l-phen'yl·al'a·nine'
l-sar'co·ly'sin
Lu'barsch' crystals
Lu'barsch-Pick' syndrome
lubb
lubb-dupp'
lu·can'thone'
Lu'cas-Cham'pion·nière'
disease
Lu'cas-Mur'ray operation
Lu'cas sign
lu'cen·cy
lu'cent
Lu'ci·a'ni triad
lu'cid
lu'cid'i·ty
lu·cif'u·gal
Lu·cil'i·a
Lu·ci'o leprosy
Lück'en·schä'del
Lud'loff
—operation
—sign
Lud'wig
—angina
—angle
—filtration theory
—muscle
lu'es'
lu·et'ic
lu'e·tin
Luft
—disease
—syndrome
Lu'gol solution
lu'ic
Lu'kens test
lum·ba'go'
lum'bar
lum'bar·i·za'tion
lum'bo·co·los'to·my
lum'bo·co·lot'o·my
lum'bo·cos'tal
lum'bo·dor'sal

lum'bo·dyn'i·a
lum'bo·in'gui·nal
lum'bo·is'chi·al
lum'bo·sa'cral
lum'bo·ver'te·bral
lum'bri·cal
lum'bri·coid'
lum·bri'cus
lum'bus pl. -bi'
lu'men pl. -mi·na or -mens
lu'mi·chrome'
lu'mi·fla'vin
lu'mi·nal
lu'mi·nance
lu'mi·nesce'
lu'mi·nes'cence
lu'mi·nes'cent
lu'mi·nif'er·ous
lu'mi·nos'i·ty
lu'mi·nous
lu'mi·rho·dop'sin
lu·mis'ter·ol'
lump
lump·ec'to·my
lu'na·cy
lu'nar
lu'nate'
lu'na·tic
lu'na·to·ma·la'ci·a
lung
lung'worm'
lu'nu·la pl. -lae'
lu'nu·lae'
—val'vu·lar'um sem'i·lu·
nar'i·um a·or'tae'
—valvularum semilunarium
trun'ci' pul·mo'nis
lu'pi·form'
lu'pine
lu'pi·no'sis
lu'poid'
lu'pus
—crus'to'sus
—en·dem'i·cus
—er'y·the'ma·to'sus
—ex·ce'dens
—hy'per·troph'i·cus
—lym·phat'i·cus
—mac'u·lo'sus
—mil'i·ar'is dis·sem'i·na'-
tus fa·ci·e'i'
—per'ni·o'
—pernio of Bes'ni·er

—se·ba'ce·us
—ser·pig'i·no'sus
—su·per·fi'ci·a'lis
—tu'mi·dus
—veg'e·tans'
—ver·ru·co'sus
—vul·gar'is
Lusch'ka
—bursa
—cartilage
—cricotracheal ligament
—crypt
—duct
—fibers
—foramen
—fossa
—ganglion
—glands
—joint
—muscle
—nerve
—subpharyngeal cartilage
—tonsil
—tubercle
Lust
—phenomenon
—reflex
lu'sus na·tu'rae'
lute
lu'te·al
lu'te·in
lu'te·in'ic
lu'te·in·i·za'tion
lu'te·in·ize', -ized', -iz'ing
Lu'tem·bach'er
—complex
—disease
—syndrome
lu'te·o·lin
lu'te·no'ma pl. -mas or -ma·ta
lu'te·o·blas'to'ma pl. -mas or
-ma·ta
lu'te·o'ma pl. -mas or -ma·ta
lu'te·o·troph'ic
lu'te·o·trop'ic
lu'te·o·tro'pin
lu·te'ti·um
Lu'ther·an blood group
Lütt'ke test
lu'tu·trin
Lutz'o·my'i·a
Lutz'-Splen·do're-
Al·mei'da disease

lux pl. lux or lux'es'
lux'ate'
lux·a'ti·o'
—con·gen'i·ta
—cox'ae'
—e·rec'ta
—im·per·fec'ta
—per·in'e·a'lis
lux·a'tion
lux·u'ri·ant
lux'us
Luys body lesion
ly'ase'
ly·can'thro·py
ly'cine'
ly'co·pene'
Ly'co·per'don
ly'co·per'don·o'sis pl. -ses'
ly'co·po'di·um
ly'co·rex'i·a
ly'di·my'cin
lye
Ly'ell syndrome
ly'go·phil'i·a
ly'ing-in'
Lyme
—arthritis
—disease
Lym·nae'a
lymph
lym'pha
lym·phad'e·nec'to·my
lym'pha·de'ni·a
lym·phad'e·ni'tis
lym·phad'e·no·cele'
lym·phad'e·no·cyst'
lym·phad'e·nog'ra·phy
lym·phad'e·noid'
lym·phad'e·no'ma pl. -mas
or -ma·ta
lym·phad'e·no·ma·to'sis
pl. -ses'
lym·phad'e·nop'a·thy
lym·phad'e·no'sis pl. -ses'
—be·nig'na cu'tis
lym·phad'e·not'o·my
lym'pha·gogue'
lym·phan'gi·al
lym·phan'gi·ec·ta'si·a
lym·phan'gi·ec·ta'sis
pl. -ses'
lym·phan'gi·ec·tat'ic
lym·phan'gi·ec·to·my

lym·phan′gi·o·en′do·the′-
li·al
lym·phan′gi·o·en′do·the′-
li·o′ma *pl.* -mas *or* -ma·ta
lym·phan′gi·o·fi·bro′ma
pl. -mas *or* -ma·ta
lym·phan′gi·o·gram′
lym·phan′gi·o·graph′ic
lym·phan′gi·og′ra·phy
lym·phan′gi·ol′o·gy
lym·phan′gi·o′ma *pl.* -mas
or -ma·ta
—cir′cum·scrip′tum
con·gen′i·ta′le′
—tu′be·ro′sum mul′ti·plex′
lym·phan′gi·o′ma·tous
lym·phan′gi·o·phle·bi′tis
lym·phan′gi·o·plas′ty
lym·phan′gi·o·sar·co′ma
pl. -mas *or* -ma·ta
lym·phan′gi·ot′o·my
lym′phan·git′ic
lym′phan·gi′tis
pl. -git′i·des′
lym·phat′ic
lym·phat′i·cos′to·my
lym′pha·tism
lym′pha·ti′tis *pl.* -tis·es *or*
-tit′i·des′
lym′pha·tol′y·sis
lym′phec·ta′si·a
lym′phe·de′ma
lym′pho·blast′
lym′pho·blas′tic
lym′pho·blas·to′ma
pl. -mas *or* -ma·ta
—ma·lig′num
lym′pho·blas′to·ma·to′sis
pl. -ses′
lym′pho·blas·to′sis *pl.* -ses′
lym′pho·cele′
lym′pho·chlo·ro′ma
pl. -mas *or* -ma·ta
lym′pho·cyte′
lym′pho·cy·the′mi·a
lym′pho·cyt′ic
lym′pho·cy′to·blast′
lym′pho·cy′to·blas′tic
lym′pho·cy′toid′
lym′pho·cy′to·ma *pl.* -mas
or -ma·ta
—cu′tis
lym′pho·cy′to·pe′ni·a

lym′pho·cy′to·poi·e′sis
pl. -ses′
lym′pho·cy′to·sis *pl.* -ses′
lym′pho·cy·tot′ic
lym′pho·der′mi·a
—per·ni′ci·o′sa
lym′pho·duct′
lym′pho·ep′i·the′li·o′ma
pl. -mas *or* -ma·ta
lym′pho·ep′i·the′li·o′ma·
tous
lym′pho·gen′e·sis *pl.* -ses′
lym′pho·gen′ic
lym·phog′e·nous
lym′pho·glan′du·la *pl.* -lae′
lym′pho·go′ni·a
lym′pho·gran′u·lo′ma
pl. -mas *or* -ma·ta
—in′gui·na′le′
—ve·ne′re·um
lym′pho·gran′u·lo′ma·to′-
sis *pl.* -ses′
—cu′tis
—of Schau′mann
lym′pho·graph′ic
lym·phog′ra·phy
lym′pho·his′ti·o·cyt′ic
lym′phoid′
lym′phoi·dec′to·my
lym′phoi′do·cyte′
lym′pho·graph′ic
lym·phog′ra·phy
lym′pho·ken′tric
lym′pho·kine′
lym′pho·ki·ne′sis
lym·phol′o·gy
lym′pho′ma *pl.* -mas *or*
-ma·ta
lym′pho′ma·toid′
lym′pho·ma·to′sis *pl.* -ses′
lym′pho′ma·tous
lym′pho·mon′o·cyte′
lym′pho·mon′o·cy·to′sis
pl. -ses′
lym′pho·no′dus *pl.* -di′
lym′pho·path′i·a
ve·ne′re·um
lym·phop′a·thy
lym′pho·pe′ni·a
lym′pho·poi·e′sis *pl.* -ses′
lym′pho·poi·et′ic
lym′pho·pro·lif′er·a·tive
lym′pho·re·tic′u·lar

lym′pho·re·tic′u·lo′ma
pl. -mas *or* -ma·ta
lym′pho·re·tic′u·lo′sis
pl. -ses′
lym′phor·rhage
lym′phor·rhe′a
lym′phor·rhoid′
lym′pho·sar·co′ma *pl.* -mas
or -ma·ta
lym′pho·sar·co′ma·to′sis
pl. -ses′
lym′pho·sar·co′ma·tous
lym′pho·sta′sis
lym′pho·tax′is
lym′phous
lym·phu′ri·a
lymph′-vas′cu·lar
lyn·es′tre·nol′
ly′o·chrome′
ly′o·en′zyme′
Ly′on hypothesis
ly′o·phile′
ly′o·phil′ic
ly·oph′i·li·za′tion
ly·oph′i·lize′
ly′o·phobe′
ly′o·pho′bic
ly′o·sol′
ly′o·sorp′tion
ly′o·trop′ic
ly·pres′sin
ly′sate′
lyse, lysed, lys′ing
ly·ser′gic
ly·ser·gide′
Lys′holm′
—grid
—line
—projection
ly′sin
ly′sine′
ly·sin′o·gen
ly′sis *pl.* -ses′
ly·so·ceph′a·lin
ly′so·chrome′
ly′so·gen
ly·sog′e·na′tion
ly·sog′e·ne·sis *pl.* -ses′
ly·sog′e·nic
ly·so·ge·nic′i·ty
ly·so·gen·i·za′tion
ly·sog′e·ny
ly′so·ki′nase′

ly'so·lec'i·thin
ly'so·so'mal
ly'so·some'
ly'so·staph'in
ly'so·type'
ly'so·zyme'
ly'so·zy·mu'ri·a
lys'sa
lys'sic
lys'soid'
lys'so·pho'bi·a
ly'syl
lyt'ic
Lyt'ta ves'i·ca·to'ri·a
lyx'o·fla'vin
lyx'ose'

M

Ma·cac'a
Mac·al'lis·ter muscle
ma·caque'
Mac·Cal'lum
—patch
—stain
Mac·chi·a·vel'lo stain
Mac·Cor'mac reflex
mac'er·ate', -at'ed, -at'ing
mac'er·a'tion
mac'er·a'tive
Mac·ew'en
—operation
—osteotomy
—sign
—triangle
Ma·cha'do-Guer·rei'ro
  reaction
Ma'che unit
ma·chine'
Mach number
Mach'o'ver test
Mac·In'tosh' operation
Mack'en·rodt' ligament
Mac·ken'zie
—amputation
—disease
—syndrome
Mac·Lean' test
Mac·Lean'-Max'well
  disease
Mac·leod' syndrome
Mac·Neal' stain
Mac·Quar'rie test

Mac'ra·can'tho·rhyn'chus
—hi·ru'di·na'ce·us
mac·rad'e·nous
mac'ren·ce·phal'ic
mac'ren·ceph'a·lous
mac'ren·ceph'a·ly
mac'ro·am'y·lase'
mac'ro·am'y·la·se'mi·a
mac'ro·bi·o'ta
mac'ro·bi·ot'ic
mac'ro·blast'
mac'ro·ble·phar'i·a
mac'ro·bra'chi·a
mac'ro·car'di·us
mac'ro·ce·pha'li·a
mac'ro·ce·phal'ic
mac'ro·ceph'a·lous
mac'ro·ceph'a·lus pl. -li'
mac'ro·ceph'a·ly
mac'ro·chei'li·a
mac'ro·chei'ri·a
mac'ro·cne'mi·a
mac'ro·co·nid'i·um pl. -i·a
mac'ro·cra'ni·a
mac'ro·cyst'
mac'ro·cyte'
mac'ro·cy·the'mi·a
mac'ro·cyt'ic
mac'ro·cy·to'sis pl. -ses'
mac'ro·dac'tyl·i·a
mac'ro·dac'tyl·ism
mac'ro·dac'ty·ly
mac'ro·dont'
mac'ro·don'ti·a
mac'ro·fol·lic'u·lar
mac'ro·gam'ete'
mac'ro·ga·me'to·cyte'
mac'ro·gen'i·to·so'mi·a
ma·crog'li·a
ma·crog'li·al
mac'ro·glob'u·lin
mac'ro·glob'u·lin·e'mi·a
mac'ro·glos'si·a
mac'ro·gna'thi·a
mac'ro·gnath'ic
mac'ro·gy'ri·a
mac'ro·lide'
mac'ro·lob'u·lar
mac'ro·lym'pho·cyte'
mac'ro·mas'ti·a
mac'ro·me'li·a
mac·rom'e·lus pl. -li
mac'ro·mere'

mac'ro·mer'o·zo'ite'
mac'ro·meth'od
mac'ro·mo·lec'u·lar
mac'ro·mol'e·cule'
mac'ro·mon'o·cyte'
mac'ro·my'e·lo·blast'
mac'ro·nod'u·lar
mac'ro·nor'mo·blast'
mac'ro·nor'mo·cyte'
mac'ro·nu'cle·us pl. -cle·i'
mac'ro·nych'i·a
mac'ro·phage'
ma·croph'a·gy
mac'roph·thal'mos'
mac'ro·pla'si·a
mac'ro·po'di·a
mac'ro·pol'y·cyte'
mac'ro·pro·so'pi·a
mac'ro·pro'so·pous
ma·crop'si·a
mac'rop'sy
mac'ro·scop'ic
mac'ros·mat'ic
mac'ro·so'mi·a
mac'ro·spore'
mac'ro·spor'ic
mac'ro·sto'mi·a
ma·cro'ti·a
Ma·cruz' index
mac'u·la pl. -lae'
—a·cu'sti·ca sac'cu·li'
—acustica u·tric'u·li'
—ad·hae'rens
—ce·ru'le·a
—com·mu'nis
—cor'ne·ae'
—cri'bro'sa inferior
—cribrosa me'di·a
—cribrosa superior
—den'sa
—fla'va
—ger'mi·na·ti'va
—lu'te·a
—sac·cu'li'
—u'tric'u·li'
mac'u·lae'
—a·cu'sti·cae'
—cri·bro'sae'
mac'u·lar
mac'ule'
mac'u·lo·an'es·thet'ic
mac'u·lo·cer'e·bral
mac'u·lo·pap'u·lar

mac'u·lo·pap'ule'
mac'u·lo·ve·sic'u·lar
mad'a·ro'sis *pl.* -ses'
mad'a·rot'ic
mad'a·rous
Mad'den repair
Mad'dox rod
Mad'e·lung' deformity
Mad'u·rel'la mycetomi
mad'u·ro·my·co'sis *pl.* -ses'
ma'fe·nide'
Maf·fuc'ci syndrome
mag'al·drate'
ma'gen·bla'se
Ma·gen'die
—foramen
—law
ma'gen·stras'se
ma·gen'ta
mag'got
mag'is·tral
mag'ma
—re·tic'u·lar'e'
Mag'nan sign
mag·ne·se'mi·a
mag·ne'si·a
mag·ne·site'
mag·ne'si·um
mag'net
mag'net'ic
mag'net·ism
mag'net·i·za'tion
mag'net·ize'
mag·ne'to·car'di·o·gram'
mag·ne'to·car'di·o·graph'
mag·ne'to·car'di·o·
  graph'ic
mag·ne'to·car'di·og'ra·phy
mag·ne'to·e·lec'tric'i·ty
mag·ne'to·en·ceph'a·lo·
  gram'
mag·ne'to·en·ceph'a·lo·
  graph'ic
mag·ne'to·en·ceph'a·log'-
  ra·phy
mag·ne'to·graph'
mag·ne'to·in·duc'tion
mag'ne·tom'e·ter
mag·ne'to·stric'tion
mag'ne·tron'
mag'ni·fi·ca'tion
mag'ni·fy', -fied', -fy'ing
mag'no·cel'lu·lar

mag'num
Mag'nus-de Kleijn' reflexes
Mag'nu·son-Stack'
  arthrotomy
Ma·haim'
—bundle
—fibers
Mah'ler sign
maid'en·head'
maim
main
—en griffe
—en lor·gnette'
main·tain'
main·tain'er
main'te·nance
Mai'son·neuve'
—amputation
—operation
—sign
—urethrotomy
Mais·sat' band
Ma·joc'chi disease
ma'jor
mal
—de ca·de'ras
—de Ca·yenne'
—de co·ït'
—de la ro'sa
—del pin'to
—del so'le
—de Me·le'da
—de mer
—des bas·sines'
—per'fo·rant'
ma·la
Mal'a·bar' itch
mal·ab·sorp'tion
ma·la'ci·a
—cor'dis
mal'a·co'ma
mal'a·co·pla'ki·a
mal'a·cot'ic
mal'a·dap·ta'tion
mal'a·dap'tive
mal'a·die'
—bleue
—bron·zée'
—de Cap'de·pont'
—de Ni'co·las' et Fa'vre
—de plon·geurs'
—de Rog·er'
—des jam·bes'

—des tics'
—de tic con·vul·sif'
—du doute'
—du som·meil'
mal'ad·just'ed
mal'ad·jus'tive
mal'ad·just'ment
mal'a·dy
ma·laise'
mal'a·lign'ment
mal'an·gu·la'tion
ma'lar
ma·lar'i·a
ma·lar'i·al
ma·lar'i·ol'o·gy
ma·lar'i·o·ther'a·py
ma·lar'i·ous
mal·ar·tic'u·la'tion
Mal·as·se'zi·a
—fur'fur
mal·as·sim'i·la'tion
mal'ate'
mal'a·thi'on'
mal'ax·ate'
mal·ax·a'tion
mal·de·vel'op·ment
mal·di·ges'tion
male
mal'e·ate'
ma·le'ic
mal·e·rup'tion
mal·eth'a·mer
mal·for·ma'tion
mal·func'tion
Mal·gaigne'
—amputation
—fracture
Mal'i·bu' disease
mal'ic
ma·lig'nan·cy
ma·lig'nant
ma·lin'ger
ma·lin'ger·er
Mall
—formula
—technique
mal'le·a·bil'i·ty
mal'le·able
mal'le·al
mal'le·ar
mal'le·a'tion
mal'le·o·in'cu·dal
mal'le·o·lar

mal·le'o'lus *pl.* -li'
—lat'er·a'lis
—me'di·a'lis
Mal'le·o·my'ces'
—mal'le·i'
—pseu'do·mal'le·i'
mal'le·o·my·rin'go·plas'ty
mal'le·ot'o·my
mal'let
mal'le·us *pl.* -le·i'
Mal'lo·ry
—bodies
—stain
Mal'lo·ry-A'zan stain
Mal'lo·ry-Weiss'
—syndrome
—tear
mal'low
Mal·loy'-Ev'e·lyn method
mal·nour'ish
mal·nour'ish·ment
mal'nu·tri'tion
mal'oc·clu'sion
mal·o'dor·ous
mal·o'nate'
ma·lon'ic
mal'o·nyl
mal'o·nyl·u'ri·a
mal·pigh'i·an
mal·posed'
mal·po·si'tion
mal·prac'tice
mal·pre·sen·ta'tion
mal'ro·ta'tion
mal'tase'
mal'tose'
mal'to·su'ri·a
mal'um
—cox'ae'
—coxae se·ni'lis
—per'fo·rans' pe'dis
—ve·ne're·um
mal·un'ion
ma·man'pi·an'
mam'ba
mam'e·lon'
ma·mil'la *pl.* -lae'
mam'il·lar'y
mam'il·lat'ed
mam'il·la'tion
ma·mil'li·form'
ma·mil'li·plas'ty
mam'il·li·tis

mam'ma *pl.* -mae'
—a·ber'rans'
—er'rat'i·ca
—mas·cu·li'na
—vi·ri'lis
mam'mae'
—ac'ces·so'ri·ae' fem'i·ni'-
nae' et mas·cu·li'nae'
—accessoriae mu·li·e'bres'
et vi·ri'les'
mam'mal
mam'mal'gi·a
Mam·ma'li·a
mam·ma'li·an
mam'ma·plas'ty
mam'ma·ry
mam'ma·stat'in
mam·mec'to·my
mam'mi·form'
mam'mi'tis
mam'mo·gen
mam'mo·gen'e·sis *pl.* -ses'
mam'mo·gen'ic
mam'mo·gram'
mam'mo·graph'ic
mam·mog'ra·phy
mam'mo·pla'si·a
mam'mo·plas'ty
mam'mose'
mam·mot'o·my
mam'mo·troph'ic
mam'mo·tro'phin
mam'mo·trop'ic
mam'mo·tro'pin
man·cha'da
man·chette'
Manck'e-Som'mer test
Manck'e test
man'del·ate'
Man'del·baum' reaction
man·del'ic
man'di·ble
man·dib'u·la *pl.* -lae'
man·dib'u·lar
man·dib'u·lec'to·my
man·dib'u·lo·fa'cial
man·dib'u·lo·glos'sus
man·dib'u·lo·mar'gi·na'lis
man·dib'u·lo·max'il·lar'y
Mandl operation
man'drel
Man'dril'lus
man'drin

ma·neu'ver
man'ga·nese'
man·gan'ic
man'ga·nous
ma'ni·a
—à po'tu
ma'ni·ac'
ma·ni'a·cal
man'ic-de·pres'sive
man'i·fest'
man'i·kin
man'i·pha'lanx'
pl. -pha·lan'ges'
man'i·ple
ma·nip'u·la·ble
ma·nip'u·late', -lat'ed, -lat'ing
ma·nip'u·la'tion
ma·nip'u·la'tive
ma·nip'u·la'tor
ma·nip'u·la·to'ry
Mann
—palsy
—sign
man'na
man'nan
Mann'-Boll'man fistula
man'ner·ism
man'nite'
man'ni·tol'
Mann'kopf sign
man'nose'
man·no·si·do'sis
Mann'-Wil'liam·son ulcer
man'-of-war'
ma·nom'e·ter
man'o·met'ric
ma·nom'e·try
ma·nop'to·scope'
Man'son disease
Man'so·nel'la
—oz·zar'di
—per'stans
—strep'to·cer'ca
Man'so·ni·a
man'tle
Man·toux' test
man'u·al
ma·nu'bri·al
ma·nu'bri·um *pl.* -bri·a
—mal'le·i'
—ster'ni'
man'u·duc'tion
man'u·dy'na·mom'e·ter

ma'nus *pl.* ma'nus
—ca'va
—cur'ta
—ex·ten'sa
—flex'a
—val'ga
—var'a
map, mapped, map'ping
ma·pro'ti·line'
Ma·quet' technique
ma·ran'tic
ma·ras'mic
ma·ras'mus
mar'ble
mar'ble·i·za'tion
Mar'burg'
—fever
—virus
marche à pe·tit' pas
Mar'che·sa'ni syndrome
Mar'chi
—globule
—stain
Mar'chi·a·fa'va-Bi·gna'mi
—disease
—syndrome
Mar'chi·a·fa'va disease
Mar'chi·a·fa'va-Mi·che'li
syndrome
Marck'wald' operation
Mar'cus Gunn
—phenomenon
—pupillary sign
—syndrome
Mar'é·chal' test
Ma'rek disease
Mar'esch stain
Ma·rey'
—law
—reflex
Mar'fan' syndrome
mar'ga·ri·to'ma *pl.* -mas *or*
-ma·ta
Mar·gar'o·pus an'nu·la'tus
mar'gin
mar'gin·al
mar'gin·a'tion
mar'gin·o·plas'ty
mar'go' *pl.* -gi'nes'
—a·cu'tus cor'dis
—anterior fib'u·lae'
—anterior hep'a·tis
—anterior li·e'nis

—anterior pan·cre'a·tis
—anterior pul·mo'nis
—anterior ra'di·i'
—anterior tes'tis
—anterior tib'i·ae'
—anterior ul'nae'
—ax'il·lar'is scap'u·lae'
—cil'i·ar'is
—dex'ter cor'dis
—dor·sa'lis ra'di·i'
—dorsalis ul'nae'
—fal'ci·for'mis fas'ci·ae'
la'tae'
—falciformis hi·a'tus
sa·phe'ni'
—fib'u·lar'is pe'dis
—fron·ta'lis a'lae' mag'nae'
—frontalis alae ma·jo'ris
—frontalis os'sis pa·ri'e·ta'-
lis
—in'ci·sa'lis
—inferior cer'e·bri'
—inferior hep'a·tis
—inferior li·e'nis
—inferior pan·cre'a·tis
—inferior pul·mo'nis
—in'fer·o·lat'er·a'lis
cer'e·bri'
—in'fer·o·me'di·a'lis
cer'e·bri'
—in'fra·gle'noi·da'lis
—in'fra·or'bi·ta'lis
—in'ter·os'se·us fib'u·lae'
—interosseus ra'di·i'
—interosseus tib'i·ae'
—interosseus ul'nae'
—lac'ri·ma'lis max·il'lae'
—lamb·doi'de·us
—lat'er·a'lis an'te·bra'chi·i'
—lateralis hu'mer·i'
—lateralis lin'guae'
—lateralis pe'dis
—lateralis re'nis
—lateralis scap'u·lae'
—lateralis un'guis
—li'ber o·var'i·i'
—liber un'guis
—lin'guae'
—mas·toi'de·us
—me'di·a'lis an'te·bra'chi·i'
—medialis cer'e·bri'
—medialis glan'du·lae'
su'pra·re·na'lis

—medialis hu'mer·i'
—medialis pe'dis
—medialis re'nis
—medialis scap'u·lae'
—medialis tib'i·ae'
—mes'o·var'i·cus
—na·sa'lis
—na'si'
—ob·tu'sus cor'dis
—oc·cip'i·ta'lis os'sis
pa·ri'e·ta'lis
—occipitalis ossis
tem'po·ra'lis
—oc·cul'tus un'guis
—pa·ri'e·ta'lis a'lae'
ma·jo'ris
—parietalis os'sis fron·ta'lis
—parietalis ossis tem'po·ra'-
lis
—pe'dis lat'er·a'lis
—pedis me'di·a'lis
—posterior fib'u·lae'
—posterior li·e'nis
—posterior pan·cre'a·tis
—posterior par'tis pe·tro'-
sae'
—posterior ra'di·i'
—posterior tes'tis
—posterior ul'nae'
—pu'pil·lar'is i'ri·dis
—ra'di·a'lis an'te·bra'chi·i'
—sag'it·ta'lis
—sphe'noi·da'lis
—squa'mo'sus a'lae'
mag'nae'
—squamosus alae ma·jo'ris
—squamosus os'sis
pa·ri'e·ta'lis
—superior cer'e·bri'
—superior glan'du·lae'
su'pra·re·na'lis
—superior li·e'nis
—superior pan·cre'a·tis
—superior par'tis
pe·tro'sae'
—superior scap'u·lae'
—su'per·o·me'di·a'lis
cer'e·bri'
—su'pra·or'bi·ta'lis
—tib'i·a'lis pe'dis
—ul'nar'is an'te·bra'chi·i'
—u'ter·i'
—ver'te·bra'lis scap'u·lae'

—vo·lar′is ra′di·i′
—volaris ul′nae′
—zy′go·mat′i·cus a′lae′
   mag′nae′
—zygomaticus alae
   ma·jo′ris
Ma·rie′
—ataxia
—disease
—syndrome
Ma·rie′-Bam′ber′ger
  disease
Ma·rie′-Foix′ sign
Ma·rie′-Strüm′pell
—arthritis
—disease
—encephalitis
—spondylitis
Ma·rie′-Tooth′ disease
mar′i·hua′na *also* marijuana
mar′i·jua′na *var. of*
  marihuana
Ma′rin A′mat syndrome
Ma′ri·nes′co hand
Ma′ri·nes′co-Sjö′gren-
  Gar′land syndrome
Ma·ri·otte′ blind spot
mar′i·tal
Mar·jo·lin′ ulcer
mark
mark′er
mark′ing
mar′mo·rate′
mar′mo·ra′tion
mar′mo·ri·za′tion
Ma·ro·teaux′-La·my′
  syndrome
mar′row
Mar′shall Hall method
Mar′shall-Mar·chet′ti-
  Krantz′ procedure
Mar′shall vein
Marsh test
mar·su′pi·al
mar·su′pi·al·i·za′tion
mar·su′pi·um *pl.* -pi·a
—pa′tel·lar′is
Mar′tin
—disease
—operation
Mar′ti·not′ti cells
Mar·to·rell′
—syndrome

—ulcer
mas′cu·line
mas′cu·lin′i·ty
mas′cu·lin·i·za′tion
mas′cu·lin·ize′, -ized′,
  -iz′ing
mas′cu·lin·o′vo·blas·to′ma
  pl. -mas *or* -ma·ta
ma′ser
mask
masked
mask′ing
mas·o′chism
mas·o′chist
mas·o·chis′tic
Ma′son
—gastroplasty
—incision
masque′ bi·liaire′
mass
mas′sa *pl.* -sae′
—in′ter·me′di·a
—lat′er·a′lis at·lan′tis
mas·sage′
mas·se′ter
mas·se·ter′ic
mas·seur′
mas·seuse′
mas′sive
Mas·son′
—body
—trichrome stain
mast
mas′tad·e·ni′tis
mas′tad·e·no′ma *pl.* -mas *or*
  -ma·ta
mas·tal′gi·a
mas′ta·tro′phi·a
mas·tat′ro·phy
mas·taux′e′
mast·ec′chy·mo′sis *pl.* -ses′
mas·tec′to·my
Mas′ter two′-step′ test
mast′hel·co′sis *pl.* -ses′
mas′tic
mas′ti·cate′, -cat′ed, -cat′ing
mas′ti·ca′tion
mas′ti·ca·to′ry
Mas′ti·goph′o·ra
mas′ti·goph′o·ran
mas′ti·goph′o·rous
mas′ti·gote′
mas·tit′ic

mas·ti′tis
mas·to·car′ci·no′ma
  pl. -mas *or* -ma·ta
mas·to·chon·dro′ma
  pl. -mas *or* -ma·ta
mas′to·cyte′
mas′to·cy·to′ma *pl.* -mas *or*
  -ma·ta
mas′to·cy·to′sis *pl.* -ses′
mas·to·dyn′i·a
mas′toid′
mas·toi′dal
mas·toid·al′gi·a
mas·toi′de·a
mas·toid·ec′to·my
mas·toi′de·o·cen·te′sis
mas·toi′de·um
mas′toid·i′tis
mas′toid·ot′o·my
mas·ton′cus
mas′to-oc·cip′i·tal
mas′to·pa·ri′e′tal
mas′to·path′i·a cys′ti·ca
mas·top′a·thy
mas′to·pex′y
mas·to·pla′si·a
mas·to·plas′ti·a
mas·to·plas′ty
mas′top·to′sis
mas′tor·rha′gi·a
mas′to·scir′rhus *pl.* -ri′ *or*
  -rhus·es
mas·to′sis *pl.* -ses′
mas·to·squa′mous
mas·tos′to·my
mas·tot′o·my
mas′tous
MAST suit
mas′tur·bate′, -bat′ed,
  -bat′ing
mas′tur·ba′tion
Mat′as
—band
—operation
match
mate, mat′ed, mat′ing
ma·te′ri·a
—al′ba
—med′i·ca
ma·te′ri·al
ma·te′ri·es′
—mor′bi′
—pec′cans′

ma·ter'nal
ma·ter'ni·ty
mat'ri·cal
mat'ri·cec'to·my
mat'ri·cide'
mat'ri·lin'e·al
ma'trix   *pl.* -tri·ces' *or* -trix·es
  —un'guis
matt
mat'ter
Mat'tox maneuver
mat'u·rate', -rat'ed, -rat'ing
mat'u·ra'tion
mat'u·ra'tion·al
ma·ture', -tured', -tur'ing
ma·tur'i·ty
ma·tu'ti·nal
Mau·chart' ligament
Mau·noir' hydrocele
Mau'rer
  —clefts
  —dots
Mau'ri·ac' syndrome
Mau'ri·ceau' method
Mau'ri·ceau'-Smel'lie-
  Veit' maneuver
Mauth'ner sheath
max·il'la   *pl.* -lae' *or* -las
max'il·lar'y
max'il·lec'to·my
max'il·li'tis
max·il'lo·den'tal
max·il'lo·fa'cial
max·il'lo·fron·ta'le'
max·il'lo·la'bi·al
max·il'lo·lac'ri·mal
max·il'lo·man·dib'u·lar
max·il'lo·pal'a·tal
max·il'lo·pal'a·tine'
max·il'lo·pha·ryn'ge·al
max·il'lo·tot'o·my
max·il'lo·tur'bi·nal
max'i·mal
Max'i·mow'
  —fixative
  —method
  —stain
max'i·mum   *pl.* -ma
Maydl operation
May'er
  —reflex
  —stain
  —view

May'-Grün'wald' stain
May'-Heg'glin anomaly
Ma'yo operation
Ma'yo-Rob'son
  —incision
  —point
  —position
ma'za
maz'ic
maz'in·dol'
ma'zo·dyn'i·a
ma'zo·pex'y
ma'zo·pla'si·a
Maz·zi'ni test
Maz·zo'ni corpuscle
Maz·zot'ti reaction
Mc·Ar'dle syndrome
Mc·Bride'
  —bunionectomy
  —operation
Mc·Bur'ney
  —operation
  —point
  —sign
Mc·Car'thy reflex
Mc·Cort' sign
Mc·Cune'-Al'bright
  syndrome
Mc·Ell'roy' test
Mc·Gill' operation
Mc·In'tosh' test
Mc·Krae' strain of
  herpesvirus
Mc·Lean' formula
Mc·Leod' blood phenotype
Mc·Mur'ray
  —maneuver
  —sign
Mc'Ne·mar' test
Mc·Reyn'olds operation
Mc·Vay' hernia repair
meal
meal'y
mean
mea'sles
mea'sly
meas'ure
meas'ure·ment
me·a'tal
me'a·ti'tis
me'a·tor'rha·phy
me'a·tos'co·py
me'a·tot'o·my

me·a'tus   *pl.* me·a'tus *or*
  -tus·es
  —a·cu'sti·cus ex·ter'nus
  —acusticus externus
    car'ti·la·gin'e·us
  —acusticus in·ter'nus
  —na'si' com·mu'nis
  —nasi inferior
  —nasi me'di·us
  —nasi superior
  —na'so·pha·ryn'ge·us
  —u're'thrae'
me·ben'da·zole'
me·bev'er·ine'
me·bu'ta·mate'
mec'a·myl'a·mine'
me·chan'i·cal
me·chan'i·cal·ly
me·chan'ics
mech'a·nism
mech'a·no·re·cep'tor
mech'a·no·ther'a·py
mech'lor·eth'a·mine'
me'cism
Me·cis'to·cir'rus
  dig'i·ta'tus
Meck'el
  —cartilage
  —cavity
  —diverticulum
  —ganglion
  —scan
  —stalk
  —syndrome
mec'li·zine'
mec'lo·cy'cline
me·clo'fen·am'ate
mec'lo·qua'lone'
me·com'e·ter
mec'o·nate'
me·con'ic
me·co'ni·um
me·cys'ta·sis   *pl.* -ses'
mec'y·stat'ic
me·daz'e·pam'
Me·de'a complex
me'di·a
me'di·ad'
me'di·al
me'di·a·lec'i·thal
me'di·a'lis
me'di·al·ly
me'di·an

me·di·a′nus
me′di·as·ti′nal
me′di·as′ti·ni′tis
me′di·as·ti′no·gram′
me′di·as·ti′nog′ra·phy
me′di·as·ti′no·per′i·car·di′- tis
me′di·as·ti′no·scope′
me′di·as′ti·nos′co·py
me′di·as′ti·not′o·my
me′di·as·ti′num pl. -na
—an·te′ri·us
—me′di·um
—pos·te′ri·us
—su·pe′ri·us
—tes′tis
me′di·ate′, -at′ed, -at′ing
me′di·a′tion
me′di·a′tor
med′i·ca·ble
med′i·cal
me·dic′a·ment
med′i·ca·men·to′sus
med′i·ca·men′tous
med′i·cant
med′i·cate′, -cat′ed, -cat′ing
med′i·ca′tion
med′i·ca′tor
me′di·ce·phal′ic
me·dic′i·nal
med′i·cine
med′i·co·le′gal
med′i·co·psy·chol′o·gy
med′i·co·sur′gi·cal
med′i·cus pl. -ci′
Med′in disease
me′di·o·car′pal
me′di·oc·cip′i·tal
me′di·o·cen′tric
me′di·o·dor′sal
me′di·o·fron′tal
me′di·o·lat′er·al
me′di·o·ne·cro′sis pl. -ses′
—a·or′tae′ id′i·o·path′i·ca cys′ti·ca
me′di·o·plan·tar′
me′di·o·su·pe′ri·or
me′di·o·tar′sal
Med′i·ter·ra′ne·an
—anemia
—fever
me′di·um pl. -di·a
me′di·us

med·pred′ni·sone′
med′ro·ges′tone′
med′ro·nate′
me·drox′y·pro·ges′ter·one′
med′ry·sone′
me·dul′la pl. -las or -lae′
—glan′du·lae′ su′pra·re· na′lis
—no′di′ lym·phat′i·ci′
—ob′lon·ga′ta
—os′si·um
—ossium fla′va
—ossium ru′bra
—re′nis
—spi·na′lis
me·dul′lar
med′ul·lar′y
med′ul·lat′ed
med′ul·la′tion
med′ul·lec′to·my
me·dul′li·spi′nal
med′ul·li·za′tion
me·dul′lo·a·dre′nal
me·dul′lo·ar·thri′tis
me·dul′lo·blast′
me·dul′lo·blas·to′ma
  pl. -mas or -ma·ta
me·dul′lo·en′ce·phal′ic
me·dul′lo·ep′i·the′li·o′ma
  pl. -mas or -ma·ta
med′ul·loid′
Mees lines
mef′e·nam′ic
me·fen′o·rex′
me·fex′a·mide′
mef′lo·quine
mef′ru·side′
meg′a·blad′der
meg′a·car′di·a
meg′a·ce′cum pl. -ca
meg′a·ce·phal′ic
meg′a·ceph′a·lous
meg′a·ceph′a·ly
meg′a·cho·led′o·chus
  pl. -chi′
meg′a·coc′cus pl. -ci′
meg′a·co′lon
meg′a·dont′
meg′a·dont′ism
meg′a·du′o·de′num pl. -na or -nums
meg′a·dyne′
meg′a·e·soph′a·gus pl. -gi

meg′a·far′ad′
meg′a·gam′ete′
meg′a·hertz′
meg′a·kar′y·o·blast′
meg′a·kar′y·o·blas·to′ma
  pl. -mas or -ma·ta
meg′a·kar′y·o·cyte′
meg′a·kar′y·o·cyt′ic
meg′a·kar′y·o·cy′to·pe′- ni·a
meg′a·kar′y·o·cy·to′sis
meg′a·kar′y·oph·thi·sis
  pl. -ses′
meg′a·lec′i·thal
meg′a·len·ceph′a·lon′
  pl. -la
meg′a·len·ceph′a·ly
meg′a·ler′y·the′ma
me·gal′gi·a
meg′a·lo·blast′
—of Sa′bin
meg′a·lo·blas′tic
meg′a·lo·blas′toid′
meg′a·lo·car′di·a
meg′a·lo·ce·pha′li·a
meg′a·lo′ce·phal′ic
meg′a·lo·ceph′a·ly
meg′a·lo·chei′ri·a
meg′a·lo·chei′rous
meg′a·lo·cor′ne·a
meg′a·lo·cys′tis
meg′a·lo·cyte′
meg′a·lo·cyt′ic
meg′a·lo·cy·to′sis pl. -ses′
meg′a·lo·dac′ty·lous
meg′a·lo·dac′ty·ly
meg′a·lo·don′ti·a
meg′a·lo·en′ter·on′
meg′a·lo·e·soph′a·gus
meg′a·lo·gas′tri·a
meg′a·lo·glos′si·a
meg′a·lo·he·pat′i·a
meg′a·lo·kar′y·o·blast′
meg′a·lo·kar′y·o·cyte′
meg′a·lo·ma′ni·a
meg′a·lo·ma′ni·ac′
meg′a·lo·ma·ni′a·cal
meg′a·lo·mas′ti·a
meg′a·lo·me′li·a
meg′a·lo·ny·cho′sis
meg′a·lo·pe′nis
meg′a·lo·pho′bi·a
meg′a·loph·thal′mos

meg′a·lo′pi·a
meg′a·lo·po′di·a
meg′a·lop′si·a
meg′a·lo·splanch′nic
meg′a·lo·sple′ni·a
meg′a·lo·spore′
meg′a·lo·syn·dac′ty·ly
meg′a·lo·thy′mus
   pl. -mus·es *or* -mi′
meg′a·lo·u·re′ter
meg′a·nu′cle·us *pl.* -cle·i′
meg′a·pros′o·pous
meg′a·rec′tum
meg′a·sig′moid′
meg′a·spore′
meg′a·spor′ic
meg′a·u·re′ter
meg′a·vi′ta·min
meg′a·volt′
me·ges′trol′
me·glu′mine′
  —di′a·tri·zo′ate′
  —i′o·dip′a·mide′
  —i′o·tha·lam′ate′
meg′ohm
meg′oph·thal′mos
me′grim
Meh′lis gland
Mei·bo′mi·an
  —cyst
  —glands
mei·bo′mi·a·ni′tis
mei′bo·mi′tis
Meige disease
Meigs syndrome
Mei′nick·e test
mei·o′sis *(cell division),*
  pl. -ses′
  ♦ miosis
mei·ot′ic
Mei·row′sky phenomenon
Meiss′ner
  —corpuscle
  —plexus
mel
me·lag′ra
me·lal′gi·a
mel′a·mine′
mel′an·cho′li·a
  —ag′i·ta′ta
  —at·ton′i·ta
  —sim′plex′
mel′an·cho′li·ac′

mel′an·chol′ic
mel′an·chol′y
mel′a·ne′mi·a
me·lan′ic
me·lan′i·dro′sis
mel′a·nif′er·ous
mel′a·nin
mel′a·nism
mel′a·nis′tic
mel′a·ni·za′tion
mel′a·nize′, -nized′, -niz′ing
mel′a·no·am′e·lo·blas·
  to′ma *pl.* -mas *or* -ma·ta
mel′a·no·blast′
mel′a·no·blas′tic
mel′a·no·blas·to′ma
  pl. -mas *or* -ma·ta
mel′a·no·car′ci·no′ma
  pl. -mas *or* -ma·ta
mel′a·no·chro′ic
mel′a·no·cyte′
mel′a·no·cyt′ic
mel′a·no·cy·to′ma *pl.* -mas
  or -ma·ta
mel′a·no·cy·to′sis *pl.* -ses′
mel′a·no·derm′
mel′a·no·der′ma
mel′a·no·der′ma·ti′tis
  —tox′i·ca
mel′a·no·der′mi·a
mel′a·no·der′mic
mel′a·no·ep′i·the′li·o′ma
  pl. -mas *or* -ma·ta
mel′a·no·floc′cu·la′tion
me·lan′o·gen
mel′a·no·gen′e·sis *pl.* -ses′
mel′a·no·gen′ic
mel′a·no·glos′si·a
mel′a·noid′
mel′a·no·leu′ko·der′ma
  col′li′
mel′a·no′ma *pl.* -mas *or*
  -ma·ta
  —su′pra·re·na′le′
mel′a·no′ma·to′sis *pl.* -ses′
mel′a·no′ma·tous
mel′a·no·nych′i·a
mel′a·no·phage′
mel′a·no·phore′
mel′a·no·phor′ic
mel′a·no·pla′ki·a
mel′a·nor·rha′gi·a
mel′a·nor·rhag′ic

mel′a·nor·rhe′a
mel′a·no·sar·co′ma
  pl. -mas *or* -ma·ta
mel′a·no·sar·co′ma·to′sis
  pl. -ses′
mel′a·no′sis *pl.* -ses′
  —cir′cum·scrip′ta pre·blas′
    to·ma·to′sa of Du·breuilh′
  —co′li′
  —i′ri·dis
mel′a·no·some′
mel′a·not′ic
mel′a·no·trich′i·a lin′guae′
mel′a·no·trop′ic
mel′a·nu′ri·a
mel′a·nu′ric
me·lar′so·prol′
me·las′ma
me·las′mic
mel′a·to′nin
me·le′na
Me·le′ney ulcer
mel′en·ges′trol′
me·le′nic
mel′e·tin
mel′i·bi′ose′
mel′i·lo·tox′in
mel′i·oi·do′sis *pl.* -ses′
me·lis′sic
mel′i·ten′sis
me·li′tis
mel′i·tra′cen
mel′i·tu′ri·a
mel′i·tu′ric
Mel′kers·son-Ro′sen·thal′
  syndrome
mel·lit′ic
mel′o·di·dy′mi·a
mel′o·did′y·mus
me·lom′e·lus
Me·loph′a·gus
mel′o·plas′ty
mel′o·rhe′os·to′sis *pl.* -ses′
me·los′chi·sis
me·lo′ti·a
me·lo′tus
mel′pha·lan′
Melt′zer-Ly′on test
Melt′zer method
mem′ber
mem·bra′na *pl.* -nae′
  —at·lan′to·oc·cip′i·ta′lis
    anterior

—atlantooccipitalis posterior
—ba·sa′lis duc′tus
sem′i·cir′cu·lar′is
—de·cid′u·a
—de·cid′u·ae′
—e·las′ti·ca la·ryn′gis
—fi′bro·e·las′ti·ca la·ryn′gis
—fi·bro′sa cap′su·lae′ ar·tic′u·lar′is
—gran′u·lo′sa
—hy′a·loi′de·a
—hy′o·thy′re·oi′de·a
—in′ter·cos·ta′lis ex·ter′na
—intercostalis in·ter′na
—in′ter·os′se·a an′te·bra′-chi·i′
—interossea cru′ris
—mu·co′sa na′si′
—ob′tu·ra·to′ri·a
—obturatoria sta·pe′dis
—per′i·ne′i′
—pro′pri·a duc′tus
sem′i·cir′cu·lar′is
—pu′pil·lar′is
—pupillaris per·sis′tens
—qua′dran·gu·lar′is
—re·tic′u·lar′is
—spi·ra′lis
—sta·pe′dis
—stat′o·co′ni·o′rum
mac′u·lar′um
—ster′ni′
—su′pra·pleu·ra′lis
—sy′no·vi·a′lis
—tec·to′ri·a
—tectoria duc′tus
coch′le·ar′is
—thy′ro·hy·oi′de·a
—tym′pa·ni′
—tympani sec′un·dar′i·a
—ves·tib′u·lar′is
—vit′re·a
mem′brane′
mem′bra·nec′to·my
mem′bra′ni·form′
mem′bra·no·car′ti·lag′i·nous
mem′bra·noid
mem′bra·no·pro·lif′er·a·tive
mem′bra·nous

mem′brum *pl.* -bra
—in·fe′ri·us
—mu′li·e′bre′
—su·pe′ri·us
—vi·ri′le′
mem′o·ry
men·ac′me
men′a·di′ol′
men′a·di′one′
men·al′gi·a
me·nar′chal
me·nar′che
Men′del
—reaction
—reflex
Men′del-Bekh·ter′ev sign
Mé′né·trier′ disease
Men′gert index
Men′go virus
men′hi·dro′sis *pl.* -ses′
Mé·nière′ syndrome
me·nin′ge·al
me·nin′ge·or′rha·phy
me·nin′gi·o·blas·to′ma
    pl. -mas *or* -ma·ta
me·nin′gi·o·fi′bro·blas·to′ma *pl.* -mas *or* -ma·ta
me·nin′gi·o′ma *pl.* -mas *or* -ma·ta
me·nin′gi·o·ma·to′sis
me·nin′gi·o·sar·co′ma
    pl. -mas *or* -ma·ta
me·nin′gi·o·the′li·o′ma
    pl. -mas *or* -ma·ta
me·nin′gism
men′in·gis′mus
men′in·git′ic
men′in·gi′tis *pl.* -git′i·des′
—cir′cum·scrip′ta spi·na′lis
—se′ro·sa cir′cum·scrip′ta
—serosa spi·na′lis
me·nin′go·ar·ter·i′tis
me·nin′go·cele′
me·nin′go·ceph′a·li′tis
me·nin′go·cer′e·bral
me·nin′go·cer′e·bri′tis
me·nin′go·coc′cal
me·nin′go·coc·ce′mi·a
me·nin′go·coc′cic
me·nin′go·coc′cus *pl.* -ci′
me·nin′go·cor′ti·cal
me·nin′go·cyte′
me·nin′go·en·ceph′a·lit′ic

me·nin′go·en·ceph′a·li′tis
me·nin′go·en·ceph′a·lo·cele′
me·nin′go·en·ceph′a·lo·my′e·li′tis
me·nin′go·en·ceph′a·lo·my′e·lo·ra·dic′u·lo·neu·ri′tis
me·nin′go·en·ceph′a·lop′a·thy
me·nin′go·fi′bro·blas·to′ma *pl.* -mas *or* -ma·ta
me·nin′go·ma·la′ci·a
me·nin′go·my′e·li′tis
me·nin′go·my′e·lo·cele′
me·nin′go-os′te·o·phle·bi′tis
men′in·gop′a·thy
me·nin′go·ra·chid′i·an
me·nin′go·ra·dic′u·lar
me·nin′go·ra·dic′u·li′tis
me·nin′gor·rha′gi·a
me·nin′gor·rhe′a
men′in·go′sis
me·nin′go·the′li·al
me·nin′go·the′li·o′ma
    pl. -mas *or* -ma·ta
me·nin′go·the′li·om′a·tous
me·nin′go·the′li·um
me·nin′go·vas′cu·lar
men′in·gu′ri·a
me′ninx *pl.* me·nin′ges′
—prim′i·ti′va
me·nis′cal
men·is·cec′to·my
me·nis·ci′ tac′tus
men·is·ci′tis
me·nis·co·cyte′
me·nis·co·cy·to′sis
me·nis·co·fem′o·ral
me·nis·co·tome′
me·nis′cus *pl.* -ci′ *or* -cus·es
—ar·tic′u·lar′is
—lat′er·a′lis
—me′di·a′lis
—tac′tus
Menkes syndrome
Men·nell′ sign
me·noc′tone′
men′o·me′tror·rha′gi·a
men′o·pau′sal
men′o·pause′
men′o·pau′sic

men'o·pla'ni·a
men'or·rha'gi·a
men'or·rhal'gi·a
men'or·rhe'a
men'or·rhe'al
me·nos'che·sis *pl.* -ses'
men'o·sta'si·a
me·nos'ta·sis *pl.* -ses'
men'o·stax'is
men'o·tro'pins
mens
—sa'na in cor'po·re sa'no
men'ses'
men'stru·al
men'stru·ant
men'stru·ate', -at'ed, -at'ing
men'stru·a'tion
men'stru·ous
men'stru·um
men'su·al
men'su·ra'tion
men'tal
men·ta'lis
men·tal'i·ty
men'tal·ly
men·ta'tion
men'thol'
men'tho·late'
men'thyl
men'ti·cide'
men'to·an·te'ri·or
men'to·hy'oid'
men'to·la'bi·al
men'ton'
men'to·pa·ri'e·tal
men'to·pos·te'ri·or
men'tum *pl.* -ta
mep'a·crine'
mep'a·zine'
me·pen'zo·late'
me·per'i·dine'
me·phen'e·sin
meph'en·ox'a·lone'
me·phen'ter·mine'
me·phen'y·to'in
meph'o·bar'bi·tal'
me·piv'a·caine'
me·pred'ni·sone'
me·pro'ba·mate'
mep'ryl·caine'
me·pyr'a·mine'
me·pyr'a·pone'
meq'ui·dox'

me·ral'gi·a
—par'es·thet'i·ca
mer·al'lu·ride'
mer·bro'min
mer·cap'tan'
mer·cap'tide'
mer·cap'tol'
mer·cap'to·mer'in
mer·cap'to·pro'pi·o·nyl·gly'cine'
mer·cap'to·pu'rine'
mer'cap·tu'ric
Mer·ce'des Benz' sign
Mer·cier' bar
mer·cu'ri·al
mer·cu'ri·al·ism
mer·cu'ric
mer·cu'ro·phyl'line'
mer·cu'rous
mer'cu·ry
mer'er·ga'si·a
mer'er·gas'tic
mer'eth·ox'yl·line'
me·rid'i·an
me·rid'i·a'ni' bul'bi' oc'u·li'
me·rid'i·a'nus *pl.* -ni'
me·rid'i·o·nal
Mer'in·di·no procedure
mer'i·sis *pl.* -ses'
mer'i·spore'
Mer'kel
—disk
—filtrum
mer'o·a·cra'ni·a
mer'o·blas'tic
mer'o·crine
me·roc'ri·nous
mer'o·di·a·stol'ic
mer'o·en·ceph'a·ly
mer'o·gen'e·sis *pl.* -ses'
mer'o·ge·net'ic
mer'o·gon'ic
me·rog'o·ny
mer'o·me'li·a
mer'o·mi'cro·so'mi·a
mer'o·my'o·sin
me·ro'pi·a
mer'o·ra·chis'chi·sis
pl. -ses'
me·ros'mi·a
mer'o·some'
me·rot'o·my
mer'o·zo'ite'

mer'sa·lyl
mer'y·cism
Merz'bach'er-Pel'i·zae'us disease
me'sad'
me·sal'a·mine'
mes'a·me'boid'
mes·an'gi·al
mes·an'gi·um
mes·a·or·ti'tis
mes·ar·ter·i'tis
me·sat'i·ce·phal'ic
me·sat'i·pel'lic
me·sat'i·pel'vic
mes·ax'on'
mes'cal'
mes'ca·line'
mes'ec'to·derm'
mes·en'ce·phal'ic
mes·en·ceph'a·li'tis
mes·en·ceph'a·lon'
mes·en·ceph'a·lot'o·my
mes·en'chy·ma
mes·en'chy·mal
mes·en'chyme'
mes·en'chy·mo'ma
pl. -mas *or* -ma·ta
mes·en'ter·ec'to·my
mes·en'ter·ic
mes·en'ter·i·co·mes'o·co'lic
mes·en'ter·i·o'lum *pl.* -la
—pro·ces'sus ver'mi·for'mis
mes·en'ter·i·o·pex'y
mes·en'ter·i·or'rha·phy
mes·en'ter·i·pli·ca'tion
mes·en'ter·i'tis
mes·en'te'ri·um *pl.* -ri·a
—com·mu'ne'
—dor·sa'le' com·nu'ne'
mes·en'ter·on'
mes·en'ter·y
mes·en'to·derm'
mes·en'tor'rha·phy
mesh
mesh'work'
me'si·ad'
me'si·al
me'si·al·ly
me'si·o·buc'cal
me'si·o·buc'co·oc·clu'sal
me'si·o·cer'vi·cal
me'si·o·clu'sion
me'si·o·dens'

me′si·o·dis′tal
me′si·o·gin′gi·val
me′si·o·gres′sion
me′si·o·in·ci′sal
me′si·o·la′bi·al
me′si·o·lin′gual
me′si·o·lin′guo·in·ci′sal
me′si·o·lin′guo·oc·clu′sal
me′si·on′
me′si·o·oc·clu′sal
me′si·o·oc·clu′sion
me′si·o·pul′pal
me′si·o·ver′sion
mes′i′ris
mes′mer·ism
mes′na
mes′o·ap·pen′di·ce′al
mes′o·ap·pen′di·ci′tis
mes′o·ap·pen′dix
   pl. -dix·es *or* di·ces′
mes′o·bil′i·ru·bin′o·gen
mes′o·bil′i·vi·o′lin
mes′o·blast′
mes′o·blas·te′ma
mes′o·blas·tem′ic
mes′o·blas′tic
mes′o·bran′chi·al
mes′o·bron·chi′tis
mes′o·car′di·a *pl.* -ae′ *or* -as
mes′o·car′di·um
mes′o·car′pal
mes′o·ce′cal
mes′o·ce′cum
mes′o·ce·phal′ic
mes′o·ceph′a·lon
mes′o·ceph′a·ly
mes′o·col′ic
mes′o·co′lon
  —as·cen′dens
  —de·scen′dens
  —sig·moi′de·um
  —trans·ver′sum
mes′o·co·lon′ic
mes′o·co′lo·pex′y
mes′o·co′lo·pli·ca′tion
mes′o·conch′
mes′o·cord′
mes′o·cor′ne·a
mes′o·cra′ni·al
mes′o·cu′ne·i·form′
mes′o·cyst′
mes′o·cy·to′ma *pl.* -mas *or*
  -ma·ta

mes′o·derm′
mes′o·der′mal
mes′o·der′mic
mes′o·di·a·stol′ic
mes′o·dont′
mes′o·du′o·de′nal
mes′o·du′o·de′num *pl.* -na
  or -nums
mes′o·ep′i·did′y·mis *pl.*
  -mi·des′
mes′o·e·soph′a·gus
mes′o·gas′ter
mes′o·gas′tric
mes′o·gas′tri·um *pl.* -tri·a
mes′o·gle′a
me·sog′li·a
mes′o·gli·o′ma *pl.* -mas *or*
  -ma·ta
mes′o·glu′te·al
mes′o·glu′te·us *pl.* -te·i′
mes′og·nath′ic
mes′og·na′thi·on′
me·sog′na·thous
mes′o·il′e·um *pl.* -e·a
mes′o·je·ju′num *pl.* -na
mes′o·lec′i·thal
mes′o·mere′
mes′o·me·tri′um *pl.* -tri·a
mes′o·morph′
mes′o·mor′phic
mes′o·mor′phy
mes′on
mes′o·na′sal
mes′o·neph′ric
mes′o·neph′roid′
mes′o·ne·phro′ma *pl.* -mas
  or -ma·ta
  —o·var′i·i′
mes′o·neph′ron
mes′o·neph′ros′
  pl. -neph′roi′
mes′o·pex′y
mes′o·phile′
mes′o·phil′ic
mes′o·phle·bi′tis
me·soph′ry·on′ *pl.* -ry·a
me·so′pi·a
me·sop′ic
mes′o·por′phy·rin
mes′o·pro·sop′ic
mes′o·pul′mo·num
me·sor′chi·um *pl.* -chi·a
mes′o·rec′tum

mes′o·rid′a·zine′
mes′o·rop′ter
mes·or′rha·phy
mes′or·rhine′
mes′o·sal·pin′ge·al
mes′o·sal′pinx
  pl. -sal·pin′ges′
mes′o·scap′u·la *pl.* -lae′ *or*
  -las
mes′o·seme′
mes′o·sig′moid′
mes′o·some′
mes′o·ster′num *pl.* -nums *or*
  -na
mes′o·struc′ture
mes′o·sys·tol′ic
mes′o·ten·din′e·um
mes′o·ten′don
mes′o·the′li·al
mes′o·the′li·o′ma *pl.* -mas
  or -ma·ta
mes′o·the′li·um *pl.* -li·a
mes′o·the′nar′
mes′o·tho′ri·um
mes′o·tron′
mes′o·var′i·um *pl.* -i·a
mes′sen·ger
mes′tra·nol′
mes′u·prine′
mes′y·late′
me·tab′a·sis *pl.* -ses′
met′a·bi·o′sis
met′a·bi·sul′fite′
met′a·bol′ic
me·tab′o·lim′e·ter
me·tab′o·lism
me·tab′o·lite′
me·tab′o·liz′a·ble
me·tab′o·lize′, -lized′, -liz′ing
met′a·bu·teth′a·mine′
met′a·bu·tox′y·caine′
met′a·car′pal
met′a·car·pec′to·my
met′a·car′po·pha·lan′ge·al
met′a·car′pus *pl.* -pi′
met′a·cen′tric
met′a·cer·car′i·a *pl.* -ae′
met′a·chro·ma′si·a
met′a·chro·mat′ic
met′a·chro′ma·tism
met′a·chro′mo·phil
met′a·coele′
met′a·cone′

met'a·co'nid
met'a·cre'sol'
met'a·cy'e·sis *pl.* -ses'
met'a·gen'e·sis *pl.* -ses'
met'a·ge·net'ic
met'a·gen'ic
met'ag·glu'ti·nin
met'a·glob'u·lin
Met'a·gon'i·mus
—o·va'tus
—yo·ko'ga'wai
met'a·gran'u·lo·cyte'
met'a·he'mo·glo'bin
met'al
me·tal'lic
me·tal'lo·en'zyme
met'al·loid'
me·tal'lo·phil'i·a
me·tal'lo·pro'tein
met'a·mere'
met'a·mer'ic
me·tam'er·ism
met'a·mor'phic
met'a·mor·phop'si·a
met'a·mor'phose', -phosed',
   -phos'ing
met'a·mor'pho·sis *pl.* -ses'
met'a·my'e·lo·cyte'
met'a·neph'ric
met'a·neph'rine'
met'a·neph'ro·gen'ic
met'a·neph'ron'
met'a·neph'ros'
   pl. -neph'roi'
met'a·phase'
met'a·phor'ic *or*
   met'a·phor'i·cal
met'a·phos·phor'ic
met'a·phre'ni·a
me·taph'y·se'al
me·taph'y·sis *pl.* -ses'
me·taph'y·si'tis
met'a·pla'si·a
me·tap'la·sis
met'a·plasm
met'a·plas'tic
met'a·pneu·mon'ic
met'a·poph'y·sis
met'a·pro'tein'
met'a·pro·ter'e·nol'
met'a·psy·chol'o·gy
met'a·ram'i·nol'
met'a·rho·dop'sin

met'ar·te'ri·ole'
met'a·ru'bri·cyte'
met'a·sta'ble
me·tas'ta·sec'to·my
me·tas'ta·sis *pl.* -ses'
me·tas'ta·size', -sized',
   -siz'ing
met'a·stat'ic
Met'a·stron'gy·lus a'pri
met'a·tar'sal
met'a·tar·sal'gi·a
met'a·tar·sec'to·my
met'a·tar'so·pha·lan'ge·al
met'a·tar'sus *pl.* -si'
   —ad·duc'to·var'us
   —ad·duc'tus
   —pri'mus var'us
   —var'us
met'a·thal'a·mus
me·tath'e·sis *pl.* -ses'
met'a·thet'ic
met'a·throm'bin
met'a·troph'ic
me·tax'a·lone'
Met'a·zo'a
met'a·zo'an
met'a·zo'nal
Metch'ni·koff' theory
me·te'cious
met'em·pir'ic
met'en·ce·phal'ic
met'en·ceph'a·lon'
me'te·or·ism
me'ter *also* metre
me'te·or·o·path'o·log'ic
me'te·or·o·pa·thol'o·gy
me'te·or·op'a·thy
me'te·or·o·re·sis'tant
me'te·or·o·sen'si·tive
me'te·or·o·trop'ic
me'te·or·ot'ro·pism
me·tes'trus
met'for'min
meth'a·cho'line'
meth·ac'ry·late'
meth'a·cy'cline'
meth'a·done'
meth·al·le·nes'tril
meth'al·thi'a·zide'
meth'am·phet'a·mine'
meth·an'dri·ol'
meth·an'dro·sten'o·lone'
meth'ane'

meth'a·no'gen'
meth'a·no·gen'ic
meth'a·no·gen'e·sis *pl.* -ses'
meth'a·nol'
meth·an'the·line'
meth'a·pyr'i·lene'
meth'a·qua'lone'
meth·ar'bi·tal'
meth'a·zol'a·mide'
meth·dil'a·zine'
met'hem·al·bu'min
met'hem·al·bu'mi·ne'mi·a
met'heme'
met·he'mo·glo'bin
met·he'mo·glo'bin·e'mi·a
met·he'mo·glo'bi·nu'ri·a
me·the'na·mine'
meth'ene'
meth·et'o·in
meth'i·cil'lin
meth·im'a·zole'
meth'ine'
me·thi'o·dal'
me·thi'o·nine'
me·this'a·zone'
me·thix'ene'
meth'o·car'ba·mol'
meth'od
meth'od·ol'o·gy
meth'o·hex'i·tal'
meth'o·ma'ni·a
meth'o·pho'line'
meth'o·trex'ate'
meth'o·tri·mep'ra·zine'
me·thox'a·mine'
me·thox'sa·len
me·thox'y·flu'rane'
me·thox'y·phen'a·mine'
meth·sco·pol'a·mine'
meth·sux'i·mide'
meth'y·clo·thi'a·zide'
meth'yl
   —an'thra·nil'ate'
   —meth·ac'ryl·ate'
meth'yl·a·cet'y·lene'
meth'yl·al'
meth'yl·am'ine'
meth'yl·am·phet'a·mine'
meth'yl·ate'
meth'yl·a'tion
meth'yl·at'ro·pine'
meth'yl·benz'e·tho'ni·um
meth'yl·cel'lu·lose'

meth'yl·do'pa
meth'yl·do'pate'
meth'yl·ene'
meth'yl·en'o·phil'
meth'yl·e·noph'i·lous
meth'yl·er'go·no'vine'
meth'yl·glu'ca·mine'
meth'yl·gly·ox'al'
meth'yl·hex·ane·a·mine'
meth'yl·ma·lon'ic·ac'i·du'-
ri·a
meth'yl·mer·cap'tan'
meth'yl·mor'phine'
meth'yl·par'a·fy'nol'
meth'yl·phen'i·date'
meth'yl·phe'no·bar'bi·tal'
meth'yl·phe'nol'
meth'yl·phe'nyl·suc·cin'i·
mide'
meth'yl·pred·nis'o·lone'
meth'yl·pu'rine'
meth'yl·tes·tos'ter·one'
meth'yl·thi'o·u'ra·cil
meth'yl·trans'fer·ase'
meth'yl·xan'thine'
meth'y·pry'lon'
meth'y·ser'gide'
me·ti'a·pine'
met·my'o·glo'bin
met'o·clo·pram'ide'
met'o·cu'rine'
me·to'la·zone'
me·ton'y·my
me·top'ic
met'o·pim'a·zine'
me·to'pi·on'
met'o·pism
me·to'pro·lol'
met'o·qui·zine'
me·tox'e'nous
me·tox'e·ny
me·tral'gi·a
me·tra·to'ni·a
me·tra·tro'phi·a
me'tre *var. of* meter
me'trec·ta'si·a
me'trec'to·my
me'trec·to'pi·a
me·tre'mi·a
me'treu·ryn'ter
me·treu'ry·sis *pl.* -ses'
me'tri·a
met'ric

met'ri·o·ce·phal'ic
me·trit'ic
me·tri'tis
me·triz'a·mide'
me'tro·cele'
me'tro·col'po·cele'
me'tro·cys·to'sis *pl.* -ses'
me'tro·cyte'
me'tro·dyn'i·a
me'tro·ec·ta'si·a
me'tro·en'do·me·tri'tis
me'tro·fi·bro'ma *pl.* -mas *or*
-ma·ta
me'tro·leu'kor·rhe'a
me·trol'o·gy
me'tro·lym'phan·gi'tis
me'tro·ma·la'ci·a
me'tro·ni'da·zole'
me'tro·pa·ral'y·sis *pl.* -ses'
me'tro·path'i·a hem'or·
rhag'i·ca
me'tro·path'ic
me·trop'a·thy
me'tro·per'i·to·ne'al
me'tro·per'i·to·ni'tis
me'tro·pex'y
me'tro·phle·bi'tis
me'tro·plas'ty
me'trop·to'sis *pl.* -ses'
me'tror·rha'gi·a
me'tror·rhe'a
me'tror·rhex'is
me'tro·sal'pin·gi'tis
me'tro·sal'pin·gog'ra·phy
me'tro·scope'
me'tro·stax'is
me'tro·ste·no'sis *pl.* -ses'
me·trot'o·my
Mett method
met'u·re·dep'a
me·tyr'a·pone'
me·ty'ro·sine'
Meu'len·gracht'
—diet
—method
mev'a·lon'ic
mex·il'e·tin'
Mey'er
—loop
—operation
—system
Mey'nert
—bundle

—commissure
Mey·net' nodes
mez'lo·cil'lin
Mi·an'a fever
mi·an'ser·in
Mi·bel'li
—angiokeratoma
—disease
mi'ca
mi·ca'ceous
mi'ca·to'sis *pl.* -ses'
mi·celle'
Mi·chae'lis
—constant
—stain
Mi·chae'lis-Gut'mann
bodies
Mi'chel flecks
Mi·che'li syndrome
mi·con'a·zole'
mi'cra·cous'tic
mi·cran'gi·um
mi'cren·ceph'a·lon'
mi'cren·ceph'a·lous
mi'cren·ceph'a·ly
mi'cro·ab'scess'
mi'cro·ad'e·no'ma *pl.* -mas
or -ma·ta
mi'cro·ad'e·nop'a·thy
mi'cro·aer'o·phil
mi'cro·aer'o·phil'ic
mi'cro·a·nal'y·sis *pl.* -ses'
mi'cro·an·a·lyt'ic *or*
mi'cro·an·a·lyt'i·cal
mi'cro·an·a·tom'ic *or*
mi'cro·an·a·tom'i·cal
mi'cro·a·nat'o·mist
mi'cro·a·nat'o·my
mi'cro·an'eu·rysm
mi'cro·an·gi·o·graph'ic
mi'cro·an·gi·og'ra·phy
mi'cro·an·gi·o·path'ic
mi'cro·an·gi·op'a·thy
mi'cro·an·gi·o·scop'ic
mi'cro·an·gi·os'co·py
mi'cro·ar·te'ri·o·gram'
mi'cro·ar·te'ri·o·graph'ic
mi'cro·ar·te'ri·og'ra·phy
mi'cro·au'di·phone'
mi'cro·bac·te'ri·um
mi'cro·bal'ance
mi'cro·bar'
mi'crobe'

mi·cro′bi·al
mi·cro′bi·an
mi·cro′bic
mi·cro′bi·cid′al
mi·cro′bi·cide′
mi·cro·bi′o·log′ic *or*
  mi·cro·bi′o·log′i·cal
mi′cro·bi′o·log′i·cal·ly
mi′cro·bi·ol′o·gist
mi′cro·bi·ol′o·gy
mi′cro·bi·ot′ic
mi′crob·ism
mi′cro·blast′
mi′cro·ble·phar′i·a
mi′cro·bleph′a·rism
mi′cro·bleph′a·ron′
mi′cro·bleph′a·ry
mi′cro·bod′y
mi′cro·bra′chi·a
mi′cro·bra′chi·us
mi′cro·bren′ner
mi′cro·bub′ble
mi′cro·bu·ret′
mi′cro·cal′ci·fi·ca′tion
mi′cro·cal′cu·lus *pl.* -li′
mi′cro·cal′o·rie
mi′cro·cal′o·rim′e·try
mi′cro·cap′su·lar
mi′cro·cap′sule
mi′cro·car′di·a
mi′cro·car′di·us
mi′cro·cau′li·a
mi′cro·cav′i·ta′tion
mi′cro·cen′trum
mi′cro·ce·pha′li·a
mi′cro·ce·phal′ic
mi′cro·ceph′a·lism
mi′cro·ceph′a·lous
mi′cro·ceph′a·lus *pl.* -li′
mi′cro·ceph′a·ly
mi′cro·chei′li·a
mi′cro·chei′lus
mi′cro·chei′ri·a
mi′cro·chei′rus
mi′cro·chem′i·cal
mi′cro·chem′is·try
mi′cro·cin′e·mat′o·graph′ic
mi′cro·cin′e·ma·tog′ra·phy
mi′cro·cir′cu·la′tion
mi′cro·cir′cu·la·to′ry
mi′cro·cli′mate
Mi′cro·coc·ca′ce·ae′
mi′cro·coc′cal

mi′cro·coc′cus *pl.* -ci′
Mi′cro·coc′cus
—al′bus
—au′re·us
—cat′ar·rha′lis
—cit′re·us
—ga·zog′e·nes′
—gon′or·rhe′ae′
—in′tra·cel′lu·lar′is
  men′in·git′i·dis
—lan′ce·o·la′tus
—mel′i·ten′sis
—men′in·git′i·dis
—par′vu·lus
—pneu·mo′ni·ae′
—py′og′e·nes′
—te·trag′e·nus
mi′cro·co′lon
mi′cro·col′o·ny
mi′cro·co·nid′i·um *pl.* -i·a
mi′cro·co′ri·a
mi′cro·cor′ne·a
mi′cro·cou′lomb
mi′cro·cous′tic
mi′cro·cra′ni·a
mi′cro·crys′tal·line′
mi′cro·cul′tur·al
mi′cro·cul′ture
mi′cro·cu′rie
mi′cro·cu′rie-hour′
mi′cro·cyst′
mi′cro·cys′tic
mi′cro·cy′tase′
mi′cro·cyte′
mi′cro·cy·the′mi·a
mi′cro·cy·the′mic
mi′cro·cyt′ic
mi′cro·cy·to′sis
mi′cro·dac·tyl′i·a
mi′cro·dac′ty·lous
mi′cro·dac′ty·ly
mi′cro·dis·sec′tion
mi′cro·dont′
mi′cro·don′ti·a
mi′cro·dont′ism
mi′cro·drep′a·no·cyt′ic
mi′cro·drep′a·no·cy·to′sis
mi′cro·e·col′o·gy
mi′cro·e′co·sys′tem
mi′cro·e·lec′trode′
mi′cro·e·lec′tro·pho·re′sis
  pl. -ses′
mi′cro·e·lec′tro·pho·ret′ic

mi′cro·em′bo·lus *pl.* -li′
mi′cro·en·ceph′a·ly
mi′cro·e·ryth′ro·cyte′
mi′cro·far′ad′
mi′cro·fau′na
mi′cro·fi′bril
mi′cro·fib′ril·lar
mi′cro·fi·bro·ad′e·no′ma
  pl. -mas *or* -ma·ta
mi′cro·fiche′
mi′cro·fil′a·ment
mi′cro·fil′a·re′mi·a
mi′cro·fi·lar′i·a *pl.* -i·ae′
mi′cro·fi·lar′i·al
mi′cro·flo′ra
mi′cro·fo′cal
mi′cro·fo′cus
mi′cro·fol·lic′u·lar
mi′cro·frac′ture
mi′cro·gam′ete′
mi′cro·ga·me′to·cyte′
mi′crog′a·my
mi′cro·gas′tri·a
mi′cro·gen′e·sis
mi′cro·ge′ni·a
mi′cro·gen′i·tal·ism
mi′crog′li·a
mi′crog′li·al
mi′crog′li·o·cyte′
mi′crog′li·o·ma *pl.* -mas *or*
  -ma·ta
mi′crog′li·o·ma·to′sis
  pl. -ses′
mi′cro·glob′u·lin
mi′cro·glob′u·lin·e′mi·a
mi′cro·glos′si·a
mi′cro·gna′thi·a
mi′cro·gnath′ic
mi′crog′na·thous
mi′cro·go′ni·o·scope′
mi′cro·gram′
mi′cro·graph′
mi′cro·graph′ic
mi′crog′ra·phy
mi′cro·gy′ri·a
mi′cro·gy′rus
mi′cro·he·pat′i·a
mi′cro·hertz′
mi′crohm′
mi′cro·in·cin′er·a′tion
mi′cro·in′farct′
mi′cro·in·jec′tion
mi′cro·in·jec′tor

mi'cro·in·va'sion
mi'cro·ker'a·tome'
mi'cro·len'ti·a
mi'cro·le'sion
mi'cro·leu·ko·blast'
mi'cro·li'ter
mi'cro·lith'
mi'cro·li·thi'a·sis
—al've·o·lar'is pul·mo'-
num
mi'cro·ma'ni·a
mi'cro·ma·nip'u·la'tion
mi'cro·ma·nip'u·la'tor
mi'cro·ma·nom'e·ter
mi'cro·mas'ti·a
mi'cro·max·il'la *pl.* -lae' *or*
-las
mi'cro·ma'zi·a
mi'cro·me·le'na
mi'cro·me'li·a
mi'cro·mel'ic
mi·crom'e·lus
mi'cro·mere'
mi'cro·me·tas'ta·sis *pl.* -ses'
mi·crom'e·ter
mi·crom'e·try
mi'cro·mi'cron'
mi'cro·mil'li·gram'
mi'cro·mo'to·scope'
mi'cro·move'ment
mi'cro·my·e'li·a
mi'cro·my'e·lo·blast'
mi'cro·my'e·lo·blas'tic
mi'cro·my'e·lo·lym'pho·
cyte'
mi'cron' *pl.* -crons' *or* -cra
mi'cro·nee'dle
mi'cron'e·mous
mi'cro·nod'u·lar
mi'cro·nod'u·la'tion
mi'cro·nu'cle·us *pl.* -cle·i'
mi'cro·nu'tri·ent
mi'cro·nych'i·a
mi'cro·or'chism
mi'cro·or·gan'ic
mi'cro·or'gan·ism
mi'cro·pap'u·lar
mi'cro·par'a·site'
mi'cro·pa·thol'o·gy
mi'cro·pe'nis
mi'cro·per·fu'sion
mi'cro·phage'

mi'cro·pha'ki·a
mi'cro·phal'lus
mi'cro·pho'bi·a
mi'cro·phone'
mi'cro·pho'ni·a
mi'cro·pho'no·graph'
mi'cro·pho'no·scope'
mi'cro·pho'to·graph'
mi'cro·pho'to·graph'ic
mi'cro·pho·tog'ra·phy
mi'croph·thal'mi·a
mi'croph·thal'mic
mi'croph·thal'mos'
mi'croph·thal'mus
mi'cro·phys'ics
mi'cro·pi·a
mi'cro·pi·pet'
mi'cro·pla'si·a
mi'cro·pleth'ys·mog'ra·
phy
mi'cro·po'di·a
mi·crop'o·dy
mi'cro·po·lar'i·scope'
mi'cro·probe'
mi'cro·pro·jec'tion
mi'cro·pro·so'pi·a
mi'cro·pro·so'pus
mi'cro·pros'o·py
mi·crop'si·a
mi·crop'tic
mi'cro·punc'ture
mi'cro·pus
mi'cro·pyk·nom'e·ter
mi'cro·pyle'
mi'cro·ra'di·o·graph'
mi'cro·ra'di·o·graph'ic
mi'cro·ra'di·og'ra·phy
mi'cror·chid'i·a
mi'cro·re·frac·tom'e·ter
mi'cro·res·pi·rom'e·ter
mi'cro·res·pi·ro·met'ric
mi'cror·rhi'ni·a
mi'cro·scel'ous
mi'cro·scope'
mi'cro·scop'ic *or*
mi'cro·scop'i·cal
mi'cro·scop'i·cal·ly
mi·cros'co·pist
mi·cros'co·py
mi'cro·sec'ond
mi'cro·sec'tion
mi'cros·mat'ic
mi'cro·so'mal

mi'cro·so'ma·tog·no'si·a
mi'cro·some'
mi'cro·so'mi·a
mi'cro·spec·trog'ra·phy
mi'cro·spec'tro·pho·tom'e·
try
mi'cro·spec'tro·scope'
mi'cro·sphe'ro·cyte'
mi'cro·sphe'ro·cy·to'sis
mi'cro·sphyg'mi·a
mi'cro·sphyg'my
mi'cro·splanch'nic
mi'cro·sple'ni·a
mi'cro·splen'ic
mi'cro·sponge'
mi'cro·spor'id
Mi'cro·spo·rid'i·a
mi'cro·spo·ro'sis *pl.* -ses'
Mi·cros'po·rum
—au'dou'i·ni'
—ca'nis
—fur'fur
—gyp'se·um
—la'no'sum
—mi'nu·tis'si·mus
mi'cro·steth'o·phone'
mi'cro·steth'o·scope'
mi'cro·sto'mi·a
mi'cro·sur'ger·y
mi'cro·sur'gi·cal
mi'cro·sy·ringe'
mi'cro·the'li·a
mi'cro·ti·a
mi'cro·ti'tri·met'ric
mi'cro·ti·trim'e·try
mi'cro·tome'
mi'cro·tom'ic *or*
mi'cro·tom'i·cal
mi·crot'o·my
mi'cro·to·nom'e·ter
mi'cro·to·pos'co·py
mi'cro·trans·fu'sion
mi'cro·trau'ma
mi'cro·tu'bu·lar
mi'cro·tu'bule'
mi'cro·u'nit
mi'cro·vas'cu·lar
mi'cro·vas'cu·la·ture
mi'cro·vil'lus *pl.* -li'
mi'cro·volt'
mi'cro·wave'
mi·crox'y·cyte'
mi·crox'y·phil

mi'cro·zo'on' *pl.* -zo'a
mi'cro·zo'o·sper'mi·a
mi'crur·gy
Mi'cru·roi'des
   eu'ry·ox·an'thus
Mi'cru'rus ful'vi·us
mic'tion
mic'tu·rate', -rat'ed, -rat'ing
mic'tu·ri'tion
mid'ab·dom'i·nal
mi'da·flur'
mid'ax·il'la
mid·ax'il·lar'y
mi·daz'o·lam
mid'bod'y
mid'brain'
mid·car'pal
mid·cir'cum·flex'
mid'cla·vic'u·lar
mid'di'a·stol'ic
mid'ep·i·gas'tric
mid'e·soph'a·ge'al
mid'e·soph'a·gus
mid'fe·mur
mid'foot'
mid·fron'tal
midge
midg'et
mid'gut'
mid'head'
mid·lat'er·al
mid'life'
mid'line'
mid'oc·cip'i·tal
mid'pain'
mid·pal'mar
mid'pa·tel'lar
mid'plane'
mid'riff
mid·sag'it·tal
mid'sec'tion
mid'shaft'
mid·ster'nal
mid·tar'sal
mid'thigh'
mid·ven'tral
mid·ves'i·cal
mid'wife'
mid'wife'ry
Mie'scher
   —granuloma
   —tubes
mi·fe'pri·stone'

Mi'gnon' delusion
mi'graine'
mi'grain·oid'
mi'grain·ous
mi'grant
mi'grate', -grat'ed, -grat'ing
mi·gra'tion
mi'gra·to'ry
Mik'u·licz
   —angle
   —cell
   —disease
   —operation
mil
mil·am'me'ter
Mi·lan'-Mark'ley technique
Milch operation
mil'dew'
Miles operation
mile'stones'
Mil'i·an
   —erythema
   —sign
mil'i·ar'i·a
   —crys'tal·li'na
   —pro·fun'da
   —pus'tu·lo'sa
mil'i·ar'y
mi·lieu' *pl.* -lieux' *or* -lieus'
   —ex·té'rieur'
   —in·té'rieur'
mil'i·per'tine'
mil'i·tate'
mil'i·um *pl.* -i·a
milk
Milk'man' syndrome
Mil'lar asthma
Mil'lard-Gub'ler syndrome
mil'li·am'me'ter
mil'li·am'pere'
mil'li·bar'
mil'li·cu'rie
mil'li·e·quiv'a·lent
mil'li·gram'
mil'li·joule'
Mil'li·kan rays
mil'li·li'ter
mil'li·me'ter
mil'li·mi'cro·cu'rie
mil'li·mi'cro·gram'
mil'li·mi'cron'
mil'li·mi'cro·sec'ond
mil'li·mol'

mil'li·mo'lar
mil'li·os'mol'
mil'li·rad'
mil'li·roent'gen
mil'li·sec'ond
mil'li·u'nit
mil'li·volt'
Mil'lon reagent
Mills
   —disease
   —test
mil'phae'
mil·pho'sis
mil'ri·none'
Mil'roy
   —disease
   —edema
Mil'ton edema
Mil'ton-Quinck'e edema
mim'bane'
mi·me'sis
mi·met'ic
mim'ic
mim'ic·ry
mim·ma'tion
Min·a·ma'ta disease
mind
min'er·al
min'er·al·i·za'tion
min'er·al·o·cor'ti·coid'
min'i·lap'a·ro·scope'
min'i·lap'a·ros'co·py
min'im
min'i·mal
min'i·mal·ly
min'i·mum *pl.* -ma
   —cog'no·scib'i·le'
   —dis'cer·nib'i·le'
   —le·gib'i·le'
   —sep'a·rab'i·le'
   —vi·sib'i·le'
Min·kow'ski-Chauf·fard'
   syndrome
Min'ne·so'ta Mul'ti·pha'-
   sic Per'son·al'i·ty In'ven·
   to'ry
min'o·cy'cline'
mi·nom'e·ter
mi'nor
Mi'nor
   —disease
   —sign
   —tremor

Mi'not-Mur'phy diet
mi·nox'i·dil
mi'o·car'di·a
mi'o·did'y·mus
mi'o·lec'i·thal
mi'o·pus
mi·o'sis *(contraction of the pupil of the eye)*, *pl.* -ses'
  ♦ *meiosis*
mi·ot'ic
Mi·rault' operation
mire
mir'ror
mir·ya'chit
mis'ad·min'i·stra'tion
mis·an'thrope'
mis·an'throp'ic
mis·an'thro·py
mis·car'riage
mis·car'ry, -ried, -ry·ing
mis'ce
mis·ce·ge·na'tion
mis'ci·bil'i·ty
mis'ci·ble
mis·di·ag·nose'
mis·di·ag·no'sis *pl.* -ses'
mis'o·cai'ne·a
mi·sog'a·mist
mi·sog'a·my *(aversion to marriage)*
  ♦ *misogyny*
mi·sog'y·nist
mi·sog'y·ny *(hatred of women)*
  ♦ *misogamy*
mis'o·lo'gi·a
mis'o·ne'ism
mi'so·nid'a·zole'
mis·o·pe'di·a
mis·o·pros'tol'
miss
mis·sense'
mis·shap'en
Mitch'ell
  —disease
  —osteotomy
mite
mith'ra·my'cin
mith'ri·da'tism
mi'ti·cid'al
mi'ti·cide'
mit'i·gate', -gat'ed, -gat'ing
mit'i·ga'tion
mi'tis

mi'to·chon'dri·a *sing.*
  -dri·on
mi'to·chon'dri·al
mi'to·chon'dri·on' *pl.* -dri·a
mi'to·cro'min
mi'to·gen
mi'to·gen'e·sis *pl.* -ses'
mi'to·ge·net'ic
mi'to·gen'ic
mi'to·gil'lin
mi'to·mal'cin
mi'tome'
mi'to·my'cin
mi'to·plasm
mi·to'sis *pl.* -ses'
mi'to·some'
mi'to·spore'
mi'to·tane'
mi·tot'ic
mi'to·xan'trone'
mi'tral
mi'tral·i·za'tion
mi'troid
Mit·su'da reaction
mit'tel·schmerz'
Mit'ten·dorf' dot
Mit'tle·meir' broach
mix
mix·o·sco'pi·a
mix·o·scop'ic
mix'ture
M'Nagh'ten rule
mne'mas·the'ni·a
mne'mic
mne'mo·der'mi·a
mne·mon'ic
mne·mon'ics
mne'mo·tech'nics
mo'bile
mo·bil'i·ty
mo·bi·li·za'tion
mo'bi·lize', -lized', -liz'ing
Mo'bitz heart block
Mö'bi·us
  —disease
  —sign
  —syndrome
Mö'bi·us-Ley'den
  dystrophy
moc'ca·sin
mod'al
mod'a·line'
mo·dal'i·ty

mode
mod'er·ate', -at'ed, -at'ing
mod'er·a'tor
mod'i·fi·ca'tion
mod'i·fied'
mo·di'o·lus *pl.* -li'
mod'u·la'tion
mod'u·la'tor
mod'u·lus
Moel'ler
  —fluid
  —glossitis
Moel'ler-Bar'low disease
Mo·ë'na anomaly
mog'i·graph'i·a
mog'i·la'li·a
mog'i·pho'ni·a
Mohr salt
Mohs
  —chemosurgery
  —excision
moi'e·ty
mo'lal
mo·lal'i·ty
mo'lar
mo·lar'i·form'
mo·lar'i·ty
mold
mold'y
mole
mo·lec'to·my
mo·lec'u·lar
mol'e·cule'
mo·li'men *pl.* -lim'i·na
mo·lin'a·zone'
mo·lin'done'
Mo'lisch test
Mol'la·ret' meningitis
Mol'ler test
Moll glands
mol·li'ti·es'
  —os'si·um
Mol·lus'ca
mol·lus'cum
  —con·ta'gi·o'sum
  —ep'i·the'li·a'le'
  —fi'bro'sum
  —se·ba'ce·um
mol'lusk
Mo·lo'ney test
mol·si·do'mine'
molt *also* moult
mo·lyb'date'

mo·lyb′de·no′sis
mo·lyb′de·num
mo·lyb′dic
mo·lyb′dous
mo′ment
mo·men′tum
mo·met′a·sone′
mo′nad′
Mon′a·kow′
  —bundle
  —nucleus
  —striae
  —syndrome
Mo·nal′di drainage
mon·am′ide′
mon·am′ine′
mon·ar′thric
mon′ar·thri′tis
mon′ar·tic′u·lar
mon·as′ter
mon′ath·e·to′sis *pl.* -ses′
mon′a·tom′ic
mon·au′ral
mon′ax·on′ic
Mönck′e·berg′
  arteriosclerosis
Mon·dor′
  —disease
  —syndrome
mo·nen′sin
mon′es·thet′ic
mon′es·trous
Mon′ge disease
mon′gol·ism
mon′gol·oid′
mo·nil′e·thrix′
Mo·nil′i·a
mo·nil′i·al
Mo·nil′i·a′les′
mon′i·li·a·sis *pl.* -ses′
mo·nil′i·id
mo·nil′i·form′
Mo·nil′i·for′mis
mo′nism
mon′i·tor
Mo·niz′ sign
mon′key
Mon′ne·ret′ pulse
mon′o·am′ine
mon′o·ar·tic′u·lar
mon′o·az′o
mon′o·bac′tam
mon′o·bal′lism

mon′o·ba′sic
mon′o·ben′zone′
mon′o·blast′
mon′o·blep′si·a
mon′o·blep′sis
mon′o·bra′chi·a
mon′o·bra′chi·us
mon′o·bro′mat′ed
mon′o·car′box·yl′ic
mon′o·car′di·an
mon′o·cel′lu·lar
mon′o·ceph′a·lus *pl.* -li′
mon′o·chord′
mon′o·cho·re′a
mon′o·cho·ri·on′ic
mon′o·chro′ic
mon′o·chro·ma′si·a
mon′o·chro′ma·sy
mon′o·chro′mat′
mon′o·chro·mat′ic
mon′o·chro·ma·tism
mon′o·chro·mat′o·phil′
mon′o·chro′ma·tor
mon′o·chro′mic
mon′o·clo′nal
mon′o·con·tam′i·nate
mon′o·con·tam′i·na′tion
mon′o·cra′ni·us
mon′o·crot′ic
mo·noc′u·lar
mo·noc′u·lus
mon′o·cy·e′sis *pl.* -ses′
mon′o·cys′tic
mon′o·cyte′
mon′o·cyt′ic
mon′o·cy′toid′
mon′o·cy·to′ma *pl.* -mas *or*
  -ma·ta
mon′o·cy′to·pe′ni·a
mon′o·cy·to′sis *pl.* -ses′
mon′o·dac′tyl·ism
mon′o·dac′ty·ly
mon′o·der·mo′ma
mon′o·di·plo′pi·a
mon′o·eth′a·nol′a·mine′
mon′o·fac·to′ri·al
mon′o·fil′a·ment
mo·nog′a·my
mon′o·gas′tric
mon′o·gen′e·sis *pl.* -ses′
mon′o·ge·net′ic
mon′o·gen′ic
mo·nog′e·nous

mon′o·ger′mi·nal
mon′o·graph′
mon′o·hy′brid
mon′o·hy′drate′
mon′o·hy′drat′ed
mon′o·hy′dric
mon′o·i·de′ism
mon′o·i·de·is′tic
mon′o·i·o′do·ty′ro·sine′
mon′o·lay′er
mon′o·lep′sis *pl.* -ses′
mon′o·lob′u·lar
mon′o·loc′u·lar
mon′o·ma′ni·a
mon′o·mas′ti·gote′
mon′o·mel′ic
mon′o·mer
mon′o·mer′ic
mon′o·mo·lec′u·lar
mon′o·mo′ri·a
mon′o·mor′phic
mon′o·mor′phism
mon′o·mor′phous
mon·om′pha·lus
mon′o·my′o·ple′gi·a
mon′o·neph′rous
mon′o·neu′ral
mon′o·neu·ri′tis
mon′o·neu·rop′a·thy
mon′o·nu′cle·ar
mon′o·nu′cle·ate′
mon′o·nu·cle·o′sis *pl.* -ses′
mon′o·nu′cle·o·tide′
mon′o·pa·re′sis *pl.* -ses′
mon′o·par·es·the′si·a
mon′o·path′o·pho′bi·a
mon′o·pha′gi·a
mon′o·pha′si·a
mon′o·pha′sic
mon′o·phe′nol′
mon′o·pho′bi·a
mon′o·phos′phate′
mon′oph·thal′mi·a
mon′oph·thal′mic
mon′oph·thal′mus
mon′o·phy·let′ic
mon′o·phy′le·tism
mon′o·ple′gi·a
  —fa′ci·a′lis
mon′o·ple′gic
mon′o·ploid′
mon′o·po′di·a
mon′o·po′lar

mon'ops'
mo·nop'si·a
mon'o·pty'chi·al
mon'o·pus
mon·or'chid
mon·or'chid·ism
mon·or'chis *pl.* -chi·des
mon·or'chism
mon'o·sac'cha·ride'
mon'o·scel'ous
mon'ose'
mon'o·sex'u·al
mon'o·so'di·um
mon'o·so'ma·tous
mon'o·some'
mon'o·so'mic
mon'o·so'my
mon'o·spasm
Mon'o·spo'ri·um
mon'os·tot'ic
mon'o·stra'tal
mon'o·symp'to·mat'ic
mon'o·sy·nap'tic
mon'o·ter'pene'
mon'o·ther'mi·a
mo·not'ic
mon'o·treme'
mo·not'ri·chate'
mon'o·trich'ic
mo·not'ri·chous
mon'o·trop'ic
mon'o·typ'ic
mon'o·va'lent
mon'o·vu·lar
mon'o·xen'ic
mon·ox'e·nous
mon·ox'ide'
mon'o·zy·got'ic
Mon·ro'
—bursa
—foramen
mons *pl.* mon'tes'
—pu'bis
—ven'er·is
Mon'son curve
mon'ster
mon·stros'i·ty
mon'strum *pl.* -stra
Mon·teg'gi·a fracture
Mon'te·ne'gro test
Mon'ter·caux' fracture
Mont·gom'er·y
—glands

—tubercles
mon·tic'u·lus
Moon molars
moor
Moore
—fracture
—lightning streaks
—syndrome
Moor'en ulcer
Moo'ser
—bodies
—reaction
—test
mo·pi'da·mol'
mo·rale'
mo·ran'tel
Mo'rax-Ax'en·feld'
—bacillus
—conjunctivitis
Mo'rax·el'la
—lac'u·na'ta
mor'bid
mor·bid'i·ty
mor·bif'ic
mor·bil'li'
mor·bil'li·form'
mor'bus *pl.* -bi'
—an'gli·cus
—ca·du'cus
—cae·ru'le·us
—car·di'a·cus
—cas·tren'sis
—coe·li'a·cus
—cor'dis
—cox'ae'
—cu·cul·lar'is
—di·vi'nus
—gal'li·cus
—hem'or·rhag'i·cus
ne'o·na·to'rum
—hun·gar'i·cus
—mac'u·lo'sus ne'o·na·to'-
rum
—maculosus Werl·hof'i·i'
—mag'nus
—major
—med'i·co'rum
—mi·ser'i·ae'
—Pa·get'i' pa·pil'lae'
—phlyc'te·noi'des'
—pu'li·car'is
—re'gi·us
—sa'cer

—sal'ta·to'ri·us
—ve·sic'u·lar'is
—vir·gin'e·us
—vul'pis
mor'cel·la'tion
mor'dant
Mo·rel'
—ear
—syndrome
Mo·rel'-Krae'pe·lin disease
Mo·rel'-Moore' syndrome
Mor·ga'gni
—caruncle
—concha
—crypt
—disease
—foramen
—glands
—hernia
—sinuses
—syndrome
—ventricle
Mor·ga'gni-Ad'ams-
Stokes' syndrome
Mor·ga'gni·an
—cataract
—cyst
—globules
Mor·ga'gni-Stew'art-
Mo·rel' syndrome
Mor'gan bacillus
morgue
mo'ri·a
mor'i·bund
mo·ric'i·zine'
Mor'i·son
—method
—pouch
Mor'i·son-Tal'ma
operation
Mör'ner
—reagent
—test
Mo'ro
—reaction
—reflex
—test
mo'ron'
mor'phe·a *(scleroderma)*
♦ *morphia*
mor'phi·a *(morphine)*
♦ *morphea*
mor'phine'

mor·phin'ic
mor'phin·ism
mor'phi·no·ma'ni·a
mor'pho·bi·om'e·try
mor'pho·gen'e·sis
mor'pho·ge·net'ic
mor'pho·gen'ic
mor·phog'e·ny
mor'pho·line'
mor'pho·log'ic *or*
  mor'pho·log'i·cal
mor'pho·log'i·cal·ly
mor·phol'o·gist
mor·phol'o·gy
mor·phom'e·try
mor·pho'sis *pl.* -ses'
mor'phot'ic
Mor·qui'o
  —dystrophy
  —sign
  —syndrome
Mor·qui'o-Ull'rich
  disease
mor'rhu·ate'
Mor'ris method
mors
  —pu'ta·ti'va
  —su'bi·ta
mor'sal
mor'sel
mor'sel·ize'
mor'sus
  —stom'a·chi'
  —ven·tric'u·li'
mor'tal
mor·tal'i·ty
mor'tal·ly
mor'tar
mor'ti·fi·ca'tion
mor'ti·fy', -fied', -fy'ing
mor'tise
Mor'ton
  —foot
  —metatarsalgia
  —syndrome
  —toe
mor'tu·ar'y
mor'u·la
Mor'van disease
mo·sa'ic
mo·sa'i·cism
Mosch'co·witz'
  —disease

—operation
—test
Mo'sen·thal' test
mos·qui'to *pl.* -toes *or* -tos
Mos'se syndrome
Moss groups
Moss'man fever
Mo'tais' operation
moth'er
mo'tile
mo·til'i·ty
mo'tion
mo'ti·vate'
mo'ti·va'tion
mo'ti·va'tion·al
mo'ti·va'tion·al·ly
mo'tive
mo'to·neu'ron'
mo'to·neu'ro·ni'tis
mo'tor
mo·to'ri·al
mo·tor'ic
mo·to'ri·us
Mott law
mot'tle, -tled, -tling
mouches' vo·lantes'
mou·lage'
moult *var. of* molt
mound
mount
mount'ant
mouse
mouth
mouth'wash'
mouve·ment' de ma·nège'
move'a·ble
move'ment
mox'a
mox'a·lac'tam
mox'i·bus'tion
moy'a·moy'a disease
Mu·cam'bo fever
Mu'cha-Ha'ber·mann
  disease
Much granules
mu'cic
mu'ci·car'mine
mu·cif'er·ous
mu'ci·fi·ca'tion
mu'ci·form'
mu'ci·gen
mu·cig'e·nous
mu'ci·lage

mu'ci·lag'i·nous
mu'ci·la'go' *pl.* -lag'i·nes'
mu'cin
mu'cin·ase'
mu'ci·no·blast'
mu·cin'o·gen
mu'ci·noid'
mu·ci·no·lyt'ic
mu·ci·no'sis
mu'ci·nous
mu·ci·nu'ri·a
mu·cip'a·rous
mu·co·al·bu'mi·nous
mu'co·buc'cal
mu'co·cele'
mu'co·cil'i·ar'y
mu'co·co·li'tis
mu'co·col'pos
mu'co·cu·ta'ne·ous
mu'co·derm'
mu'co·en·ter·i'tis
mu'co·ep'i·der'moid'
mu'co·gin'gi·val
mu'coid'
mu·co'i·tin·sul·fu'ric
mu'co·la'bi·al
mu'co·lip'i·do'sis *pl.* -ses'
mu'co·lyt'ic
mu'co·mem'bra·nous
mu'co·per'i·os'te·al
mu'co·per'i·os'te·um
  pl. -te·a
mu'co·pol'y·sac'cha·ride'
mu'co·pol'y·sac'cha·ri·do'-
  sis *pl.* -ses'
mu'co·pol'y·sac'cha·ri·du'-
  ri·a
mu'co·pro'tein'
mu'co·pu'ru·lent
mu'co·pus
Mu'cor'
Mu'co·ra'ce·ae'
Mu'co·ra'les'
mu'cor·my·co'sis *pl.* -ses'
mu·co'sa
mu·co'sal
mu·co'sal'pinx
  pl. -sal·pin'ges
mu'co·san·guin'e·ous
mu'co·se'rous
mu·co'sin
mu·co'sis *pl.* -ses'
mu·co·si'tis

mu·cos'i·ty
mu'co·stat'ic
mu'cous (*pertaining to mucus*)
♦*mucus*
mu'co·vis'ci·do'sis *pl.* -ses'
mu'cro *pl.* mu·cro'nes'
mu'cro·nate'
mu'cus (*the secretion of mucous membranes*)
♦*mucous*
Muehrck'e lines
Muel'ler maneuver
mu·guet'
mu·laire'
mu·lat'to
mul'ber'ry
Mules operation
mu·li·e'bri·a
mu·li·eb'ri·ty
mull
Mül'ler
—duct
—fibers
—fixing fluid
—hillock
—law
—muscle
—sign
—syndrome
—test
—tubercle
Mül'ler-Hil'lis maneuver
mül·le'ri·an
mul·tan'gu·lar
mul·tan'gu·lum *pl.* -la
—ma'jus
—mi'nus
mul'ti·ar·tic'u·lar
mul'ti·cap'su·lar
mul'ti·cel'lu·lar
mul'ti·cen'tric
mul'ti·cen·tric'i·ty
Mul'ti·ceps
—mul'ti·ceps
—ser'i·a'lis
mul'ti·cip'i·tal
mul'ti·clo'nal
mul'ti·cos'tate'
mul'ti·cus'pid
mul'ti·cus'pi·date'
mul'ti·cys'tic
mul'ti·den'tate'
mul'ti·dig'i·tate'

mul'ti·fac'et·ed
mul'ti·fac·to'ri·al
mul'ti·fa·mil'i·al
mul'ti·fe·ta'tion
mul'ti·fid
mul·tif'i·dus *pl.* -di'
mul'ti·flag'el·late'
mul'ti·fo'cal
mul'ti·form'
mul'ti·gan'gli·on·ate'
mul'ti·gat'ed
mul'ti·glan'du·lar
mul'ti·grav'i·da
mul'ti·gra·vid'i·ty
mul'ti·he'ma·tin'ic
mul·ti-in·fec'tion
mul'ti·lay'ered
mul'ti·lo'bar
mul'ti·lobed'
mul'ti·lob'u·lar
mul'ti·loc'u·lar
mul'ti·loc'u·lat'ed
mul'ti·mam'mae'
mul'ti·mere'
mul'ti·min'er·als
mul'ti·nod'u·lar
mul'ti·nu'cle·ar
mul'ti·nu'cle·ate'
mul'ti·nu'cle·at'ed
mul·tip'a·ra
mul'ti·par'i·ty
mul'tip'a·rous
mul'ti·par'tite'
mul'ti·pen'nate'
mul'ti·pha'sic
mul'ti·pla'nar
mul'ti·ple
mul'ti·plex'
mul'ti·plic'i·ty
mul'ti·po'lar
mul'ti·pol'y·poid'
mul'ti·pur'pose
mul'ti·sep'tate'
mul'ti·sys'tem
mul'ti·ter'mi·nal
mul'ti·va'lent
mul'ti·var'i·ate'
mul'ti·vi'ta·mins
Mum'ford-Gurd'
    procedure
mum'mi·fi·ca'tion
mum'mi·fied'
mumps

Mun'chau'sen syndrome
Münch'mey'er disease
mun·dif'i·cant
mu·pir'o·cin
mu'ral
mu·ram'ic
mu·ram'i·dase'
mu·ri·at'ic
mu'rine'
mur'mur
mu'ro·mo'nab-CD3
Mur'phy
—button
—sign
Mur'phy-Sturm'
    lymphosarcoma
mur·ri'na
Mu'ru·tu'cu fever
Mus
Mus'ca
—do·mes'ti·ca
—vet·us·tis'si·ma
—vi·ci'na
mus'cae' vol·i·tan'tes'
mus'ca·rine'
mus'ca·rin'ic
mus'ca·rin·ism
mus'ci·cide'
mus'cle
—of Bell
—of Gant'zer
—of Geg'en·baur'
—of Gru'ber
—of Hall
—of Hen'le
—of Hor'ner
—of Hous'ton
—of Jung
—of Klein
—of Land'ström
—of Lud'wig
—of Ma·cal'lis·ter
—of Mül'ler
—of Raux
—of Ri'o·lan'
—of San'to·ri'ni
—of Sap'pey
—of Treitz
—of Wood
mus'cle-bound'
mus'cu·lar
mus'cu·lar'is
—mu·co'sae'

mus′cu·lar′i·ty
mus′cu·lar·ly
mus′cu·la′tion
mus′cu·la·ture
mus′cu·li′
—ab·dom′i·nis
—ar′rec·to′res′ pi·lo′rum
—bul′bi′
—cap′i·tis
—coc·cyg′e·i′
—col′li′
—dor′si′
—ex·trem′i·ta′tis in·fe′ri·o′-
ris
—extremitatis su·pe·ri·o′ris
—in′ci·si′vi′ la′bi·i′ in·fe′ri·
o′ris
—incisivi labii su·pe′ri·o′ris
—in′fra·hy·oi′de·i′
—in′ter·cos·ta′les′ ex·ter′ni′
—intercostales in·ter′ni′
—intercostales in′ti·mi′
—in′ter·os′se·i′ dor·sa′les′
ma′nus
—interossei dorsales pe′dis
—interossei pal·mar′es′
—interossei plan·tar′es′
—interossei vo·lar′es′
—in′ter·spi·na′les′
—interspinales cer′vi·cis
—interspinales lum·bo′rum
—interspinales tho·ra′cis
—in′ter·trans·ver·sar′i·i′
—intertransversarii
an·te′ri·o′res′
—intertransversarii
anteriores cer′vi·cis
—intertransversarii
lat′er·a′les′
—intertransversarii
lat′er·a·les lum·bo′rum
—intertransversarii
me′di·a′les′
—intertransversarii
mediales lum·bo′rum
—intertransversarii
pos·te′ri·o′res′
—intertransversarii
posteriores cer′vi·cis
—intertransversarii
tho·ra′cis
—la·ryn′gis
—lev′a·to′res′ cos·tar′um

—levatores costarum
brev′es′
—levatores costarum lon′gi′
—lin′guae′
—lum′bri·ca′les′
—lumbricales ma′nus
—lumbricales pe′dis
—mem′bri′ in·fe′ri·o′ris
—membri su·pe′ri·o′ris
—mul·tif′i·di′
—oc′u·li′
—os·sic′u·lo′rum au·di′tus
—os′sis hy·oi′de·i′
—pa·la′ti′ et fau′ci·um
—pap′il·lar′es′
—papillares sep·ta′les′
—pec·ti·na′ti′
—per′i·ne′i′
—ro′ta·to′res′
—rotatores brev′es′
—rotatores cer′vi·cis
—rotatores lon′gi′
—rotatores lum·bo′rum
—rotatores tho·ra′cis
—sub′cos·ta′les′
—su′pra·hy·oi′de·i′
—tho·ra′cis
mus′cu·lo·ap′o·neu·rot′ic
mus′cu·lo·cu·ta′ne·ous
mus′cu·lo·der′mic
mus′cu·lo·fas′ci·al
mus′cu·lo·fi′brous
mus′cu·lo·in·tes′ti·nal
mus′cu·lo·mem′bra·nous
mus′cu·lo·phren′ic
mus′cu·lo·skel′e·tal
mus′cu·lo·spi′ral
mus′cu·lo·ten′di·nous
mus′cu·lo·trop′ic
mus′cu·lus *pl.* -li′
—ab·duc′tor dig′i·ti′
min′i·mi′
—abductor digiti quin′ti′
—abductor hal′lu·cis
—abductor pol′li·cis brev′is
—abductor pollicis lon′gus
—ad·duc′tor brev′is
—adductor hal′lu·cis
—adductor lon′gus
—adductor mag′nus
—adductor min′i·mus
—adductor pol′li·cis
—an·co′nae·us

—an·co′ne·us
—an′ti·trag′i·cus
—ar·tic′u·lar′is
—articularis cu′bi·ti′
—articularis ge′nu′
—articularis ge′nus
—ar′y·ep′i·glot′ti·cus
—ar′y·tae·noi′de·us ob·li′-
quus
—arytaenoideus trans·ver′-
sus
—ar′y·te·noi′de·us ob·li′-
quus
—arytenoideus trans·ver′-
sus
—au·ric′u·lar′is anterior
—auricularis posterior
—auricularis superior
—bi′ceps′ bra′chi·i′
—biceps fem′o·ris
—bi′pen·na′tus
—bra·chi·a′lis
—bra′chi·o·ra′di·a′lis
—bron′cho·e′so·phag′e·us
—bron′cho·oe·so′phag′e·us
—buc′ci·na′tor
—buc′co·pha·ryn′ge·us
—bul′bo·cav′er·no′sus
—bul′bo·spon·gi·o′sus
—ca·ni′nus
—cer′a·to·cri·coi′de·us
—cer′a·to·pha·ryn′ge·us
—chon′dro·glos′sus
—chon′dro·pha·ryn′ge·us
—cil′i·ar′is
—coc·cyg′e·us
—con·stric′tor pha·ryn′gis
inferior
—constrictor pharyngis
me′di·us
—constrictor pharyngis
superior
—co′ra·co·bra·chi·a′lis
—cor′ru·ga′tor su′per·cil′i·i′
—cre·mas′ter
—cri·co·ar′y·tae·noi′de·us
lat′er·a′lis
—cricoarytaenoideus
posterior
—cri′co·ar′y·te·noi′de·us
lat′er·a′lis
—cricoarytenoideus
posterior

—cri·co·pha·ryn'ge·us
—cri·co·thy're·oi'de·us
—cri·co·thy·roi'de·us
—cu·ta'ne·us
—del·toi'de·us
—de·pres'sor an'gu·li' o'ris
—depressor la'bi·i' in·fe'ri·o'ris
—depressor sep'ti' na'si'
—depressor su·per·cil'i·i'
—di·gas'tri·cus
—dil·a·ta'tor pu·pil'lae'
—di·la'tor pu·pil'lae'
—ep'i·cra'ni·us
—ep'i·troch'le·o·an·co'nae·us
—e·rec'tor spi'nae'
—ex·ten'sor car'pi' ra·di·a'lis brev'is
—extensor carpi radialis lon'gus
—extensor carpi ul·nar'is
—extensor dig'i·ti' min'i·mi'
—extensor digiti quin'ti' pro'pri·us
—extensor dig·i·to'rum
—extensor digitorum brev'is
—extensor digitorum com·mu'nis
—extensor digitorum lon'gus
—extensor hal'lu·cis brev'is
—extensor hallucis lon'gus
—extensor in'di·cis
—extensor indicis pro'pri·us
—extensor pol'li·cis brev'is
—extensor pollicis lon'gus
—fib·u·lar'is brev'is
—fibularis lon'gus
—fibularis ter'ti·us
—fix·a'tor ba·se·os' sta·pe'dis
—flex'or ac'ces·so'ri·us
—flexor car'pi' ra'di·a'lis
—flexor carpi ul·nar'is
—flexor dig'i·ti' min'i·mi' brev'is
—flexor digiti quin'ti' brev'is
—flexor dig·i·to'rum brev'is
—flexor digitorum lon'gus
—flexor digitorum pro·fun'dus

—flexor digitorum sub·li'mis
—flexor digitorum su'per·fi'ci·a'lis
—flexor hal'lu·cis brev'is
—flexor hallucis lon'gus
—flexor pol'li·cis brev'is
—flexor pollicis lon'gus
—fron·ta'lis
—fu'si·for'mis
—gas'troc·ne'mi·us
—ge·mel'lus inferior
—gemellus superior
—ge·ni·o·glos'sus
—ge·ni·o·hy·oi'de·us
—glos'so·pal·a·ti'nus
—glos'so·pha·ryn'ge·us
—glu'tae·us max'i·mus
—glutaeus me'di·us
—glutaeus min'i·mus
—glu'te·us max'i·mus
—gluteus me'di·us
—gluteus min'i·mus
—grac'i·lis
—hel'i·cis major
—helicis minor
—hy'o·glos'sus
—i·li'a·cus
—il'i·o·coc·cyg'e·us
—il'i·o·cos·ta'lis
—iliocostalis cer'vi·cis
—iliocostalis dor'si'
—iliocostalis lum·bo'rum
—iliocostalis tho·ra'cis
—il'i·o·pso'as
—in'ci·su'rae' hel'i·cis
—in'fra·spi·na'tus
—is'chi·o·cav'er·no'sus
—la·tis'si·mus dor'si'
—le·va'tor an'gu·li' o'ris
—levator a'ni'
—levator glan'du·lae' thy're·oi'de·ae'
—levator glandulae thy·roi'de·ae'
—levator la'bi·i' su·pe'ri·o'ris
—levator labii superioris a·lae'que' na'si'
—levator pal'pe'brae' su·pe'ri·o'ris
—levator pros'ta·tae'
—levator scap'u·lae'

—levator ve'li' pal·a·ti'ni'
—lon·gis'si·mus
—longissimus cap'i·tis
—longissimus cer'vi·cis
—longissimus dor'si'
—longissimus tho·ra'cis
—lon·gi·tu'di·na'lis inferior lin'guae'
—longitudinalis superior lin'guae'
—lon'gus cap'i·tis
—longus col'li'
—mas·se'ter
—men·ta'lis
—mul·tif'i·dus
—my'lo·hy·oi'de·us
—my'lo·pha·ryn'ge·us
—na·sa'lis
—ob·li'quus au·ric'u·lae'
—obliquus cap'i·tis inferior
—obliquus capitis superior
—obliquus ex·ter'nus ab·dom'i·nis
—obliquus inferior bul'bi'
—obliquus inferior oc'u·li'
—obliquus in·ter'nus ab·dom'i·nis
—obliquus superior bul'bi'
—obliquus superior oc'u·li'
—ob·tu'ra·tor ex·ter'nus
—obturator in·ter'nus
—ob·tu'ra·to'ri·us ex·ter'nus
—obturatorius in·ter'nus
—oc·cip'i·ta'lis
—oc·cip'i·to·fron·ta'lis
—o'mo·hy·oi'de·us
—op·po'nens dig'i·ti' min'i·mi'
—opponens digiti quin'ti' ma'nus
—opponens digiti quinti pe'dis
—opponens pol'li·cis
—or·bic'u·lar'is
—orbicularis oc'u·li'
—orbicularis o'ris
—or'bi·ta'lis
—pal·a·to·glos'sus
—pal·a·to·pha·ryn'ge·us
—pal·mar'is brev'is
—palmaris lon'gus
—pap·il·lar'is anterior ven·tric'u·li' dex'tri'

—papillaris anterior
ventriculi si·nis'tri'
—papillaris posterior
ventriculi dex'tri'
—papillaris posterior
ventriculi si·nis'tri'
—pec·tin'e·us
—pec'to·ra'lis major
—pectoralis minor
—per'o·nae'us brev'is
—peronaeus lon'gus
—peronaeus ter'ti·us
—per'o·ne'us brev'is
—peroneus lon'gus
—peroneus ter'ti·us
—pha·ryn'go·pal'a·ti'nus
—pir'i·for'mis
—plan·tar'is
—pleu'ro·e'so·phag'e·us
—pleu'ro·oe'so·phag'e·us
—pop·lit'e·us
—pro·ce'rus
—pro·na'tor qua·dra'tus
—pronator te'res'
—pros·tat'i·cus
—pso'as major
—psoas minor
—pter'y·goi'de·us ex·ter'-
nus
—pterygoideus in·ter'nus
—pterygoideus lat'er·a'lis
—pterygoideus me'di·a'lis
—pter'y·go·pha·ryn'ge·us
—pu'bo·coc·cyg'e·us
—pu'bo·pros·tat'i·cus
—pu'bo·rec'ta'lis
—pu'bo·vag'i·na'lis
—pu'bo·ves'i·ca'lis
—py·ram'i·da'lis
—pyramidalis au·ric'u·lae'
—qua·dra'tus fem'o·ris
—quadratus la'bi·i' in·fe'ri·
o'ris
—quadratus labii su·pe'ri·
o'ris
—quadratus lum·bo'rum
—quadratus plan'tae'
—qua'dri·ceps' fem'o·ris
—rec'to·coc·cyg'e·us
—rec'to·u're·thra'lis
—rec'to·u'ter·i'nus
—rec'to·ves'i·ca'lis
—rec'tus ab·dom'i·nis

—rectus cap'i·tis anterior
—rectus capitis lat'er·a'lis
—rectus capitis posterior
major
—rectus capitis posterior
minor
—rectus fem'o·ris
—rectus inferior bul'bi'
—rectus inferior oc'u·li'
—rectus lat'er·a'lis bul'bi'
—rectus lateralis oc'u·li'
—rectus me'di·a'lis bul'bi'
—rectus medialis oc'u·li'
—rectus superior bul'bi'
—rectus superior oc'u·li'
—rhom·boi'de·us major
—rhomboideus minor
—ri·so'ri·us
—sa'cro·coc·cyg'e·us
anterior
—sacrococcygeus dor·sa'lis
—sacrococcygeus posterior
—sacrococcygeus ven·tra'lis
—sa'cro·spi·na'lis
—sal·pin'go·pha·ryn'ge·us
—sar·to'ri·us
—sca·le'nus anterior
—scalenus me'di·us
—scalenus min'i·mus
—scalenus posterior
—sem'i·mem'bra·no'sus
—sem'i·spi·na'lis
—semispinalis cap'i·tis
—semispinalis cer'vi·cis
—semispinalis dor'si'
—semispinalis tho·ra'cis
—sem'i·ten'di·no'sus
—ser·ra'tus anterior
—serratus posterior inferior
—serratus posterior superior
—skel'e·ti'
—so'le·us
—sphinc'ter
—sphincter am·pul'lae'
—sphincter ampullae
hep'a·to·pan·cre·at'i·cae'
—sphincter a'ni' ex·ter'nus
—sphincter ani in·ter'nus
—sphincter duc'tus cho·
led'o·chi'
—sphincter pu·pil'lae'
—sphincter py·lo'ri'
—sphincter u·re'thrae'

—sphincter urethrae
mem'bra·na'ce·ae'
—spi·na'lis
—spinalis cap'i·tis
—spinalis cer'vi·cis
—spinalis dor'si'
—spinalis tho·ra'cis
—sple'ni·us cap'i·tis
—splenius cer'vi·cis
—sta·pe'di·us
—ster·na'lis
—ster'no·clei'do·mas·toi'-
de·us
—ster'no·hy·oi'de·us
—ster'no·thy·re·oi'de·us
—ster'no·thy·roi'de·us
—sty'lo·glos'sus
—sty'lo·hy·oi'de·us
—sty'lo·pha·ryn'ge·us
—sub·cla'vi·us
—sub·scap'u·lar'is
—su'pi·na'tor
—su'pra·spi·na'tus
—sus'pen·so'ri·us du'o·
de'ni'
—tar·sa'lis inferior
—tarsalis superior
—tem'po·ra'lis
—tem'po·ro·pa·ri'e·ta'lis
—ten'sor fas'ci·ae' la'tae'
—tensor tym'pa·ni'
—tensor ve'li' pal'a·ti'ni'
—te'res' major
—teres minor
—thy're·o·ar'y·tae·noi'de·us
—thy're·o·ar'y·te·noi'de·us
—thy're·o·ep'i·glot'ti·cus
—thy're·o·hy·oi'de·us
—thy're·o·pha·ryn'ge·us
—thy'ro·ar'y·te·noi'de·us
—thy'ro·ep'i·glot'ti·cus
—thy'ro·hy·oi'de·us
—tib'i·a'lis anterior
—tibialis posterior
—tra'che·a'lis
—trag'i·cus
—trans·ver'so·spi·na'lis
—trans·ver'sus ab·dom'-
i·nis
—transversus au·ric'u·lae'
—transversus lin'guae'
—transversus men'ti'
—transversus nu'chae'

—transversus per'i·ne'i' pro·fun'dus
—transversus perinei su'per·fi'ci·a'lis
—transversus tho·ra'cis
—tra·pe'zi·us
—tri·an'gu·lar'is
—tri'ceps' bra'chi·i'
—triceps su'rae'
—u'ni·pen'na'tus
—u'vu·lae'
—vas'tus in·ter·me'di·us
—vastus lat'er·a'lis
—vastus me·di·a'lis
—ven·tric'u·lar'is
—ver'ti·ca'lis lin'guae'
—vis'ce·rum
—vo·ca'lis
—zy'go·mat'i·cus
—zygomaticus major
—zygomaticus minor
mush'room'
mu'si·cal
mu'si·co·ther'a·py
mus'si·ta'tion
mus'tard
Mus'tard atrial operation
Mus'tar·dé' otoplasty
mus'tine'
mu'ta·cism
mu'ta·gen
mu'ta·gen'e·sis
mu'ta·gen'ic
mu'ta·ge·nic'i·ty
mu'tant
mu'ta·ro·ta'tion
mu'tase'
mu'tate'
mu·ta'tion
mu·ta'tion·al
mute
mu'ti·late', -lat'ed, -lat'ing
mu'ti·la'tion
mut'ism
mu'ton
mu'tu·al·ism
mu'tu·al·ist
muz'zle
my·al'gi·a
my·al'gic
my'as·the'ni·a
—grav'is
my'as·then'ic

my'a·to'ni·a *(absence of muscle tone)*
♦myotonia
—con·gen'i·ta
my·at'ro·phy
my·ce'li·al
my·ce'li·oid'
my·ce'li·um *pl.* -li·a
my'cete'
my·ce'tes'
my·ce·the'mi·a
my·ce'tis'mus *pl.* -mi'
my·ce·to·gen'ic
my·ce·tog'e·nous
my·ce'toid'
my·ce·to'ma
My·ce·to·zo'a
My·co·bac·te'ri·a'ce·ae'
my'co·bac·te'ri·al
my'co·bac·te'ri·o'sis *pl.* -ses'
my'co·bac·te'ri·um *pl.* -a
My·co·bac·te'ri·um
—a'vi·um
—bo'vis
—in'tra·cel'lu·la're
—lep'rae'
—par'a·tu·ber'cu·lo'sis
—phle'i'
—tu·ber'cu·lo'sis
—tuberculosis var. mu'ris
—ul'cer·ans'
my'co·ci'din
my'co·der'ma
my'coid'
my·col'o·gist
my·col'o·gy
my'co·myr'in·gi'tis
my'coph·thal'mi·a
My'co·plas'ma
—ar·thrit'i·dis
—in'cog'ni'tus
—my'coi'des'
—pneu·mo'ni·ae'
—pul·mo'nis
my'co·plas'mal
My'co·plas'ma·ta'ce·ae'
my'co·plas·mo'sis *pl.* -ses'
my'cose'
my·co'sis *pl.* -ses'
—fun·goi'des'
—fungoides d'em·blée'
my'co·stat'ic

my'co·sub'til·in
my·cot'ic
—o·ti'tis ex·ter'na
my'co·tox'ic
my'co·tox·ic'i·ty
my'co·tox'in
myc·ter'ic
my·de'sis
my·dri'a·sis *pl.* -ses'
myd'ri·at'ic
my·ec'to·my
my'ec·to'pi·a
my·ec'to·py
my'e·lal'gi·a
my'e·lap'o·plex'y
my'e·la·te'li·a
my'e·lat'ro·phy
my'e·laux'e
my'e·le'mi·a
my'e·len·ce·phal'ic
my'e·len·ceph'a·li'tis
my'e·len·ceph'a·lon'
my·el'ic
my'e·lin
my'e·li·nat'ed
my'e·li·na'tion
my'e·lin'ic
my'e·lin·i·za'tion
my'e·lin·oc'la·sis
my'e·lin·o'gen·e·sis
my'e·li·nol'y·sis *pl.* -ses'
my'e·li·nop'a·thy
my'e·li·no'sis
my'e·lit'ic
my'e·li'tis
my'e·lo·blast'
my'e·lo·blas·te'mi·a
my'e·lo·blas'tic
my'e·lo·blas·to'ma *pl.* -mas *or* -ma·ta
my'e·lo·blas·to'sis
my'e·lo·cele'
my'e·lo·cyst'
my'e·lo·cys'tic
my'e·lo·cys'to·cele'
my'e·lo·cys·tog'ra·phy
my'e·lo·cys'to·me·nin'go·cele'
my'e·lo·cyte'
my'e·lo·cy·the'mi·a
my'e·lo·cyt'ic
my'e·lo·cy·to'ma *pl.* -mas *or* -ma·ta

my'e·lo·cy·to'sis pl. -ses'
my'e·lo·di·as'ta·sis
my'e·lo·dys·pla'si·a
my'e·lo·dys·plas'tic
my'e·lo·en'ce·phal'ic
my'e·lo·en·ceph'a·li'tis
my'e·lo·fi·bro'sis pl. -ses'
my'e·lo·fi·brot'ic
my'e·lo·gen'e·sis
my'e·lo·gen'ic
my'e·log'e·nous
my'e·log'e·ny
my'e·lo·gone'
my'e·lo·gram'
my'e·lo·graph'ic
my'e·log'ra·phy
my'e·loid'
my'e·lo·ken'tric
my'e·lo·li·po'ma pl. -mas or
   -ma·ta
my'e·lo·lym·phan'gi·o'ma
my'e·lo·lym'pho·cyte'
my'e·lol'y·sis pl. -ses'
my'e·lo'ma pl. -mas or
   -ma·ta
my'e·lo·ma·la'ci·a
my'e·lo·ma·to'sis pl. -ses'
my'e·lo·me'ni·a
my'e·lo·men'in·gi'tis
my'e·lo·me·nin'go·cele'
my'e·lo·mere'
my'e·lo·mon'o·cyte'
my'e·lo·mon'o·cyt'ic
my'e·lon'
my'e·lo·neu·ri'tis
my'e·lo·pa·ral'y·sis pl. -ses'
my'e·lo·path'ic
my'e·lop'a·thy
my'e·lo·per·ox'i·dase'
my'e·lop'e·tal
my'e·lo·phthi'sis pl. -ses'
my'e·lo·plaque'
my'e·lo·plast'
my'e·lo·ple'gi·a
my'e·lo·poi·e'sis pl. -ses'
my'e·lo·poi·et'ic
my'e·lo·pore'
my'e·lo·pro·lif'er·a·tive
my'e·lo·ra·dic'u·li'tis
my'e·lo·ra·dic'u·lo·dys·
   pla'si·a
my'e·lo·ra·dic'u·lop'a·thy
my'e·lor·rha'gi·a

my'e·lo·sar·co'ma pl. -mas
   or -ma·ta
my'e·los'chi·sis pl. -ses'
my'e·lo·scin'to·gram'
my'e·lo·scin·tog'ra·phy
my'e·lo·scle·ro'sis pl. -ses'
my'e·lo·scle·rot'ic
my'e·lo'sis pl. -ses'
my'e·lo·spon'gi·um
   pl. -gi·a
my'e·lo·sy·rin'go·cele'
my'e·lot'o·my
my'e·lo·tox'ic
my'e·lo·tox'in
my'en·ta'sis
my'en·ter'ic
my·en'ter·on'
My'ers method
My'er·son reflex
my'es·the'si·a
my·i'a·sis pl. -ses'
my'io·des·op'si·a
my·i'tis
my·o·al·bu'min
my'o·ar'chi·tec·ton'ic
my'o·as·the'ni·a
my'o·blast'
my'o·blas'tic
my'o·blas·to'ma pl. -mas or
   -ma·ta
my'o·bra'di·a
my'o·car'di·al
my'o·car'di·o·graph'
my'o·car'di·op'a·thy
my'o·car·di'tis
my'o·car'di·um pl. -di·a
my'o·car·do'sis pl. -ses'
my'o·cele'
my'o·ce'li·al'gi·a
my'o·cel'lu·li'tis
my'o·ce·li'tis
my'o·cep'tor
my'o·ce·ro'sis
my'o·chor·di'tis
my'o·clo'ni·a
my'o·clon'ic
my'o·clo'nus
my'o·coele'
my'o·col·pi'tis
my'o·cyte'
my'o·cy·tol'y·sis
my'o·cy·to'ma pl. -mas or
   -ma·ta

my'o·de·gen'er·a'tion
my'o·di·as'ta·sis
my'o·dy·nam'ics
my'o·dyn'i·a
my'o·dys·to'ni·a
my'o·dys'to·ny
my'o·dys·tro'phi·a
   —fe·ta'lis
my'o·dys'tro·phy
my'o·e·de'ma
my'o·e·las'tic
my'o·en·do·car·di'tis
my'o·ep'i·the'li·al
my'o·ep'i·the'li·o'ma
   pl. -mas or -ma·ta
my'o·ep'i·the'li·um
my'o·fas'ci·al
my'o·fas·ci'tis
my'o·fi'bril
my'o·fi·bril'la
my'o·fi·bro'ma pl. -mas or
   -ma·ta
my'o·fi·bro·sar·co'ma
   pl. -mas or -ma·ta
my'o·fi·bro'sis pl. -ses'
my'o·fi·bro·si'tis
my'o·fil'a·ment
my'o·ge·lo'sis pl. -ses'
my'o·gen
my'o·gen'ic
my'og'e·nous
my'og'li·a
my'o·glo'bin
my'o·glo'bi·nu'ri·a
my'o·glob'u·lin
my'og'na·thus
my'o·gram'
my'o·graph'
my'o·graph'ic
my'og'ra·phy
my'o·he'ma·tin
my'o·he'mo·glo'bin
my'o·he'mo·glo'bi·nu'ri·a
my'o·hy'per·tro'phi·a
   —ky'mo·par'a·lyt'i·ca
my'oid'
my'o·is·che'mi·a
my'o·ke·ro'sis
my'o·ki'nase'
my'o·ki·ne·sim'e·ter
my'o·ki·ne·si·o·gram'
my'o·ki·ne·si·og'ra·phy
my'o·ki·net'ic

my·o·ky'mi·a
my·o·lei·ot'ic
my·o·li·po'ma *pl.* -mas *or*
　-ma·ta
my·o·lo'gi·a
my·o·log'ic *or* my·o·log'i·cal
my·ol'o·gy
my·ol'y·sis
my·o'ma *pl.* -mas *or* -ma·ta
　—stri·o·cel'lu·lar'e'
　—tel·an·gi·ec'to·des'
my·o·ma·la'ci·a
　—cor'dis
my·o·ma·to'sis
my·om·a'tous
my·o·mec'to·my
my·o·mel'a·no'sis *pl.* -ses'
my·o·mere'
my·o·mer'ic
my·om'e·ter
my·o·me'tri·al
my·o·me·tri'tis
my·o·me'tri·um
my·o·ne·cro'sis
my·o·neme'
my·o·neu'ral
my·o·neu·ral'gi·a
my·o·neu·ras·the'ni·a
my·o·neu·rec'to·my
my·o·neu·ro'ma *pl.* -mas *or*
　-ma·ta
my·o·pa·chyn'sis
my·o·pal'mus
my·o·pa·ral'y·sis *pl.* -ses'
my·o·pa·re'sis *pl.* -ses'
my·o·path'i·a
　—ra·chit'i·ca
my·o·path'ic
my·op'a·thy
my·ope'
my·o·per'i·car·di'tis
my·o·pha'gi·a
my·oph'a·gism
my·o'pi·a
my·op'ic
my·o·plasm
my·o·plas'tic
my·o·plas'ty
my·o·por·tho'sis
my·o·pro'tein'
my·o·psy·chop'a·thy
my·o·psy·cho'sis *pl.* -ses'
my·or'rha·phy

my·or·rhex'is
my·or·rhyth'mi·a
my·or·rhyth'mic
my·o·sal'gi·a
my·o·sal·pin·gi'tis
my·o·sal'pinx'
　pl. -sal·pin'ges'
my·o·san'
my·o·sar·co'ma *pl.* -mas *or*
　-ma·ta
my·o·schwan·no'ma
　pl. -mas *or* -ma·ta
my·o·scle·ro'sis *pl.* -ses'
my·o·seism
my·o·sep'tum
my·o·sin
my·o·sin'o·gen
my·o·sis *pl.* -ses'
my·o·sit'ic
my·o·si'tis
　—fi·bro'sa
　—os·sif'i·cans
　—ossificans pro·gres·si'va
my·o·spa'si·a
my·o·spasm
my·o·spas'mi·a
my·os·te·o'ma *pl.* -mas *or*
　-ma·ta
my·o·su'ture
my·o·syn·o·vi'tis
my·o·tac'tic *(pertaining to*
　muscular sense)
　♦myotatic
my·ot'a·sis
my·o·tat'ic *(pertaining to*
　stretching of a muscle)
　♦myotactic
my·o·ten'di·nous
my·o·te·non'to·plas'ty
my·o·ten·o·si'tis
my·o·te·not'o·my
my·o·tome'
my·ot'o·my
my·o·to'ni·a *(tonic muscle*
　spasm)
　♦myatonia
　—ac'qui·si'ta
　—a·troph'i·ca
　—con·gen'i·ta
　—congenita in'ter·mit'tens
　—dys·troph'i·ca
my·o·ton'ic
my·ot'o·noid'

my·ot'o·nus
my·o·troph'ic
my·ot'ro·phy
my·o·tube'
my·o·tu'bule'
Myr'i·an·gi·a'les
my·rin'ga
myr·in'gec'to·my
myr·in·gi'tis
　—bul·lo'sa
my·rin·go·dec'to·my
my·rin·go·my·co'sis
　pl. -ses'
my·rin'go·plas'tic
my·rin'go·plas'ty
my·rin·go·sta·pe'di·o·
　pex'y
my·rin'go·tome'
myr·in·got'o·my
my'rinx'
my·ris'tic
my·ris'ti·ca
myrrh
my·so·phil'i·a
my·so·phil'ic
my·so·pho'bi·a
my·so·pho'bic
myth'o·ma'ni·a
myth'o·pho'bi·a
myt'i·lo·tox'in
myt'i·lo·tox'ism
myx·ad'e·ni'tis
myx·ad'e·no'ma *pl.* -mas *or*
　-ma·ta
myx'an·gi'tis
myx'as·the'ni·a
myx·e·de'ma
　—cir'cum·scrip'tum thy'ro·
　tox'i·cum
myx·e·dem'a·toid'
myx·e·dem'a·tous
myx·i·o'sis
myx'o·ad'e·no'ma *pl.* -mas
　or -ma·ta
myx'o·chon·dro·fi'bro·sar·
　co'ma *pl.* -mas *or* -ma·ta
myx'o·chon·dro'ma
　pl. -mas *or* -ma·ta
myx'o·chon'dro·sar·co'ma
　pl. -mas *or* -ma·ta
myx'o·cys·to'ma *pl.* -mas *or*
　-ma·ta
myx'o·cyte'

myx'o·en'do·the'li·o'ma
pl. -mas *or* -ma·ta
myx'o·fi·bro'ma *pl.* -mas *or*
-ma·ta
myx'o·fi'bro·sar·co'ma
pl. -mas *or* -ma·ta
myx'o·gli·o'ma *pl.* -mas *or*
-ma·ta
myx'oid'
myx'o·li·po'ma *pl.* -mas *or*
-ma·ta
myx'o·lip'o·sar·co'ma
pl. -mas *or* -ma·ta
myx·o'ma *pl.* -mas *or* -ma·ta
—cav'er·no'sum
—fi·bro'sum
—ge·lat'i·no'sum
—lip'o·ma·to'des'
—med'ul·lar'e'
—sim'plex'
myx'o·ma·to'sis *pl.* -ses'
myx·om'a·tous
Myx'o·my·ce'tes'
myx'o·my·o'ma
myx'o·neu·ro'ma *pl.* -mas
or -ma·ta
myx'o·pap'il·lo'ma
pl. -mas *or* -ma·ta
myx'o·poi·e'sis
myx'or·rhe'a
myx'o·sar·co'ma *pl.* -mas *or*
-ma·ta
myx'o·sar·co'ma·tous
myx'o·spore'
myx'o·vi'ral
myx'o·vi'rus
My'zo·my'ia

N

Na·bo'thi·an
—cyst
—glands
na'cre·ous
na'dide'
na'dir
na'do·lol'
Nä'ge·le
—obliquity
—pelvis
Nae'ge·li
—test
—type leukemia

nae'paine'
naf'a·rel'in
na'fate'
naf·cil'lin
Naff'zi·ger
—operation
—syndrome
—test
naf·ox'i·dine'
naf'ti·fine'
Na'ga sore
Na'gel test
Na·gle'ri·a fow'ler·i'
Na'gler reaction
nail
—en ra·quette'
na'ked
nal'bu·phine'
nal'i·dix'ic
nal·mex'one'
nal'or·phine'
nal·ox'one'
nal·trex'one'
nam·ox'y·rate'
Nance analysis
nan'dro·lone'
na'nism
nan'o·ceph'a·lus *pl.* -li'
nan'o·ceph'aly
nan'o·cor'mi·a
nan'o·cor'mus
nan'o·cu'rie
nan'o·gram'
na'noid'
nan'o·me'li·a
na·nom'e·lus
nan'o·me'ter
nan'oph·thal'mi·a
nan'oph·thal'mos
Na·no'phy·e·tus
sal·min'co·la
nan'o·sec'ond
nan'o·so'ma
nan'o·so'mi·a
nan'o·so'mus
nan'o·tech·nol'o·gy
na'nous
na'nu·ka·ya'mi
na'nus
Na·pal'kov phenomenon
na'palm
nape
nap'el·line'

na'pex'
na·phaz'o·line'
naph'tha
naph'tha·lene'
naph'thol'
naph'tho·quin'one'
naph'thyl
na'pi·form'
nap'ra·path'
na·prap'a·thy
na·prox'en
Nar'ath operation
nar'ce·ine'
nar'cism
nar'cis'sine'
nar'cis·sism
nar'cis·sist
nar'cis·sis'tic
nar'co·a·nal'y·sis *pl.* -ses'
nar'co·di·ag'no·sis *pl.* -ses'
nar'co·hyp'ni·a
nar'co·hyp·no'sis *pl.* -ses'
nar'co·lep'sy
nar'co·lep'tic
nar·co'ma
nar·co'ma·tous
nar·co'sis *pl.* -ses'
nar'co·spasm
nar'co·syn'the·sis *pl.* -ses'
nar'co·ther'a·py
nar·cot'ic
nar·cot'i·co-ir'ri·tant
nar'co·tine'
nar'co·tism
nar'co·tize', -tized', -tiz'ing
nar'i·al
nar'is *pl.* -nar'es'
nar'row·ing
na·sal
na·sa'lis
nas'cent
na'si·o·al·ve'o·lar
na'si·on'
na·si'tis
Na'smyth membrane
na'so·al·ve'o·lar
na'so·an'tral
na'so·bas'i·lar
na'so·bil'i·ar'y
na'so·breg·mat'ic
na'so·cil'i·ar'y
na'so·fa'cial
na'so·fron'tal

na′so·gas′tric
na′so·gen′i·tal
na′so·je·ju′nal
na′so·la′bi·al
na′so·la′bi·a′lis
na′so·lac′ri·mal
na′so·lat′er·al
na′so·ma′lar
na′so·man·dib′u·lar
na′so·max′il·lar′y
na′so·me′di·al
na′so·me′di·an
na′so·men′tal
na′so-oc·cip′i·tal
na′so-o′ral
na′so-or′bit·al
na′so·pal′a·tal
na′so·pal′a·tine′
na′so·pal′pe·bral
na′so·pha·ryn′ge·al
na′so·phar′yn·gi′tis
na′so·pha·ryn′go·scope′
na′so·pha·ryn′go·scop′ic
na′so·phar′yn·gos′co·py
na′so·phar′ynx
   pl. -pha·ryn′ges′
na′so·scope′
na′so·scop′ic
na·sos′co·py
na′so·sep′tal
na′so·si′nus·i′tis *pl.* -tes
na′so·spi·na′le′
na′so·tra′che·al
na′so·tur′bi·nal
na′sus *pl.* -si′
  —a·dun′cus
  —car′ti·la·gin′e·us
  —ex·ter′nus
  —in·cur′vus
  —os′se·us
  —si′mus
na′tal
na·tal′i·ty
na′ta·my′cin
na′tant
na′ta·to′ry
na′tes′
na′ti·mor·tal′i·ty
na′tive
na·tre′mi·a
na′tri·um
na′tri·u·re′sis
na′tri·u·ret′ic

na′tron′
nat′u·ral
na·tur′o·path′ic
na′tur·op′a·thy
Naugh′ton exercise
  protocol
Nau′heim′ bath
nau′se·a
nau′se·ant
nau′se·ate′, -at′ed, -at′ing
nau′seous
na′vel
na·vic′u·la
na·vic′u·lar
na·vic′u·lar·thri′tis
na·vic′u·lo·cap′i·tate′
na·vic′u·lo·cu′boid′
na·vic′u·lo·cu·ne′i·form′
Nd:YAG laser
near′-miss′
near′sight′ed
near′sight′ed·ness
ne′ar·thro′sis *pl.* -ses′
ne′ben·kern
neb′ra·my′cin
neb·u′la *pl.* -lae′ *or* -las
neb′u·lar
neb′u·li·za′tion
neb′u·lize′, -lized′, -liz′ing
neb′u·liz′er
Ne·ca′tor
  —a·mer′i·ca′nus
ne·ca·to′ri·a′sis
neck
nec′ro·bac′il·lar′y
nec′ro·bac′il·lo′sis *pl.* -ses′
Nec′ro·bac·te′ri·um
  —ne·croph′o·rum
nec′ro·bi·o′sis *pl.* -ses′
  —li·poi′di·ca
  —lipoidica di·a·bet′i·co′rum
nec′ro·bi·ot′ic
nec′ro·cy·to′sis *pl.* -ses′
nec′ro·cy′to·tox′in
nec′ro·gen′ic
ne·crog′e·nous
nec′ro·log′ic
ne·crol′o·gist
ne·crol′o·gy
ne·crol′y·sis *pl.* -ses′
nec′ro·ma′ni·a
nec′ro·mi·me′sis
nec′ro·pha′gi·a

nec′ro·phag′ic
ne·croph′a·gous
nec′ro·phile′
nec′ro·phil′i·a
nec′ro·phil′ic
ne·croph′i·lism
ne·croph′i·lous
ne·croph′i·ly
nec′ro·pho′bi·a
nec′ro·pho′bic
nec′ro·pneu·mo′ni·a
nec′rop·sy
ne·crose′, -crosed′, -cros′ing
nec′ro·sin
ne·cro′sis *pl.* -ses′
nec′ro·sper′mi·a
nec′ro·sper′mic
ne·crot′ic
nec′ro·tize′, -tized′, -tiz′ing
nec′ro·tox′in
nec′ro·zo′o·sper′mi·a
nec·tar′e·ous
nec′ta·ry
nee′dle
nee′dling
Neel′sen
  —method
  —stain
Neer
  —acromioplasty
  —classification
ne′frens′ *pl.* ne·fren′des′
Nef·tel′ disease
neg′a·tive
neg′a·tiv·ism
neg′a·tiv·is′tic
Ne·gish′i encephalitis
neg′li·gence
neg′li·gi·ble
Neg′ri bodies
Neg′ri-Ja·cod′ syndrome
Ne′gro
  —sign
Neill′-Moo′ser
  —bodies
  —reaction
Neis′ser
  —coccus
  —stain
Neis·se′ri·a
  —cat′ar·rha′lis
  —fla·ves′cens
  —gon′or·rhoe′ae′

—in'tra·cel'lu·lar'is
—men'in·git'i·dis
—sic'ca
Né'la·ton'
—dislocation
—fibers
—fold
—line
—operation
—tumor
Nel'son test
nem
nem'a·line
nem'a·thel'minth
Nem'a·thel·min'thes'
nem'a·ti·za'tion
nem'a·to·cid'al
ne·mat'o·cide'
Nem'a·to'da
nem'a·tode'
nem'a·to·di'a·sis *pl.* -ses'
nem'a·toid'
nem'a·tol'o·gist
nem'a·tol'o·gy
nem'a·to'sis *pl.* -ses'
nem'a·to·sper'mi·a
nem'ic
ne'o·an'ti·gen
ne'o·ars·phen'a·mine'
ne'o·ar·thro'sis *pl.* -ses'
ne'o·blas'tic
ne'o·car'zi·no·stat'in
ne'o·cer'e·bel'lar
ne'o·cer'e·bel'lum
ne'o·cor'tex'
ne'o·cor'ti·cal
ne'o·cys·tos'to·my
ne'o·cyte'
ne'o·cy·to'sis *pl.* -ses'
ne'o·den·ta'tum
ne'o·dym'i·um
ne'o·fe'tus
ne'o·for·ma'tion
ne'o·for·ma'tive
ne·og'a·la
ne'o·gen'e·sis *pl.* -ses'
ne'o·ge·net'ic
ne'o·graph'ism
ne'o·ki·net'ic
ne'o·la'li·a
ne·ol'o·gism
ne'o·mem'brane'
ne'o·mor'phic

ne'o·mor'phism
ne'o·my'cin
ne'on'
ne'o·na'tal
ne'o·nate'
ne'o·na'ti·cide'
ne'o·na·tol'o·gy
ne'o·na·to'ri·um *pl.* -ri·a
ne'o·na'tus *pl.* -ti'
ne'o·pal'li·al
ne'o·pal'li·um
ne'o·pha'si·a
ne'o·pho'bi·a
ne'o·pho'bic
ne'o·pla'si·a
ne'o·plasm
ne'o·plas'tic
ne'o·plas'ty
ne'o·prene'
ne'o·spi'no·tha·lam'ic
ne'o·stig'mine'
ne'o·stri·a'tum
ne·ot'e·ny
Ne'o·tes·tu'di·na ro·sa'ti·i'
ne'o·thal'a·mus *pl.* -mi
ne'o·vas'cu·lar
ne'o·vas'cu·lar·i·za'tion
ne'o·vas'cu·la·ture
neph'a·lism
neph'a·list
neph'e·lom'e·ter
neph'e·lo·met'ric
neph'e·lom'e·try
neph'e·lo'pi·a
ne·phral'gi·a
ne·phral'gic
neph'ra·to'ni·a
neph'rec·ta'si·a
ne·phrec'to·mize', -mized',
  -miz'ing
ne·phrec'to·my
neph're·de'ma *pl.* -mas *or*
  -ma·ta
neph'rel·co'sis *pl.* -ses'
neph'ric
ne·phrid'i·um *pl.* -i·a
ne·phrit'ic
ne·phri'tis *pl.* -phrit'i·des' *or*
  -tis·es
neph'ri·to·gen'ic
neph'ro·ab·dom'i·nal
neph'ro·an'gi·o·scle·ro'sis
  pl. -ses'

neph'ro·blas·to'ma *pl.* -mas
  or -ma·ta
neph'ro·cal'ci·no'sis
  pl. -ses'
neph'ro·cap·sec'to·my
neph'ro·cap'su·lec'to·my
neph'ro·cap'su·lot'o·my
neph'ro·car'ci·no'ma
  pl. -mas *or* -ma·ta
neph'ro·car'di·ac'
neph'ro·cele'
neph'ro·col'ic
neph'ro·col'o·pex'y
neph'ro·co'lop·to'sis
  pl. -ses'
neph'ro·cyst'a·nas'to·mo'-
  sis *pl.* -ses'
neph'ro·cys·ti'tis
neph'ro·cys·to'sis *pl.* -ses'
neph'ro·dys'tro·phy
neph'ro·gas'tric
neph'ro·gen'e·sis *pl.* -ses'
neph'ro·gen'ic
ne·phrog'e·nous
neph'ro·gram'
neph'ro·graph'ic
ne·phrog'ra·phy
neph'ro·hy·dro'sis *pl.* -ses'
neph'ro·hy·per'tro·phy
neph'roid'
neph'ro·lith'
neph'ro·li·thi'a·sis *pl.* -ses'
neph'ro·lith'ic
neph'ro·li·thot'o·my
ne·phrol'o·gist
ne·phrol'o·gy
ne·phrol'y·sin
ne·phrol'y·sis *pl.* -ses'
neph'ro·lyt'ic
ne·phro'ma *pl.* -mas *or*
  -ma·ta
neph'ro·meg'a·ly
neph'ro·mere'
neph'ron'
neph'ron·oph'thi·sis
neph'ro·path'ic
ne·phrop'a·thy
neph'ro·pex'y
neph'ro·poi'e·tin
neph'rop·to'si·a
neph'rop·to'sis *pl.* -ses'
neph'ro·py'e·li'tis
neph'ro·py'e·log'ra·phy

neph′ro·py′e·lo·li· thot′o·my

neph′ro·py′e·lo·plas′ty

neph′ro·py·o′sis

neph′ror·rha′gi·a

ne·phror′rha·phy

neph′ros′ *pl.* neph′roi′

neph′ro·scle·ro′sis *pl.* -ses′

neph′ro·sid′er·o′sis

ne·phro′sis *pl.* -ses′

ne·phro·so·ne·phri′tis

neph′ro·so·nog′ra·phy

ne·phros′to·gram′

ne·phros′to·ma *pl.* neph′ro·sto′ma·ta

neph′ro·sto′mal

neph′ro·stome′

ne·phros′to·my

ne·phrot′ic

neph′ro·tome′

neph′ro·to·mo·gram′

neph′ro·to·mog′ra·phy

ne·phrot′o·my

neph′ro·tox′ic

neph′ro·tox·ic′i·ty

neph′ro·tox′in

neph′ro·trop′ic

neph′ro·tu·ber′cu·lo′sis

neph′ro·u·re′ter·al

neph′ro·u·re′ter·ec′to·my

nep·tu′ni·um

Ne′ri sign

Nernst equation

nerve

—of Ar′nold

—of Bell

—of Co·tun′ni·us

—of Cru′veil·hier′

—of Cy′on′

—of Eis′ler

—of Ja′cob·son

—of Lan·ci′si

—of La′tar·jet′

—of Scar′pa

—of Vid′i·us

—of Vieus·sens′

—of Wris′berg′

ner′vi′

—al′ve·o·lar′es′ su·pe′ri·o′- res′

—a′no·coc′cyg·e′i′

—au·ric′u·lar′es′ an·te′ri·o′- res′

—car·di′a·ci′ tho·ra′·ci·ci′

—ca·rot′i·ci′ ex·ter′ni′

—ca·rot′i·co·tym·pan′i·ci′

—cav′er·no′si′ cli·to′ri·dis

—cavernosi clitoridis mi· no′res′

—cavernosi pe′nis

—cavernosi penis mi·no′res′

—cer′e·bra′les′

—cer′vi·ca′les′

—cil′i·ar′es′ brev′es′

—ciliares lon′gi′

—clu′ni·um in·fe′ri·o′res′

—clunium me′di·i′

—clunium su·pe′ri·o′res′

—cra′ni·a′les′

—dig′i·ta′les′ dor·sa′les′ hal′lu·cis lat·er·a′lis et dig′i·ti′ se·cun′·di′ me′di·a′lis

—digitales dorsales ner′vi′ ra′di·a′lis

—digitales dorsales nervi ul′nar·is

—digitales dorsales pe′dis

—digitales pal·mar′es′ com·mu′nes′ ner′vi′ me′di·a′ni′

—digitales palmares communes nervi ul·nar′is

—digitales palmares pro′- pri·i′ ner′vi′ me′di·a′ni′

—digitales palmares proprii nervi ul·nar′is

—digitales plan·tar′es′ com·mu′nes′ ner′vi′ plan·tar′is lat·er·a′lis

—digitales plantares communes nervi plantaris me′di·a′lis

—digitales plantares pro′- pri·i′ ner′vi′ plan·tar′is lat·er·a′lis

—digitales plantares proprii nervi plantaris me′di·a′lis

—digitales vo·lar′es′ com· mu′nes′ ner′vi′ me′di· a′ni′

—digitales volares communes nervi ul·nar′is

—digitales volares pro′pri·i′ ner′vi′ me′di·a′ni′

—digitales volares proprii

nervi ul·nar′is

—er′i·gen′tes′

—haem′or·rhoi·da′les′ in·fe′ri·o′res′

—haemorrhoidales me′di·i′

—haemorrhoidales su·pe′ri·o′res′

—in′ter·cos′ta′les′

—in′ter·cos′to·bra′chi·a′les′

—la′bi·a′les′ an·te′ri·o′res′

—labiales pos·te′ri·o′res′

—lum·ba′les′

—ner′vo′rum

—ol′fac′to′ri·i′

—pal′a·ti′ni′

—palatini mi·no′res′

—per′i·ne·a′les′

—per′i·ne′i′

—phren′i·ci′ ac′ces·so′ri·i′

—pter′y·go·pal′a·ti′ni′

—rec·ta′les′ in·fe′ri·o′res′

—sa·cra′les′

—scro·ta′les′ an·te′·ri·o′res′

—scrotales pos·te′·ri·o′res′

—sphe·no·pal′a·ti′ni′

—spi·na′les′

—splanch′ni·ci′ lum·ba′les′

—splanchnici pel·vi′·ni′

—splanchnici sa·cra′les′

—sub·scap′u·lar′es′

—su′pra·cla·vic′u·lar′es′

—supraclaviculares in′ter·me′di·i′

—supraclaviculares lat·er·a′les′

—supraclaviculares me′di·a′les′

—supraclaviculares me′di·i′

—supraclaviculares pos·te′- ri·o′res′

—tem′po·ra′les′ pro·fun′di′

—ter′mi·na′les′

—tho′ra·ca′les′

—thoracales an·te′·ri·o′res′

—thoracales pos·te′·ri·o′res′

—tho·ra′ci·ci′

—vag′i·na′les′

—va·so′rum

—ves′i·ca′les′ in·fe′·ri·o′- res′ plex′us pu·den′di′

—vesicales inferiores sys·te′ma·tis sym·path′i·ci′

—vesicales su·pe'ri·o'res'
sys·te'ma·tis
sym·path'i·ci'
ner'vone'
ner·von'ic
ner'vo·sism
ner'vous *(pertaining to nerves)*
♦ *nervus*
ner'vous·ly
ner'vous·ness
ner'vus *(a nerve), pl.* -vi'
♦ *nervous*
—ab·du'cens
—ac·ces·so'ri·us
—a·cus'ti·cus
—al've·o·lar'is inferior
—am'pul·lar'is anterior
—ampullaris inferior
—ampullaris lat'er·a'lis
—ampullaris posterior
—ampullaris superior
—an'te·bra'chi·i' anterior
—antebrachii posterior
—ar·tic'u·lar'is
—au·ric'u·lar'is mag'nus
—auricularis posterior
—au·ric'u·lo·tem'po·ra'lis
—ax'il·lar'is
—buc·ca'lis
—buc'ci·na·to'ri·us
—ca'na·lis pter'y·goi'de·i'
—car·di'a·cus cer'vi·ca'lis
inferior
—cardiacus cervicalis
me'di·us
—cardiacus cervicalis
superior
—cardiacus inferior
—cardiacus me'di·us
—cardiacus superior
—ca·rot'i·co·tym·pan'i·cus
inferior
—caroticotympanicus
superior
—ca·rot'i·cus in·ter'nus
—cav'er·no'sus cli·to'ri·dis
major
—cavernosus pe'nis major
—coc·cyg'e·us
—coch'le·ae'
—cu·ta'ne·us
—cutaneus an'te·bra'chi·i'
lat'er·a'lis

—cutaneus antebrachii
me'di·a'lis
—cutaneus antebrachii
posterior
—cutaneus an'ti·bra'chi·i'
dor·sa'lis
—cutaneus antibrachii
lat'er·a'lis
—cutaneus antibrachii
me'di·a'lis
—cutaneus bra'chi·i'
lat'er·a'lis
—cutaneus brachii lateralis
inferior
—cutaneus brachii lateralis
superior
—cutaneus brachii me'di·a'-
lis
—cutaneus brachii posterior
—cutaneus col'li'
—cutaneus dor·sa'lis
in'ter·me'di·us
—cutaneus dorsalis
lat'er·a'lis
—cutaneus dorsalis
me'di·a'lis
—cutaneus fem'o·ris
lat'er·a'lis
—cutaneus femoris posterior
—cutaneus su'rae' lat'er·a'-
lis
—cutaneus surae me'di·a'lis
—dor·sa'lis cli·to'ri·dis
—dorsalis pe'nis
—dorsalis scap'u·lae'
—eth'moi·da'lis anterior
—ethmoidalis posterior
—fa'ci·a'lis
—fem'o·ra'lis
—fib'u·lar'is com·mu'nis
—fibularis pro·fun'dus
—fibularis su·per·fi'ci·a'lis
—fron·ta'lis
—fur·ca'lis
—gen'i·to·fem'o·ra'lis
—glos'so·pha·ryn'·ge·us
—glu·tae'us inferior
—glutaeus superior
—glu·te'us inferior
—gluteus superior
—hy'po·gas'tri·cus (dex'ter
et si·nis'ter)
—hy'po·glos'sus

—il'i·o·hy'po·gas'tri·cus
—il'i·o·in'gui·na'lis
—in'fra·or·bi'ta·lis
—in'fra·troch'le·ar'is
—in'ter·me'di·us
—in'ter·os'se·us anterior
—interosseus cru'ris
—interosseus dor·sa'lis
—interosseus posterior
—interosseus vo·lar'is
—is'chi·ad'i·cus
—jug'u·lar'is
—lac'ri·ma'lis
—la·ryn'ge·us inferior
—laryngeus re·cur'rens
—laryngeus superior
—lin·gua'lis
—man·dib'u·lar'is
—mas'se·ter'i·cus
—mas'ti·ca·to'ri·us
—max'il·lar'is
—me·a'tus a·cus'ti·ci'
ex·ter'ni'
—meatus au'di'·to'ri·i'
ex·ter'ni'
—me'di·a'nus
—me·nin'ge·us me'di·us
—men·ta'lis
—mus'cu·lo·cu·ta'ne·us
—my'lo·hy·oi'de·us
—na'so·cil'i·ar'is
—na'so·pal'a·ti'nus
—ob'tu·ra·to'ri·us
—oc·cip'i·ta'lis major
—occipitalis minor
—occipitalis ter'ti·us
—oc·ta'vus
—oc·u·lo·mo·to'ri·us
—ol'fac·to'ri·us
—oph·thal'mi·cus
—op'ti·cus
—pal'a·ti'nus anterior
—palatinus major
—palatinus me'di·us
—palatinus posterior
—pec·to·ra'lis lat·er·a'lis
—pectoralis me'di·a'lis
—per·o'nae·us com·mu'nis
—peronaeus pro·fun'dus
—peronaeus
su·per·fi'ci·a'lis
—per·o'ne·us com·mu'nis
—peroneus pro·fun'dus

—peroneus su·per·fi′ci· a′lis
—pe·tro′sus major
—petrosus minor
—petrosus pro·fun′dus
—petrosus su·per·fi′ci·a′lis major
—petrosus superficialis minor
—phren′i·cus
—plan·tar′is lat′er·a′lis
—plantaris me′di·a′lis
—pre′sa·cra′lis
—pter′y·goi′de·us ex·ter′- nus
—pterygoideus in·ter′nus
—pterygoideus lat′er·a′lis
—pterygoideus me′di·a′lis
—pu·den′dus
—ra′di·a′lis
—re·cur′rens
—sac′cu·lar′is
—sa·phe′nus
—sper·mat′i·cus ex·ter′nus
—spi·no′sus
—splanch′ni·cus i′mus
—splanchnicus major
—splanchnicus minor
—sta·pe′di·us
—sub·cla′vi·us
—sub′cos·ta′lis
—sub′lin·gua′lis
—sub·oc·cip′i·ta′lis
—sub·scap′u·lar′is
—su′pra·or′bi·ta′lis
—su′pra·scap′u·lar′is
—su′pra·troch′le·ar′is
—su·ra′lis
—tem′po·ra′lis pro·fun′dus anterior
—temporalis profundus posterior
—ten·so′ris tym′pa·ni′
—tensoris ve′li pal·a·ti′ni′
—ten·to′ri·i′
—tho′ra·ca′lis lon′gus
—tho′ra·ci·cus lon′gus
—tho′ra·co·dor·sa′lis
—tib′i·a′lis
—trans·ver′sus col′li′
—tri·gem′i·nus
—troch′le·ar′is
—tym·pan′i·cus

—ul′nar′is
—u·tric′u·lar′is
—u·tric′u·lo·am′pul·lar′is
—va′gus
—vas′cu·lar′is
—ver′te·bra′lis
—ves·tib′u·li′
—ves·tib′u·lo·coch′le·ar′is
—zy·go·mat′i·cus

ne·sid′i·ec′to·my
ne·sid′i·o·blast′
ne·sid′i·o·blas·to′ma pl. -mas or -ma·ta
ne·sid′i·o·blas·to′sis
ness′ler·i·za′tion
ness′ler·ize′, -ized′, -iz′ing
Ness′ler reagent
nes′ti·a
nes′ti·at′ri·a
nes′ti·os′to·my
nes′tis
nes′ti·ther′a·py
nes′to·ther′a·py
nests of Gol′gi-Holm′gren
neth′a·lide′
net′il·mi′cin
net′work′
Neu′berg ester
Neu′ber tubes
Neu′feld′
—nail
Neu′hau′ser sign
Neu′mann
—cells
—method
—operation
—sheath
neu′rad
neu′ral
neu·ral′gi·a
neu·ral′gic
neu·ral′gi·form′
neu′ra·min′ic
neu′ra·min′i·dase′
neu′ra·poph′y·sis pl. -ses′
neu′ra·prax′i·a
neu·rar·throp′a·thy
neu′ras·the′ni·a
neu′ras·then′ic
neu′ra·tro′phi·a
neu′ra·troph′ic
neu·rat′ro·phy
neu·rax′i·al

neu·rax′is
neu′rax·it′ic
neu′rax·i′tis
neu·rax′on′
neu′rec·ta′si·a
neu·rec′ta·sis pl. -ses′
neu·rec′to·my
neu·rec′to·pi·a
neu·rec′to·py
neu·ren′ter·ic
neur·ep′i·the′li·um
neu·rer′gic
neur·ex·er′e·sis pl. -ses′
neu·ri′a·sis pl. -ses′
neu·ri′a·try
neu′ri·lem′ma
neu′ri·lem′mal
neu′ri·lem·mi′tis
neu′ri·lem·mo′ma pl. -mas or -ma·ta
neu′ri·lem′mo·sar·co′ma pl. -mas or -ma·ta
neu′ri·mo′tor
neu′rine′
neu′ri·no′ma pl. -mas or -ma·ta
neu′ri·no′ma·to′sis pl. -ses′
neu′rite′
neu′rit′ic
neu·ri′tis
neu′ro·a·nas′to·mo′sis pl. -ses′
neu′ro·a·nat′o·my
neu′ro·a·ne′mi·a
neu′ro·a·ne′mic
neu′ro·an′gi·o·graph′ic
neu′ro·an′gi·og′ra·phy
neu′ro·ar′thri·tism
neu′ro·ar·throp′a·thy
neu′ro·as·the′ni·a
neu′ro·as′tro·cy·to′ma pl. -mas or -ma·ta
neu′ro·ax′on·al
neu′ro·bi·o·log′i·cal
neu′ro·bi·ol′o·gy
neu′ro·bi′o·tax′is
neu′ro·blast′
neu′ro·blas·to′ma pl. -mas or -ma·ta
—sym′pa·thet′i·cum
—sym′path′i·cum
neu′ro·blas·to′ma·to′sis pl. -ses′

neu′ro·ca·nal′
neu′ro·car′di·ac′
neu′ro·cen′tral
neu′ro·cen′trum
neu′ro·cep′tor
neu′ro·chem′is·try
neu′ro·cho′ri·o·ret′i·ni′tis
neu′ro·cho′roi·di′tis
neu′ro·cir′cu·la·to′ry
neu·roc′la·dism
neu′ro·clon′ic
neu′ro·coele′
neu′ro·cra′ni·al
neu′ro·cra′ni·um
neu′ro·crine′
neu′ro·cu·ta′ne·ous
neu′ro·cyte′
neu′ro·cy·tol′y·sin
neu′ro·cy·tol′y·sis
neu′ro·cy·to′ma pl. -mas or
  -ma·ta
neu′ro·de·a·tro′phi·a
neu′ro·de·gen′er·a·tive
neu′ro·den′drite′
neu′ro·den′dron′
neu′ro·der′ma·ti′tis
  —cir′cum·scrip′ta
  —dis·sem′i·na′ta
neu′ro·der′ma·to′sis
  pl. -ses′
neu′ro·der′ma·tro′phi·a
neu′ro·di·as′ta·sis pl. -ses′
neu′ro·dy·nam′ic
neu′ro·dyn′i·a
neu′ro·ec′to·derm′
neu′ro·ec′to·der′mal
neu′ro·en·ceph′a·lo·my′e·
  lop′a·thy
neu′ro·en′do·crine
neu′ro·en′do·cri·nol′o·gy
neu′ro·en·ter′ic
neu′ro·ep′i·der′mal
neu′ro·ep′i·the′li·al
neu′ro·ep′i·the′li·o′ma
  pl. -mas or -ma·ta
neu′ro·ep′i·the′li·um
  pl. -li·a
neu′ro·fi′bril
neu′ro·fi′bril·lar
neu′ro·fi′bril·lar′y
neu′ro·fi·bro′ma pl. -mas or
  -ma·ta
  —gan′gli·o·cel′lu·lar′e′

—gan′gli·o′nar′e′
neu′ro·fi·bro′ma·to′sis
  pl. -ses′
neu′ro·fi′bro·myx·o′ma
  pl. -mas or -ma·ta
neu′ro·fi′bro·pha′co·ma·
  to′sis pl. -ses′
neu′ro·fi′bro·sar·co′ma pl.
  -mas or -ma·ta
neu′ro·fil′a·ment
neu′ro·fix·a′tion
neu′ro·gan′gli·i′tis
neu′ro·gan′gli·o′ma my′e·
  lin′i·cum ve′rum
neu′ro·gan′gli·on pl. -gli·a
  or -gli·ons
neu′ro·gan′gli·on·i′tis
neu′ro·gas′tric
neu′ro·gen
neu′ro·gen′e·sis pl. -ses′
neu′ro·ge·net′ic
neu′ro·gen′ic
neu·rog′e·nous
neu·rog′e·ny
neu·rog′li·a
neu·rog′li·al
neu·rog′li·ar
neu·rog′li·o·cyte′
neu·rog′li·o·cy·to′ma
  pl. -mas or -ma·ta
neu·rog′li·o′ma pl. -mas or
  -ma·ta
neu·rog′li·o′sis pl. -ses′
neu′ro·gram′
neu′ro·his·tol′o·gy
neu′ro·hor·mo′nal
neu′ro·hor′mone′
neu′ro·hu′mor
neu′ro·hu′mor·al
neu′ro·hy·poph′y·se′al
neu′ro·hy·poph′y·sec′-
  to·my
neu′ro·hy·poph′y·sis
  pl. -ses′
neu′roid′
neu′ro·im′mu·no·mod′u·
  la′tion
neu′ro·im′mu·no·mod′u·
  la′tor
neu′ro·in·duc′tion
neu·ro·ker′a·tin
neu′ro·ki′nin
neu′ro·lab′y·rin·thi′tis

neu′ro·lath′y·rism
neu′ro·lem′ma
neu′ro·lem·mi′tis
neu′ro·lem·mo′ma pl. -mas
  or -ma·ta
neu′ro·lep′rid
neu′ro·lep′tan·al·ge′si·a
neu′ro·lep′tan·al·ge′sic
neu′ro·lep′tan·es·the′si·a
neu′ro·lep′tan·es·thet′ic
neu′ro·lep′tic
neu′ro·lo′gi·a
neu′ro·log′ic or
  neu′ro·log′i·cal
neu′ro·log′i·cal·ly
neu·rol′o·gist
neu·rol′o·gy
neu′ro·lu′es′
neu′ro·lymph′
neu′ro·lym′pho·ma·to′sis
  pl. -ses′
  —gal′li·nar′um
neu·rol′y·sin
neu·rol′y·sis pl. -ses′
neu′ro·lyt′ic
neu·ro′ma pl. -mas or -ma·ta
  —cu′tis
  —gan′gli·o·cel′lu·lar′e′
  —gangliocellulare ma·lig′-
  num
  —tel·an′gi·ec·to′des′
  —ve′rum
  —verum gan′gli·o′sum
  a′my·e·lin′i·cum
neu′ro·ma·la′ci·a
neu·rom′a·toid′
neu′ro·ma·to′sis pl. -ses′
neu·rom′a·tous
neu′ro·mech′a·nism
neu′ro·mel′a·nin
neu′ro·mere′
neu′ro·mi·me′sis
neu′ro·mi·met′ic
neu′ro·mo′tor
neu′ro·mus′cu·lar
neu′ro·my′al
neu′ro·my′as·the′ni·a
neu′ro·my·e·li′tis
  —hy′per·al′bu·mi·not′i·ca
  —op′ti·ca
neu′ro·my′ic
neu′ro·my′o·ar·te′ri·al
neu′ro·my′o·path′ic

neu′ro·my′o·si′tis
neu′ron′
neu′ro·nal
neu′ro·neph′ric
neu′ro·ne′vus *pl.* -vi′
neu′ro·ni′tis
neu′ron·og′ra·phy
neu′ro·nop′a·thy
neu·ron·o·phage′
neu′ron·o·pha′gi·a
neu′ro·oph·thal′mo·log′ic
neu′ro·oph′thal·mol′o·gy
neu′ro·op′tic
neu′ro·pap′il·li′tis
neu′ro·pa·ral′y·sis *pl.* -ses′
neu′ro·par′a·lyt′ic
neu′ro·path′
neu′ro·path′ic
neu′ro·path′o·gen′e·sis
 pl. -ses′
neu′ro·path′o·ge·nic′i·ty
neu′ro·path′o·log′ic
neu′ro·pa·thol′o·gy
neu·rop′a·thy
neu′ro·pep′tide′
neu′ro·phar′ma·co·log′ic *or*
 neu′ro·phar′ma·co·log′i·cal
neu′ro·phar′ma·col′o·gy
neu′ro·pho′ni·a
neu′ro·phre′ni·a
neu′ro·phys′ine′
neu′ro·phys′i·o·log′ic
neu′ro·phys′i·ol′o·gist
neu′ro·phys′i·ol′o·gy
neu′ro·pil
neu′ro·plasm
neu′ro·plas′mic
neu′ro·plas′ty
neu′ro·ple′gic
neu′ro·plex′us
neu′ro·po′di·a *sing.* -di·um
neu′ro·pore′
neu·ro·po·ten′tial
neu′ro·psy′chi·at′ric
neu′ro·psy·chi′a·trist
neu′ro·psy·chi′a·try
neu′ro·psy′chic
neu′ro·psy·cho·log′i·cal
neu′ro·psy·chol′o·gist
neu′ro·psy·chol′o·gy
neu′ro·psy·cho·path′ic
neu′ro·psy·chop′a·thy
neu′ro·psy·cho·sis *pl.* -ses′

neu′ro·ra′di·o·log′ic
neu′ro·ra′di·ol′o·gy
neu′ro·rec′i·dive′
neu′ro·re·cur′rence
neu′ro·re·lapse′
neu′ro·ret′i·ni′tis
neu′ro·ret′i·nop′a·thy
neu′ro·roent′ge·nol′o·gy
neu·ror′rha·phy
neu·ror·rhex′is
neu′ro·sar′co·clei′sis
neu′ro·sar·co′ma *pl.* -mas *or*
 -ma·ta
neu′ro·scle·ro′sis *pl.* -ses′
neu′ro·se·cre′tion
neu′ro·se·cre′to·ry
neu′ro·seg·men′tal
neu′ro·sen′so·ry
neu·ro′sis *pl.* -ses′
neu′ro·skel′e·tal
neu′ro·skel′e·ton
neu′ro·some′
neu′ro·spasm
neu′ro·splanch′nic
neu′ro·spon·gi·o′ma
 pl. -mas *or* -ma·ta
neu′ro·spon′gi·um
Neu·ros′po·ra
neu′ro·ste′a·ric
neu′ro·sthe′ni·a
neu′ro·sthen′ic
neu·ro·sur′geon
neu′ro·sur′ger·y
neu′ro·sur′gi·cal
neu′ro·su′ture
neu′ro·syph′i·lis
neu′ro·ten′di·nal
neu′ro·ten′di·nous
 —organ of Gol′gi
 —xan·tho′ma·to′sis
neu′ro·ther′a·py
neu·rot′ic
neu·rot′i·ca
neu·rot′i·cism
neu·rot′i·gen′ic
neu·ro·ti·za′tion
neu′ro·tize′, -tized′, -tiz′ing
neu·rot·me′sis
neu′rot·o·gen′ic
neu′ro·tome′
neu·rot′o·my
neu′ro·ton′ic
neu·rot′o·ny

neu′ro·tox′ic
neu′ro·tox′i·cant
neu′ro·tox·ic′i·ty
neu′ro·tox′in
neu′ro·trans′mit′ter
neu′ro·trau′ma
neu′ro·trip′sy
neu′ro·troph′ic *(pertaining to
 neurotrophy)*
 ♦ *neurotropic*
neu·rot′ro·phy
neu′ro·trop′ic *(pertaining to
 neurotropism)*
 ♦ *neurotrophic*
neu·rot′ro·pism
neu′ro·tu′bule′
neu′ro·vac′cine
neu′ro·var′i·co′sis *pl.* -ses′
neu′ro·vas′cu·lar
neu′ro·veg′e·ta′tive
neu′ro·vir′u·lent
neu′ro·vi′rus
neu′ro·vis′cer·al
neu′ru·la *pl.* -las *or* -lae′
neu′ru·la′tion
Neus′ser granules
neu′tral
neu′tral·i·za′tion
neu′tral·ize′, -ized′, -iz′ing
neu·tri′no
neu·tro·clu′sion
neu′tro·cyte′
neu′tro·cyt′ic
neu′tron′
neu·tro·pe′ni·a
neu·tro·pe′nic
neu′tro·phil′
neu′tro·phil′i·a
heu′tro·phil′ic
neu·tro′phin
ne′vi·form′
ne′vo·car′ci·no′ma *pl.* -mas
 or -ma·ta
ne′void′
ne′vo·mel′a·no′ma *pl.* -mas
 or -ma·ta
ne′vose′
ne′vo·xan′tho·en′do·the′-
 li·o′ma *pl.* -mas *or* -ma·ta
ne′vus *pl.* -vi′
 —ac′ne·i·for′mis u′ni·lat′-
 er·a′lis
 —an′gi·o·li·po·ma·to′sus

—a·rach·noi′de·us
—a·ra′ne·us
—com′e·do′ni·cus
—ep′i·the′li·o′ma·to-
   cyl′in·dro′ma·to′sus
—flam′me·us
—fol·lic′u·lar′is
—fus′co-cae·ru′li·us oph·
   thal′mo·max′il·lar′is of
   O′ta
—li·po′ma·to′des′
—lipomatodes su′per·fi′-
   ci·a′lis
—li·po′ma·to′sus
—lum′bo·in′gui·na′lis
—pap′il·lar′is
—pap′il·lo′ma·to′sus
—pel·li′nus
—pig′men·to′sus
—pi·lo′sus
—se·ba′ce·us
—spi′lus
—spon′gi·o′sus al′bus
—u′ni·lat′er·a′lis
—u′ni·us lat′er·is
—vas′cu·lo′sus
—ver′ru·co′sus
new′born′
New′cas′tle
—disease
—virus
new′ton
nex′us *pl.* nex′us *or* -us·es
Nez′e·lof syndrome
ni′a·cin
ni′a·cin′a·mide′
ni′a·cin′a·mi·do′sis
ni·al′a·mide′
nib
ni·car′di·pine′
niche
nick′el
nick′ing
ni·clo′sa·mide′
Nic′ol prism
Ni·co·las′-Fa′vre disease
Nic′oll bone graft
nic′o·tin′a·mide′
nic′o·tin·ate′
nic′o·tine′
nic′o·tin′ic
nic′o·tin·ism
nic′o·ti·nu′ric

nic′ti·tate′, -tat′ed, -tat′ing
nic′ti·ta′tion
ni′dal
ni·da′tion
ni′dus *pl.* -di′
—a′vis cer′e·bel′li′
Niel′sen method
Nie′mann-Pick′ disease
ni·fed′i·pine′
ni·fu′ri·mide′
ni′fur·ox′ime′
nig′gle
night′guard′
night′mare′
night′shade′
ni′gra
ni′gral
ni′gri·cans′
ni·gri′ti·es′
ni·gro·re·tic′u·lar
ni·gro·ru′bral
ni′gro·sine′
ni′gro·stri·a′tal
ni′hil·ism
nik·eth′a·mide′
Ni·kol′sky sign
ni·lu′ta·mide′
ni·mo′di·pine′
nin·hy′drin
ni·o′bi·um
niph′a·blep′si·a
niph′o·typh·lo′sis
nip′pers
nip′ple
ni·rid′a·zole′
nir·va′na
ni′sin
ni·so′bam·ate′
Nis′sen fundoplication
Nissl
—bodies
—granules
—stains
—substance
ni′sus
—for′ma·ti′vus
nit
Nit′a·buch′
—membrane
—stria
ni′ti·nol
ni′ton′
ni′trate′

ni·tra′tion
ni·tra′ze·pam′
ni′tre
ni·tre′mi·a
ni′tric
ni′tride′
ni′tri·fi·ca′tion
ni′tri·fi′er
ni′tri·fy′, -fied′, -fy′ing
ni′trile
ni′trite′
ni′tri·toid′
ni·tri·tu′ri·a
ni·tro·ben′zene′
ni′tro·cel′lu·lose′
ni′tro·cy′cline′
ni′tro·dan′
ni·tro·fu′ran
ni·tro·fu′ran′to·in
ni·tro·fu′ra·zone′
ni′tro·gen
ni·trog′e·nase′
ni·trog′e·nous
ni′tro·glyc′er·in
ni·tro·mer′sol′
ni·trom′e·ter
ni′tron′
ni·tro·prus′side′
ni·tros·am′ine′
ni′tro·syl
ni′trous
ni·tro·va′so·di·la′tor
ni′tryl
ni·zat′i·dine′
Njo′ver·a
no·bel′i·um
no′ble
No′ble posture
No·car′di·a
—as′ter·oi′des′
—ma·du′rae′
no·car′di·al
no·car′di·o′sis *pl.* -ses′
no·ci·as·so·ci·a′tion
no·ci·cep′tive
no·ci·cep′tor
no·ci·fen′sor
no·ci-in′flu·ence
no·ci·per·cep′tion
noc′tal·bu′mi·nu′ri·a
noc·tam′bu·la′tion
noc·tam·bu′lic
noc′ti·pho′bi·a

noc·tu'ri·a
noc·tur'nal
nod'al
node
—of Keith and Flack
—of Ran·vi·er'
—of Vir'chow-Troi'si·er'
no'di'
—lym·phat'i·ci
—lymphatici ap'i·ca'les
—lymphatici ax'il·lar'es'
—lymphatici bron'cho·pul'-
mo·na'les'
—lymphatici buc·ca'les'
—lymphatici ce·li'a·ci'
—lymphatici cen·tra'les'
—lymphatici cer'vi·ca'les'
pro·fun'di'
—lymphatici cervicales
su'per·fi'ci·a'les'
—lymphatici co'li·ci' dex'tri'
—lymphatici colici me'di·i'
—lymphatici colicisi·nis'tri'
—lymphatici cu'bi·ta'les'
—lymphatici ep'i·gas'tri·ci'
—lymphatici gas'tri·ci'
dex'tri'
—lymphatici gastrici si·nis'-
tri'
—lymphatici gas'tro·ep'i·
plo'i·ci' dex'tri'
—lymphatici gastroepiploici
si·nis'tri'
—lymphatici he·pat'i·ci'
—lymphatici il'e·o·co'li·ci'
—lymphatici i·li'a·ci' com·
mu'nes'
—lymphatici iliaci ex·ter'ni'
—lymphatici iliaci in·ter'ni'
—lymphatici in'gui·na'les'
pro·fun'di'
—lymphatici inguinales
su'per·fi'ci·a'les'
—lymphatici in·ter·cos·ta'les'
—lymphatici lat'er·a'les'
—lymphatici lin·gua'les'
—lymphatici lum·ba'les'
—lymphatici man·dib'u·
lar'es'
—lymphatici me'di·as'-
ti·na'les' an·te'ri·o'res'
—lymphatici mediastinales
pos·te'ri·o'res'

—lymphatici mes'en·ter'i·ci'
in·fe'ri·or'es'
—lymphatici mesenterici
su·pe'ri·o'res'
—lymphatici oc·cip'i·ta'les'
—lymphatici pan'cre·at'i·
co·li'e·na'les'
—lymphatici par'a·ster·na'-
les'
—lymphatici pa·rot'i·de'i'
su'per·fi'ci·a'les' et pro·
fun'di'
—lymphatici pec'to·ra'les'
—lymphatici phren'i·ci'
—lymphatici pop'lit'e·i'
—lymphatici pul'mo·na'les'
—lymphatici py·lo'ri·ci'
—lymphatici ret'ro·au·ric'-
u·lar'es'
—lymphatici ret'ro·pha·
ryn'ge·i'
—lymphatici sa·cra'les'
—lymphatici sub'man·dib'-
u·lar'es
—lymphatici sub'men·ta'-
les'
—lymphatici sub·scap'-
u·lar'es'
—lymphatici tra'che·a'les'
—lymphatici tra'che·o·
bron'chi·a'les' in·fe'ri·o'-
res'
—lymphatici tracheobron-
chiales su·pe'ri·o'res'
no'dose'
no·dos'i·ty
nod'u·lar
nod'u·lar'i·ty
nod'u·lat'ed
nod'u·la'tion
nod'ule'
nod'u·li'
—ag'gre·ga'ti' pro·ces'sus
ver'mi·for'mis
—A·ran'ti·i'
—cu'ta·ne·i'
—lym·phat'i·ci' ag'gre·ga'ti'
—lymphatici bron'chi·a'les'
—lymphatici con·junc'ti·
va'les'
—lymphatici gas'tri·ci'
—lymphatici in·tes·ti'ni'
rec'ti'

—lymphatici la·ryn'ge·i'
—lymphatici li'e·na'les'
—lymphatici sol'i·tar'i·i'
—lymphatici tu·bar'i·i'
—lymphatici vag'i·na'les'
—lymphatici ves'i·ca'les'
—thy'mi·ci' ac'ces·so'ri·i'
—val'vu·lar'um sem'i·lu·
nar'i·um
nod'u·lous
nod'u·lus pl. -li'
—lym·phat'i·cus
no'dus pl. -di'
—a'tri·o·ven·tric'u·lar'is
—lym·phat'i·cus
—lymphaticus jug'u·lo·di·
gas'tri·cus
—lymphaticus jug'u·lo·o'-
mo·hy·oi'de·us
—lymphaticus tib'i·a'lis
anterior
—si'nu·a'tri·a'lis
no'e·gen'e·sis
no'e·mat'ic
no·e'sis
no·et'ic
no'gal·a·my'cin
no'ma
no·mad'ic
no'mad·ism
no'men·cla'ture
Nom'i·na An'a·tom'i·ca
nom'i·nal
nom'o·gram'
nom'o·graph'
nom'o·thet'ic
nom'o·top'ic
no'na
non'ab·sorb'a·ble
non'ad·dic'tive
non'ad·her'ent
no'nan
non'a'que·ous
non'ar·tic'u·lar
non·ca'se·at'ing
non·cho'le·cys'to·ki'nin
non·chro'maf·fin
non'com·mu'ni·cat'ing
non'com·pen'sa·to'ry
non'com·pli'ance
non'com·pli'ant
non com'pos men'tis
non'con·duc'tor

non'con·ges'tive
non'di·rec'tive
non'dis·crete'
non'dis·junc'tion
non'dis·junc'tion·al
non'dis·placed'
non·drink'er
non·en·cap'su·lat'ed
non·en·hanced'
non·ep'i·car'di·al
non·fen'es·trat'ed
non·func'tion·ing
non·gran'u·lar
non·ic·ter'ic
no'ni·grav'i·da
non·in·fect'ed
non·in·fec'tious
non·in·va'sive
non·i·on'ic
no·nip'a·ra
non·la·mel'lar
non·lam'el·lat'ed
non·lip'id
non·lu·et'ic
non·lym'pho·cyt'ic
non·med'ul·lat'ed
non·mo'tile
non·my'e·li·nat'ed
Non'ne disease
Non'ne-Ma·rie'
  syndrome
Non'ne-Mil'roy-Meige'
  syndrome
non-nu'cle·at'ed
non·ob·struc'tive
non·o·paque'
non·op'er·a·ble
non·op'er·a·tive
non·ose'
non·os'te·o·gen'ic
non·o'vu·la·to'ry
non·ox'y·nol'-9
non·par'ous
non·path'o·gen
non·path'o·gen'ic
non·pro·pri'e·tar'y
non·psy'chot'ic
non·pu'ru·lent
non·ra'di·at'ing
non·re·frac'tive
non·re'pro·duc'tive
non·se·cre'tor
non·seg·ment'ed

non'se·lec'tive
non'sep'tate'
non'sex'u·al
non·smok'er
non'spe·cif'ic
non·stri'at'ed
non·sup'pu·ra'tive
non·sur'gi·cal
non·ten'der
non·tox'ic
non·trop'i·cal
non·un'ion
non·va'lent
non've·ne're·al
non·vi'a·ble
non·vi'su·al·i·za'tion
non·weight'bear'ing
non'yl
Noon
  —pollen unit
  —syndrome
no'o·psy'che
nor'a·cy·meth'a·dol'
nor'a'dren'a·line
nor·bi'o·tin
nor·bol'eth·one'
Nor'dau' disease
nor'dau·ism
nor'de·frin
nor·e·phed'rine
nor·ep'i·neph'rine
nor·eth'an'dro·lone'
nor·eth'in·drone'
nor·e'thy'no'drel'
nor·flox'a·cin
nor·flu'rane'
nor·ges'trel
nor·leu'cine
norm
nor'ma *pl.* -mae'
  —anterior
  —bas'i·lar'is
  —fa'ci·a'lis
  —inferior
  —lat'er·a'lis
  —oc·cip'i·ta'lis
  —sag'it·ta'lis
  —superior
  —ven·tra'lis
  —ver'ti·ca'lis
nor'mal
nor'mal·cy
nor·mal'i·ty

nor'mal·ize'
nor'ma·tive
nor·met'a·neph'rine'
nor·mo·ac'tive
nor'mo·blast'
nor'mo·blas'tic
nor'mo·blas·to'sis
nor'mo·cal·ce'mi·a
nor'mo·cal·ce'mic
nor'mo·chro·ma'si·a
nor'mo·chro·mat'ic
nor'mo·chro'mi·a
nor'mo·chro'mic
nor'mo·cyte'
nor'mo·cyt'ic
nor'mo·cy·to'sis
nor'mo·gly·ce'mic
nor'mo·ka·le'mi·a
nor'mo·ka·le'mic
nor'mo·re·flex'i·a
nor·mo·sper'mic
nor'mo·ten'sion
nor'mo·ten'sive
nor'mo·ther'mi·a
nor'mo·to'ni·a
nor'mo·ton'ic
nor'mo·to'pi·a
nor'mo·vo·le'mi·a
nor'mo·vo·le'mic
nor·mox'i·a
nor·mox'ic
Nor'rie disease
nor·trip'ty·line'
Nor'walk' agent
Nor'wood' procedure
nos'ca·pine'
nose
nose'bleed'
No·se'ma
no'sen·ceph'a·lus
nose'piece'
nos'o·co'mi·al
nos'o·gen'e·sis
nos'o·gen'ic
no·sog'e·ny
nos'o·log'ic *or* nos'o·log'i·cal
no·sol'o·gist
no·sol'o·gy
nos'o·ma'ni·a
no·som'e·try
nos'o·my·co'sis *pl.* -ses'
nos'o·par'a·site'
nos'o·phil'i·a

nos'o·pho'bi·a
nos'o·phyte'
nos'o·poi·et'ic
Nos'o·psyl'lus
  —fas'ci·a'tus
nos'o·tax'y
nos'tril
nos'trum
no'tal
no·tal'gi·a
  —par'es·thet'i·ca
no'tan·ce·pha'li·a
no'tan·en·ce·pha'li·a
no·ta'tion
notch
  —of Ri·vi'nus
no'ten·ceph'a·lo·cele'
no'ten·ceph'a·lus pl. -li'
Noth'na'gel
  —disease
  —paralysis
  —syndrome
no'ti·fi'a·ble
no'to·chord'
no·to·gen'e·sis
no·tom'e·lus
no'vo·bi'o·cin
nox'ious
nu'bile
nu·bil'i·ty
nu'cha pl. -chae'
nu'chal
Nuck
  —canal
  —hydrocele
nu'cle·ar
nu'cle·ase'
nu'cle·at'ed
nu'cle·a'tion
nu'cle·i'
  —an·te'ri·o'res' thal'a·mi'
  —ar'cu·a'ti'
  —coch'le·ar'es' ven·tra'lis et
    dor·sa'lis
  —cor'po·ris ge·nic'u·la'ti'
    lat'er·a'lis
  —corporis mam'il·lar'is
  —corporis trap'e·zoi'de·i'
  —ha·ben'u·lae' me'di·a'lis
    et lat'er·a'lis
  —in'tra·lam'i·nar'es' thal'-
    a·mi'
  —lat'er·a'les' thal'a·mi'

  —mo·to'ri·i' ner'vi' tri·
    gem'i·ni'
  —ner'vi' a·cus'ti·ci'
  —nervi coch'le·ar'is
  —nervi glos'so·pha·ryn'ge·i'
  —nervi tri·gem'i·ni'
  —nervi va·gi'
  —nervi ves·tib'u·lar'is
  —nervi ves·tib'u·lo·coch'-
    le·ar'is
  —ner'vo'rum cer'e·bra'-
    li·um
  —nervorum cra'ni·a'li·um
  —o'ri'gi·nis
  —pon'tis
  —pul'po'si'
  —sys·te'ma·tis ner·vo'si'
    cen·tra'lis
  —teg·men'ti'
  —ter'mi·na'les'
  —ter'mi·na'ti·o'nis
  —tu'ber·a'les'
  —ves·tib'u·lar'es'
nu·cle·ic
nu'cle·ide'
nu'cle·i·form'
nu'cle·in
nu'cle·in·ase'
nu'cle·in'ic
nu'cle·o·cap'sid
nu'cle·o·chy·le'ma
nu'cle·o·chyme'
nu'cle·o·cy'to·plas'mic
nu'cle·of'u·gal
nu'cle·o·his'tone'
nu'cle·o·hy'a·lo·plasm
nu'cle·oid'
nu'cle·o·lar
nu'cle·o·li·form'
nu'cle·o·lin
nu'cle·o·loid'
nu'cle·o·lo·ne'ma
nu'cle·o·lus pl. -li'
nu'cle·o·mi'cro·some'
nu'cle·on
nu'cle·on'ic
nu'cle·on'ics
nu'cle·op'e·tal
Nu'cle·oph'a·ga
nu'cle·o·phil'ic
nu'cle·o·plasm
nu'cle·o·plas'mic
nu'cle·o·pro'tein'

nu'cle·o·re·tic'u·lum
nu'cle·o·si'dase'
nu'cle·o·side'
nu'cle·o'sis pl. -ses'
nu'cle·o·spin'dle
nu'cle·o·ti'dase'
nu'cle·o·tide'
nu'cle·o·tox'ic
nu'cle·o·tox'in
nu'cle·us pl. -cle·i'
  —ac'ces·so'ri·us
  —accessorius ner'vi'
    oc'u·lo·mo·to'ri·i'
  —a'lae' ci·ne're·ae'
  —am·big'u·us
  —a·myg'da·lae'
  —an'gu·lar'is
  —anterior thal'a·mi'
  —an'ter·o·dor·sa'lis
    thal'a·mi'
  —an'ter·o·me·di·a'lis
    thal'a·mi'
  —an'ter·o·ven·tra'lis
    thal'a·mi'
  —ba·sa'lis
  —cau·da'lis cen·tra'lis
  —cau·da'tus
  —cen·tra'lis thal'a·mi'
  —cen·tro·me·di·a'nus
  —centromedianus thal'-
    a·mi'
  —cen'trum me'di·a'num
  —coch'le·ar'is dor·sa'lis
  —cochlearis ven·tra'lis
  —col·lic'u·li' in·fe·ri·o'ris
  —con·ter'mi·na'lis
  —cor'po·ris ge·nic'u·la'ti'
    lat'er·a'lis
  —corporis geniculati
    me'di·a'lis
  —corporis mam'il·lar'is
  —cu'ne·a'tus
  —cuneatus ac'ces·so'ri·us
  —den·ta'tus cer'e·bel'li'
  —dor·sa'lis
  —dorsalis cor'po·ris
    trap'e·zoi'de·i'
  —dorsalis ner'vi' glos'so·
    pha·ryn'ge·i'
  —dorsalis nervi va·gi'
  —dor'so·lat'er·a'lis
  —dor'so·me·di·a'lis
    hy'po·thal'a·mi'

—em'bol'i·for'mis cer'e·
bel'li'
—em'i·nen'ti·ae' te're·tis
—fas·tig'i·i'
—fu·nic'u·li' cu'ne·a'ti'
—funiculi grac'i·lis
—glo'bo'sus cer'e·bel'li'
—grac'i·lis
—ha·ben'u·lae'
—hy'po·tha·lam'i·cus
—inferior pon'tis
—in'ter·ca·la'tus
—in'ter·me'di·o·lat'er·a'lis
—in'ter·me'di·o·me'di·
a'lis
—in'ter·pe·dun'cu·lar'is
—in'ter·sti'ti·a'lis
—lat'er·a'lis dor·sa'lis
thal'a·mi'
—lateralis me·dul'lae'
ob'lon·ga'tae'
—lateralis medullae spi·na'-
lis
—lateralis thal'a·mi'
—lem·nis'ci' lat'er·a'lis
—len'ti·for'mis
—len'tis
—mag'no·cel'lu·lar'is
—me'di·a'lis cen·tra'lis
thal'a·mi'
—medialis dor·sa'lis
—medialis me·dul'lae'
spi·na'lis
—medialis pon'tis
—medialis thal'a·mi'
—mo·to'ri·us ner'vi'
tri·gem'i·ni'
—ner'vi' ab'du·cen'tis
—nervi ac'ces·so'ri·i'
—nervi fa·ci·a'lis
—nervi hy'po·glos'si'
—nervi oc·u·lo·mo·to'ri·i'
—nervi troch'le·ar'is
—of Bekh'ter·ev
—of Bur'dach'
—of Dark'sche·witsch
—of Ed'in·ger-West'phal'
—of Goll
—of Mo'na'kow'
—of Per'li·a
—of Rol'ler
—of Schwal'be
—ol'i·var'is

—olivaris ac'ces·so'ri·us
dor·sa'lis
—olivaris accessorius
me'di·a'lis
—olivaris inferior
—olivaris superior
—o·ri'gi·nis
—par'a·ven·tric'u·lar'is
hy'po·thal'a·mi'
—pig'men·to'sus pon'tis
—posterior hy'po·thal'a·mi'
—posterior thal'a·mi'
—pre·pos'i·tus
—pre'tec·ta'lis
—pro'pri·us
—pul'po'sus
—rad'i·cis de'scen·den'tis
ner'vi' tri·gem'i·ni'
—re·tic'u·lar'is thal'a·mi'
—ru'ber
—sal'i·va·to'ri·us inferior
—salivatorius superior
—sen'so'ri·us inferior
ner'vi' tri·gem'i·ni'
—sensorius prin'ci·pa'lis
ner'vi' tri·gem'i·ni'
—spi·na'lis ner'vi' ac'ces·
so'ri·i'
—sub'tha·lam'i·cus
—superior pon'tis
—su'pra·op'ti·cus hy'po·
thal'a·mi'
—sym·path'i·cus lat'er·
a'lis
—teg'men'ti'
—ter'mi·na'ti·o'nis
—thal'a·mi' lat'er·a'lis
—tho'ra·ci·cus
—trac'tus mes'en·ce·phal'-
i·ci' ner'vi' tri·gem'i·ni'
—tractus sol'i·tar'i·i'
—tractus spi·na'lis ner'vi'
tri·gem'i·ni'
—ven·tra'lis anterior
—ventralis an'ter·o·lat'er·a'-
lis thal'a·mi'
—ventralis cor'po·ris
—trap'e·zoi'de·i'
—ventralis in'ter·me'di·us
thal'a·mi'
—ventralis lat'er·a'lis
—ventralis pos'ter·o·lat'er·
a'lis thal'a·mi'

—ventralis pos'ter·o·me'di·
a'lis thal'a·mi'
—ventralis thal'a·mi'
—ventralis thalami anterior
—ventralis thalami in'ter·
me'di·us
—ventralis thalami pos-
terior
—ven'tro·me'di·a'lis hy'po·
thal'a·mi'
—ves·tib'u·lar'is inferior
—vestibularis lat'er·a'lis
—vestibularis me'di·a'lis
—vestibularis superior
nu'clide'
Nu·el' space
Nuhn glands
null
nul'li·grav'i·da *pl.* -das *or*
-dae'
nul'lip'a·ra
nul'li·par'i·ty
nul'lip'a·rous
nul'li·som'ic
numb
num'ber
numb'ness
nu'mer·al
nu·mer'i·cal
num'mi·form'
num'mu·lar
num'mu·la'tion
nun·na'tion
nurse, nursed, nurs'ing
nurs'er·y
nu·ta'tion
nut'gall'
nut'meg'
nu'tri·ent
nu'tri·lite'
nu'tri·ment
nu·tri'tion
nu·tri'tion·al
nu·tri'tion·ist
nu·tri'tious
nu'tri·tive
nu'tri·ture
nux' vom'i·ca
Ny·an'do fever
nyc'tal·gi·a
nyc'ta·lope'
nyc'ta·lo'pi·a
nyc'ta·pho'ni·a

nyc′ter·ine′
nyc′ter·o·hem′er·al
nyc′to·hem′er·al
nyc′to·phil′i·a
nyc′to·pho′bi·a
nyc′to·pho′ni·a
nyc′to·typh·lo′sis
Ny′hus-Nel′son gastric
  decompression
Ny′lan′der
  —reagent
  —test
ny′li·drin
ny′lon′
nymph
nym′pha *pl.* -phae′
nym′phec′to·my
nym′phi′tis
nym′pho·ca·run′cu·lar
nym′pho·hy′me·ne′al
nym′pho·lep′sy
nym′pho·ma′ni·a
nym′pho·ma′ni·ac′
nym·phon′cus
nym·phot′o·my
nys·tag′mic
nys·tag′mi·form′
nys·tag′mo·graph′
nys·tag′mog′ra·phy
nys·tag′moid′
nys·tag′mus
  —re′trac·to′ri·us
nys′ta·tin
nys·tax′is
Nys′ten law
nyx′is *pl.* -es

O

oat′-cell′
oath of Hip·poc′ra·tes′
ob′ce·ca′tion
ob′dor·mi′tion
ob·du′cent
ob·duc′tion
o·be′li·ac′
o·be′li·ad′
o·be′li·on′ *pl.* -li·a
O′ber
  —operations
  —sign
O′ber-Barr′ procedure
O′ber·may′er test

O′ber·stei′ner-Red′lich
  area
o·bese′
o·be′si·tas
o·be′si·ty
o′bex′
ob·fus·ca′tion
ob′ject′
ob·jec′tive
ob·jec·tiv′i·ty
ob′late′
ob′li·gate′
o·blig′a·to′ry
o·blique′
o·bliq′ui·ty
o·bli′quus
o·blit′er·ate′, -at′ed, -at′ing
o·blit′er·a′tion
o·blit′er·a·tive
ob′lon·ga′ta *pl.* -tas *or* -tae′
ob′lon·ga′tal
ob·mu·tes′cence
ob·nu′bi·la′tion
ob·scure′
ob·ses′sion
ob·ses′sion·al
ob·ses′sive
ob·ses′sive-com·pul′sive
ob·ses′sive·ly
ob·ses′sive·ness
ob·so·les′cence
ob·so·les′cent
ob·stet′ric *or* ob·stet′ri·cal
ob·ste·tri′cian
ob·stet′rics
ob′sti·pa′tion
ob·struct′
ob·struct′ed
ob·struc′tion
ob·struc′tive
ob·stru′ent
ob·tund′
ob·tun·da′tion
ob·tund′ent
ob′tu·rate′, -rat′ed, -rat′ing
ob′tu·ra′tion
ob′tu·ra·tor
  —ex·ter′nus
  —in·ter′nus
ob·tuse′
ob·tu′sion
oc·cip′i·tal
oc·cip′i·ta′lis

oc·cip′i·tal·ize′, -ized′, -iz′ing
oc·cip′i·to·an·te′ri·or
oc·cip′i·to·ax′i·al
oc·cip′i·to·bas′i·lar
oc·cip′i·to·breg·mat′ic
oc·cip′i·to·cer′vi·cal
oc·cip′i·to·fa′cial
oc·cip′i·to·fron′tal
oc·cip′i·to·fron·ta′lis
oc·cip′i·to·mas′toid′
oc·cip′i·to·men′tal
oc·cip′i·to·pa·ri′e·tal
oc·cip′i·to·pon′tine′
oc·cip′i·to·pos·te′ri·or
oc·cip′i·to·scap′u·lar′is
oc·cip′i·to·tem′po·ral
oc·cip′i·to·tha·lam′ic
oc′ci·put
oc·clude′, -clud′ed, -clud′ing
oc·clud′er
oc·clu′sal
oc·clu′si·o′
  —pu′pil′lae′
oc·clu′sion
oc·clu′sive
oc·clu′so·cer′vi·cal
oc·clu·som′e·ter
oc′cult′
oc′cu·pa′tion
oc′cu·pa′tion·al
oc·cur′, -curred′, -cur′ring
o·cel′lus *pl.* -li′
och·le′sis
och′lo·pho′bi·a
o′chrom′e·ter
o′chro·no′sis *pl.* -ses′
o′chro·not′ic
Ochs′ner
  —muscle
  —ring
  —treatment
oc′tad′
oc′ta·gon
oc′ta·meth′yl py′ro·phos′-
  phor·am′ide′
oc′tane′
oc′ta·no′ic
oc′ta·pep′tide′
oc′ta·ploi′dy
oc′tar′i·us
oc′ta·va′lent
oc′ti·grav′i·da
oc·tip′a·ra

oc'to·cry'lene'
oc'to·drine'
oc'to·ge·nar'i·an
oc'tose'
oc·tox'y·nol-9
oc'tyl
oc'u·lar
oc'u·len'tum
oc'u·li' mar'ma·ry·go'des'
oc'u·list
oc'u·lo·au·ric'u·lo·ver'te·bral
oc'u·lo·car'di·ac'
oc'u·lo·ceph'a·lo·gy'ric
oc'u·lo·cer'e·bro·re'nal
oc'u·lo·cu·ta'ne·ous
oc'u·lo·den'to·dig'i·tal
oc'u·lo·fa'cial
oc'u·lo·glan'du·lar
oc'u·lo·gy'ral
oc'u·lo·gy·ra'tion
oc'u·lo·gy'ric
oc'u·lo·mo'tor
oc'u·lo·my·co'sis *pl.* -ses'
oc'u·lo·na'sal
oc'u·lo·pha·ryn'ge·al
oc'u·lo·pleth'ys·mog'ra·phy
oc'u·lo·pu'pil·lar'y
oc'u·lo·sen'so·ry
oc'u·lo·zy'go·mat'ic
oc'u·lus *pl.* -li'
　—cae'si·us
　—dex'ter
　—lac'ri·mans'
　—lep'o·ri'nus
　—pu'ru·len'tus
　—sim'plex'
　—sin'is·ter
　—u'ni·tas
　—u·ter'que'
o·cy'o·din'ic
o'dax·es'mus
Od'di sphincter
o'don·tal'gi·a
o'don·tal'gic
o'don·tec'to·my
o·don'tic
o·don'ti·noid'
o·don'ti'tis
o·don'to·am'e·lo·sar·co'ma
　pl. -mas *or* -ma·ta
o·don'to·at·lan'tal

o·don'to·blast'
o·don'to·blas'tic
o·don'to·blas·to'ma
　pl. -mas *or* -ma·ta
o·don'to·cele'
o·don'to·cla'sis *pl.* -ses'
o·don'to·clast'
o·don'to·gen
o·don'to·gen'e·sis *pl.* -ses'
o·don'to·gen'ic
o'don·tog'e·ny
o·don'to·graph'
o·don'to·graph'ic
o'don·tog'ra·phy
o·don'toid'
o·don'to·lith'
o·don'to·li·thi'a·sis *pl.* -ses'
o·don'to·log'i·cal
o'don·tol'o·gist
o'don·tol'o·gy
o·don'to·lox'ia
o'don·tol'y·sis
o'don'to·ma *pl.* -mas *or* -ma·ta
o'don·top'a·thy
o·don'to·pho'bi·a
o·don'to·plas'ty
o·don'to·pri'sis
o·don'to·scope'
o'don·tos'co·py
o·don'to·sei'sis
o'don'to·sis *pl.* -ses'
o'don·tot'o·my
o'dor
o'dor·ant
o'do·ra'tism
o'dor·if'er·ous
o'dor·im·e'ter
o'dor·im'e·try
o'dor·ous
o·dyn'a·cou'sis
o'dy·nom'e·ter
o·dyn'o·pha'gi·a
o'dy·nu'ri·a
oed'i·pal
oed'i·pism
Oed'i·pus complex
Oer'tel treatment
oesophag-. See words spelled *esophag-.*
oesophago-. See words spelled *esophago-.*
of·fi'cial

O·ga'wa serotype
O'gil·vie syndrome
Og'ston-Luc' operation
O·gu'chi disease
O·ha'ra disease
Ohl'ma·cher solution
ohm
ohm·am'me'ter
Ohm law
ohm'me'ter
o·id'i·o·my·co'sis *pl.* -ses'
oil
oil'y
oi'no·ma'ni·a
oint'ment
o'le·ag'i·nous
o'le·an'do·my'cin
o'le·ate'
o·lec'ra·nal
o·lec'ra·nar·thri'tis
o·lec'ra·nar·throc'a·ce
o·lec'ra·nar·throp'a·thy
o·lec'ra·noid'
o·lec'ra·non'
o'le·fin
o·le'ic
o'le·in
o'le·o·gran'u·lo'ma
　pl. -mas *or* -ma·ta
o'le·om'e·ter
o'le·o·res'in
o'le·o·ther'a·py
o'le·o·vi'ta·min
o'le·um *pl.* o'le·a
　—suc'ci·ni'
ol'fact'
ol·fac'tion
ol·fac·tom'e·ter
ol·fac'to·ry
ol'i·ge'mi·a
ol'i·ge'mic
ol'i·ger·ga'si·a
ol'i·go·am'ni·os'
ol'i·go·blast'
ol'i·go·blen'ni·a
ol'i·go·car'di·a *pl.* -ae' *or* -as
ol'i·go·chro·ma'si·a
ol'i·go·chro·me'mi·a
ol'i·go·clo'nal
ol'i·go·cys'tic
ol'i·go·cy·the'mi·a
ol'i·go·cy·the'mic
ol'i·go·dac'ry·a

ol'i·go·dac·tyl'i·a
ol'i·go·dac'ty·ly
ol'i·go·den'dro·blas·to'ma
  pl. -mas *or* -ma·ta
ol'i·go·den'dro·cyte'
ol'i·go·den'dro·cy·to'ma
  pl. -mas *or* -ma·ta
ol'i·go·den·drog'li·a
ol'i·go·den·drog'li·al
ol'i·go·den'dro·gli·o'ma
  pl. -mas *or* -ma·ta
ol'i·go·den'dro·gli·o·ma·
  to'sis *pl.* -ses'
ol'i·go·den·dro·ma *pl.* -mas
  or -ma·ta
ol'i·go·dip'si·a
ol'i·go·don'ti·a
ol'i·go·dy·nam'ic
ol'i·go·en·ceph'a·ly
ol'i·go·ga·lac'ti·a
ol'i·go·gen'ic
ol'i·go·gen'ics
ol'i·gog'li·a
ol'i·go·hy·dram'ni·os
ol'i·go·hy'dri·a
ol'i·go·hy·dru'ri·a
ol'i·go·hy'per·men·or·
  rhe'a
ol'i·go·hy'po·men·or·rhe'a
ol'i·go·lec'i·thal
ol'i·go·men·or·rhe'a
ol'i·go'mer
ol'i·go·mer'ic
ol'i·go·my'cin
ol'i·go·nu'cle·o·tide'
ol'i·go·phos'pha·tu'ri·a
ol'i·go·phre'ni·a
ol'i·go·phren'ic
ol'i·go·plas'mi·a
ol'i·gop·ne'a
ol'i·go·pty'a·lism
ol'i·go·py'rene'
ol'i·go·sac'cha·ride'
ol'i·go·si·al'i·a
ol'i·go·sper'mi·a
ol'i·go·trich'i·a
  —con·gen'i·ta
ol'i·go·tro'phi·a
ol'i·go·troph'ic
ol'i·got'ro·phy
ol'i·go·zo'o·sper'mi·a
ol'i·gu·re'sis *pl.* -ses'
ol'i·gu·ri·a

ol'i·gu'ric
o·lis'the·ro·chro'ma·tin
o·lis·thet'ic
o·lis'thy
o·li'va
ol'i·var'y
ol'ive
Ol'i·ver sign
ol'i·vif'u·gal
ol'i·vip'e·tal
ol'i·vo·cer'e·bel'lar
ol'i·vo·pon·to·cer'e·bel'lar
ol'i·vo·spi'nal
Ol·lier' disease
ol'o·pho'ni·a
ol·sal'a·zine'
o'ma·ceph'a·lus *pl.* -li'
o·ma'gra
o·mal'gi·a
o'mar·thral'gi·a
o'mar·thri'tis
o'ma·si'tis
o·ma'sum
o·me'ga
o·men'tal
o'men·tec'to·my
o·men·ti'tis
o'men·to·fix·a'tion
o·men'to·pex'y
o·men·tor'rha·phy
o·men·tot'o·my
o·men'tum *pl.* -ta
  —ma'jus
  —mi'nus
o·men'tum·ec'to·my
o·mep'ra·zole'
o·mi'tis
om·ma·tid'i·um *pl.* -i·a
om·niv'o·rous
o'mo·cer'vi·ca'lis
o·mo·cla·vic'u·lar
o·mo·dyn'i·a
o·mo·hy'oid'
o·mo·pha'gi·a
o·mo·plat'a
o·mo·ster'num *pl.* -nums *or*
  -na
o'mo·ver'te·bral
om'pha·lec'to·my
om·phal'ic
om'pha·li'tis
om·pha·lo·an'gi·op'a·gus
om'pha·lo·cele'

om'pha·lo·cho'ri·on'
om'pha·lo·did'y·mus
om'pha·lo·gen'e·sis *pl.* -ses'
om'pha·lo·mes'en·ter'ic
om'pha·lop'a·gus
om'pha·lo·phle·bi'tis
om'pha·lo·prop·to'sis
  pl. -ses'
om'pha·lor·rha'gi·a
om'pha·los' *pl.* -li'
om'pha·lo·site'
om'pha·lo·tax'is
om'pha·lot'o·my
o'nan·ism
On'cho·cer'ca
  —cae·cu'ti·ens
  —vol'vu·lus
on'cho·cer·ci'a·sis *pl.* -ses'
on'cho·cer·co'ma
on'cho·der·ma'ti·tis
on'co·cyte'
on'co·cy·to'ma *pl.* -mas *or*
  -ma·ta
on'co·gene'
on'co·gen'e·sis *pl.* -ses'
on'co·ge·net'ic
on'co·gen'ic
on'co·graph'
on·cog'ra·phy
on·col'o·gist
on·col'o·gy
on·col'y·sis
on'co·lyt'ic
on·co'ma *pl.* -mas *or* -ma·ta
On'co·me·la'ni·a
  —for'mo·sa'na
  —hu'pen'sis
  —hy'dro·bi·op'sis
  —no·soph'o·ra
on·co'sis *pl.* -ses'
on'co·sphere'
on'co·thlip'sis
on·cot'ic
on·cot'o·my
on'co·trop'ic
on·dan'se·tron
o·nei'ric
o·nei'rism
o·nei'ro·dyn'i·a
o'nei·rog'mus
o'nei·rol'o·gy
o'nei·ros'co·py
on·kin'o·cele'

on'lay
on'o·mat'o·ma'ni·a
on'o·mat'o·pho'bi·a
on'o·mat'o·poi·e'sis *pl.* -ses'
on'o·mat'o·poi·et'ic
on'set'
on'to·a·nal'y·sis
on'to·gen'e·sis *pl.* -ses'
on'to·ge·net'ic
on·tog'e·ny
on'y·al'ai'
on'y·chal'gi·a nervosa
on'y·cha·tro'phi·a
on'y·chat'ro·phy
on'y·chaux'is *pl.* -chaux'es'
on'y·chec'to·my
o·nych'i·a
   —cra·que·lé'
   —ma·lig'na
   —punc·ta'ta
   —sim'plex'
   —su·per·fi·ci·a'lis un·du·
      la'ta
on'y·chin
on'y·choc'la·sis
on'y·cho·dys'tro·phy
on'y·cho·gen'ic
on'y·cho·graph'
on'y·cho·gry·po'sis *pl.* -ses'
on'y·cho·het'er·o·to'pi·a
on'y·choid'
on'y·chol'y·sis
on'y·cho·ma *pl.* -mas *or*
   -ma·ta
on'y·cho·ma·de'sis
on'y·cho·ma·la'ci·a
on'y·cho·my·co'sis *pl.* -ses'
on'y·chon'o·sus
on'y·cho·os·te·o·dys·pla'si·a
on'y·cho·pac'i·ty
on'y·cho·path'ic
on'y·chop'a·thy
on'y·cho·pha'gi·a
on'y·chop·to'sis
on'y·chor·rhex'is
   pl. -rhex'es'
on'y·chor·rhi'za
on'y·cho·schiz'i·a
on'y·cho'sis *pl.* -ses'
on'y·cho·stro'ma
on'y·chot'il·lo·ma'ni·a
on'y·chot'o·my
on'y·chot'ro·phy

O'nyong'-nyong' fever
on'yx
o·nyx'is
on'yx·i'tis
o'o·blast'
o'o·ceph'a·lus
o'o·cyst'
o'o·cyte'
o'o·gen'e·sis *pl.* -ses'
o'o·ge·net'ic
o'o·go'ni·um *pl.* -ni·a
o·o·ki·ne'sis *pl.* -ses'
o·o·ki·nete'
o·o·ki·net'ic
o'o·lem'ma
o'o·pho·rec'to·mize'
o'o·pho·rec'to·my
o'o·pho·ri'tis
o·oph'o·ro·cys·tec'to·my
o·oph'o·ro·cys·to'sis
   pl. -ses'
o·oph'o·ro·cys·tos'to·my
o·oph'o·ro·hys'ter·ec'-
   to·my
o·oph'o·ro·ma *pl.* -mas *or*
   -ma·ta
   —fol·lic'u·lar'e'
o·oph'o·ro·ma·la'ci·a
o·oph'o·ron'
o·oph'o·rop'a·thy
o·oph'o·ro·pex'y
o·oph'o·ro·plas'ty
o·oph'o·ro·sal'pin·gec'-
   to·my
o·oph'o·ro·sal'pin·gi'tis
o·oph'o·ros'to·my
o·oph'o·rot'o·my
o'o·phor'rha·phy
o'o·plasm
o'o·sperm'
o'o·spore'
o'o·the'ca *pl.* -cae'
o'o·tid
o'o·type'
ooze, oozed, ooz'ing
o'pac'i·fi·ca'tion
o·pac'i·fy', -fied', -fy'ing
o·pac'i·ty
o'pal·es'cence
o'pal·es'cent
O·pal'ski cells
o'paque'
o·pei'do·scope'

o'pen
op'er·a·bil'i·ty
op'er·a·ble
op'er·ant
op'er·ate', -at'ed, -at'ing
op'er·a'tion
op'er·a'tion·al
op'er·a·tive
op'er·a·tive·ly
op'er·a'tor
o·per'cu·lar
o·per'cu·late
o·per'cu·lec'to·my
o·per'cu·lum *pl.* -la *or* -lums
   —fron·ta'le'
   —fron'to·pa·ri'e·ta'le'
   —il'e·i'
   —tem'po·ra'le'
op'er·on'
o·phi'a·sis
O·phid'i·a
o·phid'i·o·pho'bi·a
o'phid·ism
O'phi·oph'a·gus han'nah
oph·ry·i'tis
oph'ry·on'
Oph'ry·o·sco·lec'i·dae'
oph'ry·o'sis *pl.* -ses'
oph'ry·phthei·ri'a·sis
   pl. -ses'
oph·ryt'ic
oph·thal'ma·cro'sis
oph·thal'ma·gra
oph·thal·mal'gi·a
oph·thal·mec'chy·mo'sis
oph·thal·mec'to·my
oph·thal·men·ceph'a·lon'
oph·thal'mi·a
   —e·lec'tri·ca
   —ne·o'na·to'rum
   —ni·va'lis
   —no·do'sa
oph·thal·mi·at'rics
oph·thal·mic
oph·thal·mit'ic
oph·thal·mi'tis
oph·thal'mo·blen'nor·rhe'a
oph·thal'mo·cele'
oph·thal'mo·cen·te'sis
oph·thal'mo·co'pi·a
oph·thal'mo·di'as·tim'e·ter
oph·thal'mo·do·ne'sis
   pl. -ses'

oph·thal'mo·dy'na·mom'e·
ter

oph·thal'mo·dy'na·mom'e·
try

oph·thal'mo·dyn'i·a

oph·thal'mo·ei'ko·nom'e·
ter

oph·thal'mo·ei'ko·nom'e·
try

oph·thal'mo·graph'

oph'thal'mog'ra·phy

oph'thal'mo·gy'ric

oph'thal'mo·i'con·om'e·try

oph'thal'mo·leu'ko·scope'

oph'thal'mo·lith'

oph'thal'mo·log'ic or
   oph·thal'mo·log'i·cal

oph·thal·mol'o·gist

oph·thal·mol'o·gy

oph·thal'mo·ma·cro'sis

oph·thal'mo·ma·la'ci·a

oph·thal'mom'e·ter

oph·thal'mom'e·try

oph·thal'mo·my·co'sis
   pl. -ses'

oph·thal'mo·my·i'a·sis

oph·thal'mo·my·i'tis

oph·thal'mo·my·o·si'tis

oph·thal'mo·my·ot'o·my

oph·thal'mo·neu·ri'tis

oph·thal'mo·neu'ro·my'e·
li'tis

oph·thal'mop'a·thy

oph·thal'mo·pha·com'e·ter

oph·thal'mo·phas'ma·tos'-
co·py

oph·thal'mo·phle·bot'o·my

oph·thal'mo·pho'bi·a

oph·thal·moph'thi·sis

oph·thal'mo·phy'ma

oph·thal'mo·plas'tic

oph·thal'mo·plas'ty

oph·thal'mo·ple'gi·a

oph·thal'mo·ple'gic

oph·thal'mop·to'sis

oph·thal'mo·re·ac'tion

oph·thal'mor·rha'gi·a

oph·thal'mor·rhe'a

oph·thal'mor·rhex'is
   pl. -rhex'es'

oph·thal'mos'

oph·thal'mo·scope'

oph·thal'mo·scop'ic

oph·thal·mos'co·py

oph'thal·mos'ta·sis pl. -ses'

oph·thal'mo·stat'

oph·thal'mo·sta·tom'e·ter

oph·thal'mo·ste·re'sis

oph·thal'mo·syn'chy·sis

oph'thal'mot'o·my

oph·thal'mo·to·nom'e·ter

oph·thal'mo·to·nom'e·try

oph'thal'mo·trope'

oph·thal'mo·tro·pom'e·ter

oph·thal'mo·tro·pom'e·try

oph·thal'mo·vas'cu·lar

oph·thal'mo·xe·ro'sis
   pl. -ses'

oph·thal'mus pl. -mi'

o'pi·ate

O'pie paradox

o'pi·oid'

o'pi·o·ma'ni·a

o'pi·o·ma'ni·ac'

o'pi·o·pha'gi·a

o'pi·oph'a·gism

o'pi·oph'a·gy

o'pi·o·phile'

o·pis'then

o·pis'the·nar'

o·pis'thi·on'

o·pis'tho·cra'ni·on'

o·pis'thog'na·thism

o·pis'tho·neph'ros'

o·pis'tho·po·rei'a

o·pis'thor·chi·a'sis pl. -ses'

Op'is·thor'chis
   —fe·lin'e·us
   —no'ver·ca
   —viv'er·ri'ni'

o'pis·thot'ic

o·pis'tho·ton'ic

op'is·thot'o·noid'

op'is·thot'o·nos

o'pi·um

o'po·bal'sa·mum

op'o·ceph'a·lus pl. -li'

op'o·did'y·mus

o'pod'y·mus

Op'pen·heim'
   —disease
   —reflex
   —sign

Op'pen·heim-Ur'bach'
disease

op'pi·la'tion

op'pi·la'tive

op·po'nens
   —dig'i·ti' min'i·mi'
   —digiti quin'ti'
   —pol'li·cis

op'por·tun'ist

op'por·tun·is'tic

op'po·si'tion

op·si·al'gi·a

op·sig'e·nes'

op'sin

op·sin'o·gen

op'si·nog'e·nous

op'si·om'e·ter

op'si·o·no'sis pl. -ses'

op'si·u'ri·a

op'so·clo'ni·a

op'so·clo'nus

op'so·ma'ni·a

op'so·ma'ni·ac'

op·son'ic

op'so·nin

op'so·ni·za'tion

op'so·nize', -nized', -niz'ing

op'so·no·cy'to·phag'ic

op'so·nom'e·try

op'so·no·ther'a·py

op·tes·the'si·a

op'tic or op'ti·cal

op·ti'cian

op·ti'cian·ry

op·ti·co·chi'as·mat'ic

op·ti·co·chi'as'mic

op·ti·co·cil'i·ar'y

op·ti·coele'

op·ti·co·fa'cial

op·ti·co·ki·net'ic

op·ti·co·pu'pil·lar'y

op'tics

op'ti·mal

op'ti·mum

op'to·blast'

op'to·chi'as'mic

op'to·gram'

op'to·ki·net'ic

op'to·me'ninx

op·tom'e·ter

op·tom'e·trist

op·tom'e·try

op'to·my·om'e·ter

op'to·phone'

op'to·type'

o'ra

—ser·ra'ta
o'rad'
o'ral (pertaining to the mouth)
 ♦aural
o·ra'le'
o·ral'i·ty
o'ral·ly
Or·be'li effect
or·bic'u·lar
or·bic'u·lar'e
or·bic'u·lar'is
 —oc'u·li'
 —o'ris
 —pal'pe·brar'um
or·bic'u·lus pl. -li'
 —cil'i·ar'is
or'bit
or'bi·ta pl. -tae'
or'bi·tal
or'bi·ta'le' pl. -ta'li·a
or'bi·ta'lis
or'bi·to·na'sal
or'bi·to·nom'e·ter
or'bi·to·nom'e·try
or'bi·to·sphe'noid'
or'bi·to·stat'
or'bi·to·tem'po·ral
or'bi·tot'o·my
or'ce·in
or'che·i'tis
or·ches'tro·ma'ni·a
or'chi·al'gi·a
or'chic
or'chi·cho·re'a
or'chi·dal'gi·a
or'chi·dec'to·my
or'chid'ic
or'chi·di'tis
or'chi·do·ce'li·o·plas'ty
or'chi·do·ep'i·did'y·mec'-
 to·my
or'chi·don'cus
or'chi·dop'a·thy
or'chi·do·pex'y
or'chi·do·plas'ty
or'chi·dop·to'sis
or'chi·dor'rha·phy
or'chi·dot'o·my
or'chi·ec'to·my
or'chi·en·ceph'a·lo'ma
 pl. -mas or -ma·ta
or'chi·ep'i·did'y·mi'tis
or'chil

or'chi·o·ca·tab'a·sis pl. -ses'
or'chi·o·cele'
or'chi·o·my'e·lo'ma
 pl. -mas or -ma·ta
or'chi·on'cus
or'chi·op'a·thy
or'chi·o·pex'y
or'chi·o·plas'ty
or'chi·or'rha·phy
or'chi·o·scir'rhus pl. -rhi' or
 -rhus·es
or'chi·ot'o·my
or'chis
or·chit'ic
or·chi'tis
or·chit'o·my
or·chot'o·my
or'ci·nol'
or'der
or'der·ly
or'di·nate
o·rec'tic
o·rex'i·a
o·rex'is
orf
or'gan
 —of Cor'ti
 —of Gol'gi
 —of Ja'cob·son
or'ga·na
 —gen'i·ta'li·a fem'i·ni'na
 —genitalia mas·cu·li'na
 —genitalia mu'li·e'bri·a
 —genitalia vi·ril'i·a
 —oc'u·li' ac'ces·so'ri·a
 —sen'su·um
 —u'ro·po·ët'i·ca
or'gan·elle'
or·gan'ic
or·gan'i·cal·ly
or·gan'i·cism
or·gan'i·cist
or'gan·ism
or'ga·ni·za'tion
or'ga·nize', -nized', -niz'ing
or'ga·niz'er
or'ga·no·ax'i·al
or·gan'o·gel'
or'ga·no·gen'e·sis
or'ga·no·ge·net'ic
or'ga·no·gen'ic
or'ga·nog'e·ny
or'ga·noid'

or'ga·no·lep'tic
or'ga·nol'o·gy
or'ga·no·meg'a·ly
or·gan'o·mer·cu'ri·al
or·gan'o·me·tal'lic
or'ga·non' pl. -na
 —au·di'tus
 —gus'tus
 —ol·fac'tus
 —pa·ren'chy·ma·to'sum
 —spi·ra'le'
 —vi'sus
 —vom'er·o·na·sa'le'
or'ga·nop'a·thy
or'ga·no·pex'y
or'ga·nos'co·py
or·gan'o·sol'
or'ga·no·tax'is
or'ga·no·ther'a·py
or'ga·no·troph'ic (pertaining
 to the nutrition of organs)
 ♦organotropic
or'ga·no·trop'ic (pertaining to
 chemical affinity)
 ♦organotrophic
or'ga·not'ro·pism
or'ga·not'ro·py
organs of Zuck'er·kandl
or'ga·nule'
or'ga·num pl. -na
 —gus'tus
 —ol·fac'tus
 —spi·ra'le'
 —ves·tib'u·lo·coch'le·ar'e
 —vi'sus
 —vom'er·o·na·sa'le'
or'gasm
or·gas'mo·lep'sy
or'go·tein'
o'ri·ent
o'ri·en·ta'tion
or'i·fice
or'i·fi'cial
o·ri·fi'ci·um pl. -ci·a
 —ex·ter'num u'ter·i'
 —in·ter'num u'ter·i'
 —u·re'ter·is
 —u·re'thrae' in·ter'num
 —urethrae mu'li·e'bris
 ex·ter'num
 —urethrae vi·ri'lis ex·ter'-
 num
 —va·gi'nae'

or·i·gin
Orms'by method
or·ni·thine'
or·ni·thi·ne'·mi·a
Or·ni·thod'o·rus
or·ni·tho'sis *pl.* -ses'
or·ni·thu'ric
or·ni·thyl
o·ro·an'tral
o·ro·di·ag·no'sis *pl.* -ses'
o·ro·dig'i·to·fa'cial
o·ro·fa'cial
o·ro·gas'tric
o·ro·lin'gual
o·ro·max'il·lar·y
o·ro·na'sal
o·ro·no'sus
o·ro·pha·ryn'ge·al
o·ro·phar'ynx
  pl. -pha·ryn'ges'
o·ro·sin
o·ro·so·mu'coid'
o·rot'ic
O·roy'a fever
or·phen'a·drine'
or·rho·im·mu'ni·ty
or·rho·men·in·gi'tis
or·rho·re·ac'tion
or'rhos'
or'ris·root'
Orr'-Loygue' technique
Or'si-Groc'co method
Or·ta·la'ni sign
or·ther·ga'si·a
or·the'sis *pl.* -ses'
or·thet'ics
or·the·tist
or'tho
or·tho·ar·te·ri·ot'o·ny
or·tho·bo'ric
or·tho·car'di·ac'
or·tho·ce·phal'ic
or·tho·ceph'a·lous
or·tho·ceph'a·ly
or·tho·chlo'ro·phe'nol'
or·tho·cho·re'a
or·tho·chro·mat'ic
or·tho·chro'mi·a
or·tho·chro'mic
or·tho·cra'si·a
or·tho·cre'sol'
or·tho·cy·to'sis *pl.* -ses'
or·tho·dac'ty·lous

or·tho·den'tin
or·tho·di'a·gram'
or·tho·di'a·graph'
or·tho·di·ag'ra·phy
or·tho·dol'i·cho·ceph'a·lous
or·tho·don'ti·a
or·tho·don'tic
or·tho·don'tics
or·tho·don'tist
or·tho·drom'ic
or·tho·gen'e·sis
or·tho·ge·net'ic
or·tho·gen'ic
or·tho·gly·ce'mic
or·thog·nath'ic
or·thog'na·thism
or·thog'na·thous
or·thog'o·nal
or·tho·grade'
or·tho·hy·drox'y·ben·zo'ic
or·tho·mes·o·ceph'a·lous
or·thom'e·ter
or·tho·mo·lec'u·lar
or·tho·myx'o·vi'rus
or·tho·pae'dic *var. of*
  orthopedic
or·tho·pae'dics *var. of*
  orthopedics
or·tho·pae'dist *var. of*
  orthopedist
or·tho·pan'to·mo·gram'
or·tho·pe'dic *also*
  orthopaedic
or·tho·pe'dics *also*
  orthopaedics
or·tho·pe'dist *also*
  orthopaedist
or·tho·per·cus'sion
or·tho·phe·nan'thro·line'
or·tho·phe'no·lase'
or·tho·phen·yl·phe'nol'
or·tho·pho'ri·a
or·tho·phos'phate'
or·tho·phos·phor'ic
or·tho·plast'
or·thop·ne'a
or·thop·ne'ic
or·tho·prax'is *pl.* -prax'es'
or·tho·prax'y
or·tho·psy·chi'a·try
Or·thop'ter·a
or·thop'tic
or·thop'tics

or·thop'to·scope'
or·tho·rhom'bic
or·tho·roent'gen·og'ra·phy
or·thor·rhach'ic
or·tho·scope'
or·tho·scop'ic
or·thos'co·py
or·tho·sis *pl.* -ses'
or·tho·sta'sis
or·tho·stat'ic
or·tho·stat'ism
or·tho·ster'e·o·scope'
or·tho·ster'e·o·scop'ic
or·tho·sym'pa·thet'ic
or·tho·tast'
or·tho·te'ri·on'
or·tho·ther'a·py
or·thot'ic
or·thot'ics
or·tho·tist
or·tho·ton'ic
or·thot'o·nos *var. of*
  orthotonus
or·thot'o·nus *also*
  orthotonos
or·tho·to'pi·a
or·tho·top'ic
or·tho·trop'ic
or·thot'ro·pism
or·tho·volt'age
Orth solution
Or'to·la'ni sign
o·ry'za·min
os *(mouth), pl.* o'ra
os *(bone), pl.* os'sa
  —ac'e·tab'u·li'
  —a·cro'mi·a'le'
  —ar·tic'u·lar'e'
  —bas'i·lar'e'
  —ba'si·ot'i·cum
  —breg·mat'i·cum
  —brev'e'
  —cal'cis
  —cap'i·ta'tum
  —cen·tra'le'
  —cli·to'ri·dis
  —coc'cy·gis
  —cor'dis
  —cos·ta'le'
  —cox'ae'
  —cu·boi'de·um
  —cu'ne·i·for'me' in'ter·me'-
  di·um

—cuneiforme lat′er·a′le′
—cuneiforme me·di·a′le′
—cuneiforme pri′mum
—cuneiforme se·cun′dum
—cuneiforme ter′ti·um
—den·ta′le′
—en·to′mi·on′
—ep′i·pter′i·cum
—eth′moi·da′le′
—fal′ci·for′me′
—fron·ta′le′
—ha·ma′tum
—hy·oi′de·um
—il′i·um
—in′ci·si′vum
—in′ter·cu′ne·i·for′me′
—in′ter·fron·ta′le′
—in′ter·met′a·tar′se·um
—in′ter·pa·ri′e·ta′le′
—is′chi·i′
—ja·pon′i·cum
—lac′ri·ma′le′
—len·tic′u·lar′e′
—lon′gum
—mag′num
—met′a·car′pa′le′
—mul·tan′gu·lum ma′jus
—multangulum mi′nus
—na·sa′le′
—na·vic′u·lar′e′
—naviculare ma′nus
—naviculare pe′dis
—no′vum
—oc·cip′i·ta′le′
—o′don·toi·de′um
—or·bic′u·lar′e′
—or′bi·ta′le′
—pal′a·ti′num
—pa·ri′e·ta′le
—pe′dis
—pe′nis
—per′o·ne′um
—pi′si·for′me′
—pla′num
—pneu·mat′i·cum
—pre·ba′si·oc·cip′i·ta′le′
—pu′bis
—pu′rum
—sa′crum
—sca·phoi′de·um
—sphe·noi·da′le′
—sty·loi′de·um

—suf·frag′i·nis
—su′pra·ster·na′le′
—tem′po·ra′le′
—tib′i·a′le′ ex·ter′num
—tra·pe′zi·um
—trap′e·zoi′de·um
—tri·go′num
—tri′que′trum
—u′ter·i′
—uteri ex·ter′num
—uteri in·ter′num
—Ve·sa′li·i′
—zy′go·mat′i·cum
o′sa·mine′
o′sa·zone′
Os′borne′ wave
os·che·a
os·che·al
os·che·i′tis
os·che·o·cele′
os·che·o·hy′dro·cele′
os·che·o·lith′
os·che·o′ma   pl. -mas or
    -ma·ta
os·che·o·plas′ty
Os·cil·lar′i·a ma·lar′i·ae′
os′cil·late′, -lat′ed, -lat′ing
os′cil·la′tion
os′cil·la·tor
os′cil·la·to′ry
os·cil′lo·gram′
os·cil′lo·graph′
os·cil′lo·graph′ic
os′cil·log′ra·phy
os·cil′lo·me·ter
os·cil′lo·met′ric
os·cil′lom·e·try
os·cil′lop′si·a
os·cil′lo·scope′
os·cil′lo·scop′ic
Os·cin′i·dae′
Os′ci·nis
    —pal′li·pes′
os′ci·tan·cy
os′ci·ta′tion
os′cu·la′tion
os′cu·lum
Os·er·et′sky test
Os′good-Has′kins test
Os′good operation
Os′good-Schlat′ter disease
O′Shaugh′nes·sy operation
Os′ler

—disease
—nodes
Os′ler-Ren·du′-Web′er
disease
Os′ler-Va·quez′
—disease
—nodes
os′mate′
os·mat′ic
os·me′sis
os′mes·the′si·a
os′mic
os′mics
os′mi·dro′sis pl. -ses′
os′mi·o·phil′ic
os′mi·um
os′mo·dys·pho′ri·a
os′mol′
os·mo′lal
os·mo·lal′i·ty
os·mo′lar
os·mo·lar′i·ty
os·mol′o·gy
os′mom′e·ter
os′mom′e·try
os′mo·no·sol′o·gy
os′mo·phil′ic
os′mo·pho′bi·a
os′mo·phore′
os′mo·re·cep′tor
os′mo·reg′u·la′tor
os′mo·reg′u·la·to′ry
os′mose′
os′mo·sis
os·mot′ic
os·phre′si·ol′o·gy
os·phre′si·om′e·ter
os·phre′sis
os·phret′ic
os·phy·o·my′e·li′tis
os·phy·ot′o·my
os′sa
    —car′pi′
    —cra′ni·i′
    —dig′i·to′rum ma′nus
    —digitorum pe′dis
    —ex·trem′i·ta′tis in·fe′ri·o′-
    ris
    —extremitatis su·pe′ri·o′ris
    —fa′ci·e′i′
    —in′ter·ca·lar′i·a
    —mem′bri′ in·fe′ri·o′ris
    —membri su·pe′ri·o′ris

—met′a·car·pa′li·a
—met′a·tar·sa′li·a
—ses′a·moi′de·a
—su′pra·ster·na′li·a
—su′tu·rar′um
—tar′si′
os·se′in
os·se·o·al·bu′min·oid′
os·se·o·car·ti·lag′i·nous
os·se·o·fi′brous
os·se·o·in·te·gra′tion
os·se·o·lig′a·men′tous
os·se·o·mu′cin
os·se·o·mu′coid′
os·se′ous
os·si·cle
—of Ber·tin′
os·sic′u·la au·di′tus
os·sic′u·lar
os·sic′u·lo·plas′ty
os·si·cu·lot′o·my
os·sic′u·lum *pl.* -la
os·sif′er·ous
os·sif′ic
os·si·fi·ca′tion
os·sif′lu·ence
os·sif′lu·ent
os·si·form′
os·si·fy′, -fied′, -fy′ing
os·tal′gi·a
os·tal′gic
os′tal·gi′tis
os·te·al
os·te·al′gi·a
os′te·al′le·o′sis *pl.* -ses′
os′te·an′a·gen′e·sis *pl.* -ses′
os·tec′to·my
os·tec′to·py
os·te·ec′to·my
os·te·ec′to·pi·a
os·te′in
os·te·it′ic
os·te·i′tis
—car·no′sa
—con·den′sans il′i·i′
—cys′ti·ca
—de·for′mans′
—fi·bro′sa cys′ti·ca
—fibrosa cystica dis·sem′-
i·na′ta
—fibrosa gen′er·al·i·sa′ta
—fra·gil′i·tans′
—fun·go′sa

—pu′bis
—tu·ber′cu·lo′sa mul′ti·
plex′ cys·toi′des′
os·tem′bry·on′
os′tem·py·e′sis
os′te·o·a·cu′sis
os′te·o·an′a·gen′e·sis
pl. -ses′
os′te·o·an′es·the′si·a
os′te·o·an′eu·rysm
os′te·o·ar·threc′to·my
os′te·o·ar·thrit′ic
os′te·o·ar·thri′tis
os′te·o·ar·throp′a·thy
os′te·o·ar·thro′sis *pl.* -ses′
os′te·o·ar·throt′o·my
os′te·o·ar·tic′u·lar
os′te·o·blast′
os′te·o·blas′tic
os′te·o·blas·to′ma *pl.* -mas
or -ma·ta
os′te·o·ca·chec′tic
os′te·o·ca·chex′i·a
os′te·o·camp′
os′te·o·camp′si·a
os′te·o·car′ci·no′ma
pl. -mas *or* -ma·ta
os′te·o·car·ti·lag′i·nous
os′te·o·cele′
os′te·o·ce·men′tum *pl.* -ta
os′te·o·chon′dral
os′te·o·chon·drit′ic
os′te·o·chon·dri′tis
—de·for′mans′ cox′ae′
ju′ve·ni′lis
—deformans ju′ve·ni′lis
—dis′se·cans′
—ne·crot′i·cans
os′te·o·chon·dro·dys·pla′-
si·a
os′te·o·chon′dro·dys·tro′-
phi·a de·for′mans′
os′te·o·chon′dro·dys′tro·
phy
os′te·o·chon·drol′y·sis
os′te·o·chon·dro′ma
pl. -mas *or* -ma·ta
os′te·o·chon·dro·ma·to′sis
os′te·o·chon·dro·myx·o′ma
pl. -mas *or* -ma·ta
os′te·o·chon·dro·myx′o·
sar·co′ma *pl.* -mas *or*
-ma·ta

os′te·o·chon·drop′a·thy
os′te·o·chon′dro·phyte′
os′te·o·chon′dro·sar·co′ma
pl. -mas *or* -ma·ta
os′te·o·chon·dro′sis *pl.* -ses′
—de·for′mans′ ju′ve·ni′lis
—deformans tib′i·ae′
—dis′se·cans′
os′te·o·chon′drous
os′te·o·cla′si·a
os′te·oc′la·sis *pl.* -ses′
os′te·o·clast′
os′te·o·clas′tic
os′te·o·clas·to′ma *pl.* -mas
or -ma·ta
os′te·o·com′ma
os′te·o·cope′
os′te·o·cop′ic
os′te·o·cra′ni·um *pl.*
-ni·ums *or* -ni·a
os′te·o·cys·to′ma *pl.* -mas *or*
-ma·ta
os′te·o·cyte′
os′te·o·den′tin
os′te·o·der′ma·to·plas′tic
os′te·o·der′ma·tous
os′te·o·der′mi·a
os′te·o·des·mo′sis *pl.* -ses′
os′te·o·di·as′ta·sis *pl.* -ses′
os′te·o·dyn′i·a
os′te·o·dys·plas′ty
os′te·o·dys·tro′phi·a
—de·for′mans′
—fi·bro′sa
os′te·o·dys·tro′phy
os′te·o·en′chon·dro′ma
pl. -mas *or* -ma·ta
os′te·o·e·piph′y·sis *pl.* -ses′
os′te·o·fi′bro·chon·dro′ma
pl. -mas *or* -ma·ta
os′te·o·fi′bro·chon′dro·sar·
co′ma *pl.* -mas *or* -ma·ta
os′te·o·fi′bro·li·po′ma
pl. -mas *or* -ma·ta
os′te·o·fi′bro′ma *pl.* -mas *or*
-ma·ta
os′te·o·fi′bro·ma·to′sis
pl. -ses′
os′te·o·fi′bro·sar·co′ma
pl. -mas *or* -ma·ta
os′te·o·fi′bro·sis *pl.* -ses′
os′te·o·gen
os′te·o·gen′e·sis

—im′per·fec′ta
—imperfecta con·gen′i·ta
—imperfecta cys′ti·ca
—imperfecta tar′da
os′te·o·ge·net′ic
os′te·o·gen′ic
os′te·og′e·nous
os′te·og′e·ny
os′te·og′ra·phy
os′te·o·hal′i·ste·re′sis
   pl. -ses′
os′te·o·he′ma·chro·ma·
   to′sis *pl.* -ses′
os′te·o·hy′per·troph′ic
os′te·oid′
os′te·o·in·duc′tive
os′te·o·lath′y·rism
os′te·o·lip′o·chon·dro′ma
   pl. -mas *or* -ma·ta
os′te·o·li·po′ma *pl.* -mas *or*
   -ma·ta
os′te·o·lith′
os′te·o·lo′gi·a
os′te·o·log′ic *or*
   os′te·o·log′i·cal
os′te·ol′o·gist
os′te·ol′o·gy
os′te·ol′y·sis
os′te·o·lyt′ic
os′te·o′ma *pl.* -mas *or* -ma·ta
   —cu′tis
   —du′rum
   —e·bur′ne·um
   —med′ul·lar′e′
   —spon′gi·o′sum
os′te·o·ma·la·ci·a
os′te·o·ma·la·ci·al
os′te·o·ma·la·cic
os′te·o′ma·toid′
os′te·o′ma·to′sis
os′te·o·mere′
os′te·o·met′ric
os′te·om′e·try
os′te·o·mi·o′sis
os′te·o·mu′coid′
os′te·o·my′e·lit′ic
os′te·o·my′e·li′tis
os′te·o·my′e·lo·dys·pla′-
   si·a
os′te·o·my′e·log′ra·phy
os′te·o·myx′o·chon·dro′ma
   pl. -mas *or* -ma·ta
os′te·on′

os′te·on′al
os′te·o·ne·cro′sis
os′te·o·ne·phrop′a·thy
os′te·o·neu·ral′gi·a
os′te·o·path′
os′te·o·path′i·a
   —con′den′sans′ dis·sem′-
      i·na′ta
   —hy′per·os·tot′i·ca
      mul′ti·plex′ in·fan′ti·lis
   —stri·a′ta
os′te·o·path′ic
os′te·op′a·thy
os′te·o·pe·cil′i·a
os′te·o·pe·di′on′
os′te·o·pe·ni·a
os′te·o·per′i·os′te·al
os′te·o·per′i·os·ti′tis
os′te·o·pe·tro′sis
   —gal′li·nar′um
   —gen′er·al·i·sa′ta
os′te·o·pe·trot′ic
os′te·o·phage′
os′te·o·pha′gi·a
os′te·o·phle·bi′tis
os′te·oph′o·ny
os′te·o·phore′
os′te·o·phy′ma *pl.* -mas *or*
   -ma·ta
os′te·o·phyte′
os′te·o·phyt′ic
os′te·o·phy·to′sis
os′te·o·plaque′
os′te·o·plast′
os′te·o·plas′tic
os′te·o·plas′ty
os′te·o·poi′ki·lo′sis *pl.* -ses′
os′te·o·po·ro′sis *pl.* -ses′
os′te·o·po·rot′ic
os′te·op·sath′y·ro′sis
   pl. -ses′
os′te·o·pul′mo·nar′y
os′te·o·ra′di·o·ne·cro′sis
os′te·or·rha′gi·a
os′te·or′rha·phy
os′te·o·sar·co′ma *pl.* -mas *or*
   -ma·ta
os′te·o·sar·co′ma·tous
os′te·o·scle·ro′sis *pl.* -ses′
   —frag′i·lis gen′er·al·i·sa′ta
os′te·o·scle·rot′ic
os′te·o′sis
   —cu′tis

os′te·o·spon′gi·o′ma
   pl. -mas *or* -ma·ta
os′te·o·stix′is
os′te·o·su′ture
os′te·o·syn′o·vi′tis
os′te·o·syn′the·sis *pl.* -ses′
os′te·o·ta′bes′
os′te·o·te·lan′gi·ec·ta′si·a
os′te·o·throm′bo·phle·bi′-
   tis
os′te·o·throm·bo′sis
   pl. -ses′
os′te·o·tome′
os′te·o·to′mo·cla′si·a
os′te·ot′o·moc′la·sis *pl.* -ses′
os′te·ot′o·my
os′te·o·tribe′
os′te·o·trite′
os′te·ot′ro·phy
Os′ter·berg′ test
os′ti·a
   —a′tri·o·ven·tric′u·lar′i·a
      dex′trum et si·nis′trum
   —ve·nar′um pul′mo·na′-
      li·um
os′ti·al
os′ti·tis
os′ti·um *pl.* -ti·a
   —ab·dom′i·na′le′ tu′bae′
      u′ter·i′nae′
   —a·or′tae′
   —ap·pen′di·cis ver′mi·for′-
      mis
   —ar·te′ri·o′sum cor′dis
   —a′tri·o·ven·tric′u·lar′e′
   —atrioventriculare
      dex′trum
   —atrioventriculare
      si·nis′trum
   —il′e·o·ce·ca′le′
   —max′il·lar′e′
   —pha·ryn′ge·um tu′bae′
      au′di·ti′vae′
   —py·lo′ri·cum
   —trun′ci′ pul′mo·na′lis
   —tym·pan′i·cum tu′bae′
      au′di·ti′vae′
   —u′re′ter·is
   —u′re′thrae′ fem′i·ni′nae′
      ex·ter′num
   —urethrae in·ter′num
   —urethrae mas·cu′li·nae′
      ex·ter′num

—u′ter·i′
—u′ter·i′num tu′bae′
—va·gi′nae′
—ve′nae′ ca′vae′ in·fe′ri·o′-
    ris
—venae cavae su·pe′ri·o′ris
—ve·no′sum cor′dis
os′to·mate′
os′to·my
os·to′sis
os′tre·o·tox′ism
o·tal′gi·a
o·tal′gic
O′ta nevus
o·tec′to·my
o′thel·co′sis pl. -ses′
ot·he′ma·to′ma pl. -mas or
    -ma·ta
ot·hem′or·rha′gi·a
ot·hem′or·rhe′a
o′tic
o′ti·co·din′i·a
o·tit′ic
o·ti′tis
—ex·ter′na
—in·ter′na
—lab′y·rin′thi·ca
—mas·toi′de·a
—me′di·a
—par′a·sit′i·ca
—scle·rot′i·ca
o′to·ac′a·ri′a·sis
o′to·blen′nor·rhe′a
o′to·ce·phal′ic
o′to·ceph′a·lus pl. -li′
o′to·ceph′a·ly
o′to·cer′e·bri′tis
o′to·clei′sis
o′to·co′ni·a sing. -ni·um
o′to·cra′ni·al
o′to·cra′ni·um pl. -ums or
    -i·a
o′to·cyst′
o′to·dyn′i·a
o′to·en·ceph′a·li′tis
o′to·gan′gli·on pl. -gli·a or
    -gli·ons
o′to·gen′ic
o·tog′e·nous
o′to·hem′i·neu′ras·the′ni·a
o′to·lar′yn·go·log′i·cal
o′to·lar′yn·gol′o·gist
o′to·lar′yn·gol′o·gy

o′to·lith′
o′to·li·thi′a·sis pl. -ses′
o′to·lith′ic
o′to·log′ic or o′to·log′i·cal
o·tol′o·gist
o·tol′o·gy
o′to·mas′toid·i′tis
o′to·mu′cor·my·co′sis
o′to·my′as·the′ni·a
o′to·my·co′sis pl. -ses′
o′to·neu·ral′gi·a
o′to·neu′ras·the′ni·a
o·top′a·thy
o′to·pha·ryn′ge·al
o′to·plas′ty
o′to·pol′y·pus
o′to·py′or·rhe′a
o′to·py·o′sis
o′to·rhi′no·lar′yn·gol′o·gy
o′to·rhi·nol′o·gy
o′tor·rha′gi·a
o′tor·rhe′a
o′to·sal′pinx pl. -sal·pin′ges′
o′to·scle·rec′to·my
o′to·scle·ro′sis pl. -ses′
o′to·scle·rot′ic
o′to·scope′
o′to·scop′ic
o·tos′co·py
o·to′sis pl. -ses′
o′to·spon·gi·o′sis pl. -ses′
o·tos′te·al
o·tos′te·on′
o·tot′o·my
o′to·tox′ic
o′to·tox·ic′i·ty
Ot′to
—disease
—pelvis
Ott precipitation test
oua·ba′in
Ouch′ter·lo′ny technique
ou′loid′
ounce
Out′er·bridge′
—ridge
—scale
out′flow′
out′growth′
out′let′
out′pa′tient
out′pouch′ing
out′put′

o′val
o′val·bu′min
o·va′le′
o′val·o·cyte′
o′val·o·cyt′ic
o′val·o·cy·to′sis pl. -ses′
o·var′i·al′gi·a
o·var′i·an
o·var′i·ec′to·my
o·var′i·o·cele′
o·var′i·o·cen·te′sis pl. -ses′
o·var′i·o·cy·e′sis pl. -ses′
o·var′i·o·dys·neu′ri·a
o·var′i·o·gen′ic
o·var′i·o·hys·ter·ec′to·my
o·var′i·o·lyt′ic
o·var′i·o·pex′y
o·var′i·or·rhex′is
    pl. -rhex′es′
o·var′i·o·sal′pin·gec′to·my
o·var′i·o·ste·re′sis pl. -ses′
o·var′i·os′to·my
o·var′i·ot′o·my
o·var′i·o·tu′bal
o′va·ri′tis
o·var′i·um pl. -i·a
o′va·ry
o′va·tes·tic′u·lar
o′ver·a·chieve′, -chieved′,
    -chiev′ing
o′ver·a·chiev′er
o′ver·bite′
o′ver·clo′sure
o′ver·com·pen·sate′, -sat′ed,
    -sat′ing
o′ver·com·pen·sa′tion
o′ver·cor·rec′tion
o′ver·den′ture
o′ver·de·pend′en·cy
o′ver·de·ter′mi·na′tion
o′ver·dose′
o′ver·drive′
o′ver·ex·ten′sion
o′ver·flex′ion
o′ver·growth′
o′ver·hang′
o′ver·jet′
o′ver·lap′, -lapped′, -lap′ping
o′ver·lay′
o′ver·load′
o′ver·nu·tri′tion
o′ver·pro·tec′tion
o′ver·rid′ing

o'ver·sense'
o·vert'
o'ver·toe'
O'ver·ton theory
o'ver·ven'ti·la'tion
o'ver·weight'
o'vi·cap'sule
o'vi·cid'al
o'vi·cide'
o'vi·duct'
o'vi·duc'tal
o·vif'er·ous
o'vi·fi·ca'tion
o'vi·form'
o'vi·gen'e·sis pl. -ses'
o'vi·ge·net'ic
o·vig'e·nous
o'vi·germ'
o·vig'er·ous
o·vip'a·rous
o'vi·sac'
o'vo·cen'ter
o'vo·cyte'
o'vo·fla'vin
o'vo·gen'e·sis pl. -ses'
o'vo·glob'u·lin
o'vo·go'ni·um pl. -ni·a
o'void'
o'vo·mu'cin
o'vo·mu'coid'
o'vo·plasm
o'vo·tes·tic'u·lar
o'vo·tes'tis pl. -tes'
o'vo·vi·tel'lin
o'vu·lar
o'vu·late', -lat'ed, -lat'ing
o'vu·la'tion
o'vu·la'tion·al
o'vu·la·to'ry
o'vule'
o'vu·log'e·nous
o'vu·lum pl. -la
o'vum pl. o'va
—tu·ber'cu·lo'sum
O'wen
—lines
—view
Ow'ren disease
ox'a·cil'lin
ox'a·late', -lat'ed, -lat'ing
ox'a·le'mi·a
ox·al'ic
ox'a·lism

ox'a·lo·ac'e·tate'
ox'a·lo·a·ce'tic
ox·a·lo'sis
ox·a·lo·suc·cin'ic
ox·a·lu'ri·a
ox·a·lu'ric
ox·am'ide'
ox·am'i·dine'
ox·am'ni·quine
ox·an'a·mide'
ox·an'dro·lone'
ox·a·ze·pam'
ox·a·zol'i·dine'
ox·eth'a·zaine'
ox'gall'
ox'i·con'a·zole'
ox'i·dant
ox'i·dase'
ox'i·date', -dat'ed, -dat'ing
ox'i·da'tion
ox'i·da'tive
ox·ide'
ox'i·dize', -dized', -diz'ing
ox'i·do-re·duc'tase'
ox'ime'
ox·im'e·ter
ox·im'e·try
ox'o·ges'tone'
ox·o·lin'ic
ox·o'ni·um
ox·o·phen·ar'sine'
ox·pren'o·lol'
ox'tri·phyl'line'
ox'y·a·can'thine'
ox'y·a·coi'a
ox'y·a·koi'a
ox'y·a'phi·a
ox'y·ben'zone'
ox'y·blep'si·a
ox'y·bu'ty·nin
ox'y·cal'o·rim'e·ter
ox'y·ce·phal'ic
ox'y·ceph'a·lous
ox'y·ceph'a·ly
ox'y·chlo'ride'
ox'y·chro·mat'ic
ox'y·chro'ma·tin
ox'y·ci·ne'si·a
ox'y·ci·ne'sis
ox'y·co'done'
ox'y·cor'ti·co·ster'oid'
ox'y·es·the'si·a
ox'y·gen

ox'y·gen·ase'
ox'y·gen·ate', -at'ed, -at'ing
ox'y·gen·a'tion
ox'y·gen·a'tor
ox'y·gen'ic
ox'y·geu'si·a
ox'y·he'ma·tin
ox'y·he'ma·to·por'phy·rin
ox'y·he'mo·glo'bin
ox'y·hy'per·gly·ce'mi·a
ox'y·la'li·a
ox'y·me·taz'o·line'
ox'y·meth'o·lone'
ox'y·mor'phone'
ox'y·my'o·glo'bin
ox'y·ner'von'
ox'y·neu'rine'
ox·yn'tic
ox'y·o'pi·a
ox'y·op'ter
ox'y·os'mi·a
ox'y·os·phre'si·a
ox·yp'a·thy
ox'y·per'tine'
ox'y·phen·bu'ta·zone'
ox'y·phen·cy'cli·mine'
ox'y·phen'ic
ox'y·phe·ni·sa'tin
ox'y·phe·no'ni·um
ox'y·phil'
ox'y·phil'i·a
ox'y·phil'ic
ox·yph'i·lous
ox'y·pho'ni·a
ox'y·pro'line'
ox'y·pu'ri·nol'
ox'y·quin'o·line'
ox'y·rhine'
ox·yt'a·lan'
ox'y·tet'ra·cy'cline'
ox'y·to'ci·a
ox'y·to'cic
ox'y·to'cin
ox'y·u·ri'a·sis pl. -ses'
ox'y·u'ri·cide'
ox'y·u'rid
Ox'y·u'ri·dae'
Ox'y·u'ris
o·ze'na
o'zo·chro'ti·a
o·zoch'ro·tous
o'zone'
o'zon·ide'

o'zon·ize'
o'zon·iz'er
o'zo·nol'y·sis *pl.* -ses'
o'zon·om'e·ter
o'zo·sto'mi·a

P

pab'u·lum
Pac'chi·o'ni·an bodies
pace, pac'ed, pac'ing
pace'mak'er
pa·chom'e·ter
Pa·chon'
—method
—test
pach'y·ac'ri·a
pach'y·bleph'a·ron'
pach'y·bleph'a·ro'sis
pach'y·ce·pha'li·a
pach'y·ce·phal'ic
pach'y·ceph'a·lous
pach'y·ceph'a·ly
pach'y·chei'li·a
pach'y·chro·mat'ic
pach'y·dac·tyl'i·a
pach'y·dac'ty·ly
pach'y·der'ma
pach'y·der·mat'o·cele'
pach'y·der·ma·to'sis
   pl. -ses'
pach'y·der'ma·tous
pach'y·der'mi·a
   —la·ryn'gis
   —lym·phan'gi·ec·tat'i·ca
pach'y·der'mic
pach'y·glos'si·a
pach'y·gy'ri·a
pach'y·hy·men'ic
pach'y·lep'to·men·in·gi'tis
pach'y·men'in·git'ic
pach'y·men'in·gi'tis
   —cer'vi·ca'lis hy·per'troph'-
      i·ca
   —ex·ter'na
   —in·ter'na hem'or·rha'gi·ca
pach'y·men'in·gop'a·thy
pach'y·me'ninx
   pl. -me·nin'ges
pach'y·mu·co'sa
pach'y·ne'ma
pa·chyn'sis *pl.* -ses'
pa·chyn'tic

pach'y·o·nych'i·a
   —con·gen'i·ta
pach'y·pel'vi·per'i·to·ni'tis
pach'y·per'i·os·to'sis
pach'y·per'i·to·ni'tis
pa·chyp'o·dous
pach'y·sal'pin·gi'tis
pach'y·sal·pin'go·o·o·va·ri'-
   tis
pach'y·tene'
pach'y·vag'i·ni'tis
pac'i·fi'er
pa·cin'i·an
Pa·ci'ni corpuscle
pack
pack'er
pack'ing
pad, pad'ded, pad'ding
pad'dle
Padg'ett operation
Pae·cil'o·my'ces
paed-. See words spelled *ped-*.
paedo-. See words spelled
   pedo-.
Pa·get'
   —cancer
   —cells
   —disease
   —necrosis
pag'et·oid'
pa·go·pha'gi·a
pa·go·plex'i·a
pain
pain'ful
pain'kill'er
pain'kill'ing
pain'less
Pais fracture
pa·ja'ro·el'lo
pal'a·dang'
pal'a·tal
pal'ate
pa·lat'ic
pa·lat'i·form'
pal'a·tine'
pal'a·ti'tis
pal'a·to·glos'sal
pal'a·to·graph'
pal'a·to·graph'ic
pal'a·tog'ra·phy
pal'a·to·max'il·lar'y
pal'a·to·my'o·graph'
pal'a·to·na'sal

pal'a·top'a·gus par'a·sit'-
   i·cus
pal'a·to·pha·ryn'ge·al
pal'a·to·plas'ty
pal'a·to·ple'gi·a
pal'a·to·prox'i·mal
pal'a·to·pter'y·goid'
pal'a·tor'rha·phy
pal'a·to·sal·pin'ge·us
pal'a·tos·chi'sis *pl.* -ses'
pa·la'tum *pl.* -ta
   —du'rum
   —fis'sum
   —mo'bi·le'
   —mol'le'
   —os'se·um
pa·le·en·ceph'a·lon'
pa·le·o·cer'e·bel'lar
pa·le·o·cer'e·bel'lum
pa·le·o·cor'tex *pl.* -cor'ti·ces'
pa·le·o·en·ceph'a·lon'
pa·le·o·gen'e·sis
pa·le·o·ki·net'ic
pa·le·o·log'ic
pa·le·om·ne'sis
pa·le·o·ol'ive
pa·le·o·pal'li·um
pa·le·o·pa·thol'o·gy
pa·le·o·stri·a'tal
pa·le·o·stri·a'tum
pa·le·o·thal'a·mus
pal'i·graph'i·a
pal'i·ki·ne'si·a
pal'i·ki·ne'sis
pal'i·la'li·a
pal'i·lex'i·a
pal'in·dro'mi·a
pal'in·drom'ic
pal'in·gen'e·sis
pal'in·graph'i·a
pal'i·nop'si·a
pal'in·phra'si·a
pal'i·op'sy
pal'i·phra'si·a
pal'i·sad'ing
pal'la·di·um
pal'lan·es·the'si·a
pal'les·the'si·a
pal'li·al
pal'li·ate', -at'ed, -at'ing
pal'li·a'tion
pal'li·a·tive
pal'li·dal

pal'li·do·hy'po·tha·lam'ic
pal'li·do·py·ram'i·dal
pal'li·do·re·tic'u·lar
pal'li·do·sub'tha·lam'ic
pal'li·dot'o·my
pal'li·dum
pal'lor
palm
pal'ma *pl.* -mae'
—ma'nus
pal'mar
pal'mar'is *pl.* -mar'es'
pal'mate'
pal'ma·ture
Pal'mer-Wi'den operation
pal'mi·tate'
pal'mi·tin
pal·mod'ic
pal'mo·men'tal
pal'mo·plan'tar
pal'mus *pl.* -mi'
pal'pa·ble
pal'pate', -pat'ed, -pat'ing
pal·pa'tion
pal'pa·to·per·cus'sion
pal'pa·to'ry
pal'pe·bra *pl.* -brae'
pal'pe·bral
pal'pe·brate', -brat'ed,
-brat'ing
pal'pe·bra'tion
pal'pe·bri'tis
pal'pi·tate', -tat'ed, -tat'ing
pal'pi·ta'tion
pal'sied
pal'sy
Pal'tauf' dwarfism
pal'u·dal
pal'u·dism
pa·lus'tral
pal'y·tox'in
pam'a·brom'
pam'i·dro'nate'
pam·pin'i·form'
pan'a·ce'a
pan·ac'i·nar'
pan'ag·glu'ti·nin
pan·an'gi·i'tis
pan'a·ris
pan'a·ri'ti·um *pl.* -ti·a
pan·ar'te·ri'tis
pan·ar·thri'tis
pan·at'ro·phy

pan'blas·to·trop'ic
pan'car·di'tis
Pan'coast'
—operation
—syndrome
—tumor
pan'co·lec'to·my
pan·col'po·hys'ter·ec'-
to·my
pan'cre·as *pl.* pan·cre'a·ta
—ac'ces·so'ri·um
—of A·sel'li
pan'cre·a·tec'to·my
pan'cre·at'ic
pan'cre·at'i·co·du'o·de'nal
pan'cre·at'i·co·du'o·de·
nec'to·my
pan'cre·at'i·co·du'o·de·
nos'to·my
pan'cre·at'i·co·en'ter·os'-
to·my
pan'cre·at'i·co·gas·tros'-
to·my
pan'cre·at'i·co·je'ju·nos'-
to·my
pan'cre·at'i·co·li·thot'o·my
pan'cre·at'i·co·splen'ic
pan'cre·a·tin
pan'cre·a·tism
pan'cre·a·tit'ic
pan'cre·a·ti'tis *pl.* -tit'i·des'
pan'cre·a·to·cho·lan'gi·o·
gram'
pan'cre·a·to·du'o·de·nec'-
to·my
pan'cre·a·to·du'o·de·nos'-
to·my
pan'cre·a·to·en'ter·os'-
to·my
pan'cre·a·tog'e·nous
pan'cre·at'o·gram'
pan'cre·a·tog'ra·phy
pan'cre·a·to·je'ju·nos'-
to·my
pan'cre·a·to·li'pase'
pan'cre·at'o·lith'
pan'cre·a·to·li·thec'to·my
pan'cre·a·to·li·thi'a·sis
pan'cre·a·to·li·thot'o·my
pan'cre·a·tol'y·sis
pan'cre·at'o·lyt'ic
pan'cre·a·tot'o·my
pan'cre·ec'to·my

pan'cre·li'pase'
pan'cre·o·lith'
pan'cre·o·li·thot'o·my
pan'cre·ol'y·sis
pan'cre·o·lyt'ic
pan'cre·o·path'i·a
pan'cre·op'a·thy
pan'cre·o·zy'min
pan'cu·ro'ni·um
pan'cy·to·pe'ni·a
pan'cy·to·pe'nic
pan·de'mi·a
pan·dem'ic
pan·dic'u·la'tion
Pan'dy
—reagent
—test
pan'e·lec'tro·scope'
pan·en·ceph'a·li'tis
pan·en'do·scope'
pan·en·dos'co·py
pan·es·the'si·a
Pa'neth cells
pang
pan·gen'e·sis
pan·glos'si·a
pan·he'ma·to·pe'ni·a
pan·hi·dro'sis
pan·hy'po·go'nad·ism
pan·hy'po·pi·tu'i·ta·rism
pan·hys'ter·ec'to·my
pan·hys'ter·o·col·pec'-
to·my
pan·hys'ter·o-
o·oph'o·rec'to·my
pan·hys'ter·o·sal'pin·gec'-
to·my
pan·hys'ter·o·sal'pin·go-
o·oph'o·rec'to·my
pan'ic
pan'im·mu'ni·ty
pa·niv'o·rous
pan·lob'u·lar
pan'me·tri'tis
pan·my'e·lop'a·thy
pan·my'e·loph'thi·sis
pl. -ses'
pan·my'e·lo'sis *pl.* -ses'
pan·my'e·lo·tox'i·co'sis
pan·my'o'si'tis
Pan'ner disease
pan·nic'u·li'tis
pan·nic'u·lus *pl.* -li'

—ad′i•po′sus
—car•no′sus
pan′nus *pl.* -ni′
—ca•ra′te•us
—car•no′sus
—cras′sus
—de•gen′er•a′ti′vus
—he•pat′i•cus
—sic′cus
—ten′u•is
—tra•cho′ma•to′sus
pan′o•graph′
pan′o•graph′ic
pan′o•pho′bi•a
pan′oph•thal′mi•a
pan•oph′thal•mi′tis
—pu′ru•len′ta
pan•op′tic
pan′o•ram′ic
Pan′o•rex′ x-ray
pan′os•te•i′tis
pan′o•ti′tis
pan′phle•bi′tis
pan•pho′bi•a
pan•proc′to•co•lec′to•my
pan′scle•ro′sis *pl.* -ses′
pan•si′nus•i′tis
Pan•stron′gy•lus
—ge•nic′u•la′tus
—me•gis′tus
pan′sys•tol′ic
pant
pan′ta•mor′phi•a
pan′ta•mor′phic
pan′tan•en•ce•pha′li•a
pan′tan•en•ce•phal′ic
pan′tan•en•ceph′a•lus
pan•tan′ky•lo•bleph′a•ron′
pan′ta•so′ma•tous
pan′ta•tro′phi•a
pan•tat′ro•phy
pan′te•the′ine
pan′the•nol′
pan′to•graph′
pan•to′ic
pan′to•mime′
pan′to•mim′ic
pan′to•paque′
pan′to•scop′ic
pan•to′the•nate′
pan′to•then′ic
pan′trop′ic
pan•tur′bi•nate′

Pa′num areas
pa′nus *pl.* -ni′
—fau′ci•um
—in′gui•na′lis
pan′u•ve•i′tis
pap
Pap
—smear
—test
pa•pa′in
Pa′pa•ni′co•laou′
—classes
—stains
—test
pa•pav′er•a•mine′
pa•pav′er•ine′
pa•pes′cent
Pa•pez′ circuit
pa•pil′la *pl.* -lae′
—den′tis
—du′o•de′ni′ major
—duodeni minor
—in′ci•si′va
—lac′ri•ma′lis
—mam′mae′
—ner′vi′ op′ti•ci′
—of Mor′ga′gni
—of San′to•ri′ni
—of Va′ter
—pa•rot′i•de′a
—pi′li′
pa•pil′lae′
—con′i•cae′
—co′ri•i′
—fi′li•for′mes′
—fo′li•a′tae′
—fun′gi•for′mes′
—lac′ri•ma′les′
—len′tic′u•lar′es′
—lin′gua′les′
—re′na′les′
—val′la′tae′
pap′il•lar′y
pap′il•late′
pap′il•lec′to•my
pa•pil′le•de′ma
pap′il•lif′er•ous
pa•pil′li•form′
pap′il•li′tis
pap′il•lo•car′ci•no′ma
pl. -mas *or* -ma•ta
pap′il•lo•cys•to′ma *pl.* -mas
or -ma•ta

pap′il•lo′ma *pl.* -mas *or*
-ma•ta
—cho•roi′de•um
pap′il•lo•mac′u•lar
pap′il•lo•ma•to′sis *pl.* -ses′
pap′il•lom′a•tous
Pa•pil•lon′-Le•Fèvre′
syndrome
pap′il•lo•ret′i•ni′tis
pa•po′va•vi′rus
Pap′pen•heim′ stain
pap′pose′
pap′u•la *pl.* -lae′
pap′u•lar
pap′u•la′tion
pap′ule′
pap′u•lif′er•ous
pap′u•lo•er′y•the′ma•tous
pap′u•lo•ne•crot′ic
pap′u•lo•pus′tu•lar
pap′u•lo′sis
—a•troph′i•cans′ ma•lig′na
pap′u•lo•squa′mous
pap′u•lo•ve•sic′u•lar
pap′y•ra′ceous
par′a *pl.* -as *or* -ae′
par′a-a•mi′no•ben•zo′ate′
par′a-a•mi′no•ben•zo′ic
par′a-an•al′ge•si•a
par′a-an•es•the′si•a
par′a-a•or′tic
par′a-ap•pen′di•ci′tis
par′a•bas′al
par′ab•du′cent
par′a•bi•gem′i•nal
par′a•bi•o′sis *pl.* -ses′
par′a•blep′si•a
par′a•blep′sis *pl.* -ses′
par′a•bu′li•a
pa•rac′an•tho′ma *pl.* -mas *or*
-ma•ta
pa•rac′an•tho′sis *pl.* -ses′
par′a•ca•ri′nal
par′a•car′mine
par′a•ce′cal
par′a•cen•te′sis *pl.* -ses′
—oc′u•li
par′a•cen′tral
par′a•ceph′a•lus *pl.* -li′
par′a•chlo′ro•met′a•xy′le•
nol′
par′a•chlo′ro•phe′nol′
par′a•chol′er•a

par′a·chord′al
par′a·chro′ma
par′a·chro′ma·tism
par′a·chro′ma·top′si·a
par′a·chro′ma·to′sis
   pl. -ses′
par′a·chute′
par′a·coc·cid′i·oi′dal
Par′a·coc·cid′i·oi′des
  —bra·sil′i·en′sis
par′a·coc·cid′i·oi·do·my·
  co′sis *pl.* -ses′
par′a·co·li′tis
par′a·col·pi′tis
par′a·col′pi·um
par′a·con′dy·lar
par′a·cone′
par′a·co′nid
par′a·cor·po′re·al
par′a·cu′si·a
  —a′cris
  —du′pli·ca′ta
  —lo·ca′lis
  —ob·tu′sa
  —Wil·lis′i·i′
par′a·cu′sis *pl.* -ses′
par′a·cy·e′sis *pl.* -ses′
par′a·cys′tic
par′a·cys·ti′tis
par′a·cys′ti·um *pl.* -ti·a
par′a·cyt′ic *(lying among cells)*
  ♦*parasitic*
par′ad·e·ni′tis
par′a·den′tal
par′a·den′ti·um *pl.* -a
par′a·den·to′sis *pl.* -ses′
par′a·did′y·mal
par′a·did′y·mis
  pl. -di·dym′i·des′
par′a·dox′i·a sex′u·a′lis
par′a·dox′ic *or*
  par′a·dox′i·cal
par′a·du′o·de′nal
par′a·dys′en·ter′y
par′a·ep′i·lep′sy
par′a·e·qui·lib′ri·um
par′a·e·ryth′ro·blast′
par′a·e·soph′a·ge′al
par′a·fas·cic′u·lar
par′af·fin
par′af·fin·o′ma
par′a·floc′cu·lus *pl.* -li′
par′a·fol·lic′u·lar

par′a·form′
par′a·for·mal′de·hyde′
par′a·func′tion
par′a·func′tion·al
par′a·gam′ma·cism
par′a·gan′gli·o′ma *pl.* -mas
  or -ma·ta
par′a·gan′gli·on *pl.* -gli·a *or*
  -gli·ons
  —ca·rot′i·cum
  —caroticum sar·co′ma
  —ca·rot′i·cus tumor
par′a·gan′gli·o·neu·ro′ma
  pl. -mas *or* -ma·ta
par′a·gan′gli·on′ic
par′a·gen′i·tal
par′a·gen′i·ta′lis
par′a·geu′si·a
par′a·geu′sic
par′a·geu′sis
par′ag·glu′ti·na′tion
par′a·gle·noi′dal
par′a·glob′u·lin
par′a·glob′u·li·nu′ri·a
par′a·glos′si·a
par·ag′na·thus
par′a·gon′i·mi·a·sis *pl.* -ses′
Par′a·gon′i·mus
  —wes′ter·man′i′
par′a·gram′ma·tism
par′a·gran′u·lo′ma
par′a·graph′i·a
par′a·graph′ic
par′a·he·mo·phil′i·a
par′a·he·pat′ic
par′a·hep′a·ti′tis
par′a·hex′yl
par′a·hi·a′tal
par′a·hip′po·cam′pal
par′a·hor′mone′
par′a·hyp·no′sis *pl.* -ses′
par′a·in·flu·en′za
par′a·ker′a·to′sis *pl.* -ses′
  —gon′or·rhe′i·ca
  —scu′tu·lar′is
  —var′i·e·ga′ta
par′a·ker′a·tot′ic
par′a·ki·ne′si·a
par′a·ki·ne′sis *pl.* -ses′
par′a·ki·net′ic
par′a·lac′tic
par′a·la′li·a
par′a·lamb′da·cism

par′al·bu′min
par·al′de·hyde′
par′a·lep′sy
par′a·lex′i·a
par′a·lex′ic
par′al·ge′si·a
par′al·ge′sic
par′al·lax′
par′al·lel
par′al·lel·ism
par′al·lel′o·gram′
par′al·lel·om′e·ter
par′a·lo′gi·a
par′a·log′i·cal
pa·ral′o·gism
pa·ral′y·sis *pl.* -ses′
  —ag′i·tans′
par′a·lys′sa
par′a·lyt′ic
par′a·ly′zant
par′a·lyze′, -lyzed′, -lyz′ing
par′a·lyz′er
par′a·mag·net′ic
par′a·mag′net·ism
par′a·mam′ma·ry
par′a·mas·ti′tis
par′a·mas′toid′
par′a·mas′toid·i′tis
Par′a·me′ci·um
par′a·me′di·al
par′a·me′di·an
par′a·med′ic
par′a·med′i·cal
par′a·me′ni·a
par′a·me·nis′cus *pl.* -ci′ *or*
  -cus·es
par′a·men′tal
par′a·me′si·al
pa·ram′e·ter
par′a·meth·a′di·one′
par′a·meth·a·sone′
par′a·me′tri·al
par′a·me′tric
par′a·me·trit′ic
par′a·me·tri′tis
par′a·me′tri·um *pl.* -tri·a
par′a·me·trop′a·thy
par′a·mim′i·a
par′a·mi′tome′
par·am·ne′si·a
par·am·ne′sis
par′a·mo′lar
par′a·mor′phine′

par′a·mu′cin
par′a·mu′si·a
par′a·mu·ta′tion
pa·ram′y·loi·do′sis
par′a·my·oc′lo·nus
  mul′ti·plex′
par′a·my′o·sin
par′a·my′o·sin′o·gen
par′a·my′o·to′ni·a
par′a·myx′o·vi′rus
par′a·na′sal
par′a·ne′mic
par′a·ne′o·plas′tic
par′a·neph′ric
par′a·ne·phri′tis
par′a·ne·phro′ma *pl.* -mas
  or -ma·ta
par′a·neph′ros′
  pl. -neph′roi′
par′a·neu′ral
par′a·ni′tro·sul′fa·thi′a·
  zole′
par′a·noi′a
par′a·noi′ac′
par′a·noid′
par′a·noid·ism
par′a·no′mi·a
par′a·nor′mal
par′a·nu′cle·ar
par′a·nu′cle·ate′
par′a·nu′cle·us *pl.* -cle·i′
par′a·ny′line′
par′a·oc·cip′i·tal
par′a·o′ral
par′a·os′ti·al
par′a·pan′cre·at′ic
par′a·pa·re′sis *pl.* -ses′
par′a·pa·ret′ic
par′a·pa·tel′lar
par′a·per·tus′sis
par′a·pha·ryn′ge·al
par′a·pha′si·a
par′a·pha′sic
par′a·phe′mi·a
pa·ra′phi·a
par′a·phil′i·a
par′a·phil′i·ac′
par′a·phi·mo′sis *pl.* -ses′
  —oc′u·li′
par′a·pho′bi·a
par′a·pho′ni·a
  —pu′ber·um
  —pu′bes·cen′ti·um

pa·raph′o·ra
par′a·phra′si·a
  —ve·sa′na
par′a·phre′ni·a
par′a·phre·ni′tis
pa·raph′y·se′al
pa·raph′y·sis *pl.* -ses′
par′a·pin′e·al
par′a·pla′si·a
par′a·plasm
par′a·plas′tic
par′a·plas′tin
par′a·plec′tic
par′a·ple′gi·a
par′a·ple′gic
par′a·ple′gi·form′
par′a·pleu·ri′tis
par′a·pneu·mo′ni·a
par′a·poph′y·sis *pl.* -ses′
par·ap′o·plex′y
par′a·prax′i·a
par′a·prax′is
par′a·proc·ti′tis
par′a·proc′ti·um *pl.* -ti·a
par′a·pros′ta·ti′tis
par′a·pro′tein′
par′a·pro′tein·e′mi·a
par′a·pso·ri′a·sis *pl.* -ses′
  —en plaques′
  —gut′ta′ta
  —var′i·o′li·for′mis a·cu′ta
par′a·psy·chol′o·gy
par′a·pyk′no·mor′phous
par′a·rec′tal
par′a·rho′ta·cism
par·ar·rhyth′mi·a
par·ar·rhyth′mic
par′a·sa′cral
par′a·sag′it·tal
par′a·sal′pin·gi′tis
par′a·scap′u·lar
par′a·scar′la·ti′na
par′a·se·cre′tion
par′a·sel′lar
par′a·sep′tal
par′a·sex′u·al
par′a·sex′u·al′i·ty
par′a·si·nus·oi′dal
par′a·site′
par′a·si·te′mi·a
par′a·sit′ic (*pertaining to a
  parasite*)
  ♦*paracytic*

par′a·sit′i·cid′al
par′a·sit′i·cide′
par′a·sit·ism
par′a·sit·i·za′tion
par′a·sit·ize′
par′a·si·to·gen′ic
par′a·si·tol′o·gist
par′a·si·tol′o·gy
par′a·si·to·sis *pl.* -ses′
par′a·si·to·trope′
par′a·si·to·trop′ic
par′a·si·tot′ro·pism
par′a·si·tot′ro·py
par′a·some′
par′a·som′ni·a
par′a·spa′di·as
par′a·spasm
par′a·spas′mus
par′a·spi′nal
par′a·sple′nic
par′a·ste′a·to′sis
par′a·ster′nal
par′a·stri·ate′
par′a·sym·pa·thet′ic
par′a·sym·path′i·co·to′ni·a
par′a·sym·pa·tho·lyt′ic
par′a·sym·pa·tho·mi·
  met′ic
par′a·syn·ap′sis *pl.* -ses′
par′a·syn·o′vi·tis
par′a·syph′i·lis
par′a·syph′i·lit′ic
par′a·sys′to·le
par′a·sys·tol′ic
par′a·tae′ni·al
par′a·tax′i·a
par′a·tax′ic
par′a·tax′is
par′a·ten′on
par′a·ter′mi·nal
par′a·the′li·o′ma *pl.* -mas *or*
  -ma·ta
par′a·thi′on
par′a·thor′mone′
par′a·thy′mi·a
par′a·thy′roid′
par′a·thy′roi·dal
par′a·thy′roi·dec′to·mize′
par′a·thy′roi·dec′to·my
par′a·thy′roi·din
par′a·thy′roi·do′ma
  pl. -mas *or* -ma·ta
par′a·thy′ro·pri′val

par·a·thy′ro·priv′ic
par·a·thy′ro·tox′i·co′sis
   pl. -ses′
par·a·thy′ro·trop′ic
par·a·to′ni·a
par·a·ton′sil·lar
par·a·tra′che·al
par·a·tra·cho′ma
par·a·tri·cho′sis *pl.* -ses′
par·a·tri·gem′i·nal
par·a·trip′sis *pl.* -ses′
par·a·troph′ic
pa·rat′ro·phy
par·a·tu′bal
par·a·tu·ber′cu·lin
par·a·tu·ber′cu·lo′sis
par·a·type′
par·a·typ′ic *or* par·a·typ′i·cal
par·a·typh·li′tis
par·a·ty′phoid′
par·a·um·bil′i·cal
par·a·u′re·ter′ic
par·a·u·re·ter·i′tis
par·a·u·re′thra *pl.* -thras *or*
  -thrae′
par·a·u·re′thral
par·a·u′ter·ine
par·a·vac·cin′i·a
par·a·vag′i·nal
par·a·vag′i·ni′tis
par·a·val′vu·lar
par·a·vas′cu·lar
par·a·ve′nous
par·a·ven·tric′u·lar
par·a·ver′te·bral
par·a·ves′i·cal
par·a·vi′ta·min·o′sis
   pl. -ses′
par·a·xan′thine′
par·ax′i·al
par·ax′on′
par·ec·ta′si·a
par·ec·ta′sis *pl.* -ses′
par·e·gor′ic
pa·rei′ra
par·el·e′i·din
par·en·ceph′a·lon′ *pl.* -la
par·en·ceph′a·lous
pa·ren′chy·ma
pa·ren′chy·mal
pa·ren′chy·ma·ti′tis
par·en·chym′a·tous
par′ent

pa·ren′ter·al
pa·ren′ter·al·ly
par′ep·i·did′y·mis
par′ep·i·gas′tric
pa·re′sis *pl.* -ses′
  —si′ne′ pa·re′si′
par·es·the′si·a
par·es·thet′ic
pa·ret′ic
pa·reu′ni·a
par·fo′cal
par′gy·line′
Par′ham band
par′i·es′ *pl.* pa·ri′e·tes′
  —anterior
  —anterior va·gi′nae′
  —anterior ven·tric′u·li′
  —ca·rot′i·ca ca′vi′
    tym′pa·ni′
  —ca·rot′i·cus ca′vi′
    tym′pa·ni′
  —ex·ter′nus duc′tus
    coch′le·ar′is
  —inferior
  —inferior or′bi·tae′
  —jug′u·lar′is ca′vi′
    tym′pan·i′
  —lab′y·rin′thi·ca ca′vi′
    tym′pa·ni′
  —lab′y·rin′thi·cus ca′vi′
    tym′pa·ni′
  —lat′er·a′lis
  —lateralis or′bi·tae′
  —mas·toi′de·us ca′vi′
    tym′pa·ni′
  —me′di·a′lis
  —medialis or′bi·tae′
  —mem′bra·na′ce·us ca′vi′
    tym′pa·ni′
  —membranaceus tra′che·ae′
  —posterior
  —posterior va·gi′nae′
  —posterior ven·tric′u·li′
  —superior
  —superior or′bi·tae′
  —teg′men·ta′lis ca′vi′
    tym′pa·ni′
  —tym′pan·i′cus duc′tus
    coch′le·ar′is
  —ves·tib′u·lar′is duc′tus
    coch′le·ar′is
pa·ri′e·tal
pa·ri′e·to·fron′tal

pa·ri′e·to·mas′toid′
pa·ri′e·to·oc·cip′i·tal
pa·ri′e·to·pon′tine′
pa·ri′e·to·sphe′noid′
pa·ri′e·to·splanch′nic
pa·ri′e·to·squa·mo′sal
pa·ri′e·to·tem′po·ral
pa·ri′e·to·vis′cer·al
Pa·ri·naud′
  —conjunctivitis
  —syndrome
par′i·ty
Park aneurysm
Par′ker
  —fluid
  —incision
  —method
Par′ker-Kerr′
  enteroenterostomy
Par′kin·son disease
par′kin·so′ni·an
par′kin·son·ism
par·oc·cip′i·tal
par·o·don′tal
par·o·don·ti′tis
par·o·don·ti·um *pl.* -ti·a
par·o·dyn′i·a
par·ol·fac′to·ry
par·ol′i·var′y
par′o·mo·my′cin
Pa·ro′na space
par′o·ni′ri·a
  —am′bu·lans′
par·o·nych′i·a
  —diph′the·rit′i·ca
par·o·nych′i·al
par·o·nych′i·um *pl.* -i·a
pa·ron′y·cho·my·co′sis
   pl. -ses′
pa·ron′y·cho′sis *pl.* -ses′
par′o·oph·o·ri′tis
par′o·oph′o·ron′
par′oph·thal′mi·a
par′oph·thal·mon′cus
par·op′si·a
par·op′sis
par·op′tic
par·or′chis
par·o·rex′i·a
par·os′mi·a
par·os·phre′sis
par·os′te·al
par·os′te·i′tis

par'os·ti'tis
par'os·to'sis
pa·rot'ic
pa·rot'id
pa·rot'i·de'an
pa·rot'i·dec'to·my
pa·rot'i·di'tis
pa·rot'i·do·scle·ro'sis
   pl. -ses'
par'o·tit'ic
par'o·ti'tis
par'ous
par'o·var'i·an
par'o·var'i·ot'o·my
par'o·va·ri'tis
par'o·var'i·um *pl.* -i·a
par·ox·ysm
par·ox·ys'mal
par·ox·ys'mic
Par'rot
  —atrophy
  —disease
  —nodes
Par'ry disease
pars *pl.* par'tes'
  —ab·dom'i·na'lise·soph'a·gi'
  —abdominalis et pel'vi'na
    sys·te'ma·tis au'to·
    nom'i·ci'
  —abdominalis mus'cu·li'
    pec'to·ra'lis ma·jo'ris
  —abdominalis oe·soph'a·gi'
  —abdominalis sys·te'ma·tis
    sym·path'i·ci'
  —abdominalis u·re'ter·is
  —a·lar'is mus'cu·li' na·sa'lis
  —al've·o·lar'is man·dib'-
    u·lae'
  —anterior com'mis·su'rae'
    an·te'ri·o'ris cer'e·bri'
  —anterior fa'ci·e'i'
    di'a·phrag·mat'i·cae'
    hep'a·tis
  —anterior lob'u·li'
    qua·dran'gu·lar'is
  —anterior rhi'nen·ceph'a·li'
  —an'u·lar'is va·gi'nae' fi·
    bro'sae' dig'i·to'rum ma'-
    nus
  —anularis vaginae fibrosae
    digitorum pe'dis
  —as'cen'dens du'o·de'ni'
  —ba·sa'lis

  —basalis ar·te'ri·ae' pul'-
    mo·na'lis dex'trae'
  —basalis arteriae pulmon-
    alis si·nis'trae'
  —bas·i·lar'is os'sis
    oc·cip'i·ta'lis
  —basilaris pon'tis
  —buc'ca'lis
  —buc'co·pha·ryn'ge·a
    mus'cu·li' con'stric'to'ris
    pha·ryn'gis su·pe'ri·o'ris
  —cal·ca'ne·o·cu·boi'de·a
    lig'a·men'ti' bi·fur·ca'ti'
  —cal·ca'ne·o·na·vic'u·lar'is
    lig'a·men'ti' bi·fur·ca'ti'
  —car·di'a·ca ven·tric'u·li'
  —car'ti·la·gin'e·a
  —cartilaginea sep'ti' na'si'
  —cartilaginea tu'bae' au'di·
    ti'vae'
  —cav'er'no·sa u·re'thrae'
  —cen'tra'lis ven·tric'u·li'
    lat·er·a'lis
  —ce·phal'i·ca et cer'vi·ca'lis
    sy·ste'ma·tis au'to·
    nom'i·ci'
  —cephalica et cervicalis
    systematis sym·path'i·ci'
  —cer'a·to·pha·ryn'ge·a
    mus'cu·li' con'stric'to'ris
    pha·ryn'gis me'di·i'
  —cer'vi·ca'lis e·soph'a·gi'
  —cervicalis me·dul'lae'
    spi·na'lis
  —cervicalis oe·soph'a·gi'
  —chon'dro·pha·ryn'ge·a
    mus'cu·li' con'stric'to'ris
    pha·ryn'gis me'di·i'
  —cil'i·ar'is ret'i·nae'
  —cla·vic'u·lar'is mus'cu·li'
    pec'to·ra'lis ma·jo'ris
  —coch'le·ar'is ner'vi'
    oc·ta'vi'
  —con'vo·lu'ta lob'u·li'
    cor'ti·ca'lis re'nis
  —cos'ta'lis di'a·phrag'-
    ma·tis
  —cri'co·pha·ryn'ge·a
    mus'cu·li' con'stric'to'ris
    pha·ryn'gis in·fe'ri·o'ris
  —cru'ci·for'mis va·gi'nae'
    fi·bro'sae' dig'i·to'rum
    ma'nus

  —cruciformis vaginae
    fibrosae digitorum pe'dis
  —cu'pu·lar'is re·ces'sus
    ep'i·tym·pan'i·ci'
  —de·scen'dens du'o·de'ni'
  —dex'tra fa·ci·e'i' di'a·
    phrag·mat'i·cae' hep'a·tis
  —dis·ta'lis
  —distalis lo'bi' an·te'ri·o'ris
    hy'po·phys'e·os'
  —dor·sa'lis pon'tis
  —fe·ta'lis pla·cen'tae'
  —flac'ci·da mem·bra'nae'
    tym'pa·ni'
  —fron·ta'lis cap'su·lae'
    in'ter·nae'
  —frontalis co·ro'nae'
    ra'di·a'tae'
  —frontalis o·per'cu·li'
  —frontalis ra·di·a'ti·o'nis
    cor'po·ris cal·lo'si'
  —glan'du·lar'is
  —glos'so·pha·ryn'ge·a
    mus'cu·li' con'stric'to'ris
    pha·ryn'gis su·pe'ri·o'ris
  —gris'e·a hy'po·thal'a·mi'
  —hor'i·zon·ta'lis du'o·
    de'ni'
  —horizontalis os'sis
    pal·a·ti'ni'
  —i·li'a·ca lin'e·ae' ter'mi·
    na'lis
  —inferior du'o·de'ni'
  —inferior fos'sae' rhom·
    boi'de·ae'
  —inferior gy'ri' fron·ta'lis
    me'di·i'
  —inferior par'tis ves·tib'-
    u·lar'is ner'vi' oc·ta'vi'
  —in'fra·cla·vic'u·lar'is
    plex'us bra'chi·a'lis
  —in'fun·dib'u·lar'is
  —in'ter·ar'tic'u·lar'is
  —in'ter·car'ti·la·gin'e·a
    ri'mae' glot'ti·dis
  —in'ter·me'di·a
  —intermedia fos'sae'
    rhom·boi'de·ae'
  —intermedia lo'bi' an·te'-
    ri·o'ris hy'po·phys'e·os'
  —in'ter·mem·bra'na·ce·a
    ri'mae' glot'ti·dis
  —i·rid'i·ca ret'i·nae'

—la'bi·a'lis mus'cu·li'
or·bic'u·lar'is o'ris
—lac'ri·ma'lis mus'cu·li'
or·bic'u·lar'is oc'u·li'
—la·ryn'ge·a pha·ryn'gis
—lat'er·a'lis
—lateralis ar'cus pe'dis
lon'gi·tu'di·na'lis
—lateralis mus'cu·lo'rum
in·ter·trans·ver·sar'i·o'-
rum pos·te'ri·o'rum
cer'vi·cis
—lateralis os'sis oc·cip'-
i·ta'lis
—lateralis ossis sa'cri'
—lum·ba'lis
—lumbalis di·a·phrag'-
ma·tis
—lumbalis me·dul'lae'
spi·na'lis
—mam'il·lar'is hy'po·thal'-
a·mi'
—mar'gi·na'lis mus'cu·li'
or·bic'u·lar'is o'ris
—marginalis sul'ci' cin'-
gu·li'
—mas'toi·de·a os'sis
tem'po·ra'lis
—me'di·a'lis ar'cus pe'dis
lon'gi·tu'di·na'lis
—medialis mus'cu·lo'rum
in·ter·trans·ver·sar'i·o'-
rum pos·te'ri·o'rum cer'-
vi·cis
—me'di·as'ti·na'lis fa·ci·e'i'
me'di·a'lis pul·mo'nis
—mem'bra·na'ce·a sep'ti'
a·tri·o'rum
—membranacea septi
in·ter·ven·tric'u·lar'is
cor'dis
—membranacea septi na'si'
—membranacea u·re'thrae'
mas·cu·li'nae'
—membranacea urethrae
vi·ri'lis
—mo'bi·lis sep'ti' na'si'
—mus'cu·lar'is sep'ti'
in·ter·ven·tric'u·lar'is
cor'dis
—my'lo·pha·ryn'ge·a
mus'cu·li' con·stric'to'ris
pha·ryn'gis su·pe'ri·o'ris

—na·sa'lis os'sis fron·ta'lis
—nasalis pha·ryn'gis
—ner·vo'sa
—neu·ra'lis
—o·bli'qua mus'cu·li'
cri·co·thy're·oi'de·i'
—obliqua musculi
cri·co·thy·roi'de·i'
—oc·cip'i·ta'lis cap'su·lae'
in·ter'nae'
—occipitalis co·ro'nae'
ra·di·a'tae'
—occipitalis ra·di·a'ti·o'nis
cor'po·ris cal·lo'si'
—ol'fac·to'ri·a
—o·per'cu·lar'is gy'ri'
fron·ta'lis in·fe'ri·o'ris
—op'ti·ca hy'po·thal'a·mi'
—optica ret'i·nae'
—o·ra'lis pha·ryn'gis
—or·bi·ta'lis
—orbitalis glan'du·lae'
lac'ri·ma'lis
—orbitalis gy'ri' fron·ta'lis
in·fe'ri·o'ris
—orbitalis mus'cu·li'
or·bic'u·lar'is oc'u·li'
—orbitalis os'sis fron·ta'lis
—os'se·a
—ossea sep'ti' na'si'
—ossea tu'bae' au'di·ti'vae'
—pal'pe·bra'lis
—palpebralis glan'du·lae'
lac'ri·ma'lis
—palpebralis mus'cu·li'
or·bic'u·lar'is oc'u·li'
—par'a·sym·path'i·ca
sy·ste'ma·tis ner·vo·si'
au'to·nom'i·ci'
—pa·ri·e·ta'lis co·ro'nae'
ra'di·a'tae'
—parietalis o·per'cu·li'
—parietalis ra·di·a'ti·o'nis
cor'po·ris cal·lo'si'
—pel·vi'na u·re'ter·is
—per'pen·dic'u·lar'is os'sis
pal·a·ti'ni'
—pe·tro'sa os'sis tem'po·ra'lis
—posterior com'mis·su'rae'
an·te'ri·o'ris cer'e·bri'
—posterior hep'a·tis
—posterior lob·u'li' quad·
ran'gu·lar'is

—posterior rhi'nen·ceph'-
a·li'
—pro·fun'da
—profunda glan'du·lae'
pa·rot'i·dis
—profunda mus'cu·li'
mas·se'te·ris
—profunda musculi sphinc·
te'ris a'ni' ex·ter'ni'
—pros·tat'i·ca u·re'thrae'
mas·cu·li'nae'
—prostatica urethrae vi·ri'lis
—pter'y·go·pha·ryn'ge·a
mus'cu·li' con·stric'to'ris
pha·ryn'gis su·pe'ri·o'ris
—pu'bi·ca lin'e·ae'
ter'mi·na'lis
—py'lo'ri·ca ven·tric'u·li'
—qua·dra'ta lo'bi' hep'a·tis
si·nis'tri'
—ra·di·a'ta lob·u'li' cor'ti·
ca'lis re'nis
—rec'ta mus'cu·li' cri·co·
thy're·oi'de·i'
—recta musculi cri·co·thy·
roi'de·i'
—ret'ro·len'ti·for'mis
cap'su·lae' in·ter'nae'
—sa·cra'lis lin'e·ae'
ter'mi·na'lis
—spon'gi·o'sa u·re'thrae'
mas·cu·li'nae'
—squa·mo'sa os'sis
tem'po·ra'lis
—ster·na'lis di·a·phrag'-
ma·tis
—ster'no·cos·ta'lis mus'cu·
li' pec·to·ra'lis ma·jo'ris
—sub'cu·ta'ne·a mus'cu·li'
sphinc·te'ris a'ni'
ex·ter'ni'
—sub'fron·ta'lis sul'ci'
cin'gu·li'
—sub·len'ti·for'mis
cap'su·lae' in·ter'nae'
—su'per·fi'ci·a'lis
—superficialis glan'du·lae'
pa·rot'i·dis
—superficialis mus'cu·li'
mas·se'te·ris
—superficialis musculi
sphinc·te'ris a'ni'
ex·ter'ni'

—superior du'o·de'ni'
—superior fa·ci·e'i' di'a·
  phrag·mat'i·cae' hep'a·tis
—superior fos'sae' rhom·
  boi'de·ae'
—superior gy'ri' fron·ta'lis
  me'di·i'
—superior par'tis ves·tib'-
  u·lar'is ner'vi' oc·ta'vi'
—su'pra·cla·vic'u·lar'is
  plex'us bra'chi·a'lis
—su'pra·op'ti·ca
—sym·path'i·ca sy·ste'ma·
  tis ner·vo'si' au'to·nom'-
  i·ci'
—tem'po·ra'lis co·ro'nae'
  ra'di·a'tae'
—temporalis o·per'cu·li'
—temporalis ra'di·a'ti·o'nis
  cor'po·ris cal·lo'si'
—ten'sa mem·bra'nae'
  tym'pa·ni'
—tho'ra·ca'lis me·dul'lae'
  spi·na'lis
—thoracalis oe·soph'a·gi'
—thoracalis sy·ste'ma·tis
  sym·path'i·ci'
—tho·ra'ci·ca
—thoracica e·soph'a·gi'
—thoracica me·dul'lae'
  spi·na'lis
—thoracica sy·ste'ma·tis
  au'to·nom'i·ci'
—thy'ro·pha·ryn'ge·a
  mus'cu·li' con·stric'to'ris
  pha·ryn'gis in·fe'ri·o'ris
—tib'i·o·cal·ca'ne·a
  lig'a·men'ti' me'di·a'lis
—tib'i·o·na·vic'u·lar'is
  lig'a·men'ti' me'di·a'lis
—tib'i·o·ta'lar'is anterior
  lig'a·men'ti' me'di·a'lis
—tibiotalaris posterior
  ligamenti medialis
—trans·ver'sa mus'cu·li'
  na·sa'lis
—tri·an'gu·lar'is gy'ri'
  fron·ta'lis in·fe'ri·o'ris
—tu'be·ra'lis
—tym·pan'i·ca os'sis
  tem'po·ra'lis
—u·ter·i'na pla·cen'tae'
—uterina tu'bae' u·ter·i'nae'

—ven·tra'lis pon'tis
—ver'te·bra'lis fa·ci·e'i'
  me'di·a'lis pul·mo'nis
—ves·tib'u·lar'is ner'vi'
  oc·ta'vi'
par'tal
par'tes'
—gen'i·ta'les' ex·ter'nae'
  mu'li·e'bres'
—genitales externae
  vi·ri'les'
—genitales fem'i·ni'nae'
  ex·ter'nae'
—genitales mas'cu·li'nae'
  ex·ter'nae'
par'the·no·gen'e·sis *pl.* -ses'
par'the·no·ge·net'ic
par'the·no·pho'bi·a
par'ti·cle
par·tic'u·late'
Par'ti·pi'lo gastrostomy
par·ti'tion
Partsch operation
par·tu'ri·ent
par·tu'ri·fa'cient
par·tu'ri·om'e·ter
par·tu·ri'tion
par'tus
—ag'rip·pi'nus
—cae·sar'e·us
—im'ma·tu'rus
—ma·tu'rus
—pre·cip'i·ta'tus
—pre'ma·tu'rus
—prep'a·ra'tor
—ser'o·ti'nus
—sic'cus
pa·ru'lis *pl.* -li·des'
par'um·bil'i·cal
par·u'ri·a
par'vi·cel'lu·lar
par'vi·loc'u·lar
par'vule'
pas'cal'
Pasch'en bodies
Pa·schu'tin degeneration
pas'sage
Pas'sa·vant'
—bar
—cushion
—ridge
pass'er
pas'sion

pas'sion·ate
pas'si·vat'ed
pas'si·va'tion
pas'sive
pas'sive-ag·gres'sive
pas'sive-de·pend'ent
pas'siv·ism
pas'siv·ist
paste
Pas·teur'
—effect
—treatment
pas'teur·el·lo'sis *pl.* -ses'
pas'teur·i·za'tion
pas'teur·ize', -ized', -iz'ing
pas'teur·iz'er
Pas'ti·a
—lines
—sign
Pas'teu·rel'la *pl.* -las *or* -lae'
—mul'to·ci'da
—pneu'mo·tro'pi·ca
pas·tille'
Pa·tau' syndrome
patch
patch'y
pa·tel'la *pl.* -lae'
—bi·par'ta
—cu'bi·ti'
Pa·tel'la disease
pa·tel'la·pex'y
pa·tel'lar
pat'el·lec'to·my
pa·tel'li·form'
pa·tel'lo·ad·duc'tor
pa·tel'lo·fem'o·ral
pat'en·cy
pa'tent
pa'tent·ly
pa·ter'nal
pa·ter'ni·ty
Pat'er·son
—bodies
—syndrome
Pat'er·son-Brown'-Kel'ly
  syndrome
Pat'er·son-Kel'ly
  syndrome
path
pa·the'ma
path'er·ga'si·a
path'er·gy
pa·thet'ic

path'o·clis'is
path'o·cure'
path'o·don'ti·a
path'o·gen
path'o·gen'e·sis
path'o·ge·net'ic
path'o·gen'ic
path'o·ge·nic'i·ty
path'og·nom'ic
pa·thog'no·mon'ic
pa·thog'no·my
path'og·nos'tic
path'o·log'ic *or*
  path'o·log'i·cal
pa·thol'o·gist
pa·thol'o·gy
path'o·ma'ni·a
path'o·met'ric
pa·thom'e·try
path'o·mi·me'sis *pl.* -ses'
path'o·mim'ic·ry
path'o·mor'phism
path'o·mor·phol'o·gy
path'o·neu·ro'sis *pl.* -ses'
path'o·pho'bi·a
path'o·pho·re'sis
path'o·phor'ic
pa·thoph'o·rous
path'o·phys'i·o·log'ic
path'o·phys'i·o·log'i·cal
path'o·phys'i·ol'o·gy
path'o·psy·chol'o·gy
path'o·psy·cho'sis *pl.* -ses'
pa·tho'sis *pl.* -ses'
path'way'
pa'tient
Pat'rick
  —area
  —test
pat'ri·lin'e·al
pat'ten
pat'tern
pat'tern·ing
pat'u·lin
pat'u·lous
pau'ci·ty
Paul
  —operation
  —test
  —tube
Paul Bert effect
Paul'-Bun·nell' test
Paul·lin'i·a

Paul'-Mik'u·licz operation
paunch
pause
Pau·trier' microabscess
Pauw'els operation
pave'ment·ing
pa'vex
Pav·lov'i·an
pav·lov'i·an·ism
Pav'lov' pouch
pa'vor
  —di·ur'nus
  —noc·tur'nus
Pa'vy
  —disease
  —joint
  —solution
Paw'lik
  —fold
  —triangle
  —trigone
Payr
  —method
  —sign
  —syndrome
peak
pearl
pearl'y
peau d'o·range'
pec'cant
pec'tase'
pec'ten *(a comblike structure of
  the body), pl.* -ti·nes'
  ♦pectin
pec'te·no'sis
pec'tic
pec'tin *(a substance in ripe fruit)*
  ♦pecten
pec'tin·ase'
pec'ti·nate'
pec'tin·e·al
pec'tin·es'ter·ase'
pec·tin'e·us
pec·tin'i·form'
pec'tin·ose'
pec'to·ral
pec'to·ral'gi·a
pec'to·ra'lis *pl.* -les'
pec'to·ril'o·quy
pec'tose'
pec'tus
  —car'i·na'tum
  —ex'ca·va'tum

ped'al
ped'a·tro'phi·a
pe·dat'ro·phy
ped'er·ast'
ped'er·as'tic
ped'er·as'ty
ped'i·al'gi·a
pe'di·at'ric
pe'di·a·tri'cian
pe'di·at'rics
pe'di·at'rist
pe'di·at'ry
ped'i·cel
ped'i·cel·late'
ped'i·cle
ped'i·cled
pe·dic'ter·us
pe·dic'u·lar
pe·dic'u·late'
pe·dic'u·la'tion
pe·dic'u·li·cid'al
pe·dic'u·li·cide'
Pe·dic'u·loi'des'
  —ven'tri·co'sus
pe·dic'u·lo'sis *pl.* -ses'
  —cap'i·tis
  —cor'po·ris
  —pal'pe·brar'um
  —pu'bis
pe·dic'u·lous *(lice-infested)*
  ♦pediculus, Pediculus
pe·dic'u·lus *(a stemlike
  structure; pedicle)*
  ♦pediculous, Pediculus
  —ar'cus ver'te·brae'
Pe·dic'u·lus *(louse)*
  ♦pediculous, pediculus
  —hu·ma'nus cap'i·tis
  —humanus cor'po·ris
pe·di'tis
pe'do·don'ti·a
pe'do·don'tics
pe'do·don'tist
pe'do·don·tol'o·gy
ped'o·dy'na·mom'e·ter
pe'do·gen'e·sis
pe·dol'o·gist
pe·dol'o·gy
pe·dom'e·ter
pe'do·mor'phism
pe'do·no·sol'o·gy
pe·dop'a·thy
pe'do·phil'i·a

pe′do·phil′ic
pe′do·pho′bi·a
pe′do·psy·chi′a·trist
pe′dor·thot′ics
pe′dor·tho·tist
pe·dun′cle
pe·dun′cu·lar
pe·dun′cu·late
pe·dun′cu·lat′ed
pe·dun′cu·la′tion
pe·dun′cu·lot′o·my
pe·dun′cu·lus *pl.* -li′
  —cer′e·bel·lar′is inferior
  —cerebellaris me′di·us
  —cerebellaris superior
  —ce′e·bri′
  —cor′po·ris mam′il·lar′is
  —floc′cu·li′
  —thal′a·mi′ inferior
peel
peer
Peet operation
peg
peg·ad′e·mase′
pei′no·ther′a·py
pe·lade′
pel′age
pel′a·gism
Pel crises
Pel′-Eb′stein′
  —disease
  —fever
  —syndrome
Pel′ger anomaly
Pel′ger-Hu′ët anomaly
pel′ge·roid′
pel′i·di′si
pel′i·o′sis
pel′i·ot′ic
Pel′i·zae′us-Merz′bach′er
  disease
pel·lag′ra
  —si′ne′ pellagra
pel·lag′ra·gen′ic
pel·lag′rin
pel·lag′roid′
pel·la·gro′sis
pel·lag′rous
Pel′le·gri′ni-Stie′da disease
pel′let
pel′li·cle
pel·lic′u·lar
pel·lic′u·lous

Pel′li·gri′ni disease
pel′li·to′ry
Pel·liz′zi syndrome
pel·lu′cid
pel·mat′o·gram′
pe·lo·he′mi·a
pe′loid′
pe·lol′o·gy
pe′lo·ther′a·py
pel′ta·tin
pel′vi·ab·dom′i·nal
pel′vic
pel′vi·fem′o·ral
pel′vi·fix·a′tion
pel·vim′e·ter
pel·vim′e·try
pel′vi·o·li·thot′o·my
pel′vi·o·ne′o·cys·tos·to·my
pel′vi·o·per′i·to·ni′tis
pel′vi·o·plas′ty
pel′vi·o·ra·di·og′ra·phy
pel′vi·ot′o·my
pel′vi·per′i·to·ni′tis
pel′vi·rec′tal
pel′vis *pl.* -vis·es *or* -ves′
  —ae′qua·bil′i·ter jus′to′
    major
  —aequabiliter justo minor
  —fis′sa
  —major
  —minor
  —na′na
  —re·na′lis
  —spi·no′sa
pel′vi·sa′cral
pel′vi·scope′
pel′vi·sec′tion
pel′vi·ver′te·bral
pel′vo·cal′i·ec′ta·sis *pl.* -ses′
pel′vo·cal′y·ce′al
Pem′ber·ton operation
pem′o·line′
pem′phi·goid′
pem′phi·gus *pl.* -gus·es *or*
  -gi′
  —a·cu′tus
  —chron′i·cus
  —con·ta′gi·o′sus
  —er′y·them′a·to′sus
  —fo′li·a′ce·us
  —ne′o·na·to′rum
  —trop′i·cus
  —veg′e·tans′

  —vul·gar′is
pem′pi·dine′
pe′nal·ge′si·a
pen·bu′to·lol′
pen′cil
pen′del·luft′
Pen′dred syndrome
pen′du·lar
pen′du·lous
pe·nec′to·my
pen′e·trance
pen′e·trat′ing
pen′e·tra′tion
pen′e·trom′e·ter
Pen′field′ operation
pen′i·ci′din
pen′i·cil′la·mine′
pen′i·cil′lase′
pen′i·cil′late′
pen′i·cil′lic
pen′i·cil′li·form′
pen′i·cil′li′ li·e′nis
pen′i·cil′lin
pen′i·cil′li·nase′
pen′i·cil′lin′ic
pen′i·cil′li·o′sis *pl.* -ses′
Pen′i·cil′li·um
pen′i·cil′lo′ic
pen′i·cil′loyl-pol′y·ly′sine′
pen′i·cil′lus *pl.* -li′
pe′nile′
pe′nis *pl.* -nis·es *or* -nes′
pen′nate′
pen′ni·form′
pen′ny·roy′al
pe·nol′o·gy
pe′no·scro′tal
Pen′rose′ drain
pen′ta·bam′ate′
pen′ta·ba′sic
pen′ta·chlo′ro·phe′nol′
pen′tad′
pen′ta·dac′tyl
pen′ta·e·ryth′ri·tol′
pen′ta·gas′trin
pen′ta·gen′ic
pen′tal′o·gy
  —of Fal·lot′
pen′tam′i·dine′
pen′tane′
pen′ta·starch′
Pen′ta·sto′mi·da
  —den·tic′u·la′tum

Pen'ta·trich'o·mo'nas
pen'ta·va'lent
pen·taz'o·cine
pent·dy'o·pent'
pen'tene'
pen·thi'e·nate'
pen'to·bar'bi·tal'
pen'to·bar'bi·tone'
pen'to·lin'i·um
pen'to·san'
pen·to·sa·zone'
pen'tose'
pen'to·side'
pen'to·stat'in
pen'to·su'ri·a
pen'to·thal'
pent·ox'ide'
pen'tox·if'yl·line'
pen'tyl
pen'ty·lene·tet'ra·zol'
pe·num'bra
Pen'zoldt' test
pe'o·til'lo·ma'ni·a
Pep'per
—syndrome
—treatment
—type
pep'si·gogue'
pep'sin
pep'sin·if'er·ous
pep·sin'o·gen
pep'tic
pep'ti·dase'
pep'tide'
pep'ti·do·gly'can
pep'ti·do·lyt'ic
pep'tize', -tized', -tiz'ing
pep'to·gen'ic
pep·tog'e·nous
pep·tol'y·sis *pl.* -ses'
pep'tone'
pep'to·ne'mi·a
pep·ton'ic
pep'to·nize', -nized', -niz'ing
pep'to·nu'ri·a
per'a·ceph'a·lus
per'a·ce'tic
per·ac'id
per'a·cid'i·ty
per'a·cute'
per a'num
per·cent' *or* per cent
per·cent'age

per·cen'tile'
per'cept'
per·cep'tion
per·cep'tive
per·cep·tiv'i·ty
per·cep·to'ri·um *pl.* -ri·ums *or* -ri·a
per·cep'tu·al
per·cep'tu·al·i·za'tion
per·chlo'rate'
per·chlo'ric
per·chlo'ro·eth'yl·ene'
Per'ci·for'mes
per'co·late'
per·co·la'tion
per·co·la'tor
per·cuss', -cussed', -cuss'ing
per·cus'si·ble
per·cus'sion
per·cus'sor
per'cu·ta'ne·ous
per'cu·ta'ne·ous·ly
per·en·ceph'a·ly
Pe·rez' sign
per·fec'tion
per·fec'tion·ism
per·fla'tion
per'fo·rans'
per'fo·rate', -rat'ed, -rat'ing
per·fo·ra'tion
per·fo·ra'tor
per·fo·ra·to'ri·um *pl.* -ri·a
per·form'ance
per·for'mic
per·fri·ca'tion
per·fus'ate'
per·fuse', -fused', -fus'ing
per·fu'sion
per'go·lide'
per'i·ac'i·nal
per'i·ac'i·nar
per'i·ac'i·nous
per'i·ad'e·ni'tis
—mu·co'sae' ne·crot'i·ca re·cur'rens
per'i·ad·ven'ti·tial
per'i·a·li·e·ni'tis
per'i·am'pul·lar'y
per'i·a'nal
per'i·an·gi·i'tis
per'i·an'gi·o·cho·li'tis
per'i·an'gi·o'ma *pl.* -mas *or* -ma·ta

per'i·a·or'tal
per'i·a·or'tic
per'i·a'or·ti'tis
per'i·a'pex' *pl.* -pex'es *or* -pi·ces'
per'i·ap'i·cal
per'i·ap'i·cal·ly
per'i·ap·pen'di·ci'tis
per'i·ap'pen·dic'u·lar
per'i·aq'ue·duc'tal
per'i·a·re'o·lar
per'i·ar·te'ri·al
per'i·ar·te'ri·o'lar
per'i·ar·te'ri·ti's
per'i·ar'thric
per'i·ar·thri'tis
—cal·car'e·a
per'i·ar·tic'u·lar
per'i·a'tri·al
per'i·au·ric'u·lar
per'i·ax'i·al
per'i·ax'il·lar'y
per'i·bron'chi·al
per'i·bron'chi·o'lar
per'i·bron'chi·o·li'tis
per'i·bron·chi'tis
per'i·bro'sis
per'i·bul'bar
per'i·bur'sal
per'i·cal'y·ce'al
per'i·can'a·lic'u·lar
per'i·cap'il·lar'y
per'i·car'di·ac'
per'i·car'di·al
per'i·car'di·ec'to·my
per'i·car'di·o·cen·te'sis *pl.* -ses'
per'i·car'di·ol'y·sis *pl.* -ses'
per'i·car'di·o·me'di·as'ti·ni'tis
per'i·car'di·o·phren'ic
per'i·car'di·o·pleu'ral
per'i·car'di·or'rha·phy
per'i·car'di·os'to·my
per'i·car'di·ot'o·my
per'i·car·dit'ic
per'i·car·di'tis *pl.* -dit'i·des'
—o·blit'er·ans'
per'i·car'di·um *pl.* -di·a
—fi·bro'sum
—se·ro'sum
per'i·ca'val
per'i·ce'cal

per'i·ce·ci'tis
per'i·cel'lu·lar
per'i·ce·men'tal
per'i·ce'men·ti'tis
per'i·ce·men·to·cla'si·a
per'i·ce·men'tum
per'i·cen'tral
per'i·cen'tric
per'i·cen·tri·o'lar
per'i·ce·phal'ic
per'i·cer'vi·cal
per'i·cho·lan'gi·o·lit'ic
per'i·cho·lan·git'ic
per'i·cho·lan·gi'tis
per'i·cho'le·cys'tic
per'i·cho'le·cys·ti'tis
per'i·chon'dral or
   per'i·chon'dri·al
per'i·chon·drit'ic
per'i·chon·dri'tis
per'i·chon'dri·um pl. -dri·a
per'i·chon·dro'ma pl. -mas
   or -ma·ta
per'i·chord'
per'i·chord'al
per'i·cho'roid'
per'i·cho·roi'dal
per'i·coc'cyg·e'al
per'i·co'lic
per'i·co·li'tis
per'i·co·lon'ic
per'i·co'lon·i'tis
per'i·col·pi'tis
per'i·con'chal
per'i·con·chi'tis
per'i·cor'ne·al
per'i·cor'o·nal
per'i·cor'o·ni'tis
per'i·cos'tal
per'i·cox·i'tis
per'i·cra'ni·al
per'i·cra·ni'tis
per'i·cra'ni·um pl. -ni·a
per'i·cys'tic
per'i·cys·ti'tis
per'i·cys'ti·um pl. -ti·a
per'i·cyte'
per'i·cy'ti·al
per'i·cy·to'ma pl. -mas or
   -ma·ta
per'i·dec'to·my
per'i·den'drit'ic
per'i·derm'

per'i·der'mal
per'i·des·mi'tis
per'i·des'mi·um
per'i·did'y·mis pl. -mi·des'
per'i·did'y·mi'tis
per'i·di·ver·tic'u·li'tis
per'i·duc'tal
per'i·du'o·de·ni'tis
per'i·du'ral
per'i·en·ceph'a·li'tis
per'i·en·ceph'a·log'ra·phy
per'i·en·ceph'a·lo·men·in·
   gi'tis
per'i·en·ter'ic
per'i·en·ter·i'tis
per'i·en·ter·on'
per'i·e·pen'dy·mal
per'i·ep'i·did'y·mi'tis
per'i·ep'i·glot'tic
per'i·ep'i·the'li·o·ma
   pl. -mas or -ma·ta
per'i·e·soph'a·ge'al
per'i·e·soph'a·gi'tis
per'i·fas·cic'u·lar
per'i·fis'tu·lar
per'i·fo'cal
per'i·fol·lic'u·lar
per'i·fol·lic'u·li'tis
   —cap'i·tis ab·sce'dens et
   suf·fod'i·ens
per'i·for'ni·cal
per'i·fu·nic'u·lar
per'i·gan'gli·i'tis
per'i·gan'gli·on'ic
per'i·gas'tric
per'i·gas·tri'tis
per'i·gem'mal
per'i·gen'i·tal
per'i·glan'du·lar
per'i·glos·si'tis
per'i·glot'tic
per'i·glot'tis
per'ig·nath'ic
per'i·he·pat'ic
per'i·hep'a·ti'tis
per'i·her'ni·al
per'i·hi'lar
per'i·hy·poph'y·si'al
per'i-im'plan·ti'tis
per'i·je'ju·ni'tis
per'i·kar'y·al
per'i·kar'y·on'
per'i·ke·rat'ic

per'i·ky'ma·ta sing. -ky'ma
per'i·lab'y·rinth'
per'i·lab'y·rin·thi'tis
per'i·la·ryn'ge·al
per'i·lar'yn·gi'tis
per'i·len·tic'u·lar
per'i·lig'a·men'tous
per'i·lo'bar
per'i·lymph'
per'i·lym'pha
per'i·lym·phan'ge·al or
   per'i·lym·phan'gi·al
per'i·lym'phan·gi'tis
per'i·lym·phat'ic
per'i·mac'u·lar
per'i·mas·ti'tis
per'i·med'ul·lar'y
per'i·men'in·gi'tis
pe·rim'e·ter
per'i·met'ric
per'i·me·trit'ic
per'i·me·tri'tis
per'i·me'tri·um pl. -tri·a
per'i·me·tro·sal'pin·gi'tis
pe·rim'e·try
per'i·my'e·li'tis
per'i·my'o·car·di'tis
per'i·my'o·en·do·car·di'tis
per'i·my'o·si'tis
per'i·my·si'um pl. -si·a
   —ex·ter'num
   —in·ter'num
per'i·na'tal
per'i·ne'al (pertaining to the
   perineum)
   ◆peroneal
per'i·ne'o·cele'
per'i·ne·om'e·ter
per'i·ne'o·plas'ty
per'i·ne'o·rec'tal
per'i·ne·or'rha·phy
per'i·ne'o·scro'tal
per'i·ne·ot'o·my
per'i·ne'o·vag'i·nal
per'i·ne'o·vag'i·no·
   rec'tal
per'i·ne'o·vul'var
per'i·neph'ri·al
per'i·neph'ric
per'i·ne·phrit'ic
per'i·ne·phri'tis
per'i·neph'ri·um pl. -ri·a
per'i·ne'um pl. -ne·a

per'i·neu'ral
per'i·neu'ri·al
per'i·neu·ri'tis
per'i·neu'ri·um *pl.* -ri·a
per'i·neu'ro·nal
per'i·ne'void'
per'i·nu'cle·ar
per'i·oc'u·lar
pe'ri·od
per'i·o·date'
pe'ri·od'ic
pe'ri·o·dic'i·ty
per'i·o·don'tal
per'i·o·don'tic
per'i·o·don'tics
per'i·o·don'tist
per'i·o·don·ti'tis
per'i·o·don'ti·um *pl.* -ti·a
per'i·o·don·to·cla'si·a
per'i·o·don·tol'o·gy
per'i·o·don·to'sis *pl.* -ses'
pe'ri·od'o·scope'
per'i·om·phal'ic
per'i·o·nych'i·a
per'i·o·nych'i·um *pl.* -i·a
per'i·on'yx
per'i·o·oph'o·ri'tis
per'i·o·oph'or·o·sal'pin·
  gi'tis
per'i·o'o·the·ci'tis
per'i·oph·thal'mic
per'i·oph'thal·mi'tis
per'i·op·tom'e·try
per'i·o'ral
per'i·or'bit
per'i·or'bi·ta
per'i·or'bit·al
per'i·or'bi·ti'tis
per'i·or·chi'tis
per'i·or'chi·um
per'i·ost'
per'i·os'te·al
per'i·os'te·i'tis
per'i·os'te·o'ma *pl.* -mas *or*
  -ma·ta
per'i·os'te·o·my'e·li'tis
per'i·os'te·o·phyte'
per'i·os'te·o·tome'
per'i·os'te·ot'o·my
per'i·os'te·ous
per'i·os'te·um *pl.* -te·a
  —al've·o·lar'e'
per'i·os·ti'tis

per'i·os·to'ma *pl.* -mas *or*
  -ma·ta
per'i·os·to'sis *pl.* -ses'
per'i·o'tic
per'i·o'va·ri'tis
per'i·o'vu·lar
per'i·pach'y·men'in·gi'tis
per'i·pan'cre·at'ic
per'i·pan'cre·a·ti'tis
per'i·pap'il·lar'y
per'i·pa·tel'lar
per'i·pe·dun'cu·lar
per'i·pha'kus
per'i·pha·ki'tis
per'i·pha·ryn'ge·al
pe·riph'er·ad'
pe·riph'er·al
pe·riph'er·al·ly
pe·riph'er·a·phose' *(an*
  aphose)
  ♦ *peripherophose*
pe·riph'er·o·phose' *(a phose)*
  ♦ *peripheraphose*
pe·riph'er·y
per'i·phle·bit'ic
per'i·phle·bi'tis
pe·riph'ra·sis *pl.* -ses'
Per'i·pla·ne'ta
  —a·mer'i·ca'na
  —aus·tra·la'si·ae
per'i·pleu'ral
per'i·pleu·ri'tis
Pe·rip'lo·ca
pe·rip'lo·cin
per'i·pneu'mo·ni'tis
per'i·po·ri'tis
per'i·por'tal
per'i·proc'tal
per'i·proc'tic
per'i·proc·ti'tis
per'i·pros·tat'ic
per'i·pros'ta·ti'tis
per'i·py'e·li'tis
per'i·py·e'ma
per'i·py'le·phle·bi'tis
per'i·py·lor'ic
per'i·ra·dic'u·lar
per'i·rec'tal
per'i·rec·ti'tis
per'i·re'nal *(around a kidney)*
  ♦ *perirhinal*
per'i·rhi'nal *(around the nose)*
  ♦ *perirenal*

per'i·sal'pin·gi'tis
per'i·sal·pin'go-o'va·ri'tis
per'i·sal'pinx *pl.* -sal·pin'-
  ges'
per'i·scop'ic
per'i·sig'moid·i'tis
per'i·sin'u·ous
per'i·si'nus·i'tis
per'i·si'nu·soi'dal
per'i·sper·ma·ti'tis
per'i·sple'nic
per'i·sple·ni'tis
  —car'ti·la·gin'e·a
per'i·spon·dyl'ic
per'i·spon'dy·li'tis
per'i·stal'sis *pl.* -ses'
per'i·stal'tic
per'i·staph'y·line'
per'i·sta'sis
per'i·stat'ic
per'i·stol'ic
pe·ris'to·ma *pl.* -mas *or*
  -ma·ta
per'i·sto'mal
per'i·stome'
per'i·sy·no'vi·al
per'i·sys·tol'ic
per'i·tec'to·my
per'i·ten·din'e·um *pl.* -e·a
per'i·ten·di·ni'tis
  —cal·car'e·a
per'i·ten'on
per'i·ten·o·ne'um
per'i·ten·o·ni'tis
per'i·the'li·al
per'i·the'li·o'ma *pl.* -mas *or*
  -ma·ta
per'i·the'li·um *pl.* -li·a
per'i·tho·rac'ic
per'i·thy'roid·i'tis
pe·rit'o·my
per'i·to·ne'al
per'i·to·ne'a·li·za'tion
per'i·to·ne'a·lize', -lized',
  -liz'ing
per'i·to·ne'o·cen·te'sis
  pl. -ses'
per'i·to·ne·op'a·thy
per'i·to·ne'o·per'i·car'di·al
per'i·to·ne'o·pex'y
per'i·to·ne'o·plas'ty
per'i·to·ne'o·scope'
per'i·to·ne·os'co·py

per'i·to·ne'o·tome'
per'i·to·ne·ot'o·my
per'i·to·ne'um *pl.* -ne'ums
  or -ne'a
  —pa·ri'e·ta'le'
  —vis'cer·a'le'
per'i·to·nit'ic
per'i·to·ni'tis
per'i·to·nize', -nized',
  -niz'ing
per'i·ton'sil·lar
per'i·ton'sil·li'tis
per'i·tor'cu·lar
per'i·tra'che·al
per'i·tra'che·i'tis
pe·rit'ri·chal
per'i·trich'i·al
pe·rit'ri·chous
per'i·tu'bal
per'i·typh'lic
per'i·typh·li'tis
per'i·um·bil'i·cal
per'i·un'gual
per'i·u·re'ter·al
per'i·u're·ter'ic
per'i·u·re·ter·i'tis
per'i·u·re'thral
per'i·u·re·thri'tis
per'i·u'ter·ine
per'i·u'vu·lar
per'i·vag'i·nal
per'i·vag'i·ni'tis
per'i·vas'cu·lar
per'i·vas'cu·li'tis
per'i·ve'nous
per'i·ven·tric'u·lar
per'i·ver'te·bral
per'i·ves'i·cal
per'i·ve·sic'u·lar
per'i·ve·sic'u·li'tis
per'i·vis'cer·al
per'i·vis'cer·i'tis
per'i·vi·tel'line'
per'i·vul'var
per'i·xe·ni'tis
per·lèche'
Per'li·a nucleus
Perls reaction
perl'sucht
per·ma·nent
per'man·ga·nate'
per'man·gan'ic
per·me·a·bil'i·ty

per'me·a·ble
per'me·ase'
per'me·ate', -at'ed, -at'ing
per'me·a'tion
per·mis'sive
per·mis'sive·ness
per·ni'cious
per'ni·o' *pl.* per'ni·o'nes'
per·ni·o'sis
per·o·bra'chi·us
per·o·ceph'a·lus
per·o·chi'rus
per·o·cor'mus
per·o·dac'tyl'i·a
per·o·dac'ty·lus *pl.* -li'
per·o·me'li·a
pe·rom'e·lus
pe·rom'e·ly
per·o·ne'al *(of the fibular side of
  the leg)*
  ♦*perineal*
per·o·ne'o·cal·ca'ne·us
  —ex·ter'nus
  —in·ter'nus
per·o·ne'o·cu·boi'de·us
per·o·ne'o·tib'i·a'lis
per·o·ne'us
  —ac'ces·so'ri·us
  —accessorius dig'i·ti'
    min'i·mi'
  —accessorius quar'tus
  —accessorius ter'ti·us
  —brev'is
  —lon'gus
  —ter'ti·us
pe·ro'ni·a
pe'ro·pla'si·a
pe'ro·pus
per·o'ral
per os
pe'ro·so'mus
pe'ro·splanch'ni·a
per·os'se·ous
per·ox'i·dase'
per·ox'ide'
per·ox'i·dize', -dized', -diz'ing
per·ox'i·some'
per·phen'a·zine'
per pri'mam
per rec'tum
Per·rin'-Fer·ra·ton' disease
per·sev'er·a'tion
per·sis'tence

per·sis'tent
per'son
per·so'na *pl.* -nae'
per'son·al
per'son·al'i·ty
per·son'i·fi·ca'tion
per·spi·ra'ti·o' in'sen·sib'-
  i·lis
per·spi·ra'tion
per·spi'ra·to'ry
per·spire', -spired', -spir'ing
per·sua'sion
per·sul'fate'
per·sul'fide'
per·tech'ne·tate'
Per'thes'
  —disease
  —test
Per'tik diverticulum
per'tur·ba'tion
per·tus'sal
per·tus'sis
per·tus'soid'
per' va·gi'nam
per·ver'sion
per·vert' *v.*
per'vert *n.*
per·vi·gil'i·um
per·vi'ous
pes *pl.* pe'des'
  —an'se·ri'nus
  —ca'vus
  —con·tor'tus
  —gi'gas
  —pe·dun'cu·li'
  —pla'no·val'gus
  —pla'nus
pes'sa·ry
pes'su·lum *pl.* -la
pes'sum *pl.* -sa
pest
pes'ti·cid'al
pes'ti·cide'
pes·tif'er·ous
pes'ti·lence
pes'ti·len'tial
pes'tis *pl.* -tes'
pes'tle
pe·te'chi·a *pl.* -ae'
pe·te'chi·al
pe·te'chi·om'e·ter
Pe'ters
  —embryo

—method
Pe′ter·sen
—bag
—operation
peth′i·dine′
pet′i·ole′
pe·ti′o·lus *pl.* -li′
—ep′i·glot′ti·dis
pe·tit′ mal′
Pe·tit′ triangle
Pe′tri
—dish
—plate
pet′ri·fac′tion
pet′ri·fi·ca′tion
pé′tris·sage′
pet′ro·bas′i·lar
pet′ro·chem′i·cal
pet′ro·la′tum
pe·tro′le·um
pet′ro·mas′toid′
pet′ro·oc·cip′i·tal
pet′ro·pha·ryn′ge·us
  pl. -ge·i′
pe·tro′sa *pl.* -sae′
pe·tro′sal
pet′ro·si′tis
pet′ro·sphe′noid′
pet′ro·squa·mo′sal
pet′ro·squa′mous
pet′ro·tym·pan′ic
pet′rous
Pet′te-Dö′ring
—disease
—panencephalitis
Pet′ten·kof′er test
Pet′ze·ta′ki disease
Peutz′-Je′ghers syndrome
pex′is
Pey′er
—glands
—patches
pe·yo′te
Pey·ro·nie′ disease
Pey·rot′ thorax
Pfan′nen·stiel′ incision
Pfeif′fer
—bacillus
—disease
Pflü′ger
—laws
—tube
phac′o·an′a·phy·lac′tic

phac′o·an′a·phy·lax′is
phac′o·cele′
phac′o·cyst′
phac′o·cys·tec′to·my
phac′o·cys·ti′tis
phac′o·e·mul′si·fi·ca′tion
phac′o·er′y·sis
phac′oid′
pha·col′y·sis *pl.* -ses′
phac′o·lyt′ic
pha·co′ma *pl.* -mas *or* -ma·ta
pha·co′ma·to′sis *pl.* -sis′
—of Bourne′ville
phac′o·met′a·cho·re′sis
  pl. -ses′
phac′o·met′e·ce′sis *pl.* -ses′
pha·com′e·ter
phac′o·pla·ne′sis *pl.* -ses′
phac′o·scle·ro′sis *pl.* -ses′
phac′o·scope′
pha·cos′co·py
phac′o·sco·tas′mus
phac′o·ther′a·py
phac′o·tox′ic
phage
phag′e·de′na
phag′e·den′ic
phag′o·cyt′a·ble
phag′o·cy′tal
phag′o·cyte′
phag′o·cyt′ic
phag′o·cy·tize′, -tized′,
  -tiz′ing
phag′o·cy′to·blast′
phag′o·cy′to·lit′ic
phag′o·cy·tol′y·sis
phag′o·cy·tose′, -tosed′,
  -tos′ing
phag′o·cy·to′sis *pl.* -ses′
phag′o·dy′na·mom′e·ter
phag′o·kar′y·o′sis
pha·gol′y·sis *pl.* -ses′
phag′o·ma′ni·a
phag′o·pho′bi·a
phag′o·some′
phag′o·ther′a·py
pha·ki′tis
pha·ko′ma *pl.* -mas *or* -ma·ta
pha′ko·ma·to′sis *pl.* -ses′
phal′a·cro′sis
pha·lan′ge·al
phal′an·gec′to·my
pha·lan′ges′

—dig′i·to′rum ma′nus
—digitorum pe′dis
phal′an·gi′tis
pha·lan′gi·za′tion
pha·lan′go·pha·lan′ge·al
pha′lanx′ *pl.* pha·lan′ges′
—dis·ta′lis dig′i·to′rum
  ma′nus
—distalis digitorum pe′dis
—me′di·a dig′i·to′rum
  ma′nus
—media digitorum pe′dis
—pri′ma dig′i·to′rum
  ma′nus
—prima digitorum pe′dis
—prox′i·ma′lis dig′i·to′rum
  ma′nus
—proximalis digitorum
  pe′dis
—se·cun′da dig′i·to′rum
  ma′nus
—secunda digitorum pe′dis
—ter′ti·a dig′i·to′rum
  ma′nus
—tertia digitorum pe′dis
Pha′len
—maneuver
—sign
—test
phal′lic
phal′li·form′
phal′lin
phal′lo·cryp′sis
phal′lo·dyn′i·a
phal′loid′
phal·loi′din
phal·lon′cus
phal′lo·plas′ty
phal·lot′o·my
phal′lus *pl.* -li′ *or* -lus·es
phan′er·o·gam′
phan′er·o·gen′ic
phan′er·o·ma′ni·a
phan′er·o′sis *pl.* -ses′
phan′quone′
phan′tasm
phan·tas′ma·to·mo′ri·a
phan′to·geu′si·a
phan′tom
phar′ci·dous
phar′ma·cal
phar′ma·ceu′tic *or*
  phar′ma·ceu′ti·cal

phar'ma·ceu'ti·cal·ly
phar'ma·ceu'tics
phar'ma·cist
phar'ma·co·chem'is·try
phar'ma·co·dy·nam'ic
phar'ma·co·dy·nam'ics
phar'ma·co·ge·net'ics
phar'ma·cog'no·sist
phar'ma·cog·nos'tic
phar'ma·cog·nos'tics
phar'ma·cog'no·sy
phar'ma·co·ki·net'ic
phar'ma·co·ki·net'ics
phar'ma·co·log'ic or
   phar'ma·co·log'i·cal
phar'ma·co·log'i·cal·ly
phar'ma·col'o·gist
phar'ma·col'o·gy
phar'ma·co·ma'ni·a
phar'ma·co·pe'di·a
phar'ma·co·pe'dic
phar'ma·co·pe'dics
phar'ma·co·pe'ia
phar'ma·co·pe'ial
phar'ma·co·pho'bi·a
phar'ma·co·phore'
phar'ma·co·psy·cho'sis
   pl. -ses'
phar'ma·co·ther'a·peu'tic
phar'ma·co·ther'a·peu'tics
phar'ma·co·ther'a·py
phar'ma·cy
phar'yn·gal'gi·a
pha·ryn'ge·al
phar'yn·gec·ta'si·a
phar'yn·gec'to·my
phar'yn·gem·phrax'is
pha·ryn'ge·us
phar'yn·gism
phar'yn·gis'mus
phar'yn·git'ic
phar'yn·gi'tis *pl.* -git'i·des'
   —sic'ca
pha·ryn'go·bran'chi·al
pha·ryn'go·cele'
pha·ryn'go·con·junc·ti'val
pha·ryn'go·con·junc'ti·vi'-
   tis
pha·ryn'go·dyn'i·a
pha·ryn'go·ep'i·glot'tic
pha·ryn'go·ep'i·glot'ti·cus
   pl. -ci'
pha·ryn'go·e·soph'a·ge'al

pha·ryn'go·e·soph'a·gus
   pl. -gi'
pha·ryn'go·glos'sal
pha·ryn'go·glos'sus *pl.* -si'
pha·ryn'go·ker'a·to'sis
   pl. -ses'
pha·ryn'go·la·ryn'ge·al
pha·ryn'go·lar'yn·gi'tis
pha·ryn'go·lith'
phar'yn·gol'y·sis *pl.* -ses'
pha·ryn'go·max'il·lar'y
pha·ryn'go·my·co'sis
   pl. -ses'
pha·ryn'go·na'sal
pha·ryn'go·pal'a·tine'
pha·ryn'go·pa·ral'y·sis
   pl. -ses'
phar'yn·gop'a·thy
pha·ryn'go·pe·ris'to·le
pha·ryn'go·plas'ty
pha·ryn'go·ple'gi·a
pha·ryn'go·rhi·ni'tis
pha·ryn'go·rhi·nos'co·py
pha·ryn'gor·rha'gi·a
pha·ryn'gor·rhe'a
pha·ryn'go·sal'pin·gi'tis
pha·ryn'go·scle·ro·ma
pha·ryn'go·scope'
phar'yn·gos'co·py
pha·ryn'go·spasm
pha·ryn'go·spas·mod'ic
pha·ryn'go·ste·no'sis
   pl. -ses'
phar'yn·gos'to·ma *pl.* -mas
   or -ma·ta
phar'yn·gos'to·my
pha·ryn'go·tome'
phar'yn·got'o·my
pha·ryn'go·ton'sil·li'tis
pha·ryn'go·tra'che·al
pha·ryn'go·tym·pan'ic
pha·ryn'go·xe·ro'sis
   pl. -ses'
phar'ynx *pl.* pha·ryn'ges'
phase
pha·se'o·lin
pha'sic
pha'sin
phas'mid
phel·lan'drene'
Phelps operation
Phem'is·ter operation
phem'i·tone'

phen'a·caine'
phe·nac'e·mide'
phe·nac'e·tin
phe·nac'e·tu'ric
phen'a·gly'co·dol'
phen'a·kis'to·scope'
phe·nan'threne'
phe·naph'tha·zine'
phe'nate'
phen·az'o·cine'
phen'a·zone'
phen·az'o·pyr'i·dine'
phen·car'ba·mide'
phen·cy'cli·dine'
phen·di·met'ra·zine'
phene
phen'el·zine'
phen·eth'i·cil'lin
phen·eth'yl
phe·net'i·din
phe·net'i·di·nu'ri·a
phen·for'min
phen·go·pho'bi·a
phe·nin'da·mine'
phen·in·di'one'
phen·ir'a·mine
phen·met'ra·zine'
phe'no·bar·bi'tal'
phe'no·bar·bi·tone'
phe'no·cop'y
phe'no·din
phe'nol'
phe'no·late'
phe'no·lic
phe'no·log'ic *or* phe'no·log'-
   i·cal
phe·nol'o·gist
phe·nol'o·gy
phe'nol·phthal'e·in
phe'nol·sul·fon'ic
phe'nol·sul'fon·phthal'e·in
phe'nol·tet'ra·chlo'ro·
   phthal'e·in
phe'nol·u'ri·a
phe·nom'e·nal
phe·nom'e·non *pl.* -na
phe'no·pho'bi·a
phe'no·pro'pa·zine'
phe'no·thi'a·zine'
phe'no·type'
phe'no·typ'ic
phe·nox'y
phe·nox'y·ben'za·mine·

phe·noz′y·gous
phen′pro·cou′mon′
phen′sux′i·mide′
phen′ter·mine′
phen·te′ti·o·thal′e·in
phen′tol·a·mine′
phen′yl
phen′yl·a·ce′tic
phen′yl·a·ce′tyl·u·re′a
phen′yl·al′a·nine′
phen′yl·al′a·ni·ne′mi·a
phen′yl·bu′ta·zone′
phen′yl·car′bi·nol′
phen′yl·ene′
phen′yl·eph′rine′
phen′yl·hy′dra·zine′
phen′yl·hy′dra·zone′
phe·nyl′ic
phen′yl·ke′to·nu′ri·a
phen′yl·ke′to·nu′ric
phen′yl·mer·cu′ric
phen′yl·pro′pa·nol′a·mine′
phen′yl·py·ru′vic
phen′yl·thi′o·car′ba·mide′
phen′yl·thi′o·u′re·a
phen′yl·to·lox′a·mine′
phen′y·to′in
phe′o·chrome′
phe′o·chro′mo·blast′
phe′o·chro′mo·blas·to′ma
  pl. -mas *or* -ma·ta
phe′o·chro′mo·cyte′
phe′o·chro′mo·cy·to′ma
  pl. -mas *or* -ma·ta
Phi′a·loph′o·ra
  —jean·sel′me·i′
  —ver′ru·co′sa
Phil′a·del′phi·a chromo-
  some
phi·mo′si·ec′to·my
phi·mo′sis *pl.* -ses′
phi·mot′ic
phle·bal′gi·a
phleb·an′gi·o′ma *pl.* -mas *or*
  -ma·ta
phleb′ar·te′ri·ec·ta′si·a
phleb·ec·ta′si·a
phle·bec′ta·sis
phle·bec′to·my
phleb·ec·to′pi·a
phleb′em·phrax′is
phleb′ex·er′e·sis
phleb′hep·a·ti′tis

phle·bis′mus
phle·bit′ic
phle·bi′tis
phleb′o·car′ci·no′ma
  pl. -mas *or* -ma·ta
phle·boc′ly·sis *pl.* -ses′
phleb′o·gram′
phleb′o·graph′
phleb′o·graph′ic
phle·bog′ra·phy
phleb′oid′
phleb′o·lith′
phleb′o·li·thi′a·sis *pl.* -ses′
phleb′o·lith′ic
phleb′o·ma·nom′e·ter
phleb′o·phle·bos′to·my
phleb′o·plas′ty
phleb′o·rhe·og′ra·phy
phleb′or·rha′gi·a
phle·bor′rha·phy
phleb′or·rhex′is *pl.* -rhex′es′
phleb′o·scle·ro′sis *pl.* -ses′
phleb′o·scle·rot′ic
phle·bo′sis *pl.* -ses′
phle·bos′ta·sis *pl.* -ses′
phleb′o·ste·no′sis *pl.* -ses′
phleb′o·throm·bo′sis
  pl. -ses′
phleb′o·tome′
phle·bot′o·mist
phle·bot′o·mize′, -mized′,
  -miz′ing
Phle·bot′o·mus *pl.* -mi′
  —ar·gen′ti·pes
  —chi·nen′sis
  —fla·vis′cu·tel′la·tus
  —in′ter·me′di·us
  —ma·ce·do′ni·cum
  —mar·ti′ni
  —no·gu′chi
  —o′ri·en·ta′lis
  —pa·pa·ta′si·i′
  —per·ni′ci·o′sus
  —pes·soi′a
  —ser·gen′ti′
  —ver′ru·ca′rum
  —vex′a·tor
phle·bot′o·my
phlegm
phleg·ma′si·a
  —ad′e·no′sa
  —al′ba do′lens
  —cel′lu·lar′is

  —ce·ru′le·a do′lens
  —mem·bra′nae′ mu·co′sae′
  gas′tro·pul′mo·na′lis
  —my·o′i·ca
phleg·mat′ic
phleg′mon′
phleg′mo·na dif·fu′sa
phleg′mon·ous
phlo′em
phlo·gis′tic
phlog·o′gen′ic
phlo·gog′e·nous
phlo·go′sis *pl.* -ses′
phlo′re·tin
phlo′ro·glu′cine′
phlo′ro·glu′ci·nol′
phlox′ine′
phlox·i′no·phil′ic
phlyc·te′na *pl.* -nae′
phlyc′te·nar
phlyc·ten′u·la *pl.* -lae′
phlyc·ten′u·lar
phlyc·ten′ule′
phlyc·ten′u·lo′sis
pho′bi·a
pho′bic
pho′bo·dip′si·a
pho′bo·pho′bi·a
Pho·cas′ disease
pho′co·me′li·a
pho′co·mel′ic
pho·com′e·lus *pl.* -li′
pho·com′e·ly
phol′co·dine′
Pho′ma
pho′nal
phon′ar·te′ri·o·gram′
phon′as·the′ni·a
pho′nate′, -nat′ed, -nat′ing
pho·na′tion
pho′na·to′ry
phone
pho′neme′
pho·nen′do·scope′
pho·net′ic
pho·net′ics
phon′ic
phon′ics
pho′nism
pho′no·an′gi·og′ra·phy
pho′no·aus′cul·ta′tion
pho′no·car′di·o·gram′
pho′no·car′di·o·graph′

pho'no·car'di·o·graph'ic
pho'no·car'di·og'ra·phy
pho'no·gram'
pho·nol'o·gy
pho·nom'e·ter
pho·nom'e·try
pho'no·my·oc'lo·nus
pho'no·my·og'ra·phy
pho'no·pa·thy
pho'no·pho'bi·a
pho'no·pho·tog'ra·phy
pho·nop'si·a
pho'no·re·cep'tor
phor'bin
pho'ri·a
Phor'i·dae'
phor'o·blast'
phor'o·cyte'
pho·rol'o·gy
pho·rom'e·ter
phor'o·met'ric
phor·rom'e·try
pho'ro·op·tom'e·ter
phor'o·scope'
phor'o·tone'
phose
phos·gen'ic
phos'pha·gen
phos'pha·tase'
phos'phate'
phos'pha·te'mi·a
phos·phat'ic
phos'pha·tide'
phos'pha·tid'ic
phos'pha·ti·do'sis
phos'pha·ti'dyl·cho'line'
phos'pha·ti'dyl·i·no'si·tol'
phos'pha·tu'ri·a
phos'phene'
phos'phide'
phos'phine'
phos'phite'
phos'pho·am'i·dase'
phos'pho·ar'gi·nine'
phos'pho·cre'a·tine'
phos'pho·di·es'ter·ase'
phos'pho·e'nol·py·ru'vic
phos'pho·fruc'to·ki'nase'
phos'pho·fruc'to·mu'tase'
phos'pho·ga·lac'tose'
phos'pho·glob'u·lin
phos'pho·glu'co·ki'nase'
phos'pho·glu'co·mu'tase'

phos'pho·glu·con'ic
phos'pho·glu'cose'
phos'pho·glyc'er·al'de·
hyde'
phos'pho·gly·cer'ic
phos'pho·glyc'er·o·mu'tase'
phos'pho·hex'o·i·som'er·
ase'
phos'pho·hex'o·ki'nase'
phos'pho·i·no'si·tide'
phos'pho·ki'nase'
phos'pho·li'pase'
phos'pho·lip'id
phos'pho·lip'i·de'mi·a
phos'pho·lip'in
phos'pho·mo·lyb'dic
phos'pho·mon'o·es'ter·ase'
phos'pho·ne·cro'sis
phos·pho'ni·um
phos'pho·pe'ni·a
phos'pho·pro'tein'
phos'pho·py·ru'vic
phos'phor
phos'pho·rat'ed
phos'pho·resce', -resced',
 -resc'ing
phos'pho·res'cence
phos'pho·res'cent
phos'phor·hi·dro'sis
 pl. -ses'
phos'pho·ri'bo·mu'tase'
phos'phor'ic
phos'pho·rism
phos'phor·ol'y·sis *pl.* -ses'
phos'pho·rus
phos'pho·ryl
phos'pho·ryl·ase'
phos'pho·ry·la'tion
phos'pho·trans'fer·ase'
phos'pho·tri'ose'
phos'pho·tung'stic
phos·vi'tin
phot
pho·tal'gi·a
pho·tau'gi·o·pho'bi·a
pho·tes·the'si·a
pho·tes·the'sis
pho'tic
pho'tism
pho'to·ac'tin'ic
pho'to·al·ler'gic
pho'to·al'ler·gy
pho'to·bac·te'ri·um *pl.* -ri·a

pho'to·bi·ot'ic
pho'to·ca·tal'y·sis *pl.* -ses'
pho'to·chem'i·cal
pho'to·chem'is·try
pho'to·che'mo·ther'a·py
pho'to·chro·mat'ic
pho'to·chro'mo·gen
pho'to·chro'mo·gen'ic
pho'to·co·ag'u·la'tion
pho'to·co·ag'u·la'tor
pho'to·col'or·im'e·ter
pho'to·con·duc'tive
pho'to·con·duc·tiv'i·ty
pho'to·con·junc'ti·vi'tis
pho'to·cu·ta'ne·ous
pho'to·der'ma·ti'tis
pho'to·der'ma·to'sis
 pl. -ses'
pho'to·dis·in'te·gra'tion
pho'to·dy·nam'ic
pho'to·dyn'i·a
pho'to·dys·pho'ri·a
pho'to·e·lec'tric
pho'to·e·lec'tron'
pho'to·e·mis'sion
pho'to·fluor'o·graph'ic
pho'to·fluo·rog'ra·phy
pho'to·fluo·ros'co·py
pho'to·gene'
pho'to·gen'e·sis *pl.* -ses'
pho'to·gen'ic
pho'to·gram'
pho'to·ki·ne'sis *pl.* -ses'
pho'to·ki·net'ic
pho'to·ky'mo·graph'
pho'to·ky'mo·graph'ic
pho'to·lu'mi·nes'cence
pho·tol'y·sis *pl.* -ses'
pho'to·lyte'
pho'to·lyt'ic
pho'to·ma'ni·a
pho·tom'e·ter
pho'to·met'ric
pho·tom'e·try
pho'to·mi'cro·graph'
pho'to·mi'cro·graph'ic
pho'to·mi·crog'ra·phy
pho'to·mi'cro·scope'
pho'to·mi·cros'co·py
pho'to·mo'tor
pho'to·mul'ti·pli·er
pho'ton'
pho'to·par·es·the'si·a

pho'to·path'ic
pho'to·path'o·log'ic
pho·top'a·thy
pho'to·per·cep'tive
pho'to·phil'ic
pho'to·pho'bi·a
pho'to·pho'bic
pho'to·phore'
pho'toph·thal'mi·a
pho·to'pi·a
pho·top'ic
pho'to·ple·thys'mo·graph'
pho'to·pleth'ys·mog'ra·
   phy
pho'to·prone'
pho'to·phos'pho·ry·la'tion
pho'to·pro'ton
pho·top'si·a
pho·top'sin
pho'top·tom'e·ter
pho'top·tom'e·try
pho'to·re·ac'ti·va'tion
pho'to·re·cep'tive
pho'to·re·cep'tors
pho'to·ret'i·ni'tis
pho'to·scan'
pho'to·sen'si·tive
pho'to·sen'si·tiv'i·ty
pho'to·sen'si·ti·za'tion
pho'to·sen'si·tize'
pho'to·sta'ble
pho'to·stim'u·la·ble
pho'to·syn'the·sis *pl.* -ses'
pho'to·syn'the·size'
pho'to·syn'thet'ic
pho'to·tac'tic
pho'to·tax'is
pho'to·ther'a·py
pho'to·ther'mal
pho'to·ther'mic
pho'to·tim'er
pho'to·ton'ic
pho·tot'o·nus
pho'to·to'pi·a
pho'to·tox'ic
pho'to·tox·ic'i·ty
pho'to·troph'ic
pho'to·trop'ic
pho·tot'ro·pism
pho·tu'ri·a
phrag'mo·plast'
phren *pl.* phre'nes
phre·nal'gi·a

phre·nec'to·my
phren'em·phrax'is
   pl. -phrax'es'
phre·net'ic *also* frenetic
phren'ic
phren'i·cec'to·my
phren'i·cla'si·a
phren'i·cla'sis *pl.* -ses'
phren'i·co·co'lic
phren'i·co·cos'tal
phren'i·co·e·soph'a·ge'al
phren'i·co·ex·er'e·sis
phren'i·co·gas'tric
phren'i·co·neu·rec'to·my
phren'i·co·splen'ic
phren'i·cot'o·my
phren'i·co·trip'sy
phre·ni'tis
phren'o·car'di·a
phren'o·car'di·ac'
phren'o·col'ic
phren'o·co'lo·pex'y
phren'o·dyn'i·a
phren'o·e·soph'a·ge'al
phren'o·gas'tric
phren'o·glot'tic
phren'o·he·pat'ic
phren'o·lep'si·a
phren'o·pa·ral'y·sis *pl.* -ses'
phren'o·ple'gi·a
phren'o·prax'ic
phren'o·sin
phren'o·spasm
phren'o·splen'ic
phren'o·trop'ic
phric'to·path'ic
phro·ne'ma
phry'nin
phryn'o·der'ma
phry·nol'y·sin
phthal'ic
phthal'yl·sul'fa·cet'a·mide'
phthal'yl·sul'fa·thi'a·zole'
phthin'oid'
phthi'o·col'
phthi·ri'a·sis *pl.* -ses'
Phthir'i·us
   —pu'bis
phthis'ic *or* phthis'i·cal
phthi'sis *pl.* -ses'
   —bul'bi'
   —cor'ne·ae'
phy'co·bil'in

phy'co·cy'a·nin
phy'co·e·ryth'rin
Phy'co·my·ce'tes
phy'co·my·co'sis *pl.* -ses'
phy'go·ga·lac'tic
phy·lac'tic
phy·lax'is
phy·let'ic
phyl'lo·er'y·thrin
phyl'loid'
phyl'lo·por'phy·rin
phyl'lo·quin'one'
phy'lo·gen'e·sis *pl.* -ses'
phy·lo·ge·net'ic
phy·log'e·ny
phy'lum *pl.* -la
phy'ma *pl.* -mas *or* -ma·ta
phy'ma·toid'
phy'ma·to'sis *pl.* -ses'
phys'a·lif'er·ous
phy·sal'i·form'
phy·sal'i·phore'
phy'sa·liph'o·rous
phys'a·lis
Phy'sa·lop'ter·a
   —cau·cas'i·ca
phys·co'ni·a
phys'i·at'rics
phys'i·at'rist
phys'ic *(a cathartic)*
   ◆*physique*
phys'i·cal
phy·si'cian
phys'i·cist
Phy'sick operation
phys'i·co·chem'i·cal
phys'i·co·gen'ic
phys'ics
phys'i·no'sis *pl.* -ses'
phys'i·o·chem'i·cal
phys'i·o·gen'ic
phys'i·og·nom'ic
phys'i·og'no·my
phys'i·og·no'sis *pl.* -ses'
phys'i·o·log'ic *or*
   phys'i·o·log'i·cal
phys'i·o·log'i·cal·ly
phys'i·o·log'i·co·an'a·
   tom'ic
phys'i·ol'o·gist
phys'i·ol'o·gy
phys'i·o·path'o·log'ic
phys'i·o·pa·thol'o·gy

phys'i·o·ther'a·peu'tic
phys'i·o·ther'a·pist
phys'i·o·ther'a·py
phy·sique' *(body)*
  ♦*physic*
phy'so·he·ma·to·me'tra
phy'so·hy'dro·me'tra
phy'so·me'tra
phy'so·py'o·sal'pinx
  pl. -sal·pin'ges'
phy'so·stig'mine'
phy·tan'ic
phy'tic
phy'to·be'zoar
phy'to·chem'is·try
phy'to·chrome'
phy'to·gen'e·sis *pl.* -ses'
phy'to·ge·net'ic
phy'to·he'mag·glu'ti·nin
phy'to·hor'mone'
phy'toid'
phy'tol'
phy'to·na·di'one'
phy'to·par'a·site'
phy'to·path'o·gen
phy'to·pa·thol'o·gy
phy·toph'a·gous
phy'to·phar'ma·col'o·gy
phy'to·pho'to·der'ma·ti'tis
phy'to·pre·cip'i·tin
phy'to'sis *pl.* -ses'
phy'to·ste'a·rin
phy·tos'ter·in
phy·tos'ter·ol'
phy·tos'ter·o·lin
phy'to·throm'bo·ki'nase'
phy'to·tox'ic
phy'to·tox·ic'i·ty
phy'to·tox'in
phy'to·tron'
pi'a
  —ma'ter
    —mater en·ceph'a·li'
    —mater spi·na'lis
pi'a-a·rach'noid'
pi'al
pi'a·ma'tral
pi·an'
pi·as'tre·ne'mi·a
pib·lok'to
pi'ca
Pic'co·lo·mi'ni striae
Pick

—apraxia
—body
—bundle
—cell
—disease
—syndrome
—vision
pick'ling
Pick·wick'i·an syndrome
pi'co·cu'rie
pi'co·gram'
pic'o·lin'ic
pi'co·pi'co·gram'
pi·cor'na·vi'rus
pi'co·sec'ond
pic·ram'ic
Pic·ras'ma
pic'rate'
pic'ric
pic'ro·car'mine
pic'ro·lon'ic
pic'ro·ni'gro·sin
pic'ro·pod'o·phyl'lin
pic'ro·tox'in
pic'ro·tox'i·nin
pic'ryl
pic'to·graph'
pie'bald'
pie'bald·ism
pi·e'dra
Pi·erre' Ro·bin' syndrome
pi·e'ses·the'si·a
pi'e·sim'e·ter
pi'e·zo·e·lec'tric
pi'e·zo·e·lec'tri·cal
pi'e·zo·e·lec·tric'i·ty
pig'bel'
pi'geon-toed'
pig'ment
pig'men·tar'y
pig'men·ta'tion
pig'ment'ed
pig·men'to·gen'e·sis
pig·men'to·phage'
pig·men'tum ni'grum
Pi·gnet' index
pi·i'tis
pi'lar
pi'la·ry
pi·las'ter
pi·las'tered
Pilcz reflex
piles

pi'le·us
pi'li'
  —an'nu·la'ti'
  —in'car·na'ti'
  —mul'ti·gem'i·ni'
  —tac'ti·les'
  —tor'ti'
pi'li·a'tion
pi'li·form'
pi'li·mic'tion
pill
pil'lar
pil'let
pil'low
pill'-roll'ing
pi'lo·car'pine'
pi'lo·car'pus *pl.* -pi
pi'lo·cys'tic
pi'lo·e·rec'tion
pi'lo·ma'tri·co'ma *pl.* -mas
  or -ma·ta
pi'lo·ma'trix·o'ma *pl.* -mas
  or -ma·ta
pi'lo·mo'tor
pi'lo·ni'dal
pi'lose'
pi'lo·se·ba'ceous
pi·lo'sis
pil'u·la *pl.* -lae'
pil'u·lar
pil'ule'
pi'lus *pl.* -li'
  —cu'nic·u·la'tus
  —in'car·na'tus
  —incarnatus re·cur'vus
pi'mel'ic
pim·e·li'tis
pim'e·lo'ma *pl.* -mas *or*
  -ma·ta
pim'e·lo·pte·ryg'i·um
pim'e·lor·rhe'a
pim'e·lor'thop·ne'a
pim'e·lu'ri·a
pi·men'ta
pi·min'o·dine'
pim'o·zide'
pim'pi·nel'la
pim'ple
pin
pin·ac'i·dil
pin'a·coid'
pi·nac'o·lone'
pin'a·cy'a·nol'

Pi·nard'
—maneuver
—sign
pince·ment'
pin'cers
pinch
pin'do·lol'
pin'e·al
pin'e·a·lec'to·my
pin'e·al·ism
pin'e·a·lo'ma *pl.* -mas *or*
-ma·ta
Pi·nel' system
pi'nene'
pin'e·o·blas·to'ma *pl.* -mas
or -ma·ta
pin'e·o·cy·to'ma *pl.* -mas *or*
-ma·ta
pin·guec'u·la *pl.* -lae'
pi'ni·form'
pink'eye'
pin'na *pl.* -nae' *or* -nas
pin'nal
pin'o·cyte'
pin'o·cy·to'sis *pl.* -ses'
pin'o·cy·tot'ic
pin'o·some'
pin·ox'e·pin
pin'prick'
Pins sign
pint
pin'ta
pin'tid
pin'worm'
pi'o·ep'i·the'li·um *pl.* -li·a
pi'o·ne'mi·a
Pi·oph'i·la ca'se·i
pi'or·thop·ne'a
Pi'o·trow'ski
—reflex
—sign
pi·pam'a·zine'
pi·pam'per·one'
pi·paz'e·thate'
pip'e·cu·ro'ni·um
pi·pen'zo·late'
pip'er·a·cet'a·zine'
pip'er·a·cil'lin
pip'er·a·mide'
pi·per'a·zine'
pi·per'i·dine'
pip'er·i·do'late'
pip'er·ine'

pip'er·o·caine'
pi·pe'ro·nyl
pip'er·ox'an'
pi·pet' *also* pipette
pi·pette' *var. of* pipet
pip'o·bro'man'
pip'o·sul'fan'
pip'ra·drol'
pip'ro·zol'in
pip'syl
pip'to·nych'i·a
piq'ui·zil
pir·bu'ter·ol'
pi·ren'ze·pine'
Pir'ie bone
pir'i·form' *also* pyriform
pir'i·for'mis
Pi·ro'goff' amputation
pi·rox'i·cam
Pir·quet' test
Pir'y fever
pi'si·an'nu·lar'is
pi'si·form'
pi'si·met'a·car'pus
pi'so·ha'mate'
pi'so·met'a·car'pal
pi'so·tri·que'tral
pis'ton
pit, pit'ted, pit'ting
pitch
pitch'blende'
pith'e·coid'
pith'i·a·tism
pith'i·at'ric
Pi·tot' tube
Pi·tres' sections
pi·tu'i·cyte'
pi·tu'i·cy·to'ma *pl.* -mas *or*
-ma·ta
pi·tu'i·ta·rism
pi·tu'i·tar'i·um
—an'te'ri·us
—pos·te'ri·us
—to'tum
pi·tu'i·tar'y
pi·tu'i·tec'to·my
pi·tu'i·tous
pi·tu'i·trism
pit'y·ri'a·sic
pit'y·ri'a·sis *pl.* -ses'
—cap'i·tis
—cir'ci·na'ta
—li'che·noi'des' chron'i·ca

—lichenoides et var'i·o'li·
for'mis a·cu'ta
—lin'guae'
—ni'gra
—pi·lar'is
—ro'se·a
—ru'bra
—rubra pi·lar'is
—sim'plex'
—ste'a·toi'des'
—ver'si·col'or
pit'y·roid'
Pit'y·ros'po·rum
—or'bic'u·lar'e
—o'va'le'
pi·val'ic
piv'ot
pix'el
pla·ce'bo
pla·cen'ta *pl.* -tas *or* -tae'
—ac·cre'ta
—cir·soi'de·a
—dif·fu'sa
—ex'tra·cho'ri·a'la
—fen'es·tra'ta
—foe·ta'lis
—in·cre'ta
—mem'bra·na'ce·a
—nep'pi·for'mis
—per·cre'ta
—pre'vi·a
—previa cen·tra'lis
—previa mar'gi·na'lis
—previa par'ti·a'lis
—re·flex'a
—ren'i·for'mis
—spu'ri·a
—suc'cen·tu'ri·a'ta
—u'ter·i'na
pla·cen'tal
plac'en·ta'tion
plac'en·ti'tis *pl.* -tit'i·des'
plac'en·tog'ra·phy
pla·cen'toid'
plac'en·to'ma *pl.* -mas *or*
-ma·ta
plac'en·to'sis *pl.* -ses'
pla·cen'to·ther'a·py
Pla·ci'do disk
pla·co'dal
plac'ode'
plad'a·ro'ma *pl.* -mas *or*
-ma·ta

plad'a·ro'sis *pl.* -ses'
pla·fond'
pla·gi·o·ce·phal'ic
pla·gi·o·ceph'a·lism
pla·gi·o·ceph'a·lous
pla·gi·o·ceph'a·ly
plague
plain
plak'al·bu'min
pla'nar
plan'chet
plane
pla'ni·gram'
pla·nig'ra·phy
pla·nim'e·ter
plan'ing
plank'ton
pla'no·cel'lu·lar
pla'no·con'cave'
pla'no·con'ic
pla'no·con'vex'
pla'no·cyte'
pla'no·val'gus
plan'ta *pl.* -tae'
plan'tar
plan·tar'is
plan·ta'tion
plan'ti·grade'
plan'u·la *pl.* -lae'
pla'num *pl.* -na
—nu·cha'le'
—oc·cip'i·ta'le'
—or'bi·ta'le'
—pop·lit'e·um
—ster·na'le'
—tem'po·ra'le'
plaque
—jaune
plasm
plas'ma
plas'ma·blast'
plas'ma·cyte'
plas'ma·cyt'ic
plas'ma·cy'toid'
plas'ma·cy·to'ma *pl.* -mas
or -ma·ta
plas'ma·cy·to'sis *pl.* -ses'
plas'ma·gel'
plas'ma·gene'
plas'mal
plas·ma·lem'ma
plas·mal'o·gen
plas'ma·pher'e·sis *pl.* -ses'

plas'ma·sol'
plas'ma·some'
plas'ma·ther'a·py
plas'mat'ic
plas'ma·tog'a·my
plas'ma·tor·rhex'is *pl.* -es
plas'ma·to'sis
plas'mic
plas'mid
plas'min
plas·min'o·gen
plas'mo·cyte'
plas'mo·cyt'ic
plas'mo·cy·to'ma *pl.* -mas
or -ma·ta
plas·mo·di·al
plas·mo'di·blast'
plas·mod'ic
plas·mo'di·cide'
Plas·mo'di·i·dae'
plas·mo'di·tro'pho·blast'
Plas·mo'di·um
—fal·cip'a·rum
—ma·lar'i·ae'
—o'va'le'
—vi'vax'
plas·mog'a·my
plas'mo·gen
plas·mol'y·sis *pl.* -ses'
plas'mo·lyt'ic
plas'mo·lyze', -lyzed',
-lyz'ing
plas·mo'ma *pl.* -mas or
-ma·ta
plas'mon'
plas'mo·nu·cle'ic
plas·mop'ty·sis *pl.* -ses'
plas'mor·rhex'is *pl.*
-rhex'es'
plas·mos'chi·sis *pl.* -ses'
plas'mo·sin
plas'mo·some'
plas'mot'o·my
plas'mo·trop'ic
plas·mot'ro·pism
plas'te·in
plas'ter
—of Par'is
plas'tic
plas·tic'i·ty
plas'ti·ciz'er
plas'tics
plas'tid

plas'ti·dule'
plas'tin
plas'to·dy·nam'i·a
plas'tog'a·my
plas'to·gene'
plas'to·some'
plate
pla·teau' *pl.* -teaus' or -teaux'
plate'let
plate'let·phe·re'sis
plat'ode'
plat'oid'
pla·ton'ic
pla'to·ni·za'tion
plat'o·nych'i·a
plat'y·ba'si·a
plat'y·ce'lous
plat'y·ce·phal'ic
plat'y·ceph'a·lous
plat'y·ceph'a·ly
plat'y·cne'mi·a
plat'y·cne'mic
plat'y·co'ri·a
plat'y·co·ri'a·sis
plat'y·cra'ni·a
plat'y·hel'minth
plat'y·hel·min'thes'
plat'y·hi·er'ic
plat'y·mer'ic
plat'y·mor'phi·a
plat'y·mor'phic
plat'y·o'pi·a
plat'y·op'ic
plat'y·pel'lic
plat'y·pel'loid'
plat'yr·rhine'
plat'yr·rhi'ny
pla·tys'ma *pl.* -ma·ta or -mas
—my·oi'des'
pla·tys'mal
plat'ys·ten·ce·pha'li·a
plat'ys·ten·ce·phal'ic
plat'ys·ten·ceph'a·ly
pledg'et
plei'o·trop'ic
plei·ot'ro·pism
plei·ot'ro·py
ple'o·chro'ic
ple·och'ro·ism
ple'o·chro·mat'ic
ple'o·co'ni·al
ple'o·cy·to'sis *pl.* -ses'
ple'o·kar'y·o·cyte'

ple'o·mas'ti·a
ple'o·ma'zi·a
ple'o·mor'phic
ple'o·mor'phism
ple'o·mor'phous
ple'o·nasm
ple'o·nas'tic
ple'o·nec'tic
ple'o·nex'i·a
ple'o·nex'y
ple'on·os'te·o'sis
 —of Lé·ri'i
ple'o·no'tus
ple·op'tics
ple'ro·cer'coid'
ple·ro'sis
ple'si·og'na·thus
ple'si·o·mor'phism
ples'ses·the'si·a
ples·sim'e·ter
ples'sor
ples'sus
pleth'o·ra
 —ap'o·cop'ti·ca
pleth'o·ric
ple·thys'mo·gram'
ple·thys'mo·graph'
ple·thys'mo·graph'ic
pleth'ys·mog'ra·phy
pleu'ra *pl.* -rae'
 —cos·ta'lis
 —di'a·phrag·mat'i·ca
 —me'di·as'ti·na'lis
 —pa·ri'e·ta'lis
 —per'i·car·di'a·ca
 —pul'mo·na'lis
pleu'ra·cen·te'sis *pl.* -ses'
pleu'ra·cot'o·my
pleu'ral
pleu·ral'gi·a
pleu·ral'gic
pleur·am'ni·on'
pleur'a·po·phys'i·al
pleur'a·poph'y·sis
pleu'ra·tome'
pleu·rec'to·my
pleu'ri·sy
pleu·rit'ic
pleu·ri'tis
pleu'ro·bron·chi'tis
pleu'ro·cele'
pleu'ro·cen·te'sis *pl.* -ses'
pleu'ro·cen'tral

pleu'ro·cen'trum
pleu'ro·cho'le·cys·ti'tis
pleu'ro·cu·ta'ne·ous
pleu·rod'e·sis
pleu'ro·dyn'i·a
pleu'ro·gen'ic
pleu·rog'e·nous
pleu·rog'ra·phy
pleu'ro·hep'a·ti'tis
pleu'ro·lith'
pleu·rol'y·sis *pl.* -ses'
pleu'ro·ma *pl.* -mas *or* -ma·ta
pleu'ro·me'lus
pleu'ro·per'i·car'di·al
pleu'ro·per'i·car·di'tis
pleu'ro·per'i·to·ne'al
pleu'ro·per'i·to·ne'um
 pl. -ne'a
pleu'ro·pneu·mo'ni·a
pleu'ro·pneu·mo·nol'y·sis
 pl. -ses'
pleu'ro·pros'o·pos'chi·sis
 pl. -ses'
pleu'ro·pul'mo·nar'y
pleu·ros'co·py
pleu'ro·so'ma
pleu'ro·so·ma·tos'chi·sis
 pl. -ses'
pleu'ro·so'mus
pleu'ro·spasm
pleu'ro·thot'o·nos
pleu'ro·tome'
pleu·rot'o·my
pleu'ro·ty'phoid'
pleu'ro·vis'cer·al
plex'al
plex·ec'to·my
plex'i·form'
plex·im'e·ter
plex'i·met'ric
plex·im'e·try
plex'or
plex'us *pl.* plex'us *or* -us·es
 —a·or'ti·cus ab·dom'i·na'lis
 —aorticus tho'ra·ca'lis
 —aorticus tho'ra·ci'cus
 —ar·te'ri·ae' cer'e·bri'
  an·te'ri·o'ris
 —arteriae cerebri me'di·i'
 —arteriae cho'ri·oi'de·ae'
 —arteriae o·var'i·cae'
 —au·ric'u·lar'is posterior
 —au'to·nom'i·ci'

 —ax'il·lar'is
 —bas'il·lar'is
 —bra'chi·a'lis
 —car·di'a·cus
 —ca·rot'i·cus com·mu'nis
 —caroticus ex·ter'nus
 —caroticus in·ter'nus
 —cav'er·no'si' con·char'um
 —cav'er·no'sus cli·to'ri·dis
 —cavernosus pe'nis
 —ce·li'a·cus
 —cer·vi·ca'lis
 —cho'ri·oi'de·us ven·tric'-
  u·li' lat'er·a'lis
 —chorioideus ventriculi
  quar'ti'
 —chorioideus ventriculi
  ter'ti·i'
 —cho·roi'de·us ven·tric'-
  u·li' lat'er·a'lis
 —choroideus ventriculi
  quar'ti'
 —choroideus ventriculi
  ter'ti·i'
 —coc·cyg'e·us
 —coe·li'a·cus
 —co·ro·nar'i·us cor'dis
  anterior
 —coronarius cordis
  posterior
 —def·er·en'ti·a'lis
 —den·ta'lis inferior
 —dentalis superior
 —en·ter'i·cus
 —e'so·phag'e·us
 —fem'o·ra'lis
 —gan'gli·o'sus cil'i·ar'is
 —gas'tri·ci'
 —gas'tri·cus anterior
 —gastricus inferior
 —gastricus posterior
 —gastricus superior
 —haem'or·rhoi·da'lis
  me'di·us
 —haemorrhoidalis superior
 —haemorrhoidalis ve·no'-
  sus
 —he·pat'i·cus
 —hy'po·gas'tri·cus
 —hypogastricus inferior
 —hypogastricus superior
 —i·li'a·ci'
 —i·li'a·cus

—iliacus ex·ter′nus
—in′gui·na′lis
—in′ter·mes′en·ter′i·cus
—jug′u·lar′is
—li′e·na′lis
—lin·gua′lis
—lum·ba′lis
—lum′bo·sa·cra′lis
—lym·phat′i·cus
—mam·mar′i·us
—mammarius in·ter′nus
—max′il·lar′is ex·ter′nus
—maxillaris in·ter′nus
—me·nin′ge·us
—mes·en·ter′i·cus inferior
—mesentericus superior
—my′en·ter′i·cus
—ner·vo′rum spi·na′li·um
—oc·cip′i·ta′lis
—oe·soph′a·ge′us anterior
—oesophageus posterior
—of Cru·veil·hier′
—oph·thal′mi·cus
—o·var′i·cus
—pam·pin′i·for′mis
—pan·cre·at′i·cus
—pa·rot′i·de′us
—pel·vi′nus
—per·i·ar·ter′i·a′lis
—pha·ryn′ge·us
—pharyngeus as·cen′dens
—pharyngeus ner′vi′ va′gi′
—phren′i·cus
—pop·lit′e·us
—pros·tat′i·cus
—pter′y·goi′de·us
—pu′den·da′lis ve·no′sus
—pu′den′dus ner·vo′sus
—pul·mo·na′lis
—pulmonalis anterior
—pulmonalis posterior
—rec·ta′lis inferior
—rectalis me′di·us
—rectalis superior
—re′na·lis
—sa·cra′lis
—sacralis anterior
—sacralis me′di·us
—sper·mat′i·cus
—sub·cla′vi·us
—sub′mu·co′sus
—sub′se·ro′sus
—su′pra·re·na′lis

—sym·path′i·ci′
—tem′po·ra′lis su′per·fi′-
  ci·a′lis
—tes·tic′u·lar′is
—thy′re·oi′de·us im′par′
—thyreoideus inferior
—thyreoideus superior
—thy·roi′de·us im′par′
—tym·pan′i·cus
—u·re′ter′i·cus
—u′ter·o·vag′i·na′lis
—uterovaginalis ve·no′sus
—vas′cu·lo′sus
—ve·no′si′ ver′te·bra′les′
  an·te′ri·o′res′
—venosi vertebrales
  ex·ter′ni′ anterior et
  posterior
—venosi vertebrales
  in·ter′ni′ anterior et
  posterior
—venosi vertebrales
  pos·te′ri·o′res′
—ve·no′sus
—venosus ar′e·o·lar′is
—venosus ca·na′lis
  hy′po·glos′si′
—venosus ca·rot′i·cus
  in·ter′nus
—venosus fo·ram′i·nis
  o·va′lis
—venosus ma·mil′lae′
—venosus pros·tat′i·cus
—venosus rec·ta′lis
—venosus sa·cra′lis
—venosus sem′i·na′lis
—venosus sub′oc·cip′i·ta′lis
—venosus u′ter·i′nus
—venosus vag′i·na′lis
—venosus ves′i·ca′lis
—ver′te·bra′lis
—ves′i·ca′lis

pli′a·ble
pli′ca *pl.* -cae′
  —ar′y·ep′i·glot′ti·ca
  —ax′il·lar′is anterior
  —axillaris posterior
  —cae·ca′lis
  —ce·ca′lis vas′cu·lar′is
  —chor′dae′ tym′pa·ni′
  —du′o·de·na′lis inferior
  —duodenalis superior
  —du′o·de·no·je′ju·na′lis

—du′o·de′no·mes′o·col′-
  i·ca
—ep′i·gas′tri·ca
—fim′bri·a′ta
—gas′tro·pan′cre·at′i·ca
—glos′so·ep′i·glot′ti·ca
  lat′er·a′lis
—glossoepiglottica
  me′di·a′na
—il′e·o·cae·ca′lis
—il′e·o·ce·ca′lis
—in′cu·dis
—in′gui·na′lis
—in·ter′u·re·ter′i·ca
—lac′ri·ma′lis
—lon′gi·tu′di·na′lis
  du′o·de·ni′
—mal′le·ar′is anterior
  mem·bra′nae′ tym′pa·ni′
—mallearis anterior tu′ni·
  cae′ mu·co′sae′ ca′vi′
  tym′pa·ni′
—mallearis posterior
  mem·bra′nae′ tym′pa·ni′
—mallearis posterior tu′ni·
  cae′ mu·co′sae′ ca′vi′
  tym′pa·ni′
—mal′le·o·lar′is anterior
  mem·bra′nae′ tym′pa·ni′
—malleolaris anterior
  tu′ni·cae′ mu·co′sae′
  tym′pan′i·cae′
—malleolaris posterior
  mem·bra′nae′ tym′pa·ni′
—malleolaris posterior
  tu′ni·cae′ mu·co′sae′
  tym′pan′i·cae′
—mu·co′sa
—pal′pe·bro·na·sa′lis
—par′a·du′o·de·na′lis
—po·lon′i·ca
—pu′bo·ves′i·ca′lis
—rec′to·u′ter·i′na
—sal·pin′go·pal′a·ti′na
—sal·pin′go·pha·ryn′ge·a
—sem′i·lu·nar′is
—semilunaris con′junc·ti′-
  vae′
—se·ro′sa
—spi·ra′lis
—sta·pe′dis
—sub′lin·gua′lis
—sy·no′vi·a′lis

—synovialis in'fra·pat'el·
  lar'is
—synovialis pat'el·lar'is
—tri·an'gu·lar'is
—um·bil'i·ca'lis lat'er·a'lis
—umbilicalis me'di·a
—umbilicalis me'di·a'lis
—umbilicalis me'di·a'na
—u're·ter'i·ca
—ve'nae' ca'vae' si·nis'trae'
—ven·tric'u·lar'is
—ves'i·ca'lis trans·ver'sa
—ves·tib'u·lar'is
—vo·ca'lis
pli'cae'
—ad'i·po'sae' pleu'rae'
—a·lar'es'
—am'pul·lar'es' tu'bae'
  u'ter·i'nae'
—cae·ca'lis'
—ce·ca'les'
—cil'i·ar'es'
—cir'cu·lar'es'
—gas'tri·cae'
—gas'tro·pan'cre·at'i·cae'
—i'ri·dis
—isth'mi·cae' tu'bae'
  u'ter·i'nae'
—pal'a·ti'nae' trans·ver'sae'
—pal·ma'tae'
—sem'i·lu·nar'es' co'li'
—trans'ver·sa'les' rec'ti'
—tu·bar'i·ae'
—tu'ni·cae' mu·co'sae'
  ve·si'cae' fel'le·ae'
—vil·lo'sae' ven·tric'u·li'
pli'ca·my'cin
pli'cate', -cat'ed, -cat'ing
pli'ca'tion
pli·cot'o·my
pli'ers
plomb
plom·bage'
plop
plug
plug'ger
plum·ba'go
plum'bic
plum'bism
plum'bum
Plum'mer
—disease
—sign

—treatment
Plum'mer-Vin'son
  syndrome
plump
plump'er
plu'ral
plu'ri·cy'to·pe'ni·a
plu'ri·de·fi'cient
plu'ri·fo'cal
plu'ri·glan'du·lar
plu'ri·grav'i·da
plu'ri·loc'u·lar
plu'ri·men'or·rhe'a
plu·rip'a·ra
plu'ri·par'i·ty
plu'ri·po'tent
plu'ri·po·ten'ti·al'i·ty
plu'ton·ism
plu·to'ni·um
pne'o·dy·nam'ics
pne'o·graph'
pne·om'e·ter
pneu'mar·throg'ra·phy
pneu'mar·thro'sis
pneu·mat'ic
pneu·mat'i·cal·ly
pneu·mat'ics
pneu'ma·ti·za'tion
pneu'ma·tize', -tized',
  -tiz'ing
pneu'ma·to·car'di·a
pneu·mat'o·cele'
pneu'ma·to·dysp'ne·a
pneu·mat'o·gram'
pneu·mat'o·graph'
pneu'ma·tom'e·ter
pneu'ma·tom'e·try
pneu'ma·tor'ra·chis
pneu'ma·to'sis pl. -ses'
  —cys·toi'des' in·tes'ti·na'lis
pneu·ma·tu'ri·a
pneu'ma·type'
pneu·mec'to·my
pneu'mo·an'gi·og'ra·phy
pneu'mo·ar'thro·gram'
pneu'mo·ar·throg'ra·phy
pneu'mo·ba·cil'lus pl. -li'
pneu'mo·bul'bar
pneu'mo·car'di·og'ra·phy
pneu'mo·cele'
pneu'mo·cen·te'sis pl. -ses'
pneu'mo·ceph'a·lus
pneu'mo·cho'le·cys·ti'tis

pneu'mo·coc'cal
pneu'mo·coc·ce'mi·a
pneu'mo·coc'cic
pneu'mo·coc·cid'al
pneu'mo·coc·co'sis pl. -ses'
pneu'mo·coc·co·su'ri·a
pneu'mo·coc'cus pl. -ci'
pneu'mo·co'lon
pneu'mo·co·ni·o'sis pl. -ses'
pneu'mo·cra'ni·um
pneu'mo·cys'tic
Pneu'mo·cys'tis
—ca·ri'ni·i'
pneu'mo·cys'to·gram'
pneu'mo·cys·tog'ra·phy
pneu'mo·cys'to·sis pl. -ses'
pneu'mo·cys'to·to·mog'ra·
  phy
pneu'mo·cyte'
pneu'mo·der'ma
pneu'mo·dy·nam'ics
pneu'mo·en·ceph'a·li'tis
pneu'mo·en·ceph'a·lo·cele'
pneu'mo·en·ceph'a·lo·
  gram'
pneu'mo·en·ceph'a·log'ra·
  phy
pneu'mo·en·ceph'a·lo·
  my'e·lo·gram'
pneu'mo·en·ceph'a·lo·
  my'e·log'ra·phy
pneu'mo·en·ter'ic
pneu'mo·en·ter'i'tis
pneu'mo·gas'tric
pneu'mo·gas·trog'ra·phy
pneu'mo·gas·tros'co·py
pneu'mo·gram'
pneu'mo·graph'
pneu'mo·graph'ic
pneu·mog'ra·phy
pneu'mo·gy'no·gram'
pneu'mo·he'mi·a
pneu'mo·he'mo·per'i·
  car'di·um
pneu'mo·he'mo·tho'rax'
pneu'mo·hy'dro·per'i·
  car'di·um
pneu'mo·hy'dro·tho'rax'
pneu'mo·hy'po·der'ma
pneu'mo·lip'i·do'sis
pneu'mo·lith'
pneu'mo·li·thi'a·sis pl. -ses'
pneu·mol'o·gy

pneu·mol′y·sis *pl.* -ses′
pneu′mo·ma·la′ci·a
pneu′mo·me′di·as′ti·nog′-
 ra·phy
pneu′mo·me′di·as′ti′num
pneu·mom′e·try
pneu′mo·my·co′sis *pl.* -ses′
pneu′mo·my′e·log′ra·phy
pneu′mo·nec′to·my
pneu·mo′ni·a
 —al′ba
pneu·mon′ic
pneu·mo·ni′tis
pneu·mon′o·cele′
pneu·mo′no·cen·te′sis
 pl. -ses′
pneu·mo′no·cir·rho′sis *pl.*
 -ses′
pneu·mon′o·cyte′
pneu·mo′nol′y·sis *pl.* -ses′
pneu·mo′no·mel′a·no′sis
 pl. -ses′
pneu·mo′no·my·co′sis
 pl. -ses′
pneu′mo·no·nop′a·thy
pneu·mo′no·pex′y
pneu·mo′nor′rha·phy
pneu·mo′no·sis *pl.* -ses′
pneu·mo′not′o·my
pneu·mo·per′i·car·di′tis
pneu·mo·per′i·car′di·um
pneu·mo·per′i·to·ne′um
 pl. -ums *or* -ne′a
pneu·mo·per′i·to·ni′tis
pneu·mo·pex′y
pneu·mo·pleu·ri′tis
pneu·mo·py′e·lo·gram′
pneu·mo·py′e·log′ra·phy
pneu·mo·py′o·per′i·car′-
 di·um
pneu·mo·ra′chis
pneu·mo·ra′di·og′ra·phy
pneu·mo·roent′gen·o·
 gram′
pneu·mor·rha′gi·a
pneu·mo·sid′er·o′sis
pneu·mo·tax′ic
pneu·mo·tax′is
pneu·mo·ther′a·py
pneu·mo·tho′rax′ *pl.* -rax′es
 or -ra·ces′
pneu·mot′o·my
pneu·mo·tox′ic

pneu′mo·tox′in
pneu′mo·trop′ic
pneu′mo·ty′phoid′
pneu′mo·ty′phus
pneu′mo·ven′tri·cle
pneu′mo·ven·tric′u·log′ra·
 phy
pneu′sis
pni′ger·o·pho′bi·a
pnig′ma
pni′go·pho′bi·a
pock
pocked
pock′et
pock′mark′
po·dag′ra
pod·a′gral
po·dag′ric
po·dal′gi·a
po·dal′ic
pod′ar·thri′tis
pod·e·de′ma
pod·el′co·ma
pod·en·ceph′a·lus
po·di′a·trist
po·di′a·try
pod·o·bro′mi·dro′sis
pod′o·cyte′
pod′o·cyt′ic
pod′o·dyn′i·a
pod′o·phyl′lin
pod′o·phyl′lum *pl.* -li′
Poe·cil′i·a
po·go′ni·on
poi′ki·lo·blast′
poi′ki·lo·cyte′
poi′ki·lo·cy·the′mi·a
poi′ki·lo·cy·to′sis *pl.* -ses′
poi′ki·lo·der′ma
 —a·troph′i·cans′ vas′cu·
  lar′e′
 —con·gen′i·ta′le′
 —of Ci·vatte′
 —re·tic′u·lar′e′ of Ci·vatte′
poi′ki·lo·der′ma·to·my′o·
 si′tis
poi·kil′o·therm′
poi′ki·lo·ther′mal
poi′ki·lo·ther′mic
poi′ki·lo·ther′mism
poi′ki·lo·ther′mous
poi′ki·lo·ther′my
poi′ki·lo·throm′bo·cyte′

poi′ki·lo·zo′o·sper′mi·a
point
poin′til·lage′
points′ dou·lou·reux′
poise
Poi·seuille′ layer
poi′son
poi′son·ing
poi′son·ous
Pois·son′ distribution
Po′land syndrome
po′lar
po′la·rim′e·ter
po·lar′i·met′ric
po′la·rim′e·try
po·lar′i·scope′
po·lar′i·scop′ic
po·lar′i·stro·bom′e·ter
po·lar′i·ty
po·lar·i·za′tion
po′lar·ize′, -ized′, -iz′ing
po′lar·iz′er
po·lar′o·gram′
po·lar′o·graph′
po·lar′o·graph′ic
po·la·rog′ra·phy
pole
po′li·en·ceph′a·li′tis
po′li·o·dys·tro′phi·a
 —cer′e·bri′ pro′gres·si′va
  in·fan′ti·lis
po′li·o·en·ceph′a·li′tis
 —a·cu′ta
 —hem·or′rha·gi′ca
po′li·o·en·ceph′a·lo·me·
 nin′go·my′e·li′tis
po′li·o·en·ceph′a·lo·my′e·
 li′tis
po′li·o·en·ceph′a·lop′a·thy
po′li·o·my′el·en·ceph′a·li′-
 tis
po′li·o·my′e·li′tis
po′li·o·my′e·lop′a·thy
po′li·o·my′o·si′tis
po′li·o·plasm
po′li·o′sis *pl.* -ses′
po′li·o·thrix′
po′li·o·vi′rus
pol′ish
Po′lit·zer
 —cone
 —maneuver

—test
po'lit·zer·i·za'tion
pol'la·ki·u'ri·a
pol'len
pol'lex' *pl.* -li·ces'
—val'gus
—var'us
pol'li·ci·za'tion
pol'li·cize', -cized', -ciz'ing
pol'li·no'sis *pl.* -ses'
pol·lu'tion
po'lo·cyte'
po·lo'ni·um
po·lox'a·lene'
po·lox'al·kol'
pol·toph'a·gy
po'lus *pl.* -li'
—anterior bul'bi' oc'u·li'
—anterior len'tis
—fron·ta'lis
—oc·cip'i·ta'lis
—posterior bul'bi' oc'u·li'
—posterior len'tis
—tem'po·ra'lis
pol'y
pol'y·ac'id
pol'y·a·cryl'a·mide'
pol'y·ad'e·ni'tis
pol'y·ad'e·no'ma *pl.* -mas *or* -ma·ta
pol'y·ad'e·nop'a·thy
pol'y·ad'e·no'sis *pl.* -ses'
pol'y·ad'e·nous
pol'y·am'ide
pol'y·am'ine'
pol'y·a·mi'no
pol'y·an'dry
pol'y·an·gi·i'tis
Pol'ya operation
pol'y·ar'te·ri'tis
—no·do'sa
pol'y·ar'thric
pol'y·ar·thri'tis
pol'y·ar·throp'a·thy
pol'y·ar·tic'u·lar
pol'y·a·tom'ic
pol'y·ax'on'
pol'y·ax·on'ic
pol'y·ba'sic
pol'y·blast'
pol'y·ble·phar'i·a
pol'y·bleph'a·ron'
pol'y·bleph'a·ry

pol'y·car'bo·phil'
pol'y·cel'lu·lar
pol'y·cen'tric
pol'y·chei'ri·a
pol'y·che'mo·ther'a·py
pol'y·cho'li·a
pol'y·chon·dri'tis
pol'y·chro'ism
pol'y·chro·ma'si·a
pol'y·chro·ma'ti·a
pol'y·chro·mat'ic
pol'y·chro·mat'o·cyte'
pol'y·chro'ma·to·phil
pol'y·chro'ma·to·phil'i·a
pol'y·chro'ma·to·phil'ic
pol'y·chro'ma·to'sis
pl. -ses'
pol'y·chrome'
pol'y·chro'mi·a
pol'y·chro'mo·cy·to'sis
pl. -ses'
pol'y·chy'li·a
pol'y·clin'ic
pol'y·clo'nal
pol'y·clo'ni·a
pol'y·co'ri·a
pol'y·crot'ic
pol'y·cy'clic
pol'y·cy·e'sis
pol'y·cys'tic
pol'y·cys·to'ma *pl.* -mas *or* -ma·ta
pol'y·cyte'
pol'y·cy·the'mi·a
—hy'per·ton'i·ca
—ru'bra ve'ra
—ve'ra
pol'y·cy·the'mic
pol'y·dac·tyl'i·a
pol'y·dac'tyl·ism
pol'y·dac'ty·lous
pol'y·dac'ty·ly
pol'y·de·fi·cien'cy
pol'y·de·fi'cient
pol'y·dip'si·a
pol'y·dys·pla'si·a
pol'y·dys'troph'ic
pol'y·dys'tro·phy
pol'y·e·lec'tro·lyte'
pol'y·em'bry·o·ny
pol'y·e'mi·a
pol'y·ene'
pol'y·es·the'si·a

pol'y·es'tra·di·ol'
pol'y·es'trous
pol'y·eth'a·dene'
pol'y·eth'yl·ene'
pol'y·ga·lac'ti·a
pol'y·ga·lac'tu·ro·nase'
pol'y·gam'ic
po·lyg'a·mist
po·lyg'a·mous
po·lyg'a·my
pol'y·gene'
pol'y·gen'ic
pol'y·glan'du·lar
pol'y·glo·bu'li·a
pol'y·glob'u·lism
pol'y·glot'
po·lyg'na·thus
pol'y·graph'
pol'y·graph'ic
po·lyg'y·nist
po·lyg'y·nous
po·lyg'y·ny
pol'y·gy'ri·a
pol'y·he'dral
pol'y·he'mi·a
pol'y·hi·dro'sis *pl.* -ses'
pol'y·hy'brid
pol'y·hy·dram'ni·os
pol'y·hy'dric
pol'y·hy·drox'y
pol'y·hy·drox'yl·eth'yl·meth·ac'ry·late'
pol'y·hy·dru'ri·a
pol'y·i·dro'sis *pl.* -ses'
pol'y·in·fec'tion
pol'y·lec'i·thal
pol'y·lep'tic
pol'y·lob'u·lar
pol'y·mas'ti·a
Pol'y·mas'ti·gi'da
pol'y·mas'ti·gote'
pol'y·ma'zi·a
pol'y·me'li·a
po·lym'e·lus *pl.* -li'
pol'y·me'ni·a
pol'y·men'or·rhe'a
pol'y·mer
po·lym'er·ase'
pol'y·me'ri·a
pol'y·mer'ic
po·lym'er·ism
po·lym'er·i·za'tion
po·lym'er·ize' -ized', -iz'ing

pol′y·met′a·car′pal·ism
pol′y·met′a·car′pi·a
pol′y·met′a·tar′si·a
pol′y·mi·cro′bi·al
pol′y·mi·cro′bic
pol′y·mi′cro·gy′ri·a
pol′y·mix′in
pol′y·morph′
pol′y·mor′phic
pol′y·mor′phism
pol′y·mor′pho·cel′lu·lar
pol′y·mor′pho·cyte′
pol′y·mor′pho·nu′cle·ar
pol′y·mor′phous
pol′y·my·al′gi·a
  —rheu·mat′i·ca
pol′y·my·oc′lo·nus
pol′y·my·op′a·thy
pol′y·my′o·si′tis
pol′y·myx′in
pol′y·ne′sic
pol′y·neu′ral
pol′y·neu·ral′gi·a
pol′y·neu′ric
pol′y·neu·rit′ic
pol′y·neu·ri′tis
pol′y·neu·ro·my′o·si′tis
pol′y·neu·rop′a·thy
pol′y·neu·ro·ra·dic′u·li′tis
pol′y·nu′cle·ar
pol′y·nu′cle·ate′
pol′y·nu′cle·o′sis *pl.* -ses′
pol′y·nu′cle·o·ti′dase′
pol′y·nu′cle·o·tide′
pol′y·o·don′ti·a
pol′y·o′ma *pl.* -mas *or* -ma·ta
pol′y·o·nych′i·a
pol′y·o′pi·a
  —mon′oph·thal′mi·ca
pol′y·op′tic
pol′y·or′chi·dism
pol′y·or′chis
pol′y·o·rex′i·a
pol′y·or′rho·men′in·gi′tis
pol′y·or′rhy·me·ni′tis
pol′y·os·tot′ic
pol′y·o′ti·a
pol′y·o′vu·lar
pol′y·o′vu·la·to′ry
pol′y·ox′yl
pol′yp
pol′y·pap′il·lo′ma *pl.* -mas
  or -ma·ta

pol′y·pa·re′sis *pl.* -ses′
pol′y·path′i·a
pol′y·pec′to·my
pol′y·pep′ti·dase′
pol′y·pep′tide′
pol′y·pep′ti·de·mi·a
pol′y·pep′ti·dor·rha′chi·a
pol′y·per′i·os·ti′tis hy′per·
  es·thet′i·ca
pol′y·pha·gi·a
pol′y·pha′gous
pol′y·pha·lan′gism
pol′y·phar′ma·cy
pol′y·pha′sic
pol′y·phe′nol
pol′y·pho′bi·a
pol′y·phy·let′ic
pol′y·phy′le·tism
pol′y·phy′o·dont′
pol′yp·if′er·ous
pol′y·plast′
pol′y·plas′tic
pol′y·ple′gi·a
pol′y·ploid′
pol′y·ploi′dy
pol′yp·ne′a
pol′y·po′di·a
pol′y·poid′
pol′y·poi′dal
pol′y·poi·do′sis
po·lyp′o·rous
Po·lyp′o·rus
pol′y·po′sis *pl.* -ses′
  —co′li′
  —ven·tric′u·li′
pol′y·pous
pol′y·pro′pyl·ene′
pol′y·pty′chi·al
pol′y·pus *pl.* -pi′ *or* -pus·es
pol′y·ra·dic′u·li′tis
pol′y·ra·dic′u·lo·neu·ri′tis
pol′y·ra·dic′u·lo·neu·
  rop′a·thy
pol′y·ri′bo·nu′cle·o·tide′
pol′y·ri′bo·some′
pol′yr·rhe′a
pol′y·sac′cha·ride′
pol′y·sce′li·a
po·lys′ce·lus
pol′y·scle·ro′sis *pl.* -ses′
pol′y·scope′
pol′y·scop′ic
pol′y·se·ro·si′tis

pol′y·si′nus·i′tis
pol′y·so′ma·tous
pol′y·some′
pol′y·so′mi·a
pol′y·so′mic
pol′y·so′mus
pol′y·so′my
pol′y·sor′bate′
pol′y·sper′mi·a
pol′y·sper′mic
pol′y·sperm′ism
pol′y·sper′my
pol′y·stich′i·a
pol′y·sto′ma·tous
pol′y·sty′rene′
pol′y·sus·pen′soid′
pol′y·syn·ap′tic
pol′y·syn·dac′tyl·ism
pol′y·syn·dac′ty·ly
pol′y·syn·o·vi′tis
pol′y·tene′
pol′y·the′li·a
pol′y·the′lism
pol′y·thi′a·zide′
po·lyt′o·cous
pol′y·trich′i·a
pol′y·tri·cho′sis
pol′y·tro′phi·a
po·lyt′ro·phy
pol′y·trop′ic
pol′y·typ′ic
pol′y·un·sat′u·rat′ed
pol′y·u′re·thane′
pol′y·u′ri·a
pol′y·u′ric
pol′y·va′lent
pol′y·vi′nyl
pol′y·vi′nyl·chlo′ride′
pol′y·vi′nyl·pyr·rol′i·done′
po·made′
Pom·pe′ disease
pom′pho·ly·he′mi·a
pom′pho·lyx′
pom′phus
po′mum A·da′mi′
pon·ceau′
  —de xy′li·dine′
Pon·cet′
  —disease
  —operation
Pon′fick shadow
Pon′gi·dae′
Pon′ka

—herniorrhaphy
—technique
pons pl. pon'tes'
—Va·ro'li·i'
Pon'ti·ac' fever
pon'tic
pon·tic'u·lar
pon·tic'u·lus
pon'tile'
pon'tine'
pon'to·bul'bar
pon'to·cer'e·bel'lar
pool'ing
Pool'-Schles'in·ger sign
pop'les'
pop·lit'e·al
pop·lit'e·us pl. -e·i'
pop'pet
por·ad·e·ni'tis
por·ad·e·no·lym·phi'tis
por'ce·lain
por'cine'
pore
—of Kohn
por'en·ce·pha'li·a
por'en·ce·phal'ic
por'en·ceph'a·li'tis
por'en·ceph'a·lus pl. -li'
por'en·ceph'a·ly
por'fi·ro·my'cin
po'ri·o·ma·ni·a
po'ri·on' pl. -ri·a or -ri·ons'
por'no·graph'ic
por·nog'ra·phy
po'ro·ceph'a·li'a·sis pl. -ses'
Po'ro·ce·phal'i·dae'
Po'ro·ceph'a·lus
po'ro·ker'a·to'sis pl. -ses'
po·ro'ma pl. -ma·ta
po'ro·plas'tic
po·ro'sis pl. -ses'
po·ros'i·ty
po·rot'ic
po'rous
por'phin
por'pho·bi'lin
por'pho·bi·lin'o·gen
por'phyr'i·a
—cu·ta'ne·a tar'da he·red'i·
tar'i·a
—cutanea tarda symp'to·
mat'i·ca
—e·ryth'ro·poi·et'i·ca

—he'ma·to·poi·et'i·ca
—he'pat'i·ca
—var'i·e·ga'ta
por'phy·rin
por'phy·rin·e'mi·a
por'phy·ri·nu'ri·a
por'phy·ri·za'tion
por'phy·rop'sin
Por'ro operation
por·rop'si·a
port
por'ta pl. -tae'
—hep'a·tis
—ves·tib'u·li'
port'a·ble
por'ta·ca'val
por'tal
porte·pol'ish·er
Por'ter sign
Por'ter-Sil'ber reaction
Por·tes' operation
Por'te·us maze
por'ti·o' pl. por'ti·o'nes'
—major ner'vi' tri·gem'i·ni'
—minor nervi tri·gem'i·ni'
—su'pra·vag'i·na'lis cer'vi·
cis
—vag'i·na'lis cer'vi·cis
—vaginalis u'ter·i'
por'tion
por'to·ca'val
por'to·en·ter·os'to·my
por'to·gram'
por·tog'ra·phy
por'to·sys·tem'ic
por'to·ve'no·gram'
por'to·ve·nog'ra·phy
po'rus pl. -ri'
—a·cus'ti·cus ex·ter'nus
—acusticus in·ter'nus
—cro'ta·phit'i·co·buc'ci·
na·to'ri·us
—gus'ta·to'ri·us
—op'ti·cus
—su'do·rif'e·rus
po·si'tion
po·si'tion·al
po·si'tion·er
pos'i·tive
pos'i·tron'
pos·i·tro'ni·um
po'so·log'ic
po·sol'o·gy

post
post'a·bor'tal
post'am·biv'a·lent
post·a'nal
post'an·es·thet'ic
post·an'gi·o·plas'ty
post·ap·o·plec'tic
post·au'di·to'ry
post·ax'i·al
post·bra'chi·al
post·cap'il·lar'y
post·car'di·ac'
post·car'di·al
post'car·di·ot'o·my
post·ca'va
post·ca'val
post·cen'tral
post·chrom'ing
post·ci'bal
post'cla·vic'u·lar
post·co'i·tal
post'con·cep'tu·al
post·con·cus'sion
post·con'dy·lar
post·con·i·za'tion
post·con·nu'bi·al
post'con·vul'sive
post·cor'di·al
post·cor'nu
post·cos'tal
post·cra'ni·al
post·cri'coid'
post·cu'bi·tal
post·dam'ming
post·di·a·stol'ic
post·di·crot'ic
post·di·ges'tive
post'diph·the·rit'ic
post·dor'mi·tal
post'em·bry·on'ic
post'en·ceph'a·lit'ic
post'ep·i·lep'tic
pos·te'ri·ad'
pos·te'ri·or
pos·te'ri·or·ly
pos'ter·o·an·te'ri·or
pos'ter·o·ex·ter'nad'
pos'ter·o·ex·ter'nal
pos'ter·o·in·ter'nad'
pos'ter·o·in·ter'nal
pos'ter·o·lat'er·ad'
pos'ter·o·lat'er·al
pos'ter·o·mar'gi·nal

pos'ter·o·me'di·ad'
pos'ter·o·me'di·al
pos'ter·o·me'di·an
pos'ter·o·su·pe'ri·or
pos'ter·o·tem'po·ral
pos'ter·o·trans·verse'
post'e·soph'a·ge'al
post'e·vac'u·a'tion
post·feb'rile
post'gan·gli·on'ic
post'gas·trec'to·my
post·gle'noid'
post·grav'id
post'hem·i·ple'gic
post'hem·or·rhag'ic
post·he·pat'ic
post'hep'a·tit'ic
post'her·pet'ic
pos·thet'o·my
pos·thi'tis
pos·tho·lith'
post·hu'mous
post'hu·mous·ly
post'hyp·not'ic
post·ic'tal
post'ic·ter'ic
pos·ti'cus
post'in·farc'tion
post'in·fec'tious
post'in·fec'tive
post'in·flu·en'zal
post·is'chi·al
post'ma·lar'i·al
post·mam'ma·ry
post'mas·tec'to·my
post·mas'toid'
post'ma·ture'
post'ma·tu'ri·ty
post·me'di·an
post'me·di·as'ti·nal
post'men·ar'che'
post'men·o·pau'sal
post'men'stru·al
post·mor'tal
post·mor'tem
post·nar'is
post·na'sal
post·na'tal
post'ne·crot'ic
post·neu·rit'ic
post·nod'u·lar
post·oc'u·lar
post·ol'i·var'y

post·op'er·a·tive
post·o'ral
post·or'bit·al
post·pal'a·tine'
post·pa·lu'dal
post·par·a·lyt'ic
post·par'tum
post'pha·ryn'ge·al
post'phle·bit'ic
post'pi·tu'i·tar'y
post·pran'di·al
post'pros·tat'ic
post·pu'ber·al
post'pu·bes'cent
post'pyc·not'ic
post·py·ram'i·dal
post·ra·di·a'tion
post·re·duc'tion
post·re'nal
post·rhi'nal
post'ro·lan'dic
post·scap'u·lar
post'scar·la·ti'nal
post·sphe'noid'
post·sphyg'mic
post'sple·nec'to·my
post·ste·not'ic
post·syn·ap'tic
post'syph·i·lit'ic
post'throm·bot'ic
post'trans·verse'
post'trau·mat'ic *(relating to trauma)*
post·treat'ment
post'-tre·mat'ic *(relating to brachial cleft)*
post·tus'sive
post·ty'phoid'
pos'tu·late', -lat'ed, -lat'ing
pos'tur·al
pos'ture
post·vac'ci·nal
post·ves'i·cal
po'ta·ble
Po·tain'
—disease
—syndrome
Pot'a·mon
pot'ash
pot'as·se'mi·a
po·tas'sic
po·tas'si·um
po'ten·cy

po'tent
po·ten'ti·a con·cep'i·en'di
po·ten'tial
po·ten'ti·ate', -at'ed, -at'ing
po·ten'ti·a'tion
po·ten'ti·a'tor
po·ten'ti·om'e·ter
po·ten'ti·o·met'ric
po'tion
po'to·ma'ni·a
Pott
—curvature
—disease
—fracture
—gangrene
—puffy tumor
Potts
—anastomosis
—operation
Potts'-Smith'
—anastomosis
—operation
Pö'tzel syndrome
pouch
—of Doug'las
—of Mor'i·son
pou·drage'
Pou·let' disease
poul'tice
pound
Pou·part' ligament
pov'er·ty
po'vi·done'
pow'der
pow'er
Pow'er test
pox
pox·vi'rus
P pul'mo·na'le'
prac'tice, -ticed, -tic'ing
prac·ti'tion·er
Pra'der-Wil'li syndrome
prae'cox'
prae·pu'ti·um *pl.* -ti·a, *var. of* preputium
prae'vi·a *var. of* previa
prag'mat·ag·no'si·a
prag'mat·am·ne'si·a
Prague maneuver
pral'i·dox'ime'
pra·mox'ine'
pran'di·al
pran'di·al·i·ty

pran'o·bex
pra'se·o·dym'i·um
Praus'nitz-Küst'ner
—reaction
—test
prav'a·stat'in
prax'i·ol'o·gy
prax'is pl. -prax'es'
pra'ze·pam'
pra'zi·quan'tel
pra'zo·sin
pre'ad·o·les'cence
pre'ad·o·les'cent
pre·ag'o·nal
pre'al·bu'mi·nu'ric
pre·am'pul·lar'y
pre·a'nal
pre'an·es·the'si·a
pre'an·es·thet'ic
pre'an·ti·sep'tic
pre'a·or'tic
pre'a·tax'ic
pre'au·ric'u·lar
pre·ax'i·al
pre'be·ta·lip'o·pro'tein'
pre'be·ta·lip'o·pro'tein·e'-
    mi·a
pre·can'cer·ous
pre·cap'il·lar'y
pre·car'ci·nom'a·tous
pre·car'di·ac'
pre·car'di·nal
pre·car'ti·lage
pre·ca'va
pre·ca'val
pre·cen'tral
pre·cer'vi·cal
pre·ces'sion
pre·ces'sion·al
pre·chord'al
pre·cip'i·ta·ble
pre·cip'i·tant
pre·cip'i·tate', -tat'ed, -tat'ing
pre·cip'i·ta'tion
pre·cip'i·ta·tor
pre·cip'i·tin
pre·cip'i·tin'o·gen
pre·cip'i·tin·oid'
pre'cir·rho'sis
pre·cla·vic'u·lar
pre·clin'i·cal
pre'clot'
pre'coc·cyg'e·al

pre·co'cious
pre·coc'i·ty
pre'cog·ni'tion
pre·co'i·tal
pre·col·lag'e·nous
pre·com'a·tose'
pre·com·mis'sur·al
pre·com'mis·sure
pre·con'scious
pre·con'scious·ly
pre'con·vul'sant
pre'con·vul'sive
pre·cor'di·al
pre·cor'di·um pl. -di·a
pre·cor'nu
pre·cos'tal
pre·cri'coid'
pre·crit'i·cal
pre·cu'ne·us pl. -ne·i'
pre·cur'sor
pred'a·tor
pre'de·men'ti·a
pre·den'tin
pre·di'a·be'tes'
pre·di·as'to·le
pre·di·a·stol'ic
pre'di·crot'ic
pre·dic'tive
pre·di·gest'ed
pre·di·ges'tion
pre'dis·pose', -posed',
    -pos'ing
pre'dis·po·si'tion
pred'ni·car'bate'
pred·nis'o·lone'
pred'ni·sone'
pred'ni·val
pre·dom'i·nance
pre·dom'i·nant
pre·dor'mi·tal
pre·dor'mi'tion
pre·dor'mi·tum
pre·duc'tal
pre'e·clamp'si·a
pre'e·clamp'tic
pre·ep'i·glot'tic
pre'e·rup'tive
pre'ex·ci·ta'tion
pre'ex·trac'tion
pre·fab'ri·cate'
pre'fi·brot'ic
pre'for·ma'tion
pre·fron'tal

pre'gan·gli·on'ic
pre·gan'gre·nous
pre·gen'i·tal
pre·gle'noid'
preg'nan·cy
preg'nane'
preg'nane·di'ol'
preg'nant
preg'nene'
preg'nen·in'o·lone'
preg·nen'o·lone'
pre·gran'u·lar
pre·hal'lux
pre'hem·i·ple'gic
pre·hen'sile
pre·hen'sion
pre·he·pat'ic
pre·ic'tal
pre·ic·ter'ic
pre'in·va'sive
Prei'ser disease
pre·kal'li·kre'in
pre·lac'ri·mal
pre·lar'val
pre·leu·ke'mi·a
pre·leu·ke'mic
pre·lo·co·mo'tion
pre·log'i·cal
pre'lum
    —ab·dom'i·na'le'
pre·ma·lig'nant
pre·mam'mil·lar'y
pre·ma·ni'a·cal
pre·mar'i·tal
pre'ma·ture'
pre'ma·tur'i·ty
pre·max·il'la
pre·max'il·lar'y
pre·med'i·cal
pre·med'i·cant
pre·med'i·cate', -cat'ed,
    -cat'ing
pre·med'i·cat'ed
pre·med'i·ca'tion
pre·mel'a·no·some'
pre·men'o·paus'al
pre·men'stru·al
pre·men'stru·al·ly
pre·mo'lar
pre·mon'i·to'ry
pre·mon'o·cyte'
pre·mor'bid
pre·mor'tal

pre·mo'tor
pre'mu·ni'tion
pre'my'e·lo·blast'
pre'my'e·lo·cyte'
pre·nal'te·rol'
pre'nar·co'sis *pl.* -ses'
pre·na'ris *pl.* -res
pre·na'tal
pre·na'tal·ly
pre'ne·o·plas'tic
pre·nid'a·to'ry
pre·nod'u·lar
pre·nyl'a·mine'
pre'oc·cip'i·tal
pre·oc'cu·pa'tion
pre·oed'i·pal
pre·op'er·a·tive
pre·op'er·a·tive·ly
pre·op'tic
pre·o'ral
pre·o'ral·ly
pre·o'vu·la·to'ry
prep, prepped, prep'ping
pre·pal'a·tal
pre·par·a·lyt'ic
prep'a·ra'tion
pre·pa·ret'ic
pre·par'tal
pre·par'tum
pre·pa·tel'lar
pre·pat'ent
pre·pel'vic
pre'per·cep'tion
pre'per·cep'tive
pre'per·i·to·ne'al
pre·phe'nic
pre·pla·cen'tal
pre·pol'lex' *pl.* -li·ces'
pre·pon'der·ance
pre·po'tent
pre·pran'di·al
pre'psy·chot'ic
pre·pu'ber·al
pre·pu'ber·ty
pre·pu'bes'cence
pre·pu'bes'cent
pre·puce'
pre·pu·cot'o·my
pre·pu'tial
pre·pu'ti·um *pl.* -ti·a, *also*
    praeputium
    —cli·to'ri·dis
    —pe·nis

pre'py·lor'ic
pre·rec'tal
pre·re'nal
pre're·pro·duc'tive
pre·ret'i·nal
pre·sa'cral
pres'by·a·cu'si·a
pres'by·at'rics
pres'by·car'di·a
pres'by·cu'sis *pl.* -ses'
pres'by·der'ma
pres'by·e·soph'a·gus
pres'by·ope'
pres'by·o·phre'ni·a
pres'by·o·phren'ic
pres'by·o'pi·a
pres'by·op'ic
pres'by·o·sphac'e·lus
pres'by·ti·a
pres·byt'ic
pres'by·tism
pre·sca'lene'
pre'schiz·o·phren'ic
pre'scle·ro'sis *pl.* -ses'
pre'scle·rot'ic
pre·scribe', -scribed,
    -scrib'ing
pre·scrip'tion
pre·se·nile'
pre'se·nil'i·ty
pre·sent'
pres'en·ta'tion
pre·ser'va·tive
pre·so'mite'
pre·spas'tic
pre·sphe'noid'
pre·sphe·noi'dal
pre·sphyg'mic
pres'sor
pres'so·re·cep'tor
pres'so·sen'si·tive
pres'sure
pre·ster'nal
pre·ster'num *pl.* -nums *or*
    -na
pre'su·bic'u·lum
pre·sump'tive
pre·sup'pu·ra·tive
pre·sur'gi·cal
pre·syl'vi·an
pre'symp·to·mat'ic
pre'syn·ap'tic
pre·syn'co·pal

pre·sys'to·le
pre'sys·tol'ic
pre·tec'tal
pre·ter'mi·nal
pre'ter·nat'u·ral
pre'thy·roi'de·an
pre·tib'i·al
pre·tra'che·al
pre·tra'gal
pre·treat'ment
pre·tre·mat'ic
pre'tu·ber'cu·lous
pre'u·re·thri'tis
prev'a·lence
pre·ven'ta·tive
pre·ven'tion
pre·ven'tive
pre·ven·to'ri·um *pl.* -ri·a *or*
    -ri·ums
pre·ven·tric'u·lus *pl.* -li'
pre·ver'bal
pre·ver'te·bral
pre·ver'tig'i·nous
pre·ves'i·cal
pre·vi·a *also* praevia
Prey'er
    —reflex
    —test
pre'zone'
pre·zo'nu·lar
pre·zyg'a·poph'y·sis
    pl. -ses'
pri'a·pism
pri'a·pus *pl.* -pi'
Price'-Jones' curve
pril'o·caine'
pri'mal
pri'ma·quine
pri'mar·y
pri'mate'
Pri·ma'tes
pri'mi·done'
pri'mi·grav'i·da *pl.* -das *or*
    -dae'
pri·mip'a·ra *pl.* -ras *or*
    -rae'
pri·mi·par'i·ty
pri·mip'a·rous
pri'mite'
pri·mi'ti·ae'
prim'i·tive
pri·mor'di·al
pri·mor'di·um *pl.* -di·a

prin'ceps'
prin'ci·pal (foremost)
♦principle
prin'ci·ple (a chemical
    component; a rule)
♦principal
Prin'gle disease
Prinz'met'al angina
pri'on
Pri'o·nu'rus
    —aus·tra'lis
    —ci·tri'nus
prism
pris'ma pl. -ma·ta
pris'ma·ta ad'a·man·ti'na
pris·mat'ic
pris'moid'
pris'mop·tom'e·ter
pris'mo·sphere'
pro·ac·cel'er·i
pro·ac'ro·so'mal
pro·ac'ti·va'tor
pro·ac'tive
pro'ag·glu'ti·noid'
pro'al
pro·am'ni·on'
pro'ar·rhyth'mi·a
pro·at'las
pro'bac·te'ri·o·phage'
pro'band'
pro'bang'
pro·bar'bi·tal'
probe, probed, prob'ing
pro·ben'e·cid
pro'bit
prob'lem
pro·bos'cis pl. -cis·es or
    -ci·des'
pro'bu·col'
pro'cain·am'ide'
pro'caine'
pro·cal'lus
pro·car'ba·zine'
pro·ce'dure
pro·ce'lous
pro·cen'tri·ole'
pro·ce·phal'ic
pro·cer'coid'
pro·ce'rus pl. -ri' or -rus·es
proc'ess
pro·ces'sus pl. pro·ces'sus
    —ac'ces·so'ri·us ver'te·
        brar'um lum·ba'li·um

—a·lar'is os'sis eth'moi·da'-
    lis
—al've·o·lar'is max·il'lae'
—anterior mal'le·i'
—ar·tic'u·lar'es' in·fe'ri·o'-
    res' ver'te·brae'
—articulares su·pe'ri·o'res'
    ver'te·brae'
—ar·tic'u·lar'is inferior
—articularis superior
—articularis superior os'sis
    sa'cri'
—articularis superior
    zyg'a·poph'y·sis
—cau·da'tus hep'a·tis
—cil'i·ar'es'
—cli·noi'de·us anterior
—clinoideus me'di·us
—clinoideus posterior
—coch'le·ar'i·for'mis
—con'dy·lar'is
—con'dy·loi'de·us
    man·dib'u·lae'
—co'ra·coi'de·us
—co'ro·noi'de·us man·dib'-
    u·lae'
—coronoideus ul'nae'
—cos·tar'i·us ver'te·brae'
—eth'moi·da'lis
—fal'ci·for'mis lig'a·men'ti'
    sa·cro·tu·be·ro'si'
—fron·ta'lis max·il'lae'
—frontalis os'sis zy'go·
    mat'i·ci'
—fron'to·sphe·noi'da'lis
    os'sis zy·go·mat'i·ci'
—grac'i·lis
—in'tra·jug·u·lar'is os'sis
    oc·cip'i·ta'lis
—intrajugularis ossis
    tem'po·ra'lis
—jug·u·lar'is os'sis oc·cip'i·
    ta'lis
—lac'ri·ma'lis
—lat'er·a'lis mal'le·i'
—lateralis ta'li'
—lateralis tu'ber·is
    cal·ca'ne·i'
—len'tic'u·lar'is in·cu'dis
—mam'il·lar'is
—mar'gi·na'lis os'sis
    zy'go·mat'i·ci'
—mas·toi'de·us

—max'il·lar'is con'chae'
    na·sa'lis in·fe'ri·o'ris
—me'di·a'lis tu·ber'is
    cal·ca'ne·i'
—mus'cu·lar'is car'ti·lag'-
    i·nis ar'y·tae·noi'de·i'
—muscularis cartilaginis
    ar'y·te·noi'de·i'
—or'bi·ta'lis os'sis pal'a·ti'ni'
—pal'a·ti'nus max·il'lae'
—pap'il·lar'is hep'a·tis
—par'a·mas·toi'de·us os'sis
    oc·cip'i·ta'lis
—posterior sphe·noi'da'lis
—posterior ta'li'
—pter'y·goi'de·us os'sis
    sphe·noi·da'lis
—pter'y·go·spi·no'sus
—py·ram'i·da'lis os'sis
    pal'a·ti'ni'
—ret'ro·man·dib'u·lar'is
    glan'du·lae' pa·rot'i·dis
—sphe·noi'da'lis os'sis
    pal'a·ti'ni'
—sphenoidalis sep'ti'
    car'ti·la·gin'e·i'
—spi·no'sus
—sty·loi'de·us os'sis
    met'a·car·pa'lis III
—styloideus ossis ra'di·i'
—styloideus ossis
    tem'po·ra'lis
—styloideus ul'nae'
—su'pra·con'dy·lar'is
—su'pra·con'dy·loi'de·us
—tem'po·ra'lis os'sis
    zy'go·mat'i·ci'
—trans·ver'sus
—troch'le·ar'is cal·ca'ne·i'
—un'ci·na'tus os'sis
    eth'moi·da'lis
—uncinatus pan·cre'a·tis
—vag'i·na'lis os'sis
    sphe·noi·da'lis
—vaginalis per'i·to·nae'i'
—vaginalis per'i·to·ne'i'
—ver'mi·for'mis
—vo·ca'lis
—xi·phoi'de·us
—zy'go·mat'i·cus max·il'-
    lae'
—zygomaticus os'sis
    fron·ta'lis

—zygomaticus ossis
   tem′po·ra′lis
pro·chei′li·a
pro·chei′lon′
pro′chlor·per′a·zine′
pro·chon′dral
pro·chord′al
pro′cho·re′sis
Pro·chow′nick method
pro·ci·den′ti·a
pro′clo·nol′
pro′co·ag′u·lant
pro′con′dy·lism
pro′con·ver′tin
pro·cras′ti·na′tion
pro′cre·ate′, -at′ed, -at′ing
pro′cre·a′tion
pro′cre·a′tive
proc·tag′ra
proc·tal′gi·a
  —fu′gax′
proc·ta·tre′si·a
proc′tec·ta′si·a
proc·tec′to·my
proc·ten′cli·sis *pl.* -ses′
proc·teu·ryn′ter
proc·ti′tis
proc′to·cele′
proc·toc′ly·sis *pl.* -ses′
proc′to·co·lec′to·my
proc′to·co·li′tis
proc′to·co′lon·os′co·py
proc′to·col′po·plas′ty
proc′to·cys′to·plas′ty
proc′to·cys·tot′o·my
proc′to·de′um *pl.* -de′a *or*
  -de′ums
proc′to·dyn′i·a
proc′to·gram′
proc′to·log′ic
proc·tol′o·gist
proc·tol′o·gy
proc′to·pa·ral′y·sis *pl.* -ses′
proc′to·pex′y
proc′to·phil′i·a
proc′to·pho′bi·a
proc′to·plas′ty
proc′to·ple′gi·a
proc·top·to′si·a
proc·top·to′sis *pl.* -ses′
proc·tor·rha′gi·a
proc·tor·rha·phy
proc·tor·rhe′a

proc′to·scope′
proc′to·scop′ic
proc·tos′co·py
proc′to·sig′moid′
proc′to·sig·moid·ec′to·my
proc′to·sig·moid·i′tis
proc′to·sig·moi′do·scop′ic
proc′to·sig′moid·os′co·py
proc′to·spasm
proc·tos·ta′sis *pl.* -ses′
proc′to·ste·no′sis *pl.* -ses′
proc·tos′to·my
proc′to·tome′
proc·tot′o·my
pro′cum′ben·cy
pro′cum′bent
pro·cur′sive
pro·cur·va′tion
pro·cy′cli·dine′
pro·dig′i·o′sin
pro·dil′i·dine′
pro·dro′ma *pl.* -mas *or*
  -ma·ta
pro·dro′mal
pro′drome′
pro·drom′ic
prod′ro·mous
pro′drug′
prod′uct
pro·duc′tive
pro·e′mi·al
pro′en·ceph′a·lus *pl.* -li′
pro′en·ceph′a·ly
pro·en′zyme′
pro′e·ryth′ro·blast′
pro′e·ryth′ro·cyte′
pro·es′tro·gen
pro·es′trum
pro·es′trus
Proetz treatment
pro·fen′a·mine′
pro·fer′ment
pro·fes′sion·al
pro·fi·bri·nol′y·sin
Pro·fi·chet′ syndrome
pro′file′
pro·fla′vine
pro·flu·vi′um *pl.* -vi·a *or*
  -vi·ums
  —al′vi′
  —lac′tis
pro·fun′da *pl.* -dae′
pro·fun′da·plas′ty

pro·fun′dus
pro·gas′ter
pro·gen′i·tor
prog′e·ny
pro·ge′ri·a
pro′ges·ta′tion·al
pro·ges′ter·one′
pro·ges′tin
pro·ges′to·gen
pro·glot′tid
pro·glot′tis
prog·nath′ic
prog′na·thism
prog′na·thous
prog·nose′, -nosed′, -nos′ing
prog·no′sis *pl.* -ses′
prog·nos′tic
prog·nos′ti·cate′, -cat′ed,
  -cat′ing
prog′nos·ti·cian
pro′go·no′ma *pl.* -mas *or*
  -ma·ta
pro′gram
pro′gram′ma·bil′i·ty
pro′gram′ma·ble
pro·gran′u·lo·cyte′
pro·grav′id
pro·gress′ *v.*
prog′ress *n.*
pro·gres′sion
pro·gres′sive
pro·gua′nil
pro·hor′mone′
pro·in′su·lin
pro·i′o·sys′to·le
pro·jec′tile
pro·jec′tion
pro·jec′tive
pro·kar′y·o·cyte′
pro·kar′y·ote′
pro·kar′y·ot′ic
pro·ki′nase′
pro·la′bi·um *pl.* -bi·a
pro·lac′tin
pro·lac′ti·no′ma *pl.* -mas *or*
  -ma·ta
pro·lam′ine′
pro·lan′
pro·lapse′, -lapsed′, -laps′ing
pro·lap′sus
  —a′ni′
  —u′ter·i′
pro·late′

pro·lep'sis *pl.* -ses'
pro·lep'tic
pro·leu'ko·cyte'
pro·lif'er·ate', -at'ed, -at'ing
pro·lif'er·a'tion
pro·lif'er·a·tive
pro·lif'er·ous
pro·lif'ic
pro·lig'er·ous
pro·lin·ase'
pro'line'
pro'li·ne'mi·a
pro·lin'tane'
pro·lon·ga'tion
pro·lo·ther'a·py
pro'lyl
pro·lym'pho·cyte'
pro·lym'pho·cyt'ic
pro·ma·zine'
pro·meg'a·kar'y·o·cyte'
pro·meg'a·lo·blast'
pro·meg'a·lo·kar'y·o·cyte'
pro·met'a·phase'
pro·meth'a·zine'
pro·meth'es·trol'
pro·me'thi·um
prom'i·nence
prom'i·nen'ti·a *pl.* -ae'
—ca·na'lis fa·ci·a'lis
—canalis sem'i·cir'cu·lar'is
lat'er·a'lis
—la·ryn'ge·a
—mal'le·ar'is
—mal'le·o·lar'is
—spi·ra'lis
—sty·loi'de·a
pro·mon'o·cyte'
prom'on·to'ri·um *pl.* -ri·a
—ca'vi' tym'pa'ni'
—os'sis sa'cri'
prom'on·to'ry
pro·mot'er
pro·my'e·lo·cyte'
pro·my'e·lo·cyt'ic
pro'nase'
pro'nate', -nat'ed, -nat'ing
pro·na'tion
pro'na·tor
—ra'di·i' te'res'
prone
pro·neph'ric
pro·neph'ron
pro·neph'ros' *pl.* -neph'roi'

pro·neth'al·ol'
pro'no·grade'
pro'nor'mo·blast'
pro'nor'mo·cyte'
pro·nounced'
pro·nu'cle·us *pl.* -cle·i'
pro·o'tic
pro'ö·var'i·um
pro'pa·di·ene'
pro·paf'e·none'
prop'a·gate', -gat'ed, -gat'ing
prop'a·ga'tion
prop'a·ga'tive
pro·pal'i·nal
pro'pam'i·dine'
pro'pane'
pro·pan'i·did
pro'pa·no'ic
pro'pa·nol
pro·pan'the·line'
pro·par'a·caine'
pro'pa·tyl
pro'pene'
pro'pe·nyl
pro·pen'zo·late'
pro·pep'sin
pro·pep'tone'
pro·pep'to·nu'ri·a
pro·per'din
pro'per·i·to·ne'al
pro'phage'
pro'phase'
pro·phen'py·rid'a·mine'
pro·phy·lac'tic
pro·phy·lac'ti·cal·ly
pro·phy·lax'is *pl.* -es'
pro'pi·cil'lin
pro'pi·o·lac'tone'
pro'pi·o·ma·zine'
pro'pi·o·nate'
Pro·pi·on'i·bac·te'ri·um
ac'nes
pro'pi·on'ic
pro·pit'o·caine'
pro·plas'ma·cyte'
pro'po·fol'
pro·pos'i·tus *pl.* -ti
pro·pox'y·caine'
pro·pox'y·phene'
pro·pran'o·lol'
pro·pri'e·tar'y
pro·pri·o·cep'tion
pro·pri·o·cep'tive

pro·pri·o·cep'tor
pro·pri·o·spi'nal
pro·pri·us
prop·tom'e·ter
prop·to'sis *pl.* -ses'
prop·tot'ic
pro·pul'sion
pro·pul'sive
pro'pyl
pro'pyl·ene'
pro·pyl·hex'e·drine'
pro·pyl·i'o·done'
pro·pyl·par'a·ben
pro·pyl·thi'o·u'ra·cil
pro'pyne'
pro re na'ta
pro·ren'nin
pro·ru'bri·cyte'
pro·scil·lar'i·din
pro·sco'lex *pl.* -li·ces'
pro·se·cre'tin
pro·sect'
pro·sec'tor
pros'en·ce·phal'ic
pros'en·ceph'a·lon'
pros'o·coele'
pros'o·dem'ic
pros'op·ag·no'si·a
pro·sop'a·gus
pros'o·pal'gi·a
pros'o·pal'gic
pro·sop'ic
pros'o·pla'si·a
pros'o·plas'tic
pros'o·po'a·nos'chi·sis
pl. -ses'
pros'o·po·di·ple'gi·a
pros'o·po·dyn'i·a
pros'o·po·neu·ral'gi·a
pros'o·pop'a·gus *pl.* -gi'
pros'o·po·ple'gi·a
pros'o·po·ple'gic
pros'o·pos'chi·sis *pl.* -ses'
pros'o·po·spasm
pros'o·po·ster'no·did'y·
mus
pros'o·po·ster'no·dym'i·a
pros'o·po·tho'ra·cop'a·gus
pl. -gi'
pro·spec'tive
pros'ta·glan'din
pros'ta·noid'
pros'ta·ta

pros'tate' *(gland)*
   ◆*prostrate*
pros·ta·tec'to·my
pros·tat'ic
pros·tat'i·co·ves'i·cal
pros'ta·tism
pros'ta·tit'ic
pros'ta·ti'tis
pros·ta·to·cys·ti'tis
pros·ta·to·cys·tot'o·my
pros·ta·to·dyn'i·a
pros·tat'o·gram'
pros'ta·tog'ra·phy
pros·tat'o·lith'
pros'ta·to·li·thot'o·my
pros'ta·to·meg'a·ly
pros'ta·to·my'o·mec'to·my
pros'ta·tor·rhe'a
pros'ta·tot'o·my
pros'ta·to·tox'in
pros'ta·to·ve·sic'u·lec'-
   to·my
pros'ta·to·ve·sic'u·li'tis
pros'ter·na'tion
pros·the'sis *pl.* -ses'
pros·thet'ic
pros·thet'i·cal·ly
pros·thet'ics
pros'the·tist
pros'thi·on'
pros·tho·don'ti·a
pros·tho·don'tics
pros·tho·don'tist
pros·tig'mine'
pros'ti·tute'
pros'ti·tu'tion
pros'trate' *(to bow down)*,
   -trat'ed, -trat'ing
   ◆*prostate*
pros·tra'tion
pro·tac·tin'i·um
pro·tag'o·nist
pro'tal
pro·tal'bu·mose'
pro·ta·mine'
pro·ta·nom'a·ly
pro·ta·nope'
pro·ta·no'pi·a
pro·ta·nop'ic
pro'te·an *(changing form)*
   ◆*protein*
pro'te·ase'
pro·tec'tion

pro·tec'tive
pro·tec'tor
pro·te'ic
pro·te'id
pro·te'i·form'
pro'tein' *(substance)*
   ◆*protean*
pro'tein·a'ceous
pro'tein·ase'
pro'tein·e'mi·a
pro·tein'ic
pro'tein·o'sis *pl.* -ses'
pro'tein·o·ther'a·py
pro'tein·u'ri·a
pro'tein·u'ric
pro·te·o·lip'id
pro'te·ol'y·sis *pl.* -ses'
pro·te·o·lyt'ic
pro'te·o·met'a·bol'ic
pro·te·o·me·tab'o·lism
pro·te·o·pep'sis *pl.* -ses'
pro·te·o·pep'tic
pro'te·ose'
pro·te·o·su'ri·a
Pro'ter·o·glyph'a
pro'te·u'ri·a
Pro'te·us
   —mi·rab'i·lis
   —mor·gan'i·i'
   —rett'ger·i'
   —vul·gar'is
pro·throm'base'
pro·throm'bin
pro·throm'bin·ase'
pro·throm'bin·e'mi·a
pro·throm'bi·no·gen'ic
pro·throm'bi·no·pe'ni·a
pro·throm'bo·gen'ic
pro'throm'bo·ki'nase'
pro·thy'mi·a
pro'ti·de'
pro'ti're·lin
pro'tist
Pro·tis'ta
pro'tis·tol'o·gist
pro'tis·tol'o·gy
pro'ti·um
pro'to·al'bu·mose'
pro'to·blast'
pro'to·blas'tic
pro'to·cat'e·chu'ic
pro'to·chlo'ride'
pro'to·col'

pro'to·cone'
pro·to·co'nid
pro'to·cop'ro·por·phyr'i·a
   he·red'i·tar'i·a
pro'to·derm'
pro·to·di·a·stol'ic
pro'to·e·las'tose'
pro·to·fi'bril
pro·to·fil'a·ment
pro'to·gen
pro·to·glob'u·lose'
pro·tok'y·lol'
pro'to·leu'ko·cyte'
pro·tol'y·sis *pl.* -ses'
pro·tom'e·ter
pro'to·me'tro·cyte'
pro'ton'
pro'to·neu'ron'
pro·to-on'co·gene'
pro·to·path'ic
pro·to·pec'tin
pro·to·pep'si·a
pro'to·phyte'
pro·to·pla'sis
pro'to·plasm
pro·to·plas·mat'ic
pro·to·plas'mic
pro'to·plast'
pro·to·por·phyr'i·a
pro·to·por'phy·rin
pro·to·por'phy·ri·nu'ri·a
pro·to·pro'te·ose'
pro·top'sis
pro'to·spasm
pro·to·sul'fate'
pro·to·syph'i·lis
pro'to·troph'
pro·to·troph'ic
pro·tot'ro·py
pro'to·type'
pro'to·ver'a·trine'
pro'to·ver·ine'
pro'to·ver'te·bra
pro'to·ver'te·bral
pro·tox'ide'
pro·tox'in
Pro'to·zo'a
pro'to·zo'a·cide'
pro'to·zo'al
pro'to·zo'an
pro'to·zo·i'a·sis *pl.* -ses'
pro'to·zo·ol'o·gist
pro'to·zo·ol'o·gy

pro'to·zo'on' *pl.* -zo'a
pro'to·zo'o·phage'
pro·tract'
pro·trac'tion
pro·trac'tor
pro·trip'ty·line'
pro·trude', -trud'ed,
  -trud'ing
pro·tru'si·o' ac'e·tab'u·li'
pro·tru'sion
pro·tru'sive
pro·tryp'sin
pro·tu'ber·ance
pro·tu'ber·ant
pro·tu'be·ran'ti·a
  —men·ta'lis
  —oc·cip'i·ta'lis ex·ter'na
  —occipitalis in·ter'na
Proust'-Licht'heim'
  maneuver
pro·ven'tri·cule'
pro·ven·tric'u·lus *pl.* -li'
Prov'i·den'ci·a rett'ge·ri
pro·vi'ral
pro·vi'rus
pro·vi'sion·al
pro·vi'ta·min
pro·vi'sion·al
pro·voc'a·tive
Pro'wa·zek bodies
Prow'er factor
prox'a·zole'
prox'i·mad'
prox'i·mal
prox'i·ma'lis
prox'i·mal·ly
prox'i·mate
prox'i·mo·a·tax'i·a
prox'i·mo·buc'cal
prox'i·mo·la'bi·al
prox'i·mo·lin'gual
pro'zone'
pro'zy·go'sis
pru'i·nate'
pru·rig'i·nous
pru·ri'go'
  —aes'ti·va'lis
  —ag'ri·a
  —der'mo·graph'i·ca
  —fer'ox'
  —mi'tis
  —nod'u·lar'is
  —sim'plex'

pru·rit'ic
pru·ri'tus
  —a'ni'
  —hi'e·ma'lis
  —se·ni'lis
  —vul'vae'
Prus'sak'
  —fibers
  —pouch
Prus'sian blue
prus'si·ate'
prus'sic
Pryce method
psa'lis
psal·te'ri·al
psal·te'ri·um *pl.* -ri·a
psam'mism
psam·mo'ma *pl.* -mas *or*
  -ma·ta
psam·mom'a·tous
psam·mo·sar·co'ma
  pl. -mas *or* -ma·ta
psam'mous
psel'a·phe'si·a
psel'lism
psel'lis·mus mer·cu'ri·a'lis
pseud'a·cous'ma
pseud'a·graph'i·a
pseud·al·bu·mi·nu'ri·a
Pseud'al·les·che'ri·a
  boy'di·i'
pseud'am·ne'si·a
pseud·an·gi'na
pseud·an·ky·lo'sis *pl.* -ses'
pseud·ar·thri'tis
pseud·ar·thro'sis *pl.* -ses'
Pseu·dech'is
pseu·del'minth
pseu'des·the'si·a
pseu'do·ab'scess'
pseu'do·ac'an·tho'sis
  ni'gri·cans'
pseu'do·a·ceph'a·lus *pl.* -li'
pseu'do·ac·ro·meg'a·ly
pseu'do·ac'ti·no·my·co'sis
  pl. -ses'
pseu'do·ag·glu·ti·na'tion
pseu'do·a·gram'ma·tism
pseu'do·a·graph'i·a
pseu'do·al·bu·mi·nu'ri·a
pseu'do·al'lele'
pseu'do·al·lel'ism
pseu'do·al·ve'o·lar

pseu'do·a·ne'mi·a
pseu'do·an'eu·rysm
pseu'do·an·gi'na
pseu'do·an·gi·o'ma
pseu'do·an·o·rex'i·a
pseu'do·a·pha'ki·a
pseu'do·ap'o·plex'y
pseu'do·ap·pen'di·ci'tis
pseu'do·ar·thri'tis
pseu'do·ar·thro'sis *pl.* -ses'
pseu'do·as·ter'e·og·no'sis
pseu'do·a·tax'i·a
pseu'do·ath'er·o'ma
pseu'do·ath'e·to'sis
pseu'do·at'ro·pho·der'ma
  col'li'
pseu'do·ba·cil'lus *pl.* -li'
pseu'do·blep'si·a
pseu'do·blep'sis
pseu'do·bul'bar
pseu'do·car'ti·lage
pseu'do·car'ti·lag'i·nous
pseu'do·cast'
pseu'do·cele' *also*
  pseudocoele
pseu'do·ceph'a·lo·cele'
pseu'do·chan'cre
pseu'do·cho'le·cys·ti'tis
pseu'do·cho·les'te·a·to'ma
  pl. -mas *or* -ma·ta
pseu'do·cho·lin·es'ter·ase'
pseu'do·cho·re'a
pseu'do·chro'mes·the'si·a
pseu'do·chro'mi·a
pseu'do·chro'mo·some'
pseu'do·chy'lous
pseu'do·cir·rho'sis *pl.* -ses'
pseu'do·clau'di·ca'tion
pseu'do·co·arc'ta'tion
pseu'do·coele' *var. of*
  pseudocele
pseu'do·col'loid'
pseu'do·col'o·bo'ma
  pl. -mas *or* -ma·ta
pseu'do·cox·al'gi·a
pseu'do·cri'sis *pl.* -ses'
pseu'do·croup'
pseu'do·cryp'tor·chism
pseu'do·cy·e'sis *pl.* -ses'
pseu'do·cyl'in·droid'
pseu'do·cyst'
pseu'do·de·cid'u·a
pseu'do·de·men'ti·a

pseu′do·dex′tro·car′di·a
pseu′do·di′a·stol′ic
pseu′do·diph′the′ri·a
pseu′do·di′ver·tic′u·lum
pseu′do·dys′en·ter′y
pseu′do·e·de′ma
pseu′do·en·do·me·tri′tis
pseu′do·e·o·sin′o·phil′
pseu′do·e·phed′rine
pseu′do·ep′i·lep′sy
pseu′do·e·piph′y·sis
pseu′do·es·the′si·a
pseu′do·ex·fo′li·a′tion
pseu′do·ex′o·pho′ri·a
pseu′do·ex′oph·thal′mos
pseu′do·fluc′tu·a′tion
pseu′do·fol·lic′u·lar
pseu′do·frac′ture
pseu′do·gan′gli·on
pseu′do·gene′
pseu′do·geu′ses·the′si·a
pseu′do·geu′si·a
pseu′do·glan′ders
pseu′do·gli·o′ma
pseu′do·glob′u·lin
pseu′do·gon′or·rhe′a
pseu′do·gout′
pseu′do·gy′ne·co·mas′ti·a
Pseu′do·ha′je
pseu′do·hal·lu′ci·na′tion
pseu′do·haus·tra′tion
pseu′do·hem′i·car′di·us
pseu′do·he·mo·phil′i·a
pseu′do·her·maph′ro·dite′
pseu′do·her·maph′ro·dit′ic
pseu′do·her·maph′ro·dit·
 ism
pseu′do·her·maph′ro·di·
 tis′mus
—fem′i·ni′nus
—mas′cu·li′nus
pseu′do·hy′dro·ceph′a·ly
pseu′do·hy′dro·ne·phro′-
 sis pl. -ses′
pseu′do·hy′per·al·dos′ter·
 on·ism
pseu′do·hy′per·troph′ic
pseu′do·hy′per·tro′phy
pseu′do·hy′po·al·dos′ter·
 on·ism
pseu′do·hy′po·na·tre′mi·a
pseu′do·hy′po·par′a·thy′-
 roid·ism

pseu′do·il′e·us
pseu′do·in·farc′tion
pseu′do·i′so·chro·mat′ic
pseu′do·jaun′dice
pseu′do·ke′loid′
pseu′do·ker′a·tin
pseu′do·ker′a·to′sis pl. -ses′
pseu′do·leu·ke′mi·a
pseu′do·li·po′ma pl. -mas or
 -ma·ta
pseu′do·li·thi′a·sis pl. -ses′
pseu′do·lo′gi·a fan·tas′ti·ca
pseu′do·lux·a′tion
pseu′do·lym·pho′ma pl.
 -mas or -ma·ta
pseu′do·ma·lar′i·a
pseu′do·mam′ma
pseu′do·ma′ni·a
pseu′do·mel′a·no′sis
 pl. -ses′
pseu′do·mem′brane′
pseu′do·mem′bra·nous
pseu′do·men′in·gi′tis
pseu′do·men′stru·a′tion
pseu′do·met·he′mo·glo′bin
pseu′do·mi′cro·ceph′a·ly
pseu′dom·ne′si·a
pseu′do·mo′nad′
Pseu′do·mo′na·da·ce·ae′
Pseu′do·mo′nas
—ae·ru′gi·no′sa
—mal′to·phil′i·a
—pseu′do·mal′le·i′
—py′o·cy·a′ne·a
pseu′do·mu′cin
pseu′do·mu′cin·ous
pseu′do·my′as·then′ic
pseu′do·myx·o′ma pl. -mas
 or -ma·ta
—per′i·to·ne′i′
pseu′do·myx·om′a·tous
pseu′do·nar′co·tism
pseu′do·ne′o·plasm
pseu′do·ne′o·plas′tic
pseu′do·neu·ri′tis
pseu′do·neu·ro′ma pl.
 -mas or -ma·ta
pseu′do·nu′cle·o′lus pl. -li′
pseu′do·nys·tag′mus
pseu′do-ob·struc′tion
pseu′do·oph·thal′mo·ple′-
 gi·a
pseu′do·os′te·o·ma·la′ci·a

pseu′do·pap′il·le·de′ma
pseu′do·pa·ral′y·sis pl. -ses′
pseu′do·par′a·ple′gi·a
pseu′do·par′a·site′
pseu′do·pa·re′sis pl. -ses′
pseu′do·pe′lade′
pseu′do·pep′tone′
pseu′do·per′i·car′di·al
pseu′do·per′i·to·ni′tis
pseu′do·pha′ki·a
pseu′do·pho′tes·the′si·a
Pseu′do·phyl·lid′e·a
pseu′do·ple′gi·a
pseu′do·pneu·mo′ni·a
pseu′do·pock′et
pseu′do·pod′
pseu′do·po′di·o·spore′
pseu′do·po′di·um pl. -di·a
pseu′do·pol′y·co′ri·a
pseu′do·pol′yp
pseu′do·pol′y·po′sis
 pl. -ses′
pseu′do·por′en·ceph′a·ly
pseu′do·preg′nan·cy
pseu′do·pseu′do·hy′po·
 par′a·thy′roid·ism
pseu·dop′si·a
pseu′do·psy′cho·path′ic
pseu′do·pte·ryg′i·um
 pl. -i′ums or -i·a
pseu′do·pto′sis pl. -ses′
pseu′do·ra′bies′
pseu′do·re·ac′tion
pseu′do·re·tar·da′tion
pseu′do·ret′i·ni′tis
—pig′men′to′sa
pseu′do·rhon′cus pl. -chi
pseu′do·rick′ets
pseu′do·ro·sette′
pseu′do·ru·bel′la
pseu′do·sar·co′ma pl. -mas
 or -ma·ta
pseu′do·scar′la·ti′na
pseu′do·scle·re′ma
pseu′do·scle·ro′sis pl. -ses′
—of West′phal′ and
 Strüm′pell
pseu′do·se′rous
pseu′do·small′pox′
pseu′dos′mi·a
pseu′do·sto′ma
pseu′do·stra·bis′mus
pseu′do·strat′i·fied

pseu'do·struc'ture
pseu'do·ta'bes'
pseu'do·tet'a·nus
pseu'do·tho'rax' *pl.* -rax'es
  or -ra·ces'
pseu'do·tin·ni'tus
pseu'do·tol'er·ance
pseu'do·trich'i·no'sis
  pl. -ses'
pseu'do·trun'cus
  ar·te'ri·o'sus
pseu'do·tu'ber·cle
pseu'do·tu·ber'cu·lo'sis
pseu'do·tu·ber'cu·lous
pseu'do·tu'mor
  —cer'e·bri'
pseu'do·tym'pa·ni'tes'
pseu'do·tym'pa·ny
pseu'do·ty'phoid'
pseu'do·u·re'mi·a
pseu'do·vac'u·ole'
pseu'do·vag'i·nal
pseu'do·ven'tri·cle
pseu'do·vom'it·ing
pseu'do·xan·tho'ma
  e·las'ti·cum
psi
psil'o·cin
psil'o·cy'bin
psi·lo'sis *pl.* -ses'
psit'ta·co'sis *pl.* -ses'
pso'as *pl.* -ai' *or* -ae'
psod'y·mus
pso·i'tis
pso'mo·pha'gi·a
pso'mo·phag'ic
pso·moph'a·gy
pso'ra·len
pso·ri'a·si·form'
pso·ri'a·sis *pl.* -ses'
  —buc·ca'lis
  —cir'ci·na'ta
  —dif·fu'sa
  —dis·coi'de·a
  —fol·lic'u·lar'is
  —gut·ta'ta
  —gy·ra'ta
  —in·vet'er·a'ta
  —num'mu·lar'is
  —or·bic'u·lar'is
  —pal·mar'is
  —punc·ta'ta
  —ru'pi·oi'des'

  —u'ni·ver·sa'lis
pso·ri'at'ic
psor'oph·thal'mi·a
Pso·rop'tes
psy'chal'gi·a
psy'chal'gic
psy'cha·go'gy
psy'cha'li·a
psych'as·the'ni·a
psych'as·then'ic
psych'a·tax'i·a
psych·au'di·to'ry
psy'che
psy'che·del'ic
psy'che·ism
psy'chi·at'ric
psy'chi·at'ri·cal
psy'chi·at'rics
psy·chi'a·trist
psy·chi'a·try
psy'chic
psy'chi·cal
psy'chics
psy'chi·no'sis *pl.* -ses'
psy'cho·a·cous'tic
psy'cho·a·cous'tics
psy'cho·ac'ti·va'tor
psy'cho·ac'tive
psy'cho·an·al'ge'si·a
psy'cho·a·nal'y·sis *pl.* -ses'
psy'cho·an'a·lyst
psy'cho·an'a·lyt'ic
psy'cho·an'a·lyt'i·cal
psy'cho·an'a·lyze'
psy'cho·au'di·to'ry
psy'cho·bi·o·log'ic *or*
  psy'cho·bi'o·log'i·cal
psy'cho·bi·ol'o·gist
psy'cho·bi·ol'o·gy
psy'cho·cor'ti·cal
psy'cho·cu·ta'ne·ous
psy'cho·del'ic
psy'cho·di·ag·no'sis
  pl. -ses'
psy'cho·di·ag·nos'tic
psy'cho·di·ag·nos'tics
Psy·cho'di·dae'
psy'cho·dom'e·ter
psy'cho·dom'e·try
psy'cho·dra'ma
psy'cho·dy·nam'ic
psy'cho·dy·nam'i·cal·ly
psy'cho·dy·nam'ics

psy'cho·gal·van'ic
psy'cho·gal'va·nom'e·ter
psy'cho·gen'e·sis *pl.* -ses'
psy'cho·ge·net'ic
psy'cho·gen'ic
psy·chog'e·ny
psy'chog·no'sis *pl.* -ses'
psy'chog·nos'tic
psy'cho·gram'
psy'cho·graph'ic
psy·chog'ra·phy
psy'cho·ki·ne'si·a
psy'cho·ki·ne'sis *pl.* -ses'
psy'cho·lag'ny
psy'cho·lep'sy
psy'cho·lep'tic
psy'cho·log'ic *or*
  psy'cho·log'i·cal
psy'cho·log'i·cal·ly
psy·chol'o·gist
psy·chol'o·gy
psy'cho·met'ric
psy'cho·me·tri'cian
psy'cho·met'rics
psy·chom'e·try
psy'cho·mo'tor
psy'cho·neu'ro·log'ic *or*
  psy'cho·neu'ro·log'i·cal
psy'cho·neu·ro'sis *pl.* -ses'
psy'cho·neu·rot'ic
psy'cho·nom'ic
psy'cho·nom'ics
psy'cho·pa·re'sis *pl.* -ses'
psy'cho·path'
psy'cho·path'i·a
  —chi·rur'gi·ca'lis
  —sex'u·a'lis
psy'cho·path'ic
psy'cho·path'o·log'ic *or*
  psy'cho·path'o·log'i·cal
psy'cho·pa·thol'o·gist
psy'cho·pa·thol'o·gy
psy'chop'a·thy
psy'cho·phar'ma·ceu'ti·cal
psy'cho·phar'ma·co·log'ic
  or psy'cho·phar'ma·co·
  log'i·cal
psy'cho·phar'ma·col'o·gy
psy'cho·pho'nas·the'ni·a
psy'cho·phys'i·cal
psy'cho·phys'ics
psy'cho·phys'i·o·log'ic *or*
  psy'cho·phys'i·o·log'i·cal

psy'cho·phys'i·ol'o·gy
psy'cho·ple'gi·a
psy'cho·ple'gic
psy'cho·rhyth'mi·a
psy'chor·rha'gi·a
psy'chor·rhex'is *pl.* -rhex'es'
psy'cho·sen·so'ri·al
psy'cho·sen'so·ry
psy'cho·sex'u·al
psy'cho·sine'
psy'cho·sis (*mental
  disorder*), *pl.* -ses'
  ♦*sycosis*
psy'cho·so'cial
psy'cho·so·mat'ic
psy'cho·sur'geon
psy'cho·sur'ger·y
psy'cho·sur'gi·cal
psy'cho·syn'the·sis *pl.* -ses'
psy'cho·tec'nics
psy'cho·ther'a·peu'tic
psy'cho·ther'a·peu'tics
psy'cho·ther'a·pist
psy'cho·ther'a·py
psy·chot'ic
psy·chot'o·gen
psy·chot'o·gen'ic
psy·chot'o·mi·met'ic
psy'cho·trop'ic
psy·chral'gi·a
psy'chro·es·the'si·a
psy'chrom'e·try
psy'chro·phil'ic
psy'chro·pho'bi·a
psy'chro·phore'
psy'chro·ther'a·py
psyl'li·um
ptar'mic
ptar'mus
ptel'e·or·rhine'
pter'i·dine'
pter'i·do·phyte'
pter'in
pter'i·on'
pte·ro'ic
pter'o·yl·glu·tam'ic
pte·ryg'i·al
pte·ryg'i·um *pl.* -i·ums *or*
  -i·a
  —col'li'
pter'y·goid'
pter'y·go·man·dib'u·lar
pter'y·go·max'il·lar'y

pter'y·go·pal'a·tine'
pter'y·go·pha·ryn'ge·us
pter'y·go·spi'nous
pti·lo'sis *pl.* -ses'
pto'maine'
ptosed
pto'sis *pl.* -ses'
  —i'ri·dis
  —sym'pa·thet'i·ca
ptot'ic
pty·al'a·gogue'
pty'a·lec'ta·sis *pl.* -ses'
pty'a·lin
pty'a·lism
pty'a·lith'
pty'a·lo·cele'
pty'a·lo·gen'ic
pty'a·log'ra·phy
pty'a·lo·li·thi'a·sis *pl.* -ses'
pty'a·lor·rhe'a
pty'a·lose'
pty·oc'ri·nous
pu'ber·tal
pu'ber·tas
  —ple'na
  —prae'cox'
  —pre'cox'
pu'ber·ty
pu'be·ru'lic
pu'be·ru·lon'ic
pu'bes'
pu·bes'cence
pu·bes'cent
pu'be·trot'o·my
pu'bic
pu'bi·ot'o·my
pu'bis
pu'bo·ad·duc'tor
pu'bo·cap'su·lar
pu'bo·cav'er·no'sus
pu'bo·coc·cyg'e·al
pu'bo·coc·cyg'e·us
pu'bo·fem'o·ral
pu'bo·per'i·to·ne·a'lis
pu'bo·pros·tat'ic
pu'bo·rec'tal
pu'bo·rec·ta'lis
pu'bo·scro'tal
pu'bo·tib'i·al
pu'bo·trans·ver'sa·lis
pu'bo·tu'ber·ous
pu'bo·ves'i·cal
pu'bo·ves'i·ca'lis

puck'er
pud'dling
pu'den·dag'ra
pu·den'dal
pu·den'dum *pl.* -da
  —fem'i·ni'num
  —mu'li·e'bre'
pu'dic
pu·er'i·cul'ture
pu·er'ile
pu·er'per·a *pl.* -ae'
pu·er'per·al
pu·er'per·al·ism
pu·er'per·ant
pu·er·pe'ri·um *pl.* -ri·a
Pue'stow pancreaticojeju-
  nostomy
Pu'lex'
  —ir'ri·tans'
Pu·lic'i·dae'
pu·li'cid'al
pu·li·cide'
pul'ley
pul'lu·late', -lat'ed, -lat'ing
pul'lu·la'tion
pul'mo *pl.* pul·mo'nes'
pul'mo·car'di·ac'
pul'mo·gas'tric
pul'mo·he·pat'ic
pul'mo·nal
pul'mo·nar'y
pul'mo·nate'
pul'mo·nec'to·my
pul·mon'ic
pul'mo·ni'tis
pul'mo·nol'o·gist
pul'mo·nol'o·gy
pul'mo'tor
pul'mo·vas'cu·lar
pulp
pul'pa
  —co'ro·na'le'
  —den'tis
  —li·e'nis
  —ra·dic'u·lar'is
pulp'al
pulp'ar
pul·pa'tion
pul·pec'to·my
pul'pe·fac'tion
pul·pi'tis *pl.* -pit'i·des'
pul'po·ax'i·al
pul'po·buc'co·ax'i·al

pul'po·dis'tal
pul'po·don'tics
pul'po·la·bi·al
pul'po·lin'gual
pul'po·lin'guo·ax'i·al
pul'po·me'si·al
pul·pot'o·my
pulp'stone'
pulp'y
pul'sate', -sat'ed, -sat'ing
pul'sa·tile
pul·sa'tion
pul'sa'tor
pulse, pulsed, puls'ing
pulse'less
pulse'less·ness
pul·sim'e·ter
pul'sion
pul'sus
—ab·dom'i·na'lis
—al'ter·nans'
—bi·fer'i·ens
—bi·gem'i·nus
—bis·fer'i·ens
—ce'ler
—celer et al'tus
—ce·ler'i·mus
—cor'dis
—deb'i·lis
—dif'fe·rens
—du'plex'
—du'rus
—fi'li·for'mis
—for'mi·cans
—for'tis
—fre'quens
—het'er·o·chron'i·cus
—in·con'gru·ens
—ir·reg'u·lar'is per·pet'u·us
—mag'nus
—mag'nus et ce'ler
—mol'lis
—mo·noc'ro·tus
—par'a·dox'us
—par'vus
—parvus et tar'dus
—ple'nus
—tar'dus
—tri·gem'i·nus
—vac'u·us
—ve·no'sus
pul·ta'ceous
pul'ver·i·za'tion

pul'ver·ize', -ized', -iz'ing
pul'ver·u·lent
pul·vi'nar
—thal'a·mi'
pul'vis
—an'ti·mo'ni·a'lis
pu'mex'
pum'ice
pump
pu'na
punch
punc'ta
—do'lo·ro'sa
—lac'ri·ma'li·a
—vas'cu·lo'sa
punc'tate'
punc'tat'ed
punc·tic'u·lum
punc'ti·form'
punc'tum pl. -ta
—ce'cum
—lac'ri·ma'le'
—prox'i·mum
—re·mo'tum
punc·tu'ra
—ex·plo'ra·to'ri·a
punc'ture, -tured, -tur·ing
pun'gent
Pun'ta To'ro fever
pu·nu'dos
pu'pa pl. -pae' or -pas
pu'pal (of a pupa)
  ◆pupil
pu'pil (a part of the eye)
  ◆pupal
pu·pil'la pl. -lae'
pu'pil·lar'y
pu'pil·la·to'ni·a
pu'pil·lo·con·stric'tor
pu'pil·lo·di·la'tor
pu'pil·lom'e·ter
pu'pil·lom'e·try
pu'pil·lo·mo'tor
pu'pil·lo·ple'gi·a
pu'pil·lo·sta·tom'e·ter
pu'pil·lo·to'ni·a
pu'pil·lo·ton'ic
pure
pur·ga'tion
pur'ga·tive
purge, purged, purg'ing
pu'ric
pu'ri·form'

pu'ri·fy', -fied', -fy'ing
pu'rine'
pu'ri·ne'mi·a
pu'ri·ne'mic
pu'ri·ty
Pur·kin'je
—cells
—corpuscle
—fibers
Pur·kin'je-San·son' images
Pur'mann method
pu'ro·hep'a·ti'tis pl. -tis·es
or -tit'i·des'
pu'ro·mu'cous
pu'ro·my'cin
pur'pu·ra
—an'nu·lar'is te·lan'gi·ec·
to'des'
—ful'mi·nans'
—hem'or·rhag'i·ca
—hy'per·glob'u·li·ne'mi·ca
—ne·crot'i·ca
—rheu·mat'i·ca
—se·ni'lis
—sim'plex'
—ur'ti·cans'
pur·pu'ric
pur'pu·rin
pur'pu·ri·nur'i·a
purr
purse'string'
pur·suit'
pu'ru·lence
pu'ru·len·cy
pu'ru·lent
pu'ru·loid'
pus
push'er
pus'tu·lant
pus'tu·lar
pus·tu·la'tion
pus'tule'
pus'tu·li·form'
pus'tu·lo·der'ma
pus'tu·lo'sis pl. -ses'
—pal·mar'is et plan·tar'is
pu·ta'men
Put'nam-Da'na syndrome
Put'nam sclerosis
pu'tre·fac'tion
pu'tre·fac'tive
pu'tre·fy', -fied', -fy'ing
pu·tres'cence

pu·tres′cent
pu·tres′cine′
pu′trid
pu′tro·maine′
Put′ti-Platt′ operation
Pu′us·sepp′
  —operation
  —reflex
py′ar·thro′sis *pl.* -ses′
py·ec′chy·sis *pl.* -ses′
py′e·lec′ta·si·a
py′e·lec′ta·sis *pl.* -ses′
py·el′ic
py′e·lit′ic
py′e·li′tis
  —cys′ti·ca
py′e·lo·cal′i·ce′al *or*
  py′e·lo·cal′y·ce′al
py′e·lo·cal′i·ec′ta·sis
  pl. -ses′
py′e·lo·cys·ti′tis
py′e·lo·cys′to·sto·mo′sis
  pl. -ses′
py′e·lo·gen′ic
py′e·lo·gram′
py′e·lo·graph′ic
py′e·log′ra·phy
py′e·lo·il′e·o·cu·ta′ne·ous
py′e·lo·li·thot′o·my
py′e·lom′e·try
py′e·lo·ne·phri′tis
py′e·lo·ne·phro′sis
py′e·lop′a·thy
py′e·lo·phle·bi′tis
py′e·lo·plas′ty
py′e·lo·pli·ca′tion
py′e·los′to·my
py′e·lot′o·my
py′e·lo·tu′bu·lar
py′e·lo·u·re′ter·al
py′e·lo·u·re′ter·ec′ta·sis
  pl. -ses′
py′e·lo·u′re·ter·ic
py′e·lo·u·re′ter·og′ra·phy
py′e·lo·u·re′ter·ol′y·sis
  pl. -ses′
py′e·lo·ve′nous
py·em′e·sis
py·e′mi·a
py·e′mic
py′en·ceph′a·lus
py·e′sis
py′gal

py·gal′gi·a
pyg·ma′li·on·ism
pyg′my
py′go·a·mor′phus
py′go·did′y·mus
py·gom′e·lus *pl.* -li′
py·gop′a·gus
py′ic
py′in
pyk·ne′mi·a
pyk′nic
pyk′no·cyte′
pyk′no·cy·to′ma *pl.* -mas *or*
  -ma·ta
pyk′no·cy·to′sis
pyk′no·dys·os·to′sis
  pl. -ses′
pyk′no·ep′i·lep′sy
pyk′no·lep′sy
pyk·nom′e·ter
pyk′no·mor′phous
pyk′no·phra′si·a
pyk·no′sis
pyk·not′ic
py′la *pl.* -lae′
py′lar
py′lem·phrax′is
py′le·phleb′ec·ta′si·a
py′le·phle·bec′ta·sis *pl.*
  -ses′
py′le·phle·bi′tis
py′le·throm′bo·phle·bi′tis
py′le·throm·bo′sis *pl.* -ses′
py′lic
py′lon′
py′lo·ral′gi·a
py′lo·rec′to·my
py·lor′ic
py·lo′ri·ste·no′sis
py′lo·ri′tis
py·lo′ro·col′ic
py′lo·ro·di′la·tor
py·lo′ro·di·o′sis *pl.* -ses′
py·lo′ro·du′o·de′nal
py·lo′ro·du′o·de·ni′tis
py·lo′ro·gas·trec′to·my
py·lo′ro·my·ot′o·my
py·lo′ro·plas′ty
py·lo′rop·to′si·a
py·lo′rop·to′sis
py·lo′ro·sche′sis *pl.* -ses′
py·lo′ros·co·py
py·lo′ro·spasm

py·lo′ro·ste·no′sis
py′lo·ros′to·my
py′lo·rot′o·my
py·lo′rus *pl.* -ri′ *or* -rus·es
py′o·ar·thro′sis *pl.* -ses′
py′o·blen′nor·rhe′a
py′o·ca′lix *pl.* -li·ces′
py′o·cele′
py′o·ce′li·a
py′o·ceph′a·lus
py′o·che′zi·a
py′o·coc′cus *pl.* -ci′
py′o·col′po·cele′
py′o·col′pos′
py′o·cul′ture
py′o·cy′a·nase′
py′o·cy·an′ic
py′o·cy′a·nin
py′o·cy′a·nol′y·sin
py′o·cy′a·no′sis *pl.* -ses′
py′o·cyst′
py′o·cys′tis
py′o·cyte′
py′o·der′ma
  —fa′ci·a′le′
  —gan′gre·no′sum
py′o·der·ma·ti′tis
py′o·der·ma·to′sis *pl.* -ses′
py′o·der′ma·tous
py′o·fe′ci·a
py′o·gen
py·og′e·nes′
py′o·gen′e·sis
py′o·ge·net′ic
py′o·gen′ic
py·og′e·nous
py′o·he′mi·a
py′o·he′mo·tho′rax′
py′oid′
py′o·lab′y·rin·thi′tis
py′o·me′tra
py′o·me·tri′tis
py′o·me′tri·um
py′o·my′o·si′tis
py′o·ne·phri′tis
py′o·neph′ro·li·thi′a·sis
  pl. -ses′
py′o·ne·phro′sis *pl.* -ses′
py′o·ne·phrot′ic
py′o·nych′i·a
py′o·o·var′i·um
py′o·per′i·car·di′tis
py′o·per′i·car′di·um

py′o·per′i·to·ne′um
py′o·per′i·to·ni′tis
py′o·pha′gi·a
py′oph·thal′mi·a
py′oph·thal·mi′tis
py′o·phy′lac′tic
py′o·phy′so·me′tra
py′o·pla′ni·a
py′o·pneu′mo·cyst′
py′o·pneu′mo·hep′a·ti′tis *p*
l. -tis·es *or* -tit′i·des′
py′o·pneu′mo·per′i·car·
di′tis
py′o·pneu′mo·per′i·car′-
di·um
py′o·pneu′mo·per′i·to·
ne′um
py′o·pneu′mo·per′i·to·
ni′tis
py′o·pneu′mo·tho′rax′
py′o·poi·e′sis *pl.* -ses′
py′o·poi·et′ic
py·op′ty·sis *pl.* -ses′
py′o·py′e·lec′ta·sis *pl.* -ses′
py′or·rhe′a
—al′ve·o·lar′is
py′or·rhe′al
py′o·sal′pin·gi′tis
py′o·sal·pin′go-
o′o·pho·ri′tis
py′o·sal′pinx *pl.* -sal·pin′ges′
py′o·scle·ro′sis *pl.* -ses′
py′o·sep′ti·ce′mi·a
py·o′sis
py′o·sper′mi·a
py′o·stat′ic
py′o·sto′ma·ti′tis
py′o·ther′a·py
py′o·tho′rax′ *pl.* -rax′es *or*
-ra·ces′
py′o·tox′i·ne′mi·a
py′o·um·bil′i·cus *pl.* -ci′ *or*
-cus·es
py′o·u′ra·chus
py′o·u′re′ter
py′o·ve·sic′u·lo′sis *pl.* -ses′
py′o·xan′thin
py′o·xan′those′
py′ra·hex′yl
pyr′a·mid
py·ram′i·dal
py·ram′i·da′le
py·ram′i·da′lis

—na′si′
py·ram′i·des′ re·na′les′
pyr′a·mi·dot′o·my
pyr′a·min
pyr′a·mis *pl.* py·ram′i·des′
—me·dul′lae′ ob′lon·ga′tae′
—ver′mis
—ves·tib′u·li′
py′ran
py′ra·nose′
py·ran′tel
pyr·a·zin′a·mide′
pyr′a·zine′
py·raz′o·lene′
py·rec′tic
py′rene
py′re·ne′mi·a
Py·re′no·chae′ta rom′er·oi′
py·reth′rins
py·reth′roid′
py·re′thrum
py·ret′ic
py·ret′o·gen
pyr·e·to·gen′e·sis
pyr·e·to·ge·net′ic
pyr·e·to·gen′ic
pyr·e·tog′e·nous
pyr·e·tol′o·gy
pyr·e·tol′y·sis *pl.* -ses′
pyr·e·to·ther′a·py
pyr′e·to·ty·pho′sis *pl.* -ses′
py·rex′i·a
py·rex′i·al
py·rex′ic
py·rex′in
py·rex′i·o·pho′bi·a
pyr′he·li·om′e·ter
pyr′i·dine′
pyr′i·do·stig′mine′
pyr′i·dox′al
pyr′i·dox′a·mine′
pyr′i·dox′ic
pyr′i·dox′i·lat′ed
pyr′i·dox′ine′
pyr′i·form′ *var. of* piriform
pyr·il′a·mine′
pyr′i·meth′a·mine′
pyr·rim′i·dine′
pyr·in′o·line′
pyr′i·thi′a·mine′
pyr′i·thi′one′
py′ro·cat′e·chin
py′ro·cat′e·chol′

py′ro·gal′lic
py′ro·gal′lol′
py′ro·gen
py′ro·ge·net′ic
py′ro·gen′ic
py′ro·glob′u·lin
py′ro·glob′u·lin·e′mi·a
py′ro·glos′si·a
py′ro·lag′ni·a
py′ro·lig′ne·ous
pyr·rol′y·sis *pl.* -ses′
py′ro·lyt′ic
py′ro·ma′ni·a
py′ro·ma′ni·ac′
py·rom′e·ter
py′rone′
py′ro·nine′
py′ro·nin′o·phil′ic
py′ro·pho′bi·a
py′ro·phos′pha·tase′
py′ro·phos′phate′
py′ro·phos′pho·ki′nase′
py′ro·phos′phor′ic
py′ro·phos′pho·trans′fer·
ase′
py·rop′to·thy′mi·a
py′ro·punc′ture
py′ro·scope′
py·ro′sis
py·rot′ic
py′ro·tox′in
py′ro·va·ler′one′
py·rox′a·mine′
py·rox′y·lin
pyr′ro·bu′ta·mine′
pyr′ro·caine′
pyr′role′
pyr·rol′i·done′
pyr·rol′i·phene′
pyr·rol·ni′trin
pyr′ro·lo·por·phyr′i·a
py′ru·vate′
py·ru′vic
pyr·vin′i·um pam′o·ate′
py′tho·gen′ic
py·u′ri·a
py·u′ric

Q

quack
quack′er·y
quad′ran′gle

qua·dran′gu·lar
quad′rant
quad′ran·ta·no′pi·a
quad·ran′tic
quad′rate′
quad′ra·ture
qua·dra′tus *pl.* -ti′
  —fem′o·ris
  —la′bi·i′ in·fe′ri·o′ris
  —labii su·pe′ri·o′ris
  —lum·bo′rum
  —men′ti′
quad′ri·ceps′
  —fem′o·ris
  —su′rae′
quad′ri·ceps′plas·ty
quad′ri·cus′pid
quad′ri·gem′i·na
quad′ri·gem′i·nal
quad′ri·lat′er·al
qua·drip′a·ra
quad′ri·pa·re′sis *pl.* -ses′
quad′ri·par′i·ty
qua·drip′a·rous
quad′ri·ple′gi·a
quad′ri·ple′gic
quad′ri·tu·ber′cu·lar
quad′ri·va′lence
quad′ri·va′lent
quad·ru′ple
quad·ru′plet
Quain
  —degeneration
  —fatty heart
qual′i·ta′tive
qual′i·ty
quan′tal
quan′ta·some′
quan·tim′e·ter
quan′ti·ta′tive
quan′ti·ty
quan′tum *pl.* -ta
  —lib′et
  —plac′et
  —sat′is
  —suf′fi·cit
  —vis
quar′an·tine′, -tined′,
  -tin′ing
quart
quar′tan
quar′ter
quar′tile′

quar·tip′a·ra
quar·tip′a·rous
quar·ti·ster′nal
quartz
qua·si·crys′tal
qua·si·crys′tal·line′
qua·si·pe′ri·od′ic
qua′ter in di′e
qua′ter·nar′y
qua′ze·pam
qua′zo·dine′
quea′si·ness
quea′sy
que·bra′chine′
que·bra′cho
Queck′en·stedt′
  —sign
  —test
quench
Qué·nu′-Mu′ret′ sign
Qué·nu′ operation
que′nu·tho′ra·co·plas′ty
quer′ce·tin
quer′u·lent
Quer·vain′
  —disease
  —fracture
ques′tion
ques′tion·naire′
Quey·rat′ erythroplasia
quick
quick′en
quick′lime′
quick′sil′ver
Quick test
qui·es′cence
qui·es′cent
quin′a·crine′
quin′al·bar′bi·tone′
quin′al′dine′
quin′a·pril
quin·az′o·sin
quin′bo·lone′
Quinck′e
  —disease
  —edema
  —pulse
quin·dec′a·mine′
quin·do′ni·um
quin·es′trol′
quin·eth′a·zone′
quin·ges′ta·nol′
quin·ges′trone′

quin′i·dine′
qui′nine′
qui′nin·ism
quin′i·no·der′ma
quin′ism
Quin′lan test
quin′oid′
qui·nol′o·gy
quin′o·lone′
quin′one′
qui·no′vin
quin′o·vose′
Quin·quaud′
  —disease
  —phenomenon
quin′que·tu·ber′cu·lar
quin·qui′na
quin′sy
quin′tan
quin·ter′e·nol′
quin·tip′a·ra
quin·tip′a·rous
quin′ti·ster′nal
quin·tu′plet
quip′a·zine′
quo·tid′i·an
quo′tient

R

rab′bet·ing
rab′id
ra′bies′
ra′bi·form′
race
ra′ce·mase′
ra′ce·mate′
ra·ceme′
ra·ce·me·thi′o·nine′
ra·ce′mic
ra·ce′mi·za′tion
rac′e·mose′
ra′ce·phed′rine
ra′ce·phen′i·col′
ra·chi·al
ra·chi·al′gi·a
ra·chi·an·al′ge·si′a
ra·chi·an·es·the′si·a
ra′chi·cen·te′sis *pl.* -ses′
ra·chid′i·al
ra·chid′i·an
ra′chi·graph′
ra·chil′y·sis *pl.* -ses′

ra′chi·o·camp′sis *pl.* -ses′
ra′chi·o·cen·te′sis *pl.* -ses′
ra′chi·och′y·sis
ra′chi·o·dyn′i·a
ra′chi·o·ky·pho′sis *pl.* -ses′
ra′chi·om′e·ter
ra′chi·o·my′e·li′tis
ra′chi·op′a·thy
ra′chi·o·ple′gi·a
ra′chi·o·sco′li·o′sis *pl.* -ses′
ra′chi·o·tome′
ra′chi·ot′o·my
ra·chip′a·gus *pl.* -gi′
ra′chi·re·sis′tance
ra′chis *pl.* -chis·es *or*
    rach′i·des′
ra′chi·sag′ra
ra·chis′chi·sis *pl.* -ses′
ra·chit′ic
ra·chi′tis
ra·chi′tism
ra·chit′o·gen′ic
rach′i·tome′
ra·chit′o·my
ra′cial
rad
ra′dar·ky′mo·gram′
ra′dar·ky·mog′ra·phy
ra·dec′to·my
ra′di·a·bil′i·ty
ra′di·ad′
ra′di·al
ra′di·a′le *pl.* -a′li·a
ra′di·a′lis
ra′di·an
ra′di·ant
ra′di·ate′, -at′ed, -at′ing
ra′di·a′ti·o′ *pl.* -ti·o′nes′
    —a·cus′ti·ca
    —cor′po·ris cal·lo′si′
    —corporis stri·a′ti′
    —oc·cip′i·to·tha·lam′i·ca
    —op′ti·ca
ra′di·a′tion
rad′i·cal *(basic, extreme)*
    ♦*radicle*
ra′di·ces′
    —cra·ni·a′les′ ner′vi′
        ac′ces·so′ri·i′
    —spi·na′les′ ner′vi′
        ac′ces·so′ri·i′
    —sym·path′i·cae′ gan′gli·i′
        cil′i·ar′is

—vis′cer·a′les′ ve′nae′
    ca′vae′ in·fe′ri·o′ris
rad′i·cle *(a small root)*
    ♦*radical*
rad′i·cot′o·my
ra·dic′u·lal′gi·a
ra·dic′u·lar
ra·dic′u·lec′to·my
ra·dic′u·li′tis
ra·dic′u·lo·gan′gli·on·i′tis
ra·dic′u·lo·med′ul·lar′y
ra·dic′u·lo·me·nin′go·
    my′e·li′tis
ra·dic′u·lo·my′e·lop′a·thy
ra·dic′u·lo·neu·ri′tis
ra·dic′u·lo·neu·rop′a·thy
ra·dic′u·lop′a·thy
ra·dic′u·lo·sac·cog′ra·phy
ra′di·i′
    —len′tis
ra′di·o·ac·tin′i·um
ra′di·o·ac′tive
ra′di·o·ac·tiv′i·ty
ra′di·o·al′ler′go·sor′bent
ra′di·o·ar·te′ri·o·gram′
ra′di·o·au′to·gram′
ra′di·o·au′to·graph′
ra′di·o·au·tog′ra·phy
ra′di·obe′
ra′di·o·bi·cip′i·tal
ra′di·o·bi′o·log′i·cal
ra′di·o·bi·ol′o·gist
ra′di·o·bi·ol′o·gy
ra′di·o·cal′ci·um
ra′di·o·car′bon
ra′di·o·car′ci·no·gen′e·
    sis *pl.* -ses′
ra′di·o·car′di·o·gram′
ra′di·o·car′di·og′ra·phy
ra′di·o·car′pal
ra′di·o·car′pus *pl.* -pi′
ra′di·o·chem′is·try
ra′di·o·cin′e·mat′o·graph′
ra′di·o·co′balt′
ra′di·o·col′loid′
ra′di·o·cur′a·ble
ra′di·o·cys·ti′tis
ra′di·ode′
ra′di·o·dense′
ra′di·o·der′ma·ti′tis
ra′di·o·di·ag·no′sis *pl.* -ses′
ra′di·o·di·ag·nos′tic
ra′di·o·dig′i·tal

ra′di·o·don′ti·a
ra′di·o·don′tics
ra′di·o·don′tist
ra′di·o·e·col′o·gy
ra′di·o·el′e·ment
ra′di·o·en·ceph′a·lo·gram′
ra′di·o·en·ceph′a·log′ra·
    phy
ra′di·o·fre′quen·cy
ra′di·o·gen′ic
ra′di·o·gold′
ra′di·o·gram′
ra′di·o·graph′
ra′di·og′ra·pher
ra′di·o·graph′ic
ra′di·o·graph′i·cal·ly
ra′di·og′ra·phy
ra′di·o·hu′mer·al
ra′di·o·im′mu·ni·ty
ra′di·o·im′mu·no·as′say
ra′di·o·im′mu·no·de·tec′-
    tion
ra′di·o·im′mu·no·e·lec′tro·
    pho·re′sis
ra′di·o·im′mu·no·scin·tig′-
    ra·phy
ra′di·o·i′o·dine′
ra′di·o·i′ron
ra′di·o·i′so·tope′
ra′di·o·ky′mog′ra·phy
ra′di·o·lead′
ra′di·o·log′ic
ra′di·o·log′i·cal
ra′di·o·log′i·cal·ly
ra′di·ol′o·gist
ra′di·ol′o·gy
ra′di·o·lu′cen·cy
ra′di·o·lu′cent
ra′di·o·lu′mi·nes′cence
ra′di·ol′y·sis *pl.* -ses′
ra′di·om′e·ter
ra′di·o·met′ric
ra′di·o·mi·crom′e·ter
ra′di·o·mi·met′ic
ra′di·o·ne·cro′sis
ra′di·o·ne·crot′ic
ra′di·o·neu·ri′tis
ra′di·o·ni′tro·gen
ra′di·o·nu′clide′
ra′di·o·pac′i·ty
ra′di·o·paque′
ra′di·o·pa·thol′o·gy
ra′di·o·pel·vim′e·try

ra·di·o·phar′ma·ceu′ti·cal
ra′di·o·phos′pho·rus
ra′di·o·po·ten′ti·a′tion
ra′di·o·prax′is
ra′di·o·pul′mo·nog′ra·phy
ra′di·o·re·cep′tor
ra′di·o·re·sis′tance
ra′di·o·re·sis′tant
ra′di·o·re·spon′sive
ra′di·o·scin·tig′ra·phy
ra′di·o·scin′ti·scan′
ra′di·os′co·py
ra′di·o·sen′si·tive
ra′di·o·sen′si·tiv′i·ty
ra′di·o·so′di·um
ra′di·o·ster′e·os′co·py
ra′di·o·stron′ti·um
ra′di·o·sur′ger·y
ra′di·o·te·lem′e·try
ra′di·o·ther′a·peu′tic
ra′di·o·ther′a·peu′tics
ra′di·o·ther′a·pist
ra′di·o·ther′a·py
ra′di·o·ther′my
ra′di·o·tox·e′mi·a
ra′di·o·trac′er
ra′di·o·trans·par′ent
ra′di·o·trop′ic
ra′di·o·tro′pism
ra′di·o·ul′nar
ra′di·um
ra′di·us *pl.* -di·i′ *or* -di·us·es
 —fix′us
ra′dix *pl.* -di·ces′ *or* -dix·es
 —anterior ner′vo′rum spi′na′li·um
 —a·or′tae′
 —ar′cus ver′te·brae′
 —brev′is gan′gli·i′cil′i·ar′is
 —clin′i·ca
 —coch′le·ar′is ner′vi′ a·cus′ti·ci′
 —den′tis
 —de·scen′dens ner′vi′ tri·gem′i·ni′
 —dor·sa′lis ner′vo′rum spi·na′li·um
 —fa′ci·a′lis
 —inferior an′sae′ cer′vi·ca′lis
 —inferior coch′le·ar′is
 —inferior ner′vi′ ves·tib′u·lo·coch′le·ar′is

 —lat′er·a′lis ner′vi′ me′di·a′ni′
 —lateralis trac′tus op′ti·ci′
 —lin′guae′
 —lon′ga gan′gli·i′ cil′i·ar′is
 —me′di·a′lis ner′vi′ me′di·a′ni′
 —medialis trac′tus op′ti·ci′
 —mes′en·ter′i·i′
 —mo′to′ri·a ner′vi′ tri·gem′i·ni′
 —na′si′
 —oc′u·lo·mo·to′ri·a gan′gli·i′ cil′i·ar′is
 —pe′nis
 —pi′li′
 —posterior ner′vi′ spi·na′lis
 —pul·mo′nis
 —sen·so′ri·a ner′vi′ tri·gem′i·ni′
 —superior an′sae′ cer′vi·ca′lis
 —superior ner′vi′ ves·tib′u·lo·coch′le·ar′is
 —superior ves·tib′u·lar′is
 —sym·path′i·ca gan′gli·i′ sub·max′il·lar′is
 —un′guis
 —ven′tra′lis ner·vo′rum spi′na′li·um
ra′don′
Ra·do·vi′ci reflex
Rae′der syndrome
raf′fi·nase′
raf′fi·nose′
rage
rag′o·cyte′
rag′weed′
Rail′li·e·ti′na
Rai′mist sign
Rai′ney corpuscle
raise, raised, rais′ing
Ra′ji cell assay test
rake
rale
râle
 —de re·tour′
 —mu·queux′
ra′mal
ra′mi′
 —ad pon′tem ar·te′ri·ae′ bas′i·lar′is

 —al′ve·o·lar′es′ su·pe′ri·o′res′ an·te′ri·o′res′ ner′vi in′fra·or′bi·ta′lis
 —alveolares superiores pos·te′ri·o′res′ ner′vi′ in′fra·or′bi·ta′lis
 —alveolares superiores posteriores nervi max′il·lar′is
 —a·nas′to·mot′i·ci′ ner′vi′ au·ric′u·lo·tem′po·ra′lis cum ner′vo′ fa′ci·a′li′
 —an·te′ri·o′res′ ar·te′ri·o′rum in′ter·cos′ta′li·um
 —anteriores ner′vo′rum cer′vi·ca′li·um
 —anteriores nervorum lum·ba′li·um
 —anteriores nervorum tho′ra·ca′li·um
 —ar·te′ri·o′si′ in′ter·lob′u·lar′es′ hep′a·tis
 —ar·tic′u·lar′es′ ar·te′ri·ae′ ge′nus de·scen′den·tis
 —articulares arteriae ge′nu su·pre′mae′
 —au·ric′u·lar′es′ an·te′ri·o′res′ ar·te′ri·ae′ tem′po·ra′-lis su′per·fi′ci·a′lis
 —bron′chi·a′les′ an·te′ri·o′res′ ner′vi′ va′gi′
 —bronchiales a·or′tae′ tho·ra′ci·cae′
 —bronchiales ar·te′ri·ae′ mam·mar′i·ae′ in·ter′nae′
 —bronchiales arteriae tho·ra′ci·cae′ in·ter′nae′
 —bronchiales bron·cho′rum
 —bronchiales hyp·ar·te′ri·a′les′
 —bronchiales ner′vi′ va′gi′
 —bronchiales pos·te′ri·o′res′ ner′vi′ va′gi′
 —bronchiales seg′men·to′-rum
 —buc·ca′les′ ner′vi′ fa′ci·a′lis
 —cal·ca′ne·i′ ar·te′ri·ae′ tib′i·a′lis pos·te′ri·o′ris
 —calcanei lat′er·a′les′ ar·te′ri·ae′ per′o·nae′ae′
 —calcanei laterales ner′vi′ su·ra′lis

—calcanei me′di•a′les′ ar•te′ri•
ae tib′i•a′lis pos•te′ri•o′ris
—calcanei mediales ner′vi′
tib′i•a′lis
—calcanei ra•mo′rum mal′-
le•o•lar′i•um lat′er•a′li•um
ar•te′ri•ae′ fib′u•lar′is
—calcanei ramorum
malleolarium lateralium
arteriae per′o•ne′ae′
—cap′su•lar′es′ ar•te′ri•ae′
re′nis
—car•di′a•ci′ cer′vi•ca′les′
in•fe′ri•o′res′ ner′vi′ va′gi′
—cardiaci cervicales su•pe′-
ri•o′res′ ner′vi′ va′gi′
—cardiaci in•fe′ri•o′res′
ner′vi′ rec′ur•ren′tis
—cardiaci su•pe′ri•o′res′
ner′vi′ va′gi′
—cardiaci tho•ra′ci•ci ner′vi′
va′gi′
—ca•rot′i•co•tym•pan′i•ci′
ar•te′ri•ae′ ca•rot′i•dis
in•ter′nae′
—ce•li′a•ci′ ner′vi′ va′gi′
—cen•tra′les′ ar•te′ri•ae′
cer′e•bri′ an•te′ri•o′ris
—centrales arteriae cerebri
me′di•ae′
—centrales arteriae cerebri
pos•te′ri•o′ris
—cho•roi′de•i′ pos•te′ri•o′-res′
ar•te′ri•ae′ cer′e•bri′
pos•te′ri•o′ris
—coe′li′a•ci′ ner′vi′ va′gi′
—com•mu′ni•can′tes′
—communicantes gan′gli•i′
sub′man•dib′u•lar′is cum
ner′vo′ lin•gua′li′
—communicantes ganglii
sub•max′il•lar′is cum
ner′vo′ lin•gua′li′
—communicantes ner′vi′
au•ric′u•lo•tem′po•ra′lis
cum ner′vo′ fa•ci•a′li′
—communicantes nervi
lin•gua′lis cum ner′vo′
hy′po•glos′so′
—communicantes ner•vo′-
rum spi•na′li•um
—cor′ti•ca′les′ ar•te′ri•ae′
cer′e•bri′ an•te′ri•o′ris

—corticales arteriae cerebri
me′di•ae′
—corticales arteriae cerebri
pos•te′ri•o′ris
—cu•ta′ne•i′ an•te′ri•o′res′
ner′vi′ fem′o•ra′lis
—cutanei anteriores
(pec′to•ra′les′ et ab•dom′i•
na′les′) ra•mo′rum an•te′-
ri•o′rum ar•te′ri•ar′um
in′ter•cos•ta′li•um
—cutanei ar•te′ri•ae′
man•mar′i•ae′ in•ter′nae′
—cutanei cru′ris me′di•a′les′
ner′vi′ sa•phe′ni′
—cutanei lat′er•a′les′ pec′-
to•ra′les′ et ab•dom′i•na′-
les′ ra•mo′rum an•te′ri•o′-
rum ar•te′ri•ar′um
in′ter•cos•ta′li•um
—den•ta′les′ ar•te′ri•ae′
al′ve•o•lar′is in•fe′ri•o′ris
—dentales arteriae alveolaris
su•pe′ri•o′ris pos•te′ri•o′-
ris
—dentales ar•te′ri•ar′um
al′ve•o•lar′i•um su•pe′ri•
o′rum an•te′ri•o′rum
—dentales in•fe′ri•o′res′
plex′us den•ta′lis in•fe′ri•
o′ris
—dentales su•pe′ri•o′res′
plex′us den•ta′lis su•pe′ri•
o′ris
—dor•sa′les′ ar•te′ri•ae′
in′ter•cos•ta′lis su•pre′-
mae′
—dorsales ar•te′ri•ar′um
in′ter•cos•ta′li•um pos•te′-
ri•o′rum (III-XI)
—dorsales lin′guae′
ar•te′ri•ae′ lin•gua′lis
—dorsales ner•vo′rum
cer′vi•ca′li•um
—dorsales nervorum
lum•ba′li•um
—dorsales nervorum
sa•cra′li•um
—dorsales nervorum
tho′ra•ci•co′rum
—du′o•de•na′les′ ar•te′ri•ae′
pan′cre•at′i•co•du′o•de•
na′lis su•pe′ri•o′ris

—duodenales arteriae
su′pra•du′o•de•na′les
su•pe′ri•o′res′
—ep′i•plo′i•ci′ ar•te′ri•ae′
gas′tro•ep′i•plo′i•cae′
dex′trae′
—epiploici arteriae gastro-
epiploicae si•nis′trae′
—e•soph′a•ge′i′ a•or′tae′
tho•ra′ci•cae′
—esophagei ar•te′ri•ae′
gas′tri•cae′ si•nis′trae′
—esophagei arteriae thy•
roi′de•ae′ in•fe′ri•o′ris
—esophagei ner′vi′ la•ryn′-
ge•i′ rec′ur•ren′tis
—fron•ta′les′ ar•te′ri•ae′
cer′e•bri′ an•te′ri•o′ris
—frontales arteriae cerebri
me′di•ae′
—gas′tri•ci′ an•te′ri•o′res′
ner′vi′ va′gi′
—gastrici ner′vi′ va′gi′
—gastrici pos•te′ri•o′res′
ner′vi′ va′gi′
—gin′gi•va′les′ in•fe′ri•o′-
res′ plex′us den•ta′lis
in•fe′ri•o′ris
—gingivales su•pe′ri•o′res′
plex′us den•ta′lis su•pe′-
ri•o′ris
—glan′du•lar′es′ ar•te′ri•ae′
fa•ci•a′lis
—glandulares arteriae
max′il•lar′is ex•ter′nae′
—glandulares arteriae thy′-
re•oi′de•ae′ in•fe′ri•o′ris
—glandulares arteriae
thyreoideae su•pe′ri•o′ris
—glandulares arteriae
thy•roi′de•ae′ in•fe′ri•o′ris
—glandulares gan′gli•i′
sub′man•dib′u•lar′is
—he•pat′i•ci′ ner′vi′ va′gi′
—in•fe′ri•o′res′ ner′vi′ cu•
ta′ne•i′ col′li′
—inferiores nervi trans•
ver′si′ col′li′
—in′gui•na′les′ ar•te′ri•ae′
fem′o•ra′lis
—in′ter•cos•ta′les′ an•te′ri•
o′res′ ar•te′ri•ae′ tho•ra′ci•
cae′ in•ter′nae′

—nasales posteriores inferiores (laterales) ner'vi' pal'a·ti'ni' an·te'ri·o'ris
—nasales posteriores su·pe'ri·o'res' lat·er·a'les' gan'gli·i' pter'y·go·pal'a·ti'ni'
—nasales posteriores superiores laterales ganglii sphe'no·pal'a·ti'ni'
—nasales posteriores superiores me'di·a'les' gan'gli·i' pter'y·go·pal'a·ti'ni'
—nasales posteriores superiores mediales ganglii sphe'no·pal'a·ti'ni'
—oc·cip'i·ta'les' ar·te'ri·ae' cer'e·bri' pos·te'ri·o'ris
—occipitales arteriae oc·cip'i·ta'lis
—oe·soph'a·ge'i' a·or'tae' tho'ra·ca'lis
—oesophagei ar·te'ri·ae' gas'tri·cae' si·nis'trae'
—oesophagei ner'vi' rec·ur·ren'tis
—oesophagei nervi va'gi'
—or·bi·ta'les' ar·te'ri·ae' cer'e·bri' an·te'ri·o'ris
—orbitales arteriae cerebri me'di·ae'
—orbitales gan'gli·i' pter'y·go·pal'a·ti'ni'
—orbitales ganglii sphe'no·pal'a·ti'ni'
—pal'pe·bra'les' in·fe'ri·o'res' ner'vi' in·fra·or·bi·ta'lis
—palpebrales ner'vi' in'fra·troch'le·ar'is
—pan'cre·at'i·ci' ar·te'ri·ae' li'e·na'lis
—pancreatici arteriae pan'cre·at'i·co·du'o·de·na'lis su·pe'ri·o'ris
—pancreatici arteriae su'pra·du'o·de·na'les' su·pe'ri·o'res'
—pa·ri'e·ta'les' a·or'tae' ab·dom'i·na'lis
—parietales aortae tho'ra·ca'lis

—parietales ar·te'ri·ae' cer'e·bri' an·te'ri·o'ris
—parietales arteriae cerebri me'di·ae'
—parietales arteriae hy'po· gas'tri·cae'
—pa·rot'i·de'i' ar·te'ri·ae' tem'po·ra'lis su·per·fi'ci·a'lis
—parotidei ner'vi' au·ric'u·lo·tem'po·ra'lis
—parotidei ve'nae' fa·ci·a'lis
—pec'to·ra'les' ar·te'ri·ae' tho'ra·co·a·cro'mi·a'lis
—per'fo·ran'tes' ar·te'ri·ae' mam·mar'i·ae' in·ter'nae'
—perforantes arteriae tho'ra·ci'cae' in·ter'nae'
—perforantes ar·te'ri·ar'um met'a·car·pa'li·um vo·lar'i·um
—perforantes arteriarum met'a·car·pe·ar'um pal·mar'i·um
—perforantes arteriarum met'a·tar·sa'li·um plan·tar'i·um
—perforantes arteriarum met'a·tar·se·ar'um plan·tar'i·um
—per'i·car'di·a·ci' a·or'tae' tho'ra·ca'lis
—pericardiaci aortae tho·ra·ci·cae'
—per'i·ne·a'les' ner'vi' cu·ta'ne·i' fem'o·ris pos·te'ri·o'ris
—pha·ryn'ge·i' ar·te'ri·ae'
— pha·ryn'ge·ae' as'cen·den'tis
—pharyngei arteriae thy're·oi'de·ae' in·fe'ri·o'ris
—pharyngei arteriae thy·roi'de·ae' in·fe'ri·o'ris
—pharyngei ner'vi' glos'so·pha·ryn'ge·i'
—pharyngei nervi va'gi'
—phren'i·co·ab·dom'i·na'les' ner'vi' phren'i·ci'
—pos·te'ri·o'res' ar·te'ri·ar'um in·ter·cos·ta'li·um
—posteriores ner·vo'rum cer'vi·ca'li·um

—posteriores nervorum sa·cra'li·um
—posteriores nervorum tho'ra·ca'li·um
—pter'y·goi'de·i' ar·te'ri·ae' max'il·lar'is
—pterygoidei arteriae maxillaris in·ter'nae'
—pul'mo·na'les' sys·te'ma·tis au'to·nom'i·ci'
—pulmonales systematis sym·path'i·ci'
—re·na'les' ner'vi' va'gi'
—scro·ta'les' an·te'ri·o'res' ar·te'ri·ae' fem'o·ra'lis
—scrotales pos·te'ri·o'res' ar·te'ri·ae' pu·den'dae' in·ter'nae'
—spi·na'les' ar·te'ri·ae' cer'vi·ca'lis as'cen·den'tis
—spinales arteriae il'i·o·lum·ba'lis
—spinales arteriae in'ter·cos·ta'lis su·pre'mae'
—spinales arteriae ver'te·bra'lis
—ster·na'les' ar·te'ri·ae' mam·mar'i·ae' in·ter'nae'
—sternales arteriae tho·ra'ci·cae' in·ter'nae'
—ster'no·clei'do·mas'toi'de·i' ar·te'ri·ae' oc·cip'i·ta'lis
—stri·a'ti' ar·te'ri·ae' cer'e·bri' me'di·ae'
—sub·max'il·lar'es' gan'gli·i' sub·max'il·lar'is
—sub·scap'u·lar'es ar·te'ri·ae' ax'il·lar'is
—su·pe'ri·o'res' ner'vi' cu·ta'ne·i' col'li'
—superiores nervi trans·ver'si' col'li'
—su'pra·re·na'les' su·pe'ri·o'res' ar·te'ri·ae' phren'i·cae' in·fe'ri·o'ris
—tem'po·ra'les' ar·te'ri·ae' cer'e·bri' me'di·ae'
—temporales arteriae cerebri pos·te'ri·o'ris
—temporales ner'vi' fa·ci·a'lis
—temporales su'per·fi'ci·a'les' ner'vi' au·ric'u·lo·tem'po·ra'lis

—thy•mi•ci′ ar•te′ri•ae′
tho•ra′ci•cae′ in•ter′nae′
—ton′sil•lar′es′ ner′vi′
glos′so•pha•ryn′ge•i′
—tra•che•a′les′ ar•te′ri•ae′
thy•roi′de•ae′ in•fe′ri•o′ris
—tracheales ner′vi′ la•ryn′-
ge•i′ rec′ur•ren′tis
—tracheales nervi rec•ur•
ren′tis
—tra•che•a′lis ar•te′ri•ae′
thy′re•oi′de•ae′ in•fe′ri•o′-
ris
—u′re•ter′i•ci′ ar•te′ri•ae′
duc′tus def′e•ren′tis
—ureterici arteriae o•var′-
i•cae′
—ureterici arteriae re•na′lis
—ureterici arteriae tes•tic′u•
lar′is
—ven•tra′les′ ner′vo′rum
cer′vi•ca′li•um
—ventrales nervorum
lum•ba′li•um
—ventrales nervorum
sa•cra′li•um
—ventrales nervorum
tho•ra′ci•co′rum
—ves•tib′u•lar′es′ ar•te′ri•
ae′ au′di•ti′vae′ in•ter′nae′
—vestibulares arteriae
lab′y•rin′thi′
—vis•cer•a′les′ a•or′tae′
ab•dom′i•na′lis
—viscerales aortae
tho•ra•ca′lis
—viscerales ar•te′ri•ae′
hy′po•gas′tri•cae′
—zy′go•mat′i•ci′ ner′vi′
fa′ci•a′lis
ram′i•fi•ca′tion
ram′i•fy′, -fied′, -fy′ing
ram′i•pril
ram′i•sec′tion
ram′i•sec′to•my
ra′mose′
Ram′say Hunt syndrome
Rams′den eyepiece
Ram′stedt-Fre•det′
pyloromyotomy
Ram′stedt operation
ram′u•lus *pl.* -li′
ra′mus *pl.* -mi′

—ac′e•tab′u•lar′is ar•te′ri•
ae′ cir′cum•flex′ae′
fem′o•ris me′di•a′lis
—acetabularis arteriae
ob′tu•ra•to′ri•ae′
—ac′e•tab′u•li′ ar•te′ri•ae′
cir′cum•flex′ae′ fem′o•ris
me′di•a′lis
—a•cro′mi•a′lis ar•te′ri•ae′
su′pra•scap′u•lar′is
—acromialis arteriae tho•ra•
co•a•cro′mi•a′lis
—acromialis arteriae
trans•ver′sae′ scap′u•lae′
—al′ve•o′lar′is superior
me′di•us ner′vi′ in′fra•
or′bi•ta′lis
—a•nas′to•mot′i•cus
—anastomoticus ar•te′ri•ae′
me•nin′ge•ae′ me′di•ae′
cum ar•te′ri•a lac′ri•ma′li′
—anastomoticus gan′gli•i′
o′ti•ci′ cum chor′da tym′-
pa•ni′
—anastomoticus ganglii otici
cum ner′vo′ au′ric′-
u•lo•tem′po•ra′li′
—anastomoticus ganglii otici
cum nervo spi•no′so′
—anastomoticus ner′vi′
fa′ci•a′lis cum ner′vo′
glos′so•pha•ryn′ge•o′
—anastomoticus nervi facialis
cum plex′u tym•pan′i•co′
—anastomoticus nervi glos′-
so•pha•ryn′ge•i cum ra′mo′
au′ric′u•lar′i′ ner′vi′ va′gi′
—anastomoticus nervi
lac′ri•ma′lis cum ner′vo′
zy′go•mat′i•co′
—anastomoticus nervi
la•ryn′ge•i′ su•pe′ri•o′ris
cum ner′vo′ la•ryn′ge•o′
in•fe′ri•o′re′
—anastomoticus nervi
lin•gua′lis cum ner′vo′
hy′po•glos′so′
—anastomoticus nervi
me′di•a′ni′ cum ner′vo′
ul′nar′i′
—anastomoticus nervi va′gi′
cum ner′vo′ glos′so•pha•
ryn′ge•o′

—anastomoticus per′o•
nae′us
—anastomoticus ul•nar′is
ra′mi′ su′per•fi′ci•a′lis
ner′vi′ ra′di•a′lis
—anterior ar•te′ri•ae′
ob′tu•ra•to′ri•ae′
—anterior arteriae
rec′ur•ren′tis ul•nar′is
—anterior arteriae re•na′lis
—anterior arteriae thy′-
re•oi′de•ae′ su•pe′ri•o′ris
—anterior arteriae thy•roi′-
de•ae′ su•pe′ri•o′ris
—anterior as•cen′dens
ar•te′ri•ae′ pul′mo•na′lis
dex′trae′
—anterior ascendens arteriae pulmonalis si•nis′trae′
—anterior ascendens
fis′su′rae′ cer′e•bri′
lat′er•a′lis
—anterior de•scen′dens
ar•te′ri•ae′ pul′mo•na′lis
dex′trae′
—anterior descendens
arteriae pulmonalis
si•nis′trae′
—anterior duc′tus he•pat′-
i•ci′ dex′tri′
—anterior ho•ri•zon•ta′lis
fis′su′rae′ cer′e•bri′ lat′-
er•a′lis
—anterior ner′vi′ au′ric′-
u•lar′is mag′ni′
—anterior nervi cu•ta′ne•i′
an′te•bra′chi•i′ me′di•a′lis
—anterior nervi la•ryn′ge•i′
in•fe′ri•o′ris
—anterior nervi ob′tu•ra•to′-
ri•i′
—anterior nervi spi•na′lis
—anterior ra′mi′ cu•ta′ne•i′
lat′er•a′lis ner′vo′rum
tho•ra•ca′li•um
—anterior rami cutanei
lateralis rami an•te′ri•o′ris
ar•te′ri•ae′ in′ter•cos′ta′lis
—anterior sul′ci′ lat′er•a′lis
cer′e•bri′
—anterior ve′nae′ pul′mo•
na′lis su•pe′ri•o′ris
dex′trae′

—anterior venae pulmonalis
  superioris si·nis'trae'
—ap'i·ca'lis ar·te'ri·ae'
  pul'mo·na'lis dex'trae'
—apicalis arteriae pulmo-
  nalis si·nis'trae'
—apicalis lo'bi' in·fe'ri·o'ris
  ar·te'ri·ae' pul'mo·na'lis
  dex'trae'
—apicalis lobi inferioris
  arteriae pulmonalis
  si·nis'trae'
—apicalis ve'nae' pul'mo·
  na'lis in·fe'ri·o'ris
  dex'trae'
—apicalis venae pulmonalis
  inferioris si·nis'trae'
—apicalis venae pulmonalis
  su·pe'ri·o'ris dex'trae'
—ap'i·co·pos·te'ri·or ve'-
  nae' pul'mo·na'lis su·pe'-
  ri·o'ris si·nis'trae'
—as·cen'dens ar·te'ri·ae'
  cir'cum·flex'ae' fem'o·ris
  lat'er·a'lis
—ascendens arteriae circumflexae femoris me'di·a'lis
—ascendens arteriae circumflexae il'i·i' pro·fun'dae'
—ascendens arteriae
  trans·ver'sae' col'li
—ascendens sul'ci' lat'er·a'-
  lis cer'e·bri'
—au·ric'u·lar'is ar·te'ri·ae'
  au·ric'u·lar'is pos·te'ri·o'-
  ris
—auricularis arteriae
  oc·cip'i·ta'lis
—auricularis ner'vi' va'gi'
—ba·sa'lis an·te'ri·or ar·te'-
  ri·ae' pul'mo·na'lis dex'-
  trae'
—basalis anterior arteriae
  pulmonalis si·nis'trae'
—basalis anterior ve'nae'
  pul'mo·na'lis in·fe'ri·o'ris
  dex'trae'
—basalis anterior venae
  pulmonalis inferioris
  si·nis'trae'
—basalis lat'er·a'lis ar·te'-
  ri·ae' pul'mo·na'lis
  dex'trae'

—basalis lateralis arteriae
  pulmonalis si·nis'trae'
—basalis me·di·a'lis ar·te'-
  ri·ae' pul'mo·na'lis
  dex'trae'
—basalis medialis arteriae
  pulmonalis si·nis'trae'
—basalis posterior arteriae
  pulmonalis dex'trae'
—basalis posterior arteriae
  pulmonalis si·nis'trae'
—bron'chi·a'lis ep'ar·te'-
  ri·a'lis
—car·di·a·cus
—cardiacus ar·te'ri·ae'
  pul'mo·na'lis dex'trae
—ca·rot'i·co·tym·pan'i·cus
  ar·te'ri·ae' ca·rot'is
  in·ter'-nae'
—ca·rot'i·cus
—car'pe·us dor·sa'lis
  ar·te'ri·ae' ra'di·a'lis
—carpeus dorsalis arteriae
  ul·nar'is
—carpeus pal·mar'is
  ar·te'ri·ae' ra'di·a'lis
—carpeus palmaris arteriae
  ul·nar'is
—carpeus vo·lar'is
  ar·te'ri·ae' ra'di·a'lis
—carpeus volaris arteriae
  ul·nar'is
—cho·roi'de·us ar·te'ri·ae'
  cer'e·bri' pos·te'ri·o'ris
—cir'cum·flex'us ar·te'-
  ri·ae' co'ro·nar'i'ae'
  cor'dis si·nis'trae'
—circumflexus arteriae
  coronariae si·nis'trae'
—circumflexus fib'u·lae'
  ar·te'ri·ae' tib'i·a'lis pos·
  te'ri·o'ris
—cla·vic'u·lar'is ar·te'ri·ae'
  tho'ra·co·a·cro'mi·a'lis
—coch'le·ae' ar·te'ri·ae'
  au·di·ti'vae' in·ter'nae'
—coch'le·ar'is ar·te'ri·ae'
  lab'y·rin'thi'
—col·lat'er·a'lis ar·te'ri·
  ar'um in'ter·cos·ta'li·um
  pos·te'ri·o'rum (III-XI)
—col'li' ner'vi' fa'ci·a'lis
—com·mu'ni·cans'

—communicans ar·te'ri·ae'
  fib'u·lar'is
—communicans arteriae
  per'o·nae'ae'
—communicans arteriae
  per'o·ne'ae'
—communicans fib'u·lar'is
  ner'vi' fib'u·lar'is com·
  mu'nis
—communicans gan'gli·i'
  cil'i·ar'is cum ner'vo' na'-
  so·cil'i·ar'i'
—communicans ganglii o'ti·
  ci' cum chor'da tym'pa·ni'
—communicans ganglii otici
  cum ner'vi' au·ric'u·lo·
  tem'po·ra'li'
—communicans ganglii otici
  cum ra'mo' me·nin'ge·o'
  ner've' man·dib'u·lar'is
—communicans ner'vi'
  fa'ci·a'lis cum ner'vo'
  glos'so·pha·ryn'ge·o'
—communicans nervi facia-
  lis cum plex'u tym·pan'-
  i·co'
—communicans nervi
  glos'so·pha·ryn'ge·i' cum
  ra'mo' au·ric'u·lar'i'
  ner'vi' va'gi'
—communicans nervi
  lac'ri·ma'lis cum ner'vo'
  zy'go·mat'i·co'
—communicans nervi
  la·ryn'ge·i' rec·ur'ren'tis
  cum ra'mo' la·ryn'ge·o'
  in·ter'no'
—communicans nervi laryn-
  gei su·pe'ri·o'ris cum
  ner'vo' laryn'ge·o' in·fe'-
  ri·o're'
—communicans nervi
  lin·gua'lis cum chor'da
  tym'pa·ni'
—communicans nervi
  lingualis cum ner'vo'
  hy'po·glos'so'
—communicans nervi
  me·di·a'ni' cum ner'vo'
  ul·nar'i'
—communicans nervi
  na'so·cil'i·ar'is cum
  gan'gli·o' cil'i·ar'i'

—communicans nervi
spi·na′lis
—communicans nervi va′gi′
cum ner′vo′ glos′so·pha·
ryn′ge·o′
—communicans per′o·ne′us
ner′vi′ per′o·ne′i′ com·
mu′nis
—communicans ul·nar′is
ner′vi′ ra·di·a′lis
—cos·ta′lis lat′er·a′lis
ar·te′ri·ae′
mam·mar′i·ae′ in·ter′nae′
—costalis lateralis arteriae
tho·ra′ci·cae′ in·ter′nae′
—cri′co·thy′re·oi′de·us
ar·te′ri·ae′
thy′re·oi′de·ae′
su·pe′ri·o′ris
—cri′co·thy·roi′de·us
ar·te′ri·ae′ thy·roi′de·ae′
su·pe′ri·o′ris
—cu·ta′ne·us an·te′ri·or
ner′vi′ il′i·o·hy′po·gas′-
tri·ci′
—cutaneus anterior (pec′to·
ra′lis et ab·dom′i·na′lis)
ner′vi′ in·ter′cos·ta′lis
—cutaneus anterior
(pectoralis et
abdominalis) nervi
tho·ra′ci·ci′
—cutaneus lat′er·a′lis ar·te′-
ri·ar′um in·ter′cos·ta′-
li·um pos·te′ri·o′rum (III-
XI)
—cutaneus lateralis ner′vi′
il′i·o·hy′po·gas′tri·ci′
—cutaneus lateralis
(pec′to·ra′lis et ab·dom′-
i·na′lis) ner′vi′ tho·ra′-
ci·ci′
—cutaneus lateralis (pectoralis et abdominalis) ner·
vo′rum in·ter′cos·ta′li·um
—cutaneus lateralis ra′mi′
dor·sa′lis ar·te′ri·ar′um
in·ter′cos·ta′li·um pos·te′-
ri·o′rum (III-XI)
—cutaneus lateralis
ra·mo′rum dor·sa′li·um
ner·vo′rum tho·ra·ci·co′-
rum

—cutaneus lateralis ramo-
rum pos·te′ri·o′rum
ar·te′ri·ar′um in·ter′cos·
ta′li·um
—cutaneus lateralis ramo-
rum posteriorum ner·vo′-
rum tho·ra·ca′li·um
—cutaneus me·di·a′lis
ra′mi′ dor·sa′lis ar·te′ri·
ar′um in·ter′cos·ta′li·um
pos·te′ri·o′rum (III-XI)
—cutaneus medialis
ra·mo′rum dor·sa′li·um
ner·vo′rum
tho·ra′ci·co′rum
—cutaneus medialis ra·mo′-
rum pos·te′ri·o′rum
ar·te′ri·o′rum in·ter′cos·
ta′li·um
—cutaneus medialis
ramorum posteriorum
ner·vo′rum tho·ra·ca′-
li·um
—cutaneus ner′vi′ ob′tu·ra·
to′ri·i′
—cutaneus pal·mar′is
ner′vi′ ul·nar′is
—del′toi′de·us ar·te′ri·ae′
pro·fun′dae′ bra′chi·i′
—deltoideus arteriae
tho·ra·co·a·cro′mi·a′lis
—de·scen′dens anterior
ar·te′ri·ae′ co·ro·nar′i·ae′
cor′dis si·nis′trae′
—descendens ar·te′ri·ae′
cir′cum·flex′ae′ fem′o·ris
lat′er·a′lis
—descendens arteriae
oc·cip′i·ta′lis
—descendens arteriae
trans·ver′sae col′li′
—descendens cer′vi·cis
—descendens hy′po·glos′si′
—descendens ner′vi′ hy′po·
glos′si′
—descendens posterior
ar·te′ri·ae′ cor′o·nar′i·ae′
cordis dex′trae′
—dex′ter ar·te′ri·ae′
he·pat′i·cae′ pro′pri·ae′
—dexter arteriae pul′mo·
na′lis
—dexter ve′nae′ por′tae′

—di·gas′tri·cus ner′vi′
fa′ci·a′lis
—dor·sa′lis ar·te′ri·ae′
sub′cos·ta′lis
—dorsalis ar·te′ri·ar′um
in′ter·cos·ta′li·um
pos·te′ri·o′rum (III-XI)
—dorsalis arteriarum
lum·ba′li·um
—dorsalis ma′nus ner′vi′
ul·nar′is
—dorsalis ner′vi′ coc·
cyg′e·i′
—dorsalis nervi ul·nar′is
—dorsalis ner·vo′rum
spi·na′li·um
—dorsalis ve·nar′um
in′ter·cos·ta′li·um
—dorsalis venarum inter-
costalium pos·te′ri·o′rum
(IV-XI)
—ex·ter′nus ner′vi′
ac·ces·so′ri·i′
—externus nervi la·ryn′ge·i′
su·pe′ri·o′ris
—fem′o·ra′lis ner′vi′ gen′i·
to·fem′o·ra′lis
—fib′u·lar′is ar·te′ri·ae′
tib′i·a′lis pos·te′ri·o′ris
—fron·ta′lis ar·te′ri·ae′
me·nin′ge·ae′ me′di·ae′
—frontalis arteriae tem′po·
ra′lis su·per·fi′ci·a′lis
—frontalis ner′vi′ fron·ta′lis
—gen′i·ta′lis ner′vi′ gen′i·
to·fem′o·ra′lis
—hy·oi′de·us ar·te′ri·ae′
lin·gua′lis
—hyoideus arteriae thy′re·
oi′de·ae′ su·pe′ri·o′ris
—i·li′a·cus ar·te′ri·ae′
il′i·o·lum·ba′lis
—inferior ar·te′ri·ae′ glu′-
tae·ae′ su·pe′ri·o′ris
—inferior arteriae glu′te·ae′
su·pe′ri·o′ris
—inferior ner′vi′ oc′u·lo·
mo·to′ri·i′
—inferior os′sis is′chi·i′
—inferior ossis pu′bis
—in′fra·hy·oi′de·us ar·te′ri·
ae′ thy·roi′de·ae′ su·pe′ri·
o′ris

—in′fra·pat′el·lar′is ner′vi′
sa·phe′ni′
—in′ter′nus ner′vi′ ac′ces·
so′ri·i′
—internus nervi la·ryn′ge·i′
su·pe′ri·o′ris
—in′ter·ven·tric′u·lar′is
anterior ar·te′ri·ae′ co′ro·
nar′i·ae′ si·nis′trae′
—interventricularis posterior arteriae coronariae
dex′trae′
—lat′er·a′lis ar·te′ri·ae′ pul′-
mo·na′lis dex′trae′
—lateralis duc′tus he·pat′-
i·ci′ si·nis′tri′
—lateralis ner′vi′ su′pra·or′-
bi·ta′lis
—lateralis ra′mi′ pos·te′ri·
o′ris ner·vo′rum cer′vi·
ca′li·um
—lateralis rami posterioris
nervorum lum·ba′li·um
—lateralis rami posterioris
nervorum sa·cra′li·um et
ner′vi′ coc′cyg′e·i′
—lateralis ra·mo′rum
dor·sa′li·um ner·vo′rum
cer′vi·ca′li·um
—lateralis ramorum dorsa-
lium nervorum lum·ba′-
li·um
—lateralis ramorum dorsa-
lium nervorum sa·cra′li·
um et ner′vi′ coc′cyg′e·i′
—lin·gua′lis ner′vi′ fa·ci·a′-
lis
—lin′gu·lar′is ar·te′ri·ae′
pul′mo·na′lis si·nis′trae′
—lingularis inferior arteriae
pulmonalis sinistrae
—lingularis superior arteriae pulmonalis sinistrae
—lingularis ve′nae′ pul′mo·
na′lis su·pe′ri·o′ris si·nis′-
trae′
—lo′bi′ me′di·i′ ar·te′ri·ae′
pul′mo·na′lis dex′trae′
—lobi medii ve′nae′ pul′mo·
na′lis su·pe′ri·o′ris dex′-
trae′
—lum·ba′lis ar·te′ri·ae′
il′i·o·lum·ba′lis

—man·dib′u·lae′
—mar′gi·na′lis man·dib′u·
lae′ ner′vi′ fa·ci·a′lis
—mas·toi′de·us ar·te′ri·ae′
oc·cip′i·ta′lis
—me′di·a′lis ar·te′ri·ae′
pul′mo·na′lis dex′trae′
—medialis duc′tus he·pat′-
i·ci′ si·nis′tri′
—medialis ner′vi′ su′pra·
or′bi·ta′lis
—medialis ra′mi′ pos·te′ri·
o′ris ner·vo′rum cer′vi·
ca′li·um
—medialis rami posterioris
nervorum lum·ba′li·um
—medialis rami posterioris
nervorum sa·cra′li·um et
ner′vi′ coc′cyg′e·i′
—medialis ra·mo′rum
dor·sa′li·um ner·vo′rum
cer′vi·ca′li·um
—medialis ramorum dorsa-
lium nervorum lum·ba′-
li·um
—medialis ramorum dorsa-
lium nervorum sa·cra′li·
um et ner′vi′ coc′cyg′e·i′
—mem·bra′nae′ tym′pa·ni′
ner′vi′ au·ric′u·lo·tem′-
po·ra′lis
—membrane tympani nervi
me·a′tus au′di·to′ri·i′ ex·
ter′nae′
—me·nin′ge·us ac′ces·so′-
ri·us ar·te′ri·ae′ max·il′-
lae′
—meningeus ar·te′ri·ae′
oc·cip′i·ta′lis
—meningeus arteriae ver′te·
bra′lis
—meningeus me′di·us
ner′vi′ max·il·lar′is
—meningeus ner′vi′
man·dib′u·lar′is
—meningeus nervi spi·na′lis
—meningeus nervi va′gi′
—meningeus ner·vo′rum
spi·na′li·um
—mus′cu·lar′is
—mus′cu·li′ sty′lo·pha·ryn′-
ge·i′ ner′vi′ glos′so·pha·
ryn′ge·i′

—my′lo·hy·oi′de·us
ar·te′ri·ae′ al′ve·o·lar′is
in·fe′ri·o′ris
—mylohyoideus arteriae
max·il·lar′is in·ter′nae′
—na·sa′lis ex·ter′nus ner′vi′
eth′moi·da′lis an·te′ri·o′ris
—ob′tu·ra·to′ri·us ar·te′ri·
ae′ ep′i·gas′tri·cae′ in·fe′-
ri·o′ris
—oc·cip′i·ta′lis ar·te′ri·ae′
au·ric′u·lar′is pos·te′ri·o′-
ris
—occipitalis ner′vi′ au·ric′u·
lar′is pos·te′ri·o′ris
—os′sis is′chi·i′
—o·var′i·cus ar·te′ri·ae′
u′ter·i′nae′
—o·var′i·i′ ar·te′ri·ae′
u′ter·i′nae′
—pal′mar′is ner′vi′ me′di·
a′ni′
—palmaris nervi ul·nar′is
—palmaris pro·fun′dus
ar·te′ri·ae′ ul·nar′is
—palmaris su·per·fi′ci·a′lis
ar·te′ri·ae′ ra·di·a′lis
—pal′pe·bra′lis inferior
ner′vi′ in′fra·troch′le·ar′is
—palpebralis ner′vi′ in′fra·
troch′le·ar′is
—palpebralis superior nervi
infratrochlearis
—pa·ri′e·ta′lis ar·te′ri·ae′
me·nin′ge·ae′ me′di·ae′
—parietalis arteriae tem′po·
ra′lis su·per·fi′ci·a′lis
—pa·ri′e·to·oc·cip′i·ta′lis
ar·te′ri·ae′ cer′e·bri′ pos·
te′ri·o′ris
—per′fo·rans′ ar·te′ri·ae′
fib′u·lar′is
—perforans arteriae per′o·
nae′ae′
—perforans arteriae per′o·
ne′ae′
—per′i·car′di·a′cus ner′vi′
phren′i·ci′
—pe′tro·sus ar·te′ri·ae′
me·nin′ge·ae′ me′de·ae′
—petrosus su·per·fi′ci·a′lis
ar·te′ri·ae′ me·nin′ge·ae′
me′di·ae′

—pha·ryn′ge·us gan′gli·i′
pter′·go·pal′a·ti′ni′
—plan′tar′is pro·fun′dus
ar·te′ri·ae′ dor·sa′lis ped′is
—posterior ar·te′ri·ae′ ob′-
tu·ra·to′ri·ae′
—posterior arteriae pul′mo·
na′lis si·nis′trae′
—posterior arteriae rec·ur·
ren′tis ul·nar′is
—posterior arteriae re·na′lis
—posterior arteriae thy′re·
oi′de·ae′ su·pe′ri·o′ris
—posterior arteriae thy·roi′-
de·ae′ su·pe′ri·o′ris
—posterior as·cen′dens′
ar·te′ri·ae′ pul′mo·na′lis
dex′trae′
—posterior de·scen′dens′
ar·te′ri·ae′ pul′mo·na′lis
dex′trae′
—posterior duc′tus he·pat′-
i·ci′ dex′tri′
—posterior fis·su′rae′ cer′-
e·bri′ lat′er·a′lis
—posterior ner′vi′ au·ric′-
u·lar′is mag′ni′
—posterior nervi coc·
cyg′e·i′
—posterior nervi la·ryn′ge·i′
in·fe′ri·o′ris
—posterior nervi ob·tu·ra·
to′ri·i′
—posterior nervi spi·na′lis
—posterior ra′mi′ cu·ta′ne·i′
lat′er·a′lis ner′vi′ in′ter·
cos·ta′lis
—posterior rami cutanei lateralis (pec′to·ra′les′ et
ab·dom′i·na′les′) ra·mo′-
rum an·te′ri·o′rum ar·te′-
ri·ar′um in′ter·cos·ta′-
li·um
—posterior sul′ci′ lat′er·a′lis
cer′e·bri′
—posterior ve′nae′ pul′mo·
na′lis su·pe′ri·o′ris
dex′trae′
—pro·fun′dus ar·te′ri·ae′
cer′vi·ca′lis as·cen′den′tis
—profundus arteriae cir′-
cum·flex′ae′ fem′o·ris
me·di·a′lis

—profundus arteriae
glu·te·ae′ su·pe′ri·o′ris
—profundus arteriae
plan′tar′is me′di·a′lis
—profundus arteriae
trans·ver′sae′ col′li′
—profundus ner′vi′
plan·tar′is lat′er·a′lis
—profundus nervi ra·di·a′-
lis
—profundus nervi ul·nar′is
—profundus ra′mi′ vo·lar′is
ma′nus ner′vi′ ul·nar′is
—pu′bi·cus ar·te′ri·ae′ ep′i·
gas′tri·cae′ in·fe′ri·o′ris
—pubicus arteriae ob·tu·ra·
to′ri·ae′
—re·na′lis ner′vi′ splanch′-
ni·ci′ mi·no′ris
—sa·phe′nus ar·te′ri·ae′
ge′nus de·scen′dens
—saphenus arteriae ge′nu
su·pre′mae′
—si·nis′ter ar·te′ri·ae′
he·pat′i·cae′ pro′pri·ae′
—sinister arteriae pul′mo·
na′lis
—sinister ve′nae′ por′tae′
—si′nus ca·rot′i·ci′ ner′vi′
glos′so·pha·ryn′ge·i′
—spi′na′lis ar·te′ri·ae′
il′i·o·lum·ba′lis
—spinalis arteriae sub′cos·
ta′lis
—spinalis ar·te′ri·ar′um
lum·ba′li·um
—spinalis ra′mi′ dor·sa′lis
ar·te′ri·ar′um in′ter·cos·
ta′li·um pos·te′ri·o′rum
(III-XI)
—spinalis rami pos·te′ri·o′-
ris ar·te′ri·ae′ in′ter·cos·
ta′lis
—spinalis ve·nar′um in′ter·
cos·ta′li·um
—spinalis venarum intercos-
talium pos·te′ri·o′rum
(IV-XI)
—sta·pe′di·us ar·te′ri·ae′
sty′lo·mas·toi′de·ae′
—ster′no·clei′do·mas·toi′-
de·us ar·te′ri·ae′ thy·re·
oi′de·ae′ su·pe′ri·o′ris

—sternocleidomastoideus
arteriae thy·roi′de·ae′
su·pe′ri·o′ris
—sty′lo·hy·oi′de·us ner′vi′
fa·ci·a′lis
—sty′lo·pha·ryn′ge·us
ner′vi′ glos′so·pha·ryn′-
ge·i′
—sub·ap′i·ca′lis ar·te′ri·ae′
pul′mo·na′lis dex′trae′
—subapicalis arteriae pulmonalis si·nis′trae′
—sub·su·pe′ri·or ar·te′-
ri·ae′ pul′mo·na′lis
dex′trae′
—subsuperior arteriae
pulmonalis si·nis′trae′
—su′per·fi′ci·a′lis ar·te′-
ri·ae′ cir′cum·flex·ae′
fem′o·ris me′di·a′lis
—superficialis arteriae
glu·te·ae′ su·pe′ri·o′ris
—superficialis arteriae
plan·tar′is me′di·a′lis
—superficialis arteriae
trans·ver′sae′ col′li
—superficialis ner′vi′
plan·tar′is lat′er·a′lis
—superficialis nervi ra·di·
a′lis
—superficialis nervi ul·nar′is
—superficialis ra′mi′
vo·lar′is ma′nus ner′vi′
ul·nar′is
—superior ar·te′ri·ae′
glu·te·ae′ su·pe′ri·o′ris
—superior lo′bi′ in·fe′ri·o′ris
ar·te′ri·ae′ pul′mo·na′lis
dex′trae′
—superior lobi inferioris
arteriae pulmonalis si·
nis′trae′
—superior ner′vi′ oc′u·lo·
mo·to′ri·i′
—superior os′sis is′chi·i′
—superior ossis pu′bis
—superior ve′nae′ pul′mo·
na′lis in·fe′ri·o′ris dex′-
trae′
—superior venae pulmo-
nalis inferioris si·nis′trae′
—su′pra·hy·oi′de·us
ar·te′ri·ae′ lin·gua′lis

—sym·path'i·cus ad
    gan'gli·on' cil'i·ar'e'
—sympathicus ad ganglion
    sub·man·dib'u·lar'e'
—ten·to'ri·i' ner'vi' oph·
    thal·mi·ci'
—thy're·o·hy·oi'de·us
    ner'vi' hy'po·glos'si'
—thy'ro·hy·oi'de·us an'sae'
    cer'vi·ca'lis
—ton'sil·lar'is ar·te'ri·ae'
    fa'ci·a'lis
—tonsillaris arteriae
    max'il·lar'is ex·ter'nae'
—trans·ver'sus ar·te'ri·ae'
    cir'cum·flex'ae' fem'o·ris
    lat'er·a'lis
—transversus arteriae cir-
    cumflexae femoris me'di·
    a'lis
—tu'bae' plex'us tym·
    pan'i·ci'
—tu·bar'i·us ar·te'ri·ae'
    u'ter·i'nae'
—tubarius plex'us tym·
    pan'i·ci'
—ul'nar'is ner'vi' cu·ta'ne·i'
    an'te·bra'chi·i' me'di·a'lis
—ven·tra'lis ner·vo'rum
    spi·na'li·um
—vo·lar'is ma'nus ner'vi'
    ul·nar'is
—volaris ner'vi' cu·ta'ne·i'
    an'ti·bra'chi·i' me'di·a'lis
—volaris pro·fun'dus
    ar·te'ri·ae' ul·nar'is
—volaris su'per·fi'ci·a'lis
    ar·te'ri·ae' ra'di·a'lis
—zy'go·mat'i·co·fa'ci·a'lis
    ner'vi' zy'go·mat'i·ci'
—zy'go·mat'i·co·tem'po·ra'lis
    ner'vi' zy'go·mat'i·ci'
ran'cid
ran·cid'i·ty
ran'dom
ran'dom·i·za'tion
ran'dom·ize'
range, ranged, rang'ing
ra·ni·my'cin
ra'nine'
ra·ni'ti·dine'
Ran'ke
—angle

—hypothesis
—theory
Ran'kine scale
Ran'kin operation
Ran'son pyridine silver
    stain
ran'u·la
ran'u·lar
Ran·vier' node
Ra·oult' law
rape, raped, rap'ing
ra·pha'ni·a
raph'a·nin
ra'phe'
—inferior cor'po·ris cal·lo'si'
—me·dul'lae' ob·long·ga'-
    tae'
—pa·la'ti'
—palati du'ri'
—pal'pe·bra'lis lat'er·a'lis
—pe'nis
—per'i·ne'i'
—pha'ryn'gis
—pon'tis
—post'ob·lon·ga'ta
—pter'y·go·man·dib'u·lar'is
—scro'ti'
—superior cor'po·ris cal·
    lo'si'
rap'id
rap'port'
rap'tus *pl.* -ti'
rar'e·fac'tion
rar'e·fy', -fied', -fy'ing
ra'ri·tas
ra·sce'ta
rash
Rash'kind procedure
ra'sion
Ras'mus'sen aneurysm
rasp
ras'pa·to'ry
Ra·stel'li procedure
RAST test
rate, rat'ed, rat'ing
Rath'ke
—duct
—pouch
ra'ti·o'
ra'tion
ra'tion·al
ra'tion·ale'
ra'tion·al·i·za'tion

ra'tion·al·ize', -ized', -iz'ing
rat'tle, -tled, -tling
rat'tle-snake'
Rat'tus
Rau'ber cell
rau·ce'do
Rau·wol'fi·a
rau·wol'fine'
Ra·va·ton'
—amputation
—method
ray
Ray'leigh'
—equation
—scattering
—test
Ray mania
Ray·mond'-Ces·tan'
    syndrome
Ray·mond' syndrome
Ray·naud'
—disease
—phenomenon
—syndrome
rays of Sa·gnac'
re'ab·sorp'tion
re'ac·quired'
re·ac'tance
re·ac'tant
re·ac'tion
re·ac'ti·vate', -vat'ed, -vat'ing
re·ac'ti·va'tion
re·ac'tive
re'ac·tiv'i·ty
re·ac'tor
re·ad·mis'sion
re·ad·mit', -mit'ted, -mit'ting
re·a'gent
re·ag'gre·ga'tion
re·a'gin
re·a'gin·ic
re·al·gar'
re·a'lign'
re·a'lign'ment
re·al'i·ty
real'-time'
ream
ream'er
re·am'i·na'tion
re·am'pu·ta'tion
re·a·nas'to·mo'sis *pl.* -ses'
re·an'i·mate', -mat'ed,
    -mat'ing

re′ap·prox′i·mate′, -mat′ed,
   -mat′ing
re′at·tach′ment
Ré·au·mur′ scale
re·base′
re·bel′lion
re·bleed′
re·bound′ *n.*
re·bound′ *v.*
re·breath′ing
re·cal′ci·fi·ca′tion
re·cal′ci·fy′, -fied′, -fy′ing
re·cal′ci·trant
re·call′
Ré·ca·mier′ operation
re·can′al·i·za′tion
re·can′al·ize′
re·ca·pit′u·la′tion
re·ce′men·ta′tion
re·cep·tac′u·lum *pl.* -la
   —chy′li′
re·cep′tive
re·cep′to·ma *pl.* -mas *or*
   -ma·ta
re·cep′tor
re·cess′
   —of Tröltsch
re·ces′sion
re·ces′sive
re·ces′sus *pl.* re·ces′sus
   —anterior fos′sae′ in′ter·pe·
      dun′cu·lar′is
   —coch′le·ar′is ves·tib′u·li′
   —cos′to·di·a·phrag·mat′i·cus
      pleu′rae′
   —cos′to·me′di·as·ti·na′lis
      pleu′rae′
   —du·o·de·na′lis inferior
   —duodenalis superior
   —du·o·de·no·je·ju·na′lis
   —el·lip′ti·cus ves·tib′-
      u·li′
   —ep·i·tym·pan′i·cus
   —hep′a·to·re·na′lis
   —il·e·o·cae·ca′lis inferior
   —ileocaecalis superior
   —il·e·o·ce·ca′lis inferior
   —ileocecalis superior
   —inferior o′men·ta′lis
   —in·fun·dib′u·li′
   —in′ter·sig·moi′de·us
   —lat′er·a′lis fos′sae′
      rhom·boi′de·ae′

   —lateralis ven·tric′u·li
      quar′ti′
   —li′e·na′lis
   —mem·bra′nae′ tym′pa·ni′
      anterior
   —membranae tympani
      posterior
   —membranae tympani
      superior
   —op′ti·cus
   —par′a·co′li·ci′
   —par′a·du·o·de·na′lis
   —pha·ryn′ge·us
   —phren′i·co·he·pat′i·ci′
   —pin′e·a′lis
   —pir′i·for′mis
   —pleu·ra′les′
   —posterior fos′sae′ in′ter·
      pe·dun′cu·lar′is
   —ret′ro·cae·ca′lis
   —ret′ro·ce·ca′lis
   —ret′ro·du·o·de·na′lis
   —sac′ci·for′mis ar·tic′u·la′-
      ti·o′nis cu′bi·ti′
   —sacciformis articulationis
      ra′di·o·ul′nar′is dis·ta′lis
   —sphae′ri·cus
   —sphe′no·eth′moi·da′lis
   —sphe′ri·cus ves·tib′u·li′
   —sub′he·pat′i·ci′
   —sub·phren′i·ci′
   —sub′pop′lit′e·us
   —superior o′men·ta′lis
   —su′pra·pin′e·a′lis
   —tri·an′gu·lar′is
re·cid′i·va′tion
re·cid′i·vism
re·cid′i·vist
rec′i·div′i·ty
rec′i·pe′
re·cip′i·ent
re·cip′i·o·mo′tor
re·cip′ro·cal
re·cip′ro·ca′tion
rec′i·proc′i·ty
Reck′ling·hau′sen disease
rec′li·na′ti·o′
rec′li·na′tion
Re·clus′ disease
re·coil′ *n.*
re·coil′ *v.*
re·com′bi·nant
re·com′bi·na′tion

re·com′po·si′tion
re′com·pres′sion
re·con·di′tion
re·con·stit′u·ent
re·con′sti·tute′, -tut′ed,
   -tut′ing
re·con·sti·tu′tion
re·con·struc′tion
re·con·struc′tive
re·con·tour′
rec′ord *n.*
re·cord′ *v.*
re·cov′er
re·cov′er·y
rec′re·ment
rec′re·men′tal
rec′re·men·ti′tial
rec′re·men·ti′tious
re·cru·des′cence
re·cru·des′cent
re·cruit′ment
rec′tal
rec·tal′gi·a
rec·tal·ly
rec·tec′to·my
rec·ti·fi·ca′tion
rec′ti·fy′, -fied′, -fy′ing
rec·ti·lin′e·ar
rec·ti′tis
rec′to·ab·dom′i·nal
rec′to·a′nal
rec′to·cele′
rec·toc′ly·sis *pl.* -ses′
rec′to·coc·cyg′e·al
rec′to·coc·cyg′e·us *pl.* -e·i′
rec′to·co·li′tis
rec′to·co·lon′ic
rec′to·cu·ta′ne·ous
rec′to·cys·tot′o·my
rec′to·fis′tu·la
rec′to·gen′i·tal
rec′to·la′bi·al
rec′to·per′i·ne′al
rec′to·per′i·ne·or′rha·phy
rec′to·pex′y
rec′to·plas′ty
rec′to·rec·tos′to·my
rec′to·ro′man′o·scope′
rec·tor′rha·py
rec′to·scope′
rec·tos′co·py
rec′to·sig′moid′
rec′to·sig′moid·ec′to·my

rec′to·sig·moi′do·scope′
rec′to·sig·moi′do·scop′ic
rec′to·sig′moid·os′co·py
rec′to·ste·no′sis *pl.* -ses′
rec·tos′to·my
rec′to·tome′
rec·tot′o·my
rec′to·u·re′thral
rec′to·u′re·thra′lis
rec′to·u′ter·ine
rec′to·vag′i·nal
rec′to·vag′i·no·ab·dom′i·
  nal
rec′to·ves′i·cal
rec′to·ves′i·ca′lis
rec′to·ves·tib′u·lar
rec′to·vul′var
rec′tum *pl.* -tums *or* -ta
rec′tus
  —ab·dom′i·nis
  —ac′ces·so′ri·us
re·cum′ben·cy
re·cum′bent
re·cu′per·ate′, -at′ed, -at′ing
re·cu′per·a′tion
re·cu′per·a·tive
re·cur′, -curred′, -cur′ring
re·cur′rence
re·cur′rent
re′cur·va′tion
re′cur·va′tum
red
re·dif′fer·en′ti·a′tion
re·din′te·gra′tion
re′di·rect′
re′di·rec′tion
re·dis·trib′ute′
re·dis′tri·bu′tion
red′out′
re′dox′
re·dresse′ment
re·duce′, -duced′, -duc′ing
re·duc′i·ble
re·duc′tant
re·duc′tase′
re·duc′tic
re·duc′tion
re·duc′tone′
re·dun′dan·cy
re·dun′dant
re·du′pli·cate′, -cat′ed,
  -cat′ing
re·du′pli·ca′tion

re·du′vi·id
Red′u·vi′i·dae′
Re·du′vi·us
  —per′so·na′tus
Reed′-Stern′berg′ cell
re·ed′u·ca′tion
reef
reef′ing
Reen·stier′na
  —reaction
  —test
re·en′trant
re·en′try
re·ep′i·the′li·al·i·za′tion
re·ep′i·the′li·al·ize′, -ized′,
  -iz′ing
Rees and Eck′er fluid
re·e′val′u·ate′, -at′ed, -at′ing
re·e′val′u·a′tion
re·ev′o·lu′tion
re·ex·cise′, -cised′, -cis′ing
re·ex·ci·ta′tion
re′ex·pand′
re′ex·plo·ra′tion
re·fect′
re·fec′tion
re·fer′, -ferred′, -fer′ring
re·fer′ral
re·fill′, -filled′, -fill′ing
re·fine′, -fined′, -fin′ing
re·flect′
re·flec′tance
re·flect′ed
re·flec′tion
re·flec′tor
re′flex′
re·flex′i·o′
  —pal′pe·brar′um
re·flex·o·gen′ic
re·flex·og′e·nous
re′flex·o·graph′
re·flex·ol′o·gy
re·flex·om′e·ter
re·flex′o·ther′a·py
re′flux′
re·fract′
re·frac′ta do′si′
re·frac′tile
re·frac′tion
re·frac′tion·ist
re·frac′tive
re′frac·tiv′i·ty
re′frac·tom′e·ter

re′frac·tom′e·try
re·frac′tor
re·frac′to·ry
re·frac′ture, -tured, -tur·ing
re·fran′gi·bil′i·ty
re·fran′gi·ble
re·fresh′
re·frig′er·ant
re·frig′er·a′tion
re·frin′gence
re·frin′gent
Ref′sum
  —disease
  —syndrome
re·fu′sion
re·gain′er
Re·gaud′
  —fixing fluid
  —stain
re′gel
re·gen′er·a·ble
re·gen′er·ate′, -at′ed, -at′ing
re·gen′er·a′tion
re·gen′er·a·tive
Re′gen flexion exercises
reg′i·men
re′gi·o′ *pl.* re′gi·o′nes′
  —ab·dom′i·na′lis lat′er·a′lis
  —a·cro′mi·a′lis
  —a·na′lis
  —an′te·bra′chi·i′ anterior
  —antebrachii posterior
  —an′ti·bra′chi·i′ dor·sa′lis
  —antibrachii ra′di·a′lis
  —antibrachii ul′nar′is
  —antibrachii vo·lar′is
  —au·ric′u·lar′is
  —ax′il·lar′is
  —bra′chi·i′ anterior
  —brachii lat′er·a′lis
  —brachii me′di·a′lis
  —brachii posterior
  —buc·ca′lis
  —cal·ca′ne·a
  —cla·vic′u·iar′is
  —col′li′ anterior
  —colli lat′er·a′lis
  —colli posterior
  —cos·ta′lis lat·er·a′lis
  —cox′ae′
  —cru′ris anterior
  —cruris lat′er·a′lis
  —cruris me′di·a′lis

—cruris posterior
—cu′bi•ti′ anterior
—cubiti lat′er•a′lis
—cubiti me•di•a′lis
—cubiti posterior
—del′toi′de•a
—dor•sa′lis ma′nus
—dorsalis pe′dis
—ep′i′gas′tri•ca
—fem′o•ris anterior
—femoris lat′er•a′lis
—femoris me•di•a′lis
—femoris posterior
—fron•ta′lis
—ge′nu anterior
—genu posterior
—ge′nus anterior
—genus posterior
—glu′tae•a
—glu′te•a
—hy′oi′de•a
—hy′po•chon•dri′a•ca
—hypochondriaca (dex′tra
  et si•nis′tra)
—hy′po•gas′tri•ca
—in′fra•cla•vic′u•lar′is
—in′fra•mam•ma′lis
—in′fra•or•bi•ta′lis
—in′fra•scap′u•lar′is
—in′fra•tem′po•ra′lis
—in′gui•na′lis
—inguinalis (dex′tra et
  si•nis′tra)
—in′ter′scap′u•lar′is
—la′bi•a′lis inferior
—labialis superior
—la•ryn′ge•a
—lat′er•a′lis ab•dom′i•nis
  (dex′tra et si•nis′tra)
—lum•ba′lis
—mal′le•o•lar′is lat′er•a′lis
—malleolaris me•di•a′lis
—mam•ma′lis
—mam•mar′i•a
—ma•stoi′de•a
—me•di•a′na dor′si′
—men•ta′lis
—mes′o•gas′tri•ca
—na•sa′lis
—nu′chae′
—oc•cip′i•ta′lis
—o′le•cra′ni′
—ol′fac•to′ri•a

—olfactoria tu′ni•cae′
  mu•co′sae′ na′si′
—o′ra′lis
—or•bi•ta′lis
—pal′pe•bra′lis inferior
—palpebralis superior
—pa•ri•e•ta′lis
—par•o•tid′e•o•mas•se•ter′-
  i•ca
—pat′el•lar′is
—pec′to•ris anterior
—pectoris lat′er•a′lis
—per′i•ne•a′lis
—plan•tar′is pe′dis
—pu′bi•ca
—pu′den•da′lis
—re•spi′ra•to′ri•a
—ret′ro•mal′le•o•lar′is
  lat•er•a′lis
—retromalleolaris me•di•a′-
  lis
—sa•cra′lis
—scap′u•lar′is
—ster•na′lis
—ster′no•clei′do•mas•toi′-
  de•a
—sub′hy•oi′de•a
—sub•max′il•lar′is
—sub′men•ta′lis
—su′pra•or•bi•ta′lis
—su′pra•scap•u•lar′is
—su′pra•ster•na′lis
—su•ra′lis
—tem′po•ra′lis
—thy′re•oi′de•a
—tro′chan•ter′i•ca
—um•bil′i•ca′lis
—u′ro•gen′i•ta′lis
—ver′te•bra′lis
—vo′lar′is ma′nus
—zy′go•mat′i•ca

re′gion
re′gion•al
re′gi•o′nes′
—ab•dom′i•nis
—cap′i•tis
—col′li′
—cor′po•ris
—corporis hu•ma′ni′
—dig′i•ta′les′ ma′nus
—digitales pe′dis
—dor•sa′les′ dig′i•to′rum
—dorsales digitorum pe′dis

—dor′si′
—ex•trem′i•ta′tis in•fe′ri•o′-
  ris
—extremitatis su•pe′ri•o′ris
—fa′ci•e′i′
—mem′bri′ in•fe′ri•o′ris
—membri su•pe′ri•o′ris
—pec′to•ris
—plan•tar′es′ dig′i•to′rum
  pe′dis
—un′guic′u•lar′es′ ma′nus
—unguiculares pe′dis
—vo′lar′es′ dig′i•to′rum

reg′is•ter
reg′is•trant
reg′is•trar′
reg′is•tra′tion
reg′is•try
reg′nan•cy
re•gress′
re•gres′sion
re•gres′sive
reg′u•lar
reg′u•lar′i•ty
reg′u•late′, -lat′ed, -lat′ing
reg′u•la′tion
reg′u•la′tive
reg′u•la′tor
reg′u•la•to′ry
re•gur′gi•tant
re•gur′gi•tate′, -tat′ed,
  -tat′ing
re•gur′gi•ta′tion
re•ha•bil′i•tate′, -tat′ed,
  -tat′ing
re•ha•bil′i•ta′tion
re•ha•bil′i•ta′tive
re•ha•la′tion
Reh′fuss
—method
—tube
Reh′ne-De•lorme′
  operation
re•hy′drate′
re•hy′dra′tion
Rei′chel duct
Rei′chert
—cartilage
—membrane
Rei′chert-Meissl′ number
Reich′mann
—disease
—syndrome

Reich'stein' substance
Reid base line
Reil'ly bodies
re·im'plan·ta'tion
re'in·farc'tion
re'in·fec'tion
re'in·force', -forced', -forc'ing
re'in·force'ment
re'in·forc'er
re'in·fu'sion
Rein'ke crystalloids
re·in'ner·va'tion
re'in·oc'u·late', -lat'ed, -lat'ing
re'in·oc'u·la'tion
Reinsch test
re'in·sert'
re'in·ser'tion
re·in'te·gra'tion
re·in'tu·ba'tion
re'in·ver'sion
Reiss'ner membrane
Rei'ter syndrome
Reit'man-Fran'kel test
re·jec'tion
re·ju've·nate'
re·ju've·na'tion
re·ju've·nes'cence
re·lapse', -lapsed', -laps'ing
re·late', -lat'ed, -lat'ing
re·la'tion
re·la'tion·al
re·la'tion·ship'
rel'a·tive
rel'a·tiv·is'tic
re·lax'
re·lax'ant
re·lax·a'tion
re·lax'in
re·lease'
re·leas'er
re·lief'
re·lieve', -lieved', -liev'ing
re·line'
rem
Re'mak'
—band
—fibers
—ganglion
—reflex
re·me'di·a·ble
re·me'di·al
rem'e·dy

re·min'er·al·i·za'tion
re·mis'sion
re·mit'
re·mit'tence
re·mit'tent
rem'nant
re·mod'el, -mod'eled, -mod'el·ing
re·mote'
re·move'
ren pl. re'nes'
—mo'bi·lis
—un'gui·for'mis
re'nal
—os'te·i'tis fi·bro'sa gen·er·al·i·sa'ta
re·nat'u·ra'tion
Ren·du'-Os'ler-Web'er disease
Ren·du' tremor
ren'i·cap'sule
re·nic'u·lus pl. -li'
ren'i·fleur'
ren'i·form'
re'nin
ren'i·pel'vic
ren'net
ren·nin'o·gen
re'no·cor'ti·cal
re'no·cu·ta'ne·ous
re'no·gas'tric
re'no·gram'
re'no·in·tes'ti·nal
Ré·non'-De·lille' syndrome
re·nop'a·thy
re'no·pri'val
re'no·troph'ic
re'no·trop'ic
re'no·vas'cu·lar
Ren'shaw' cell
rent
re·or'gan·i·za'tion
re'o·vi'rus
re·ox'i·da'tion
re·pair'
re·par'a·tive
re·pa'ten·cy
re·peat'
re·pel'lent
re·pel'ler
re·per'co·la'tion
re'per·cus'sion
re'per·cus'sive

re'per·fuse', -fused', -fus'ing
re'per·fu'sion
re·per'i·to·ne'a·li·za'tion
re'pe·ta'tur
rep'e·ti'tion
re·phase', -phased', -phas'ing
re·place'ment
re'plan·ta'tion
re·plete'
re·ple'tion
rep'li·ca·ble
rep'li·case'
rep'li·cate', -cat'ed, -cat'ing
rep'li·ca'tion
re·po'lar·i·za'tion
re·port'
re·po'si·tion
re·pos'i·tor
re·pos'i·to'ry
re·prep'
re·pres'sion
re·pres'sor
re'pro·duce', -duced', -duc'ing
re'pro·duc'tion
re'pro·duc'tive
re'pro·duc'tive·ly
re·prox'i·ma'tion
Rep·til'i·a
re·pul'lu·la'tion
re·pul'sion
re·route'
res·az'u·rin
res'cue
re'search'
re·search'er
res·cin'na·mine'
re·sect'
re·sect'a·bil'i·ty
re·sect'a·ble
re·sec'tion
re·sec'to·scope'
re·ser'pine'
re·serve', -served', -serv'ing
res·er·voir'
res'i·den·cy
res'i·dent
re·sid'u·al
res'i·due'
re·sid'u·um pl. -u·a
re·sil'ience
re·sil'ien·cy
re·sil'ient

res'in
res'in·oid'
res'in·ous
re·sis'tance
re·sis'tant
re·so'cial·i·za'tion
res'o·lu'tion
re·solve', -solved', -solv'ing
re·sol'vent
res'o·nance
res'o·nant
res'o·na'tor
re·sorb'
re·sorb'ent
re·sor'cin
re·sor'cin·ism
re·sor'cin·ol'
re·sor'cin·ol·phthal'ein'
re·sorp'tion
re·sorp'tive
res'pi·ra·ble
res'pi·ra'tion
res'pi·ra'tor
res'pi·ra·to'ry
re·spire', -spired', -spir'ing
res'pi·rom'e·ter
res'pi·rom'e·try
re·sponse'
re·spon'si·bil'i·ty
rest
Res'tan fever
rest'bite'
re·ste·no'sis pl. -ses'
res'ti·bra'chi·um
res'ti·form'
res'tis pl. -tes'
res'ti·tu'ti·o' ad in'te·grum
res'ti·tu'tion
rest'less
rest'less·ness
res'to·ra'tion
re·stor'a·tive
re·store', -stored', -stor'ing
re·straint'
re·sul'tant
re·su'pi·nate', -nat'ed,
  -nat'ing
re·su'pi·na'tion
re·sus'ci·tate', -tat'ed,
  -tat'ing
re·sus'ci·ta'tion
re·sus'ci·ta'tor
re·su'ture, -tured, -tur'ing

re·sym'bol·i·za'tion
re·tain'
re·tain'er
re·tar'date'
re·tar'da'tion
re·tard'ed
re·tard'er
retch
re·te' pl. re'ti·a
—a·cro'mi·a'le'
—ar·te'ri·o'sum
—ar·tic'u·lar'e' cu'bi·ti'
—articulare gen'u
—articulare ge'nus
—cal·ca'ne·um
—ca·na'lis hy'po·glos'si'
—car'pi' dor·sa'le'
—cu'ta'ne·um
—dor·sa'le' pe'dis
—fo·ra'mi·nis o·va'lis
—mal'le·o·lar'e' lat·er·a'le'
—malleolare me'di·a'le'
—mi'ra·bi·le'
—mu·co'sum
—o'le·cra'ni'
—o'var'i·ti'
—pa·tel'lae'
—sub·pap'il·lar'e'
—tes'tis
—vas'cu·lo'sum
—ve·no'sum
—venosum dor·sa'le'
  ma'nus
—venosum dorsale pe'dis
—venosum plan·tar'e'
re·ten'tion
re·te·the'li·o'ma pl. -mas or
  -ma·ta
re·throm·bo'sis pl. -ses'
re'ti·a
—ve·no'sa ver'te·brar'um
re'ti·al
ret'i·cent
re·tic'u·lar
re·tic'u·late
re·tic'u·lat'ed
re·tic'u·la'tion
re·tic'u·lin
re·tic'u·li'tis
re·tic'u·lo·bul'bar
re·tic'u·lo·cyte'
re·tic'u·lo·cyt'ic
re·tic'u·lo·cy'to·pe'ni·a

re·tic'u·lo·cy·to'sis pl. -ses'
re·tic'u·lo·en·do·the'li·al
re·tic'u·lo·en·do·the'li·
  o'ma pl. -mas or -ma'ta
re·tic'u·lo·en·do·the'li·o'sis
  pl. -ses'
re·tic'u·lo·en·do·the'li·um
re·tic'u·lo·his'ti·o·cy·to'ma
  pl. -mas or -ma'ta
re·tic'u·lo·his'ti·o·cy·to'sis
re·tic'u·loid'
re·tic'u·lo'ma pl. -mas or
  -ma·ta
re·tic'u·lo·pe'ni·a
re·tic'u·lo·po'di·um
  pl. -di·a
re·tic'u·lo·sar·co'ma
  pl. -mas or -ma·ta
re·tic'u·lose'
re·tic'u·lo'sis pl. -ses'
re·tic'u·lo·spi'nal
re·tic'u·lo·the'li·a
re·tic'u·lo·the'li·o'ma
  pl. -mas or -ma·ta
re·tic'u·lo·the'li·um
re·tic'u·lum pl. -la
ret'i·fism
ret'i·form'
ret'i·na
ret'i·nac'u·la
—cu'tis
—un'guis
ret'i·nac'u·lum pl. -la
—cau·da'le'
—ex'ten·so'rum ma'nus
—flex'o'rum ma'nus
—lig'a·men'ti' ar'cu·a'ti'
—mus'cu·lo'rum ex'ten·so'-
  rum pe'dis in·fe'ri·us
—musculorum extensorum
  pedis su·pe'ri·us
—musculorum fib'u·lar'-
  i·um in·fe'ri·us
—musculorum fibularium
  su·pe'ri·us
—musculorum flex'o'rum
  pe'dis
—musculorum per'o'nae·
  o'rum in·fe'ri·us
—musculorum peronae-
  orum su·pe'ri·us
—musculorum per'o'ne·o'-
  rum in·fe'ri·us

—musculorum peroneorum su·pe′ri·us
—pa·tel′lae′ lat′er·a′le′
—patellae me′di·a′le′
ret′i·nal
ret′i·nene′
ret′i·ni′tis
—cir′ci·na′ta
—cir′cum·pap′il·lar′is
—dis′ci·for′mis
—ex·u′da·ti′va
—ne·phrit′i·ca
—pig′men·to′sa
—pro·lif′er·ans
—punc·ta′ta al·bes′cens
—se·ro′sa
—sim′plex′
ret′i·no·blas·to′ma *pl.* -mas *or* -ma·ta
ret′i·no·cho′roid′
ret′i·no·cho′roid·i′tis
—jux′ta·pap′il·lar′is
ret′i·no·cy·to′ma *pl.* -mas *or* -ma·ta
ret′i·no·di·al′y·sis *pl.* -ses′
ret′i·no·di·en·ce·phal′ic
ret′i·no′ic
ret′i·noid′
ret′i·nol′
ret′i·no·ma·la′ci·a
ret′i·no·pap′il·li′tis
ret′i·nop′a·thy
ret′i·no·pex′y
ret′i·nos′chi·sis *pl.* -ses′
ret′i·no·scope′
ret′i·no·scop′ic
ret′i·nos′co·py
ret′i·no·sis *pl.* -ses′
re·to·the′li·al
re·to·the′li·o′ma *pl.* -mas *or* -ma·ta
re·to·the′li·o·sar·co′ma *pl.* -mas *or* -ma·ta
re·to·the′li·um
re·tract′
re·trac′tile
re·trac·til′i·ty
re·trac′tion
re·trac′tor
re·trad′
re·treat′ment
re·trench′ment
ret′ro·ac′tion

ret′ro·ac′tive
ret′ro·an′ter·o·grade′
ret′ro·au·ric′u·lar
ret′ro·bron′chi·al
ret′ro·buc′cal
ret′ro·bul′bar
ret′ro·cal·ca′ne·al
ret′ro·cal·ca′ne·o·bur·si′tis
ret′ro·car′di·ac′
ret′ro·ca′val
ret′ro·ce′cal
ret′ro·cele′
ret′ro·cer′vi·cal
ret′ro·ces′sion
ret′ro·chei′li·a
ret′ro·cla·vic′u·lar
ret′ro·cli·na′tion
ret′ro·cline′
ret′ro·col′ic *(behind the colon)*
  ♦retrocollic
ret′ro·col′lic *(pertaining to the back of the neck)*
  ♦retrocolic
ret′ro·col′lis
ret′ro·con′dy·lism
ret′ro·cop′u·la′tion
ret′ro·cru′ral
ret′ro·cur′sive
ret′ro·de·vi·a′tion
ret′ro·dis·place′ment
ret′ro·du′o·de′nal
ret′ro·e·soph′a·ge′al
ret′ro·flex′
ret′ro·flexed′
ret′ro·flex′ion
ret′ro·gas·se′ri·an
ret′ro·gna′thi·a
ret′ro·gnath′ic
ret′ro·gnath′ism
ret′ro·grade′
re·trog′ra·phy
ret′ro·gres′sion
ret′ro·gres′sive
ret′ro·in′gui·nal
ret′ro·in′su·lar
ret′ro·jec′tion
ret′ro·jec′tor
ret′ro·len′tal
ret′ro·len·tic′u·lar
ret′ro·lin′gual
ret′ro·ma′lar
ret′ro·mam′ma·ry
ret′ro·man·dib′u·lar

ret′ro·mas′toid′
ret′ro·max′il·lar′y
ret′ro·mes′en·ter′ic
ret′ro·mo′lar
ret′ro·mor·pho′sis *pl.* -ses′
ret′ro·mo′tor
ret′ro·my′o·hy′oid′
ret′ro·na′sal
ret′ro·oc′u·lar
ret′ro·or′bi·tal
ret′ro·pa·rot′id
ret′ro·per′i·to·ne′al
ret′ro·per′i·to·ne′um *pl.* -ne′ums *or* -ne′a
ret′ro·per′i·to·ni′tis
ret′ro·pha·ryn′ge·al
ret′ro·phar′yn·gi′tis
ret′ro·phar′ynx
ret′ro·pla·cen′tal
ret′ro·pla′si·a
ret′ro·posed′
ret′ro·po·si′tion
ret′ro·pros·tat′ic
ret′ro·pu′bic
ret′ro·pul′sion
ret′ro·py·ram′i·dal
ret′ro·spect′
ret′ro·spec′tion
ret′ro·spec′tive
ret′ro·stal′sis *pl.* -ses′
ret′ro·ster′nal
ret′ro·tar′sal
ret′ro·ten′di·nous
ret′ro·thy′roid′
ret′ro·ton′sil·lar
ret′ro·tra′che·al
ret′ro·u′ter·ine
ret′ro·ver·si·o·flex′ion
ret′ro·ver′sion
ret′ro·vert′ed
ret′ro·ves′i·cal
ret′ro·vi′ral
Ret′ro·vi′ri·dae′
ret′ro·vi′rus
re·trude′, -trud′ed, -trud′ing
re·tru′sion
Ret′zi·us
—lines
—striae
—veins
re·un′ion
re·vac′ci·nate′, -nat′ed, -nat′ing

re·vac'ci·na'tion
re·vas'cu·lar·ize'
re·vas'cu·lar·i·za'tion
re·vel'lent
re·ver'ber·ate', -at'ed, -at'ing
re·ver'ber·a'tion
Re·ver·din' graft
re·ver'sal
re·verse', -versed', -vers'ing
re·vers'i·ble
re·ver'sion
re·ver'tant
Re·vil·liod' sign
re·vise', -vised', -vis'ing
re·vi'sion
re·vi'tal·i·za'tion
re·vive', -vived', -viv'ing
re·viv'i·fi·ca'tion
rev'o·lute'
re·vul'sant
re·vul'sion
re·vul'sive
re·warm'
Reye syndrome
Rh
—factor
—genes
Rhab·di'tis
Rhab'di·toi'de·a
rhab'do·cyte'
rhab'doid'
rhab'do·my'o·blast'ic
rhab'do·my'o·blas·to'ma
   pl. -mas *or* -ma·ta
rhab'do·my·ol'y·sis *pl.* -ses'
rhab'do·my·o'ma *pl.* -mas
   or -ma·ta
—u'ter·i'
rhab'do·my'o·sar·co'ma
   pl. -mas *or* -ma·ta
rhab'do·pho'bi·a
rhab'do·sar·co'ma *pl.* -mas
   or -ma·ta
rhab'do·vi'rus
rha·co'ma *pl.* -mas *or* -ma·ta
rha'cous
rhag'a·des'
rha·ga'di·a
rha·gad'i·form'
rhag'i·o·crine
rham'nose'
rham'no·xan'thin
rha·thy'mi·a

rhe
rhe'bo·sce'li·a
rhe'bo·sce'lic
rhe·bo'sis *pl.* -ses'
rheg'ma
rheg'ma·tog'e·nous
rhe'ni·um
rhe'o·base'
rhe'o·ba'sic
rhe'o·en·ceph'a·log'ra·phy
rhe'o·log'ic
rhe·ol'o·gist
rhe·ol'o·gy
rhe·om'e·ter
rhe·om'e·try
rhe'o·nome'
rhe'o·pex'y
rhe'o·stat'
rhe'os·to'sis
rhe'o·ta·chyg'ra·phy
rhe'o·tax'is *pl.* -tax'es'
rhe'o·trope'
rhe·ot'ro·pism
rhes'to·cy·the'mi·a
rheum
rheu'mar·thri'tis
rheu'ma·tal'gi·a
rheu·mat'ic
rheu'ma·tism
rheu'ma·tis'mal
rheu'ma·toid'
rheu'ma·to·log'ic
rheu'ma·tol'o·gist
rheu'ma·tol'o·gy
rhex'is *pl.* rhex'es'
rhi'nal
rhi·nal'gi·a
rhi'ne·de'ma *pl.* -mas *or*
   -ma·ta
rhi'nel'cos'
rhi'nen·ce·pha'li·a
rhi'nen·ce·phal'ic
rhi'nen·ceph'a·lon' *pl.* -la
rhi'nen·chy'sis *pl.* -ses'
rhi'nes·the'si·a
rhi'neu·ryn'ter
rhin·he'ma·to'ma
rhin'i·on'
rhi'nism
rhi·ni'tis
—sic'ca
rhi'no·an·tri'tis
rhi'no·by'on'

rhi'no·can·thec'to·my
rhi'no·ce·pha'li·a
rhi'no·ceph'a·lus *pl.* -li'
rhi'no·ceph'a·ly
rhi'no·chei'lo·plas'ty
rhi'no·clei'sis *pl.* -ses'
rhi'no·coele'
rhi'no·dac'ry·o·lith'
rhi'no·der'ma
rhi'no·dym'i·a
rhi·nod'y·mus
rhi'no·dyn'i·a
Rhi'no·es'trus
rhi·nog'e·nous
rhi'no·ky·pho'sis
rhi'no·la'li·a
   —a·per'ta
   —clau'sa
rhi'no·lar'yn·gi'tis
rhi'no·lar'yn·gol'o·gy
rhi'no·lith'
rhi'no·li·thi'a·sis *pl.* -ses'
rhi'no·log'ic
rhi·nol'o·gist
rhi·nol'o·gy
rhi'no·ma·nom'e·ter
rhi·nom'e·ter
rhi'no·mi·o'sis *pl.* -ses'
rhi'nom·mec'to·my
rhi'no·my·co'sis *pl.* -ses'
rhi'no·ne·cro'sis
rhi·nop'a·thy
rhi'no·pha·ryn'ge·al
rhi'no·phar'yn·gi'tis
   —mu'ti·lans'
rhi'no·pha·ryn'go·cele'
rhi'no·pha·ryn'go·lith'
rhi'no·phar'ynx
   pl. -pha·ryn'ges'
rhi'no·pho'ni·a
rhi'no·phy'co·my·co'sis
rhi'no·phy'ma
rhi'no·plas'tic
rhi'no·plas'ty
rhi'no·pneu·mo'ni·tis
rhi'no·pol'yp
rhi'no·pol'y·pus *pl.* -pi' *or*
   -pus·es
rhi·nop'si·a
rhi'nor·rha'gi·a
rhi'nor·rha·phy
rhi'nor·rhe'a
rhi'no·sal'pin·gi'tis

rhi·nos'chi·sis
rhi'no·scle·ro'ma *pl.* -ma·ta
rhi'no·scope'
rhi'no·scop'ic
rhi·nos'co·py
rhi'no·si'nus·i'tis
rhi'no·spo·rid'i·o'sis
  pl. -ses'
Rhi'no·spo·rid'i·um
  —see'ber'i'
rhi'no·ste·no'sis *pl.* -ses'
rhi'no·thrix'
rhi·not'o·my
rhi'no·tra'che·i'tis
rhi'no·vi'rus
Rhi'pi·ceph'a·lus
  —san·guin'e·us
rhi'zo·don'tro·py
rhi'zoid'
rhi'zome'
rhi'zo·mel'ic
rhi'zo·me·nin'go·my'e·
  li'tis
rhi'zo·mor'phoid'
Rhi'zo·mu'cor'
rhi'zo·neure'
rhi'zo·nych'i·a
rhi'zo·nych'i·um
Rhi·zop'o·da
rhi·zop'ter·in
Rhi'zo·pus
  —ni'gri·cans'
rhi·zot'o·my
Rh-neg'a·tive
rho'da·mine'
rho'da·nese'
rho·dan'ic
Rho'din fixative
rho'di·um
Rhod'ni·us
Rho'do·coc'cus
rho'do·gen'e·sis
rho'do·phy·lac'tic
rho'do·phy·lax'is
rho·dop'sin
rhom'ben·ce·phal'ic
rhom'ben·ceph'a·lon'
  pl. -la
rhom'bic
rhom'bo·coele'
rhom'boid'
rhom·boi'dal
rhom·boi'de·us *pl.* -de·i'

—oc·cip'i·ta'lis
rhom'bo·mere'
rhon'chal
rhon'chi·al
rhon'chus *pl.* -chi'
rho'phe·o·cy'to'sis *pl.* -ses'
rho'ta·cism
Rh-pos'i·tive
rhy'poph'a·gy
rhy'po·pho'bi·a
rhythm
rhyth'mic
rhyth'mi·cal
rhyth'mi·cal·ly
rhyth·mic'i·ty
rhyt'i·dec'tom·y
rhyt'i·do·plas'ty
rhyt'i·do'sis *pl.* -ses'
rib
ri·bam'i·nol'
ri'ba·vi'rin
rib'bon
ri'bi·tol'
ri'bo·des'ose'
ri'bo·fla'vin
ri'bo·nu'cle·ase'
ri'bo·nu·cle'ic
ri'bo·nu'cle·o·pro'tein'
ri'bo·nu'cle·o·side'
ri'bo·nu'cle·o·tide'
ri'bo·prine'
ri'bose'
ri'bo·side'
ri'bo·so'mal
ri'bo·some'
ri'bo·syl
ri'bo·zyme'
ri'bu·lose'
Ric·cò' law
rice
Rich'ter hernia
ri'cin
ri'cin·ism
ric'in·o'le·ate'
ric'in·o·le'ic
ric'in·o'le·in
Ric'i·nus
rick'ets
rick·ett'si·a *pl.* -ae' *or* -as
Rick·ett'si·a
  —ak'a·mu'shi
  —ak'a·ri'
  —aus·tra'lis

—bur·net'i·i'
—co·no'ri·i'
—di'a·po'ri·ca
—me·loph'a·gi'
—moo'ser·i'
—or'i·en·ta'lis
—pe·dic'u·li'
—pro'wa·zek'i·i'
—psit'ta·ci'
—quin·ta'na
—rick·ett'si·i'
—ru'mi·nan'ti·um
—si·be'ri·ca
—tsu'tsu·ga·mu'shi
—wol·hyn'i·ca
Rick·ett'si·a'ce·ae'
rick·ett'si·al
rick·ett'si·al·pox'
rick·ett'si·cid'al
rick·ett'si·o'sis *pl.* -ses'
rick·ett'si·o·stat'ic
rick'et·y
Ri·cord'
  —chancre
  —method
ric'tal
ric'tus
Rid'doch
  —mass reflex
  —syndrome
Rid'e·al-Wal'ker test
ri·deau'
ridge, ridged, ridg'ing
ridge'ling
Rie'del
  —disease
  —lobe
  —struma
Rie'der cell
Rie'gel
  —pulse
  —test
Rie'ger
  —anomaly
  —syndrome
Riehl melanosis
Ries'-Clark' operation
Ries'man
  —myocardosis
  —sign
Rieux hernia
rif'a·mide'
rif'am·pi·cin

rif'am·pin
rif'a·my'cin
Rift Val'ley fever
Ri'ga
—aphthae
—disease
Ri'ga-Fe'de disease
right'-eyed'
right'-foot'ed
right'-hand'ed
rig'id
ri·gid'i·tas
—ar·tic'u·lo'rum
—cad'a·ver'i·ca
ri·gid'i·ty
rig'or
—mor'tis
Ri'ley-Day' syndrome
rim, rimmed, rim'ming
ri'ma pl. -mae'
—cor'ne·a'lis
—glot'ti·dis
—o'ris
—pal'pe·brar'um
—pu·den'di'
—ves·tib'u·li'
—vul'vae'
ri·man'ta·dine'
ri'mose'
rim'u·la
rind'er·pest'
Rind'fleisch fold
ring
ring'bin'den
Ring'er
—injection
—lactate
—solution
ring'like'
ring'worm'
Rin'ne test
ri'no·lite'
Ri·o·lan'
—arc
—bone
—muscle
—ossicles
ri·par'i·an
Rip'stein procedure
risk
Ris'ley prism
ri·so'ri·us
ris'to·ce'tin

ri'sus
—ca·ni'nus
—sar·don'i·cus
Rit'gen maneuver
ri'to·drine'
Rit'ter disease
Rit'ter-Val'li law
rit'u·al
ri'val·ry
Ri·val'ta test
Ri·vi'nus
—ducts
—gland
—notch
ri'vus pl. -vi'
—lac'ri·ma'lis
riz'i·form'
Rob'ert pelvis
Rob'erts
—reagent
—test
Rob'in·son disease
Rob'in·son-Kep'ler-
 Pow'er test
Ro·bin' syndrome
Rob'i·son ester
rob'o·rant
Ro·chelle' salt
Ro'cho·li·mae'a quin·ta'na
Ro'ci·o'
Rock'ley sign
Rock'well test
Rock'y Moun'tain fever
rod
Ro·den'ti·a
ro·den'ti·cide'
Rod'man incision
rod'-mon'o·chro'mat
rods of Cor'ti
Roe'der·er
—ecchymoses
—obliquity
Roen'ne nasal step
roent'gen
roent'gen·o·der'ma
roent'gen·o·gram'
roent'gen·o·graph'
roent'gen·o·graph'ic
roent'ge·nog'ra·phy
roent'gen·o·ky'mo·gram
roent'gen·o·ky·mog'ra·phy
roent'gen·o·log'ic
roent'ge·nol'o·gist

roent'ge·nol'o·gy
roent'gen·o·lu'cent
roent'ge·nom'e·ter
roent'ge·nom'e·try
roent'gen·o·scope'
roent'ge·nos'co·py
roent'gen·o·ther'a·py
roe'theln
ro·flu'rane'
Ro·ger'
—disease
—murmur
Rohr stria
Ro'ki·tan'sky
—disease
—diverticulum
—pelvis
Ro'ki·tan'sky-Asch'off'
—duct
—sinus
Ro'ki·tan'sky-Cush'ing
 ulcer
ro·lan'dic
Ro·lan'do
—area
—fibers
—fissure
—substance
role
ro·let'a·mide'
rolf'ing
ro'li·cy'prine'
ro'li·tet'ra·cy'cline'
roll
roll'er
Rol'ler nucleus
Rol'les·ton rule
Rol'let
—cell
—stroma
Rol·lett' disease
Rol·lier' method
ro'lo·dine'
Ro·ma'na sign
ro·man'o·scope'
Ro'ma·nov'sky stains
Rom'berg'
—disease
—sign
—spasm
—test
rom'berg·ism
Ro·mieu' reaction

ron·geur'
ro·nid'a·zole'
Rön'ne nasal step
roof
room'ing-in'
root
rop'y
Ror'schach' test
ro·sa'ce·a
ro·sa'ce·i·form'
ro·sa'li·a
ro·san'i·line'
ro'sa·ry
Rose
—operations
—position
—tamponade
rose ben'gal
ro'se·in
ro·sel'la
Ro'sen·bach'
—disease
—law
—sign
—test
Ro'sen·müel'ler
—cavity
—fossa
—gland
—node
—organ
—valve
Ro'sen·thal' canal
ro·se'o·la
—cho·ler'i·ca
—in·fan'tum
—scar'la·ti'ni·forme'
—syph'i·lit'i·ca
—ty·pho'sa
—vac·cin'i·a
ro·se'o·lous
Ro'ser sign
ro·sette'
Rose'-Waa'ler test
ros'in
ro·sol'ic
Ross'bach' disease
Ross bodies
Ross'-Jones' test
Ross'man fluid
Ros'so·li'mo reflex
Ros·tan' asthma
ros·tel'lum

ros'trad'
ros'tral
ros'trum *pl.* -tra
—cor'po·ris cal·lo'si'
—sphe'noi·da'le'
rot, rot'ted, rot'ting
ro'ta·mase'
ro·tam'e·ter
ro'ta·ry
ro'tate', -tat'ed, -tat'ing
ro·ta'tion
ro'ta'tor
ro'ta·to'res'
—spi'nae'
ro'ta·to'ri·a
ro'ta·to'ry
ro'ta·vi'rus
Rotch sign
röt'eln
ro'te·none'
ro'texed'
ro·tex'ion
Roth
—disease
—spots
—symptom complex
Roth'-Bern'hardt' disease
Roth'er·a test
Roth'mund syndrome
Roth'mund-Thom'son
  syndrome
Ro'tor syndrome
ro'to·sco'li·o'sis *pl.* -ses'
ro·tox'a·mine'
Rot'ter test
rot'u·la
rot'u·lad'
rot'u·lar
ro·tund'
Rou·get' cell
rough'age
rough'en
Rough'ton-Scho'lan·der
  method
Rou·gnon'-Heb'er·den
  disease
rou·leau' *pl.* -leaux'
round'worm'
Rous sarcoma
Rous·sy'-De·je·rine'
  syndrome
Rous·sy'-Lé·vy' disease
Roux

—gastroenterostomy
—operation
—serum
Roux en Y
—bypass
—gastroenterostomy
—loop
Roux'-Gold'thwait'
  operation
Roux'-Y'
—anastomosis
—bypass
—drainage
—gastrojejunostomy
Ro·vi'ghi sign
Rov'sing sign
Rown'tree-Ger'agh·ty test
rub
Ru'barth disease
rub'ber·y
ru'be·an'ic
ru'be·fa'cient
ru'be·fac'tion
ru·bel'la
ru·bel'li·form'
ru·be'o·la
ru·be'o·sis
—i'ri·dis
—iridis di'a·bet'i·ca
ru'ber
ru·bes'cence
ru·bes'cent
ru·bid'i·um
ru·big'i·nous
ru'bi·jer'vine'
ru'bin
Ru'bin·stein-Tay'bi
  syndrome
Ru'bin test
Rub'ner
—laws
—test
ru'bor
ru'bri·blast'
ru'bric
ru'bri·cyte'
ru'bri·u'ri·a
ru'bro·bul'bar
ru'bro·ol'i·var'y
ru'bro·re·tic'u·lar
ru'bro·spi'nal
ru'bro·sta'sis *pl.* -ses'
ru'bro·tha·lam'ic

ru'brum scar'la·ti'num
ruc·ta'tion
ruc'tus
—hys·ter'i·cus
ru'di·ment
ru'di·men·ta·ry
ru'di·men'tum *pl.* -ta
—pro·ces'sus vag'i·na'lis
Rud syndrome
Ruf·fi'ni
—cell
—corpuscle
—end organ
ru'fous
ru'ga *pl.* -gae'
—vag'i·na'les'
ru'gal
ru'gi·tus
ru'gose'
ru·gos'i·ty
ru'gous
Ru·iz'-Mo'ra operation
rule
rum'ble
ru'men *pl.* -mi·na *or* -mens
ru'men·i'tis
ru'me·not'o·my
ru'mi·nant
ru'mi·nate', -nat'ed, -nat'ing
ru'mi·na'tion
ru'mi·na'tive
Rum'mo disease
rump
Rum'pel-Leede'
—phenomenon
—sign
—test
Rumpf sign
run, ran, run, run'ning
Ru'ne·berg disease
run'off'
Ru·otte' operation
ru'pi·a
ru'pi·al
ru'po·pho'bi·a
rup'ture, -tured, -tur·ing
rush
Rus'sell
—bodies
—dwarfism
—syndrome
—traction
rust

Rust
—disease
—phenomenon
—sign
rut, rut'ted, rut'ting
ru'ta·my'cin
ru·the'ni·um
ruth'er·ford
ru'tin
ru'tin·ose'
Ruysch disease
ry
Rye classification
Ry'er·son operation
Rytz test

S

sab'a·dil'la
Sa'bin-Feld'man dye test
Sab'ou·raud
—agar
—medium
sab'u·lous
sa·bur'ra
sa·bur'ral
sac
sac·cade'
sac·cad'ic
sac'cate'
sac'cha·rase'
sac'cha·rate'
sac'cha·rat'ed
sac'char·eph'i·dro'sis
pl. -ses'
sac·char'ic
sac'cha·ride'
sac·char'i·fi·ca'tion
sac·char'i·fy', -fied', -fy'ing
sac'cha·rim'e·ter
sac'cha·rim'e·try
sac'cha·rin *(a calorie-free sweetener)*
♦saccharine
sac'cha·rine *(pertaining to sugar)*
♦saccharin
sac'cha·ro·bi'ose'
sac'cha·ro·ga·lac'tor·rhe'a
sac'cha·ro·lyt'ic
sac'cha·ro·met'a·bol'ic
sac'cha·ro·me·tab'o·lism
sac'cha·rom'e·ter

Sac'cha·ro·my'ces'
—hom'i·nis
Sac'ca·ro·my'ce·ta·ce·ae'
sac'cha·ro·my·ce'tic
sac'cha·ro·my·co'sis
pl. -ses'
sac'cha·ror·rhe'a
sac'cha·rose'
sac'cha·ro·su'ri·a
sac'ci·form'
sac·cu·lar
sac'cu·lat'ed
sac'cu·la'tion
sac'cule'
sac'cu·li'
—al've·o·lar'es'
sac'cu·lo·coch'le·ar
sac'cu·lus *pl.* -li'
—la·ryn'gis
sac'cus *pl.* -ci'
—con'junc·ti'vae'
—en'do·lym·phat'i·cus
—lac'ri·ma'lis
—om'pha·lo·en·ter'i·cus
—vag'i·na'lis
Sachs disease
Sachs'-Geor'gi test
sa'crad'
sa'cral
sa'cral'gi·a
sa'cral·i·za'tion
sa'cral·ize', -ized', -iz'ing
sa·crec'to·my
sa'cro·an·te'ri·or
sa'cro·coc·cyg'e·al
sa'cro·coc·cyg'e·us *pl.* -e·i'
—dor·sa'lis
—ven·tra'lis
sa'cro·coc'cyx *pl.* -cy'ges' *or* -cyx·es
sa'cro·cox·al'gi·a
sa'cro·cox·i'tis
sa'cro·dyn'i·a
sa'cro·gen'i·tal
sa'cro·il'i·ac'
sa'cro·il'i·i'tis
sa'cro·lis·the'sis
sa'cro·lum·ba'lis
sa'cro·lum·bar
sa'cro·per'i·ne'al
sa'cro·pos·te'ri·or
sa'cro·prom'on·to'ry
sa'cro·pu'bic

sa'cro·sci·at'ic
sa'cro·spi·na'lis
sa'cro·spi'nous
sa'cro·trans·verse'
sa'cro·tu'ber·ous
sa'cro·u'ter·ine
sa'cro·ver'te·bral
sa'crum *pl.* -cra
sac'to·sal'pinx
  pl. -sal·pin'ges'
sad'dle
sad'dle·back'
sad'dle·nose'
Sade modification
sa'dism
sa'dist
sa·dis'tic
sa'do·mas'o·chism
sa'do·mas'o·chis'tic
Saeng'er operation
safe'ty
saf'flow'er
saf'fron
saf'ra·nine
saf'ra·no·phil
saf'role'
sa'fu
sage
sag'it·ta
sag'it·tal
sag'it·ta'lis
Sah'li
  —method
  —test
Saint An'tho·ny
  —dance
  —disease
  —fire
Saint A·ver'tin disease
Saint Blaise disease
Saint E·ras'mus disease
Saint Hu'bert disease
Saint Roch disease
Saint tri'ad'
Saint Val'en·tine' disease
Saint Vi'tus dance
Saint Zach'a·ry disease
Sak'el method
sal
  —am·mo'ni·ac'
  —vol'a·tile
sal·eth'a·mide'
sal'i·cin

sal'i·cyl
sal'i·cyl·al'de·hyde'
sal'i·cyl·am'ide'
sal'i·cyl·an'i·lide'
sa·lic'yl·ase'
sa·lic'y·late'
sa·lic'y·lat'ed
sal'i·cyl·a'zo·sul'fa·pyr'i·
  dine'
sal'i·cy·le'mi·a
sal'i·cyl'ic
sal'i·cyl·ism
sal'i·cyl·ize'
sal'i·cyl·sal'i·cyl'ic
sal'i·cyl·u'ric
sa·lic'y·lyl
sa'li·ent
sal'i·fi'a·ble
sal'i·fy', -fied', -fy'ing
sa·lim'e·ter
sa'line'
sal'i·nom'e·ter
sa·li'va
sal'i·vant
sal'i·var'y
sal'i·vate', -vat'ed, -vat'ing
sal'i·va'tion
sal'i·va'tor
sal'i·va·to'ry
sal'i·vo·li·thi'a·sis *pl.* -ses'
sa·li'vous
Salk vaccine
sal'mine'
Sal'mo·nel'la
  —a·bor'ti·vo·e·qui'na
  —aer'try·cke
  —chol'e·rae·su'is
  —en·ter·it'i·dis
  —hirsch·fel'di·i'
  —o'ra·ni·en·burg'
  —par'a·ty'phi'
  —par'a·ty·pho'sa
  —schott·mül'ler·i'
  —su'i·pes'ti·fer
  —ty'phi'
  —ty'phi·mu'ri·um
  —ty·pho'sa
Sal'mo·nel'le·ae'
sal'mo·nel·lo'sis *pl.* -ses'
sal'ol'
sal'pin'ge·al
sal'pin·gec'to·my
sal'pin·gem·phrax'is

sal·pin'gi·an
sal·pin'gi·on'
sal·pin'git'ic
sal·pin·gi'tis
sal·pin'go·cath'e·ter·ism
sal·pin'go·cele'
sal·pin'go·cy·e'sis *pl.* -ses'
sal·pin'go·gram'
sal·pin·gog'ra·phy
sal·pin'go·li·thi'a·sis
  pl. -ses'
sal·pin·gol'y·sis
sal·pin'go-
  o'o·pho·rec'to·my
sal·pin'go-o·o'pho·ri'tis
sal·pin'go-o·oph'o·ro·cele'
sal·pin'go-
  o'o·the·cec'to·my
sal·pin'go-o·o'the·ci'tis
sal·pin'go-o·o'the·co·cele'
sal·pin'go·o·var'i·ec'to·my
sal·pin'go·o·var'i·ot'o·my
sal·pin'go·o·o·va·ri'tis
sal·pin'go·pal'a·tine'
sal·pin'go·per'i·to·ni'tis
sal·pin'go·pex'y
sal·pin'go·pha·ryn'ge·al
sal·pin'go·pha·ryn'ge·us
sal·pin'go·plas'ty
sal·pin·gor'rha·phy
sal·pin'go·sal'pin·gos'-
  to·my
sal·pin'go·scope'
sal·pin·gos'co·py
sal·pin'go·sten'o·cho'ri·a
sal·pin'go·sto·mat'o·my
sal·pin'go·sto·mat'o·
  plas'ty
sal·pin·gos'to·my
sal·pin'go·the'cal
sal·pin'got'o·my
sal'pinx *pl.* sal·pin'ges'
sal'sa·late'
salt
sal·ta'tion
sal'ta·tor'ic
sal'ta·to'ry
Sal'ter
  —fractire
  —lines
salt·pe'ter
sa·lu'bri·ous
sa·lu'bri·ty

sal'u·re'sis
sal'u·ret'ic
sal'u·tar'y
sal'vage, -vaged, -vag·ing
salve
sal'vi·a
sal'vo
Salz'mann dystrophy
sa·mar'i·um
sam·bu'cus
sam'ple, -pled, -pling
Samp'son cysts
San'a·rel'li virus
san'a·to'ri·um *pl.* -ri·ums *or*
-ri·a
san'a·to'ry
san'da·rac
sand'bag'
San'der disease
San'ders sign
sane
sand'fly'
Sand'hoff disease
San·fi·lip'po syndrome
Sang'er Brown ataxia
san·guic'o·lous
san·guif'er·ous
san'gui·fi·ca'tion
san'gui·nar'i·a
san'gui·nar'ine'
san'gui·nar'y
san'guine
san·guin'e·ous
san·guin'o·lent
san'gui·no·poi·et'ic
san'gui·no·pu'ru·lent
san'gui·no·se'rous
san'gui·nous
san'guis
san'gui·suc'tion
san'gui·su'ga
san·guiv'er·ous
sa'ni·es'
sa'ni·ous
san'i·tar'i·an
san'i·tar'i·um *pl.* -ri·ums *or*
-ri·a
san'i·tar'y
san'i·ta'tion
san'i·ti·za'tion
san'i·tize', -tized', -tiz'ing
san'i·ty
San Joa·quin' Val'ley fever

San'som sign
san·ton'i·ca
san'to·nin
san'to·nism
San'to·ri'ni
—cartilages
—duct
—muscle
—plexus
—tubercle
sap
sa·phe'na
saph'e·nec'to·my
sa·phe'no·fem'o·ral
sa·phe'nous
sap'id
sap'o·gen'in
sap'o·na'ceous
sap'o·nar'i·a
sap'o·nat'ed
sa·pon'i·fi'a·ble
sa·pon'i·fi·ca'tion
sa·pon'i·form'
sap'o·nin
Sap'pey' muscle
sap'phism
sa·pre'mi·a
sa·pre'mic
sap'ro·gen
sap'ro·gen'ic
sa·prog'e·nous
sa·proph'a·gous
sa·proph'i·lous
sap'ro·phyte'
sap'ro·phyt'ic
sap'ro·phy·to'sis
sap'ro·zo'ic
sa·ral'a·sin
sar'a·pus
Sar'bo sign
Sar·ci'na *pl.* -nae'
sar'co·ad·e·no'ma *pl.* -mas
or -ma·ta
sar'co·blast'
sar'co·car'ci·no'ma *pl.*
-mas *or* -ma·ta
sar'co·cele'
Sar'co·cys'tis
—lin'de·man'ni'
sar'code'
Sar'co·di'na
sar'co·en'do·the'li·o'ma
pl. -mas *or* -ma·ta

sar'co·gen'ic
sar·cog'li·a
sar'co·hy'dro·cele'
sar'coid'
sar·coi·do'sis *pl.* -ses'
sar'co·lac'tic
sar'co·lem'ma
sar'co·lem'mal
sar'co·lem'mic
sar'co·lem'mous
sar'co·leu·ke'mi·a
sar·col'y·sis *pl.* -ses'
sar'co·lyte'
sar'co·lyt'ic
sar·co'ma *pl.* -mas *or* -ma·ta
—bot'ry·oi'des'
—cap'i·tis
—col'li' u'ter·i' hy·drop'-
i·cum pap'il·lar'e'
—cu·ta'ne·um te·lan'gi·ec·
tat'i·cum mul'ti·plex'
—myx·o'ma·to'des'
—phyl·loi'des'
sar'co·ma·gen·e'sis *pl.* -ses'
sar'co·ma·gen'ic
sar'co·ma·toid'
sar'co·ma·to'sis *pl.* -ses'
sar'co·ma·tous
sar'co·mere'
sar'co·mes·o·the'li·o·ma
pl. -mas *or* -ma·ta
sar'co·my'ces'
Sar'co·phag'i·dae'
sar'co·plasm
sar'co·plas'mic
sar'co·plast'
sar'co·poi·e'sis
sar'co·poi·et'ic
Sar·cop'tes'
—sca'bie·i'
sar·cop'tic
Sar·cop'ti·dae'
sar·cop'toid'
sar'co·sine'
sar'co·si·ne'mi·a
sar'co·sis
sar'co·spo·rid'i·o'sis
pl. -ses'
sar'cos·to'sis
sar'co·style'
sar·cot'ic
sar'co·tu'bule'
sar'cous

sar·don'ic
sa·rin'
sar'men·to·cy'ma·rin
sar'men·tog'e·nin
sar'men·tose'
sar'sa·sap'o·gen'in
sar'sa·sap'o·nin
sar·to'ri·us *pl.* -ri·i'
sa'tan·o·pho'bi·a
sat'el·lite'
sat'el·li·to'sis *pl.* -ses'
sa'ti·ate', -at'ed, -at'ing
sa'ti·a'tion
sa·ti'e·ty
Sat'ter·thwaite' method
sat'u·rate', -rat'ed, -rat'ing
sat'u·ra'tion
sat'ur·nine'
sat'urn·ism
sat'y·ri'a·sis *pl.* -ses'
sat'y·ro·ma'ni·a
sau'cer
sau'cer·i·za'tion
sau'cer·ize', -ized', -iz'ing
sau'na
Saund'by test
Saun'ders disease
sau·ri'a·sis
sau'ri·o'sis
Sau·rop'si·da
sau'sag·ing
Sau·vi·neau'
  ophthalmoplegia
sav'in
Sa·vi'no test
saw
saw'tooth'
sax'i·tox'in
scab, scabbed, scab'bing
sca·bet'ic
sca·bi·cide'
sca'bies'
  —crus·to'sa
  —pap'u·li·for'mis
  —pap'u·lo'sa
  —pus'tu·lo'sa
sca·bi·et'ic
sca·bi·o·pho'bi·a
sca'bi·ous
sca·bri·ti·es'
  —un'gui·um syph'i·lit'i·ca
sca'la *pl.* -lae'
  —me'di·a

—tym'pa·ni'
—ves·tib'u·li'
sca·lar'i·form'
scald
scale
sca'lene'
sca'le·nec'to·my
sca'le·not'o·my
sca·le'nus *pl.* -ni'
  —an·ti'cus syndrome
  —min'i·mus
  —pleu·ra'lis
scal'er
scal'ing
scall
scal'lop·ing
scalp
scal'pel
scal'pri·form'
scal'prum *pl.* -pra
scal'y
scam'mo·ny
scan, scanned, scan'ning
scan'di·um
scan·og'ra·phy
scan'ner
scan·so'ri·us
Scan·zo'ni maneuver
sca'pha
scaph'o·ce·phal'ic
scaph'o·ceph'a·lism
scaph'o·ceph'a·lous
scaph'o·ceph'a·ly
scaph'oid'
scaph'oid·i'tis
scaph'o·lu'nate'
scap'u·la *pl.* -lae' *or* -las
  —a'la·ta
scap'u·lal'gi·a
scap'u·lar
scap'u·lar'y
scap'u·lec'to·my
scap'u·lo·an·te'ri·or
scap'u·lo·cla·vic'u·lar
scap'u·lo·cla·vic'u·lar'is
scap'u·lo·cos'tal
scap'u·lo·dyn'i·a
scap'u·lo·hu'mer·al
scap'u·lo·per'i·os'te·al
scap'u·lo·pex'y
scap'u·lo·pos·te'ri·or
scap'u·lo·tho·rac'ic
scap'u·lo·ver'te·bral

sca'pus *pl.* -pi'
  —pi'li'
scar, scarred, scar'ring
scar'a·bi·a·sis *pl.* -ses'
scar'i·fi·ca'tion
scar'i·fi·ca'tor
scar'i·fi'er
scar'i·fy', -fied', -fy'ing
scar'la·ti'na
scar'la·ti'nal
scar'la·ti·nel'la
scar'la·ti'ni·form'
scar'la·ti'noid'
scar'la·ti'nous
scar'let
Scar'pa
  —fascia
  —foramen
  —ganglion
  —triangle
scat'a·cra'ti·a
sca·te'mi·a
scat'o·lo'gi·a
scat'o·log'ic *or*
  scat'o·log'i·cal
sca·tol'o·gy
sca·to'ma *(fecal matter in the colon)*
  ♦scotoma
sca·toph'a·gous
sca·toph'a·gy
scat'o·phil'i·a
scat'o·pho'bi·a
sca·tos'co·py
scat'ter
scav'en·ger
scel'o·tyr'be
Scha'fer
  —method
  —syndrome
Schäf'fer reflex
Schales and Schales
  method
Scham'berg' disease
Schanz
  —disease
  —syndrome
Schar'lach' R stain
Schatz'ki ring
Schau'dinn fixing fluid
Schau'mann bodies
Schau'ta-Wert'heim'
  operation

Sche'de
—method
—operation
sched'ule, -uled, -ul·ing
Scheie syndrome
Schel'long-Stri'sow·er
    phenomenon
sche'ma *pl.* -ma·ta
sche·mat'ic
sche·mat'o·gram'
sche·mat'o·graph'
sche'mo·graph'
Schenck disease
Scher'er test
sche·ro'ma
Scheu'er·mann disease
Schick test
Schiff
—reagent
—test
Schiff'-Sher'ring·ton
    phenomenon
Schil'der-Ad'di·son
    complex
Schil'der disease
Schil'ler test
Schil'ling
—classification
—test
—type leukemia
Schim'mel·busch' disease
schin'dy·le'sis *pl.* -ses'
Schi·ötz' tonometer
Schir'mer test
schis'ta·sis
schis'ten·ceph'a·ly
schis'to·ce'li·a
schis'to·ce·phal'ic
schis'to·ceph'a·lus *pl.* -li'
schis'to·cor'mi·a
schis'to·cor'mus
schis'to·cys'tis
schis'to·cyte'
schis'to·cy·to'sis
schis'to·glos'si·a
schis·tom'e·lus
schis·tom'e·ter
schis'to·pro·so'pi·a
schis'to·pros'o·pus
schis'to·pros'o·py
schis·tor'rha·chis
schis'to·sis *pl.* -ses'
Schis'to·so'ma

—hae'ma·to'bi·um
—ja·pon'i·cum
—man·so'ni'
schis'to·so'mal
schis'to·some'
schis'to·so·mi'a·sis *pl.* -ses'
—hae'ma·to'bi·a
—ja·pon'i·ca
—man·so'ni
schis'to·so'mi·cid'al
schis'to·so'mi·cide'
schis'to·so'mus
schis'to·ster'ni·a
schis'to·tho'rax' *pl.* -rax'es
    or -ra'ces'
schis'to·tra'che·lus
schiz·am'ni·on'
schiz·ax'on'
schiz'en·ce·phal'ic
schiz'en·ceph'a·ly
schiz'o·af·fec'tive
schiz'o·ble·phar'i·a
schiz'o·cyte'
schiz'o·cy·to'sis
schiz'o·gen'e·sis *pl.* -ses'
schi·zog'e·nous
schiz'o·gon'ic
schi·zog'o·ny
schiz'o·gy'ri·a
schiz'oid'
schiz'oid'ism
schiz'o·ki·ne'sis *pl.* -ses'
schiz'o·ma'ni·a
Schiz'o·my·ce'tes'
schiz'ont'
schi·zon'ti·cide'
schiz'o·nych'i·a
schiz'o·pha'si·a
schiz'o·phre'ni·a
schiz'o·phren'ic
schiz'o·phren'i·form'
schiz'o·phren'o·gen'ic
schiz'o·the'mi·a
schiz'o·tho'rax' *pl.* -rax'es *or*
    -ra'ces'
schiz'o·thy'mi·a
schiz'o·thy'mic
schiz'o·try·pan'o·so·mi'a·
    sis *pl.* -ses'
Schiz'o·tryp'a'num cru'zi
Schla'er test
Schlat'ter disease
Schlein arthroplasty

Schlemm canal
Schle'sin·ger
—sign
—test
Schlof'fer
—operation
—tumor
Schlös'ser treatment
Schmidt
—fibrinoplastin
—syndrome
—test
Schminck'e tumor
Schmitz bacillus
Schmorl
—disease
—grooves
—nodules
Schmutz pyorrhea
Schna'bel atrophy
Schnei'der
—index
—stain
Schnei·de'ri·an membrane
Scho'ber test
Schoen'bein' test
Schoen'hei'mer and
    Sper'ry method
Scholz'-Bi'al·schow'sky-
    Hen'ne·berg' disease
Scholz disease
Schön'lein'
—disease
—purpura
Schön'lein-Hen'och
    purpura
Schott'mül'ler disease
Schre'ger-Hun'ter bands
Schre'ger lines
Schrid'de disease
Schroe'der method
Schüff'ner dots
Schül'ler
—disease
—glands
—method
—syndrome
—view
Schül'ler-Chris'tian
    syndrome
Schultz
—method
—syndrome

—test
Schultz'-Charl'ton
—test
Schultz'-Dale' test
Schult'ze
—method
—paresthesia
—placenta
Schumm test
Schwa'bach' test
Schwal'be
—fissure
—line
—nucleus
—ring
—sheath
Schwann cell tumor
schwan'no·gli·o'ma
  pl. -mas *or* -ma·ta
schwan'no'ma *pl.* -mas *or*
  -ma·ta
schwan'no·sar·co'ma
  pl. -mas *or* -ma·ta
Schwann sheath
Schwartz test
Schweig'ger-Sei'del sheath
Schwei'zer-Fo'ley Y'-
  plas'ty
Schwen'in·ger method
sci·age'
sci·at'ic
sci·at'i·ca
sci'ence
sci'en·tif'ic
sci'en·tist
sci'e·ro'pi·a
scil'la
scil'lism
scil'lo·ceph'a·lus *pl.* -li'
scil'lo·ceph'a·ly
scin'ti·gram'
scin'ti·graph'ic
scin·tig'ra·phy
scin'til·late', -lat'ed, -lat'ing
scin'til·la'tion
scin'til·la'tor
scin'ti·pho·tog'ra·phy
scin'ti·scan'
scin'ti·scan'ner
sci'on'
scir'rhoid'
scir·rho'ma *pl.* -mas *or*
  -ma·ta

scir'rhoph·thal'mi·a
scir'rhous *(hard)*
  ♦*scirrhus*
scir'rhus *(a carcinoma),*
  pl. -rhi' *or* -rhus·es
  ♦*scirrhous*
scis'sile
scis'sion
scis·si·par'i·ty
scis'sor·ing
scis'sors
scis·su'ra *pl.* -rae'
scis'sure
scle'ra *pl.* -ras *or* -rae'
scler·ac'ne
scler·ad·e·ni'tis
scle'ral
scle·ra·ti'tis
scle·ra·tog'e·nous
scler·ec·ta'si·a
scle·rec·to·ir'i·dec'to·my
scle·rec'tome'
scle·rec'to·my
scler·e·de'ma
  —ad·ul'to'rum
  —ne·o'na·to'rum
scle·re'ma
  —ad'i'po'sum
  —cu'tis
  —e'dem'a·to'sum
  —ne·o'na·to'rum
scle'ren·ce·pha'li·a
scle'ren·ceph'a·ly
scle'ren'chy·ma *pl.* -mas *or*
  scle'ren·chym'a·ta
scle'ren·chym'a·tous
scle·ri'a·sis *pl.* -ses'
scle·rit'ic
scle·ri'tis
scle'ro·ad'i·pose'
scle'ro·a·troph'ic
scle'ro·blas·te'ma *pl.* -mas
  or -ma·ta
scle'ro·blas·tem'ic
scle'ro·cho·roi·di'tis
scle'ro·con·junc·ti'val
scle'ro·con·junc·ti·vi'tis
scle'ro·cor'ne·a
scle'ro·cor'ne·al
scle'ro·dac·tyl'i·a
scle'ro·dac·ty·ly
scle'ro·der'ma
scle'ro·der'ma·ti'tis

scle'ro·der'ma·tous
scle'ro·des'mi·a
scle'ro·gen'ic
scle·rog'e·nous
scle'ro·gum'ma·tous
scle'ro·gy'ri·a
scle'roid'
scle'ro·i·ri'tis
scle'ro·ker·a·ti'tis
scle·ro'ma *pl.* -mas *or* -ma·ta
scle'ro·ma·la'ci·a
  —per'fo'rans'
scle'ro·me'ninx
  pl. -me·nin'ges'
scle'ro·mere'
scle·rom'e·ter
scle'ro·myx'e·de'ma
scle'ro·nych'i·a
scle'ro·nyx'is
scle'ro-o·o'pho·ri'tis
scle'roph·thal'mi·a
scle'ro·plas'ty
scle'ro·pro'tein'
scle·ro'sal
scle·ro'sant
scle'ro·sar·co'ma *pl.* -mas *or*
  -ma·ta
scle·rose', -rosed', -ros'ing
scle·ro'sis *pl.* -ses'
  —co'ri·i'
  —der'ma·tis
  —os'si·um
scle'ro·skel'e·ton
scle'ro·ste·no'sis *pl.* -ses'
  —cu·ta'ne·a
scle·ros'to·my
scle'ro·ther'a·py
scle'ro·thrix'
scle·rot'ic
scle·rot'i·ca
scle·rot'i·cec'to·my
scle·rot'i·co·nyx'is
scle·rot'i·co·punc'ture
scle·rot'i·cot'o·my
scle·rot'i·dec'to·my
scle'ro·ti'tis
scle·ro'ti·um *pl.* -ti·a
scle'ro·tome'
scle·rot'o·mic
scle·rot'o·my
scle'rous
sco'bi·nate
sco·lec'i·form'

sco'le·coid'
sco'lex' *pl.* sco'li·ces',
  sco·le'ces' *or* sco'lex'es
sco'li·o·lor·do'sis *pl.* -ses'
sco'li·o·ra·chit'ic
sco'li·o·si·om'e·try
sco'li·o'sis *pl.* -ses'
sco'li·o·som'e·ter
sco'li·o·som'e·try
sco'li·ot'ic
sco'li·o·tone'
Sco'lo·pen'dra
scom'broid'ism
scom'broid' poisoning
scom'bro·tox'ic
scoop
sco·par'i·us
scope
sco'pine'
sco'po·la
sco·pol'a·mine'
sco·po'li·a
sco'po·phil'i·a
sco'po·phil'ic
sco'po·pho'bi·a
Scop'u·lar'i·op'sis
  —brev'i·cau'le'
scor'a·cra'ti·a
scor·bu'tic
scor·bu'ti·gen'ic
scor·bu'tus
scor'di·ne'ma
score, scored, scor'ing
scor'e·te'mi·a
scor'ing
Scor'pi·o
scor'pi·on
Scor'pi·on'i·da
scot'o·chro'mo·gen
scot'o·din'i·a
scot'o·gram'
sco·to'ma *(an area of depressed
vision in the visual field),*
  pl. -mas *or* -ma·ta
  ♦scatoma
sco·to'ma·graph'
sco·tom'a·tous
sco·tom'e·ter
scot'o·phil'i·a
scot'o·pho'bi·a
sco·to'pi·a
sco·top'ic
sco·top'sin

sco·tos'co·py
scout
scrap'er
screen
screw
screw'driv'er
screw'worm'
scribe
scro·bic'u·late'
scro·bic'u·lus *pl.* -li'
  —cor'dis
scrof'u·la
scrof'u·lo·der'ma
scrof'u·lous
scro'tal
scro·tec'to·my
scro·ti'tis
scro'to·cele'
scro'to·plas'ty
scro'tum *pl.* -ta *or* -tums
scrub
scru'ple
scru'pu·los'i·ty
scul·te'tus
scurf
scur'vy
scu'tate'
scute
scu·tel'lum *pl.* -la
scu'ti·form'
Scu·tig'er·a
scu'tu·lar
scu'tu·late'
scu'tu·lum *pl.* -la
scu'tum *pl.* -ta
  —tym·pan'i·cum
scyb'a·la
scyb'a·lous
scyb'a·lum *pl.* -la
scy'phi·form'
scy'phoid'
Sea'bright'-Ban'tam
  syndrome
seal
seal'ant
seam
sea'sick'
sea'sick'ness
seat
seat'worm'
se·ba'ce·o·fol·lic'u·lar
se·ba'ceous
se·bac'ic

se·bif'er·ous
se·bip'a·rous
seb'o·lith'
seb'or·rha'gi·a
seb'or·rhe'a
  —cap'i·tis
  —con'ges·ti'va
  —cor'po·ris
  —fur'fu·ra'ce·a
  —ich'thy·o'sis
  —na'si'
  —ni'gri·cans'
  —o'le·o'sa
  —sic'ca
seb'or·rhe'al
seb'or·rhe'ic
seb'or·rhe'id
se'bum
  —cu·ta'ne·um
  —pal'pe·bra'le'
  —prae·pu'ti·a'le'
Seck'el syndrome
se·clu'sion
sec'o·bar'bi·tal'
sec'o·dont'
sec'on·dar'y
se·cre'ta
se·cre'ta·gogue'
Se·cré'tan' syndrome
se·crete', -cret'ed, -cret'ing
se·cre'tin
se·cre'tin·ase'
se·cre'tion
se·cre'to·gogue'
se·cre'to·in·hib'i·tor
se·cre'to·in·hib'i·to'ry
se·cre'to·mo'tor
se·cre'tor
se·cre'to·ry
sec'tile'
sec'ti·o' *pl.* sec'ti·o'nes'
sec'tion
sec'tion·al
sec'ti·o'nes'
  —cer'e·bel'li'
  —cor'po·rum qua'dri·gem'-
    i·no'rum
  —hy'po·thal'a·mi'
  —isth'mi'
  —me·dul'lae' ob'lon·
    ga'tae'
  —medullae spi·na'lis
  —mes'en·ceph'a·li'

—pe·dun'cu·li' cer'e·bri'
—pon'tis
—tel'en·ceph'a·li'
—thal'a·men·ceph'a·li
sec'tor
sec·to'ri·al
se·cun'di·grav'i·da
se·cun·di'na *pl.* -nae'
sec'un·dines'
sec'un·dip'a·ra
sec'un·di·par'i·ty
sec'un·dip'a·rous
se·cun'dum ar'tem
se·cure'
se·cu'ri·ty
se·date', -dat'ed, -dat'ing
se·da'tion
sed'a·tive
sed'en·tar'y
sed'i·ment
sed'i·men'ta·ry
sed'i·men·ta'tion
sed'i·men·tom'e·ter
se'do·hep'tu·lose'
seed
See'lig·muel'ler
—neuralgia
—sign
seg'ment *n.*
seg·ment' *v.*
seg·men'ta
—bron'cho·pul'mo·na'li·a
—re·na'li·a
seg·men'tal
seg'men·tar'y
seg'men·ta'tion
seg'men·tec'to·my
Seg'men·ti'na
seg·men'tum *pl.* -ta
—an·te'ri·us in·fe'ri·us
    re·na'lis
—anterius lo'bi' hep'a·tis
    dex'tri'
—anterius lobi su·pe'ri·o'ris
    pul·mo'nis dex'tri'
—anterius lobi superioris
    pulmonis si·nis'tri'
—anterius su·pe'ri·us re·
    na'lis
—ap'i·ca'le' lo'bi' in·fe'ri·o'-
    ris pul·mo'nis dex'tri'
—apicale lobi inferioris
    pulmonis si·nis'tri'

—apicale lobi su·pe'ri·o'ris
    pul·mo'nis dex'tri'
—ap'i·co·pos·te'ri·us lo'bi'
    su·pe'ri·o'ris pul·mo'nis
    si·nis'tri'
—ba·sa'le' an·te'ri·us lo'bi'
    in·fe'ri·o'ris pul·mo'nis
    dex'tri'
—basale anterius lobi inferi-
    oris pulmonis si·nis'tri'
—basale lat'er·a'le' lo'bi'
    in·fe'ri·o'ris pul·mo'nis
    dex'tri'
—basale laterale lobi inferio-
    ris pulmonis si·nis'tri'
—basale me·di·a'le' lo'bi'
    in·fe'ri·o'ris pul·mo'nis
    dex'tri'
—basale mediale lobi inferi-
    oris pulmonis si·nis'tri'
—basale pos·te'ri·us lo'bi'
    in·fe'ri·o'ris pul·mo'nis
    dex'tri'
—basale posterius lobi
    inferioris pulmonis
    si·nis'tri'
—car·di'a·cum lo'bi'
    in·fe'ri·o'ris pul·mo'nis
    dex'tri'
—cardiacum lobi inferioris
    pulmonis si·nis'tri'
—in·fe'ri·us re·na'lis
—lat'er·a'le' lo'bi' hep'a·tis
    si·nis'tri'
—laterale lobi me'di·i'
    pul·mo'nis dex'tri'
—lin'gu·lar'e' in·fe'ri·us
    lo'bi su·pe'ri·o'ris pul·
    mo'nis si·nis'tri'
—linguare su·pe'ri·us lo'bi'
    su·pe'ri·o'ris pul·mo'nis
    si·nis'tri'
—me·di·a'le' lo'bi' hep'a·tis
    si·nis'tri'
—mediale lobi me·di·i' pul·
    mo'nis dex'tri'
—pos·te'ri·us lo'bi' hep'a·tis
    dex'tri'
—posterius lobi su·pe'ri·o'-
    ris pul·mo'nis dex'tri'
—posterius re·na'lis
—sub·ap'i·ca'le' lo'bi' in·fe'-
    ri·o'ris pul·mo'nis dex'tri'

—subapicale lobi inferioris
    pulmonis si·nis'tri'
—sub'su·pe'ri·us lo'bi
    in·fe'ri·o'ris pul·mo'nis
    dex'tri'
—subsuperius lobi inferioris
    pulmonis si·nis'tri
—su·pe'ri·us lo'bi' in·fe'ri·
    o'ris pul·mo'nis dex'tri'
—superius lobi inferioris
    pulmonis si·nis'tri'
—superius re·na'lis
seg're·gate', -gat'ed, -gat'ing
seg're·ga'tion
seg're·ga'tion·al
seg're·ga'tor
Sé'guin' sign
sei'es·the'si·a
Sei·gnette' salt
Sei'tel·ber'ger disease
Seitz filter
sei'zure
se·junc'tion
Sel'ding·er technique
se·lec'tion
se·lec'tive
se·lec'tor
se·le'ne' *pl.* -nai'
se·le'nic
sel'e·nif'er·ous
se·le'ni·ous
sel'e·nite'
se·le'ni·um
se·le'no·dont'
se·le'no·me·thi'o·nine'
sel'e·no'sis
self
self'-ab·sorp'tion
self'-ac·cu'sa'tion
self'-al'ien·a'tion
self'-a·nal'y·sis
self'-as·pi·rat'ing
self'-a·ware'ness
self'-con'cept
self'-con·trol'
self'-de·ni'al
self'-de·struc'tive·ness
self'-dif'fer·en'ti·a'tion
self'-di·ges'tion
self'-dis'ci·pline
self'-es·teem'
self'-ex·am'i·na'tion
self'-fer'men·ta'tion

self'-fer'til·i·za'tion
self'-hyp·no'sis *pl.* -ses'
self'-in·duced'
self'-in·duc'tance
self'-in·fec'tion
self'-in·flict'ed
self'-in·oc'u·la'tion
self-lim'it·ed
self-lim'it·ing
self'-mu'ti·la'tion
self'-re·tain'ing
self'-stim'u·la'tion
self'-sus·pen'sion
Sel'i·wa'noff' test
sel'la (*a saddle*), *pl.* -lae'
   ♦*cella*
   —tur'ci·ca
sel'lar
Sel'ler stain
Sel'ter disease
Sel'ye syndrome
se·man'tic
se·man'tics
Semb operation
se'mei·og'ra·phy
se'mei·o·log'ic
se'mei·ol'o·gy
se'mei·ot'ic
se'mei·ot'ics
se'men *pl.* -mens *or* sem'i·na
sem'i·a·ceph'a·lus *pl.* -li'
sem'i·ca·nal'
sem'i·ca·na'lis *pl.* -les'
   —mus'cu·li' ten·so'ris
     tym'pa·ni'
   —tu'bae' au'di·ti'vae'
sem'i·car'ba·zone'
sem'i·car'bi·zide'
sem'i·car'ti·lag'i·nous
sem'i·cir'cu·lar
sem'i·co'ma
sem'i·com'a·tose'
sem'i·con'scious
sem'i·cris'ta *pl.* -tae'
   —in'ci·si'va
sem'i·de'cus·sa'tion
sem'i·flex'ion
sem'i·len'te
sem'i·le'thal
sem'i·lu'nar
sem'i·lux·a'tion
sem'i·mem'bra·no'sus
   pl. -si'

sem'i·mem'bra·nous
sem'i·nal
sem'i·nar·co'sis *pl.* -ses'
sem'i·na'tion
sem'i·nif'er·ous
sem'i·no'ma *pl.* -mas *or*
   -ma·ta
sem'i·nor'mal
se'mi·nu'ri·a
se'mi·ol'o·gy
se'mi·ot'ics
sem'i·pen'ni·form'
sem'i·per'me·a·ble
sem'i·pla·cen'ta
sem'i·ple'gi·a
sem'i·pro·na'tion
sem'i·prone'
sem'i·quin'one'
sem'i·re·cum'bent
se'mis
sem'i·sid'e·ra'ti·o'
sem'i·som'nus
sem'i·so'por'
sem'i·spec'u·lum *pl.* -la *or*
   -lums
sem'i·spi·na'lis
sem'i·sul'cus
sem'i·su'pi·na'tion
sem'i·syn·thet'ic
sem'i·ten'di·no'sus *pl.* -si'
sem'i·ten'di·nous
Se'mon
   —law
   —symptom
Se'mon-Ro'sen·bach' law
Sen'e·ar-Ush'er syndrome
Se·ne'ci·o
se·ne'ci·o'sis *pl.* -ses'
se·nec'ti·tude'
sen'e·ga
Sen'ek·jie medium
se·nes'cence
se·nes'cent
se'nile'
se'nil·ism
se·nil'i·ty
se'ni·um
   —prae'cox'
   —pre'cox'
Sen method
sen'na
sen'no·side'
se·no'pi·a

sen·sa'tion
sen·sa'tion·al
sense, sensed, sens'ing
sen'si·bil'i·ty
sen'si·bil·iz'er
sen·sib'i·lus pro'pri·us
   nucleus
sen'si·ble
sen·sim'e·ter
sen'si·tive
sen'si·tiv'i·ty
sen'si·ti·za'tion
sen'si·tize', -tized', -tiz'ing
sen'si·tiz'er
sen'so·mo'tor
sen'so·pa·ral'y·sis *pl.* -ses'
sen'sor
sen·so'ri·al
sen'so·ri·glan'du·lar
sen'so·ri·mo'tor
sen'so·ri·neu'ral
sen·so'ri·um *pl.* -ri·ums *or*
   -ri·a
sen'so·ri·va'so·mo'tor
sen'so·ry
sen'su·al
sen'su·al·ism
sen'su·al'i·ty
sen'sus
sen'ti·ent
sen'ti·ment
sen'ti·nel
sep'a·ra'tion
sep'a·ra'tor
sep'sis *pl.* -ses'
   —a·gran'u·lo·cyt'i·ca
sep'ta
   —in'ter·al've·o·lar'i·a
     man·dib'u·lae'
   —interalveolaria max·il'lae'
   —in'ter·ra·dic'u·lar'i·a
     man·dib'u·lae'
   —interradicularia max·il'-
     lae'
sep'tal
sep'tate'
sep'ta'tion
sep'tec'to·my
sep·te'mi·a
sep'tic
sep'ti·ce'mi·a
sep'ti·ce'mic
sep'ti·co·phle·bi'tis

sep'ti·co·py·e'mi·a
sep'ti·co·py·e'mic
sep'ti·grav'i·da
sep'tile'
sep'ti·me·tri'tis
sep·tip'a·ra
sep'to·mar'gi·nal
sep·tom'e·ter
sep'to·na'sal
sep'to·plas'ty
sep'tos'to·my
sep'to·tome'
sep·tot'o·my
sep'tu·la tes'tis
sep'tu·lum *pl.* -la
sep'tum *pl.* -tums *or* -ta
—a'tri·o'rum
—a'tri·o·ven·tric'u·lar'e'
—bul'bae' u·re'thrae'
—ca·na'lis mus'cu·lo·tu·
bar'i·i'
—car'ti·la·gin'e·um na'si'
—cer'vi·ca'le' in·ter·me'-
di·um
—cor'po·rum cav·er·no·so'-
rum
—corporum cavernosorum
cli·tor'i·dis
—cru·ra'le'
—fem'o·ra'le'
—femorale (Clo·quet'i')
—glan'dis pe'nis
—in·ter·a'tri·a'le'
—in·ter·mus·cu·lar'e'
an·te'ri·us cru'ris
—intermusculare anterius
fib'u·lar'e'
—intermusculare bra'chi·i'
lat'er·a'le'
—intermusculare brachii
me'di·a'le'
—intermusculare fem'o·ris
lat'er·a'le'
—intermusculare femoris
me'di·a'le'
—intermusculare hu'mer·i'
lat'er·a'le'
—intermusculare humeri
me'di·a'le'
—intermusculare pos·te'-
ri·us cru'ris
—intermusculare posterius
fib'u·lar'e'

—in'ter·ven·tric'u·lar'e'
—interventriculare pri'mum
—lin'guae'
—lu'ci·dum
—mem'bra·na'ce·um na'si'
—membranaceum ven·tric'-
u·lo'rum
—mo'bi·le' na'si'
—mus'cu·lar'e' ven·tric'-
u·lo'rum
—na'si'
—nasi os'se·um
—or'bi·ta'le'
—pel'lu·ci·dum
—pe'nis
—pri'mum
—rec'to·vag'i·na'le'
—rec'to·ves·i·ca'le'
—scro'ti'
—se·cun'dum
—si'nu·um fron·ta'li·um
—sinuum sphe·noi·da'li·um
—spu'ri·um
—trans·ver'sum
—ven·tric'u·lo'rum
sep·tup'let
se·quel'a *pl.* -ae'
se'quence
se·quen'tial
se·ques'ter
se·ques'tral
se·ques'trant
se'ques·tra'tion
se·ques·trec'to·my
se·ques·trot'o·my
se·ques'trum *pl.* -trums *or*
-tra
se·quoi·o'sis
ser·ac'tide'
ser'al·bu'min
se·ra·phe·re'sis
se·rem'pi·on'
Ser'gent sign
se'ri·al
se'ri·al·ly
se'ri·al'o·graph'
ser'i·cin
se'ries' *pl.* se'ries'
ser'i·flux'
ser'ine'
ser'i·scis'sion
se'ro·al·bu'mi·nous
se'ro·al·bu'mi·nu'ri·a

se·ro·an'a·phy·lax'is
pl. -lax'es'
se'ro·che
se'ro·chrome'
se'ro·co·li'tis
se'ro·con·ver'sion
se'ro·cul'ture
se'ro·cys'tic
se'ro·der'ma·ti'tis
se'ro·der'ma·to'sis *pl.* -ses'
se'ro·der·mi'tis
se'ro·di·ag·no'sis *pl.* -ses'
se'ro·di·ag·nos'tic
se'ro·en·ter'i·tis
se'ro·ep'i·de'mi·o·log'ic
se'ro·ep'i·de·mi·ol'o·gy
se'ro·fi'bri·nous
se'ro·fi'brous
se'ro·floc'cu·la'tion
se'ro·flu'id
se'ro·gas'tri·a
se'ro·gen'e·sis
se'ro·glob'u·lin
se'ro·gly'coid'
se'ro·hem'or·rhag'ic
se'ro·hep'a·ti'tis *pl.* -tis·es *or*
-tit'i·des'
se'ro·im·mu'ni·ty
se'ro·lem'ma
se'ro·li'pase'
se'ro·log'ic *or* se'ro·log'i·cal
se·rol'o·gist
se·rol'o·gy
se·rol'y·sin
se·ro'ma *pl.* -mas *or* -ma·ta
se'ro·mem'bra·nous
se'ro·mu'ci·nous
se'ro·mu'cous
se'ro·mus'cu·lar
se'ro·neg'a·tive
se'ro·neg'a·tiv'i·ty
se'ro·per'i·to·ne'um
se'ro·plas'tic
se'ro·pos'i·tive
se'ro·pos'i·tiv'i·ty
se'ro·prog·no'sis *pl.* -ses'
se'ro·pu'ru·lent
se'ro·pus
se'ro·re·ac'tion
se'ro·re·sis'tance
se'ro·re·sis'tant
se·ro'sa *pl.* -sas *or* -sae'
se·ro'sal

se′ro·sa·mu′cin
se′ro·san·guin′e·ous
se′ro·se′rous
se′ro·si′tis
se·ros′i·ty
se′ro·sy·no′vi·al
se′ro·syn′o·vi′tis
se′ro·ther′a·py
se′ro·to′nin
se′ro·tox′in
se′ro·type′
se′rous
ser′pen·tar′i·a
ser′pen·tine′
ser′pig′i·nous
ser′ra
ser′rate′, -rat′ed, -rat′ing
Ser·ra′ti·a
—mar·ces′cens
ser·ra′tion
ser·ra′tus
—mag′nus
serre·fine′
Ser′res angle
ser′ru·late′
Ser·to′li cells
se′rum *pl.* -rums *or* -ra
se′rum·al
se′rum-fast′
ser′vo·mech′a·nism
ser′yl
ses′a·me
ses′a·moid′
ses′a·moid·i′tis
ses′qui·ho′ra
ses′qui·sul′fide′
ses′qui·ter′pene′
ses′sile′
set, set, set′ting
se′ta *pl.* -tae′
se·ta′ceous
Se·tar′i·a
se′ton
set′up′
17-hy·drox′y·cor′ti·cos′-ter·one′
17-hy·drox′y-11-de·hy′dro·cor′ti·cos′ter·one′
Se′ver disease
Se′ver-L′E·pis′co·po repair
se′vum
sex
sex′i·dig′i·tal

sex′i·dig′i·tate′
sex′-lim·it·ed
sex′-linked′
sex′o·log′ic
sex·ol′o·gy
sex′ti·grav′i·da
sex·tip′a·ra
sex·tup′let
sex′u·al
sex′u·al′i·ty
sex′u·al·i·za′tion
sex′u·al·ize′, -ized′, -iz′ing
sex′u·al·ly
Sé′za·ry
—cell
—syndrome
Sgam·ba′ti
—reaction
—test
shad′ow
shad′ow-cast′ing
Shaf′fer method
shaft
shag′gy
sha·green′
shank
shark
Shar′pey fibers
shave, shaved, shav′ing
shav′er
Sha′ver disease
shears
sheath
—of Hen′le
—of Neu′mann
—of Schweig′ger-Sei′del
sheathe, sheathed, sheath′ing
shed, shed, shed′ding
Shee′han syndrome
sheet
sheet′like′
shelf
shell
shell′shock′
shelv′ing
Shep′herd fracture
Sher′man-Mun·sell′ unit
Sher′ren triangle
Sher′ring·ton law
Shev′sky test
shi·at′su
Shib′ley sign

shield
shift
Shi′ga bacillus
Shi·gel′la
—al′ka·les′cens
—am·big′u·a
—dys′en·ter′i·ae′
—flex·ne′ri
—schmitz′i·i′
shig′el·lo′sis *pl.* -ses′
shi·kim′ic
shim
shin
shin′bone′
shin′gles
shin′-splints′
Shi·rod′kar procedure
shiv′er
shock
Shock and Has′tings method
shock′y
shoe
Shohl solution
Shone
—anomaly
—syndrome
Shope papilloma
Shorr trichrome stain
short′en
short′ness
short′sight′ed
short′sight′ed·ness
shot′ty
shoul′der
Shoul′dice repair
Shrap′nell membrane
shriv′el
shrunk′en
shud′der
Shu′ni fever
shunt
Shwartz′man phenomenon
Shy′-Dra′ger syndrome
si·al′a·den
si·al′ad·e·ni′tis
si·al′ad′e·nog′ra·phy
si·al′ad′e·non′cus
si·al′a·gog′ic
si·al′a·gogue′
si·al′an·gi·og′ra·phy
si·al′a·po′ri·a
si′al·ec·ta′si·a

si'a·lem'e·sis *pl.* -ses'
si'al'ic
si'a·line'
si'a·li·thot'o·my
si'a·li'tis
si'a·lo·ad'e·nec'to·my
si'a·lo·ad'e·ni'tis
si'a·lo·ad'e·not'o·my
si'a·lo·aer'o·pha'gi·a
si'a·lo·an'gi·ec'ta·sis
   pl. -ses'
si'a·lo·an'gi·og'ra·phy
si'a·lo·an·gi'tis
si'a·lo·cele'
si'a·lo·do·chi'tis
si'a·lo·do'chi·um *pl.* -chi·a
si'a·lo·do'cho·li·thi'a·sis
si'a·lo·do'cho·plas'ty
si'a·lo·gas'trone'
si'a·log'e·nous
si·al'o·gogue'
si·al'o·gram'
si·al'o·graph'
si'a·log'ra·phy
si'a·loid'
si·al'o·lith'
si'a·lo·li·thi'a·sis
si'a·lo·li·thot'o·my
si'a·lo'ma *pl.* -mas *or* -ma·ta
si'a·lo·mu'cin
si'a·lon'
si'a·lor·rhe'a
si'a·los'che·sis
si'a·lo·se·mei·ol'o·gy
si'a·lo'sis
si'a·lo·ste·no'sis *pl.* -ses'
si'a·lo·syr'inx
   pl. -inx·es *or* -sy·rin'ges'
si'a·lot'ic
Si'a·mese' twins
Si'a water test
sib
sib'i·lant
sib'i·la'tion
sib'i·lis'mus
  —au'ri·um
sib'i·lus
sib'ling
sib'ship'
Sib'son fascia
Si·card' syndrome
sic'cant
sic'ca·tive

sic·cha'si·a
sic'cus
sick
sick'le
sick'le cell' anemia
sick'le-form'
sick'le·mi·a
sick'le·mic
sick'ling
sick'ness
Sid'bur'y syndrome
side
sid'er·a'tion
sid'er·i·nu'ri·a
sid'er·ism
Sid'er·o·bac'ter
sid'er·o·blast'
sid'er·o·blas'tic
sid'er·o·cyte'
sid'er·o·cy·to'sis *pl.* -ses'
sid'er·o·der'ma
sid'er·o·fi·bro'sis *pl.* -ses'
sid'er·o·pe'ni·a
sid'er·o·pe'nic
sid'e·ro·phage'
sid'er·o·phil'
sid'er·o·phil'i·a
sid'er·oph'i·lin
sid'er·oph'i·lous
sid'er·o·phyl'lin
sid'er·o·sil'i·co'sis *pl.* -ses'
sid'er·o'sis
  —bul'bi'
sid'er·ot'ic
side'swipe'
side'wall'
side'wind'er
Sie'gert sign
Sie'mens syndrome
sigh
sight
sig'ma
sig'ma·tism *(lisping)*
  ♦*stigmatism*
sig'moid'
sig'moid·ec'to·my
sig'moid·i'tis
sig'moi'do·pex'y
sig'moi'do·proc·tos'to·my
sig'moi'do·rec·tos'to·my
sig'moid'o·scope'
sig'moid'o·scop'ic
sig'moid·os'co·py

sig·moi'do·sig'moid·os'-
  to·my
sig'moid·os'to·my
sig'moid·ot'o·my
sig·moi'do·ves'i·cal
sign
sig'na
sig'nal
sig'na·ture
signe
  —de jour'nal'
  —de peau d'o·range'
sig'net
sig'num *pl.* -na
si·lan'drone'
si'lent
si'lex
sil'hou·ette'
sil'i·ca
sil'i·cate'
sil'i·ca·to'sis *pl.* -ses'
si·lic'ic
si·li'cious
si·li'ci·um
sil'i·co·an'thra·co'sis
  pl. -ses'
sil'i·co·fluor'ide'
sil'i·con' *(element)*
  ♦*silicone*
sil'i·cone' *(polymer)*
  ♦*silicon*
sil'i·co·sid'er·o'sis *pl.* -ses'
sil'i·co'sis *pl.* -ses'
sil'i·cot'ic
sil'i·co·tu·ber'cu·lo'sis
si·lique'
sil'i·quose'
sil'ver
Sil'ver syndrome
Sil·ves'ter method
si·meth'i·cone'
sim'i·an
si·mil'i·a si·mil'i·bus
  cu·ran'tur
si·mil'i·mum
Sim'monds disease
Sim'mons citrate agar
Si'mon
  —foci
  —operation
  —position
  —septic factor
Si'mo·nart'

—ligaments
—threads
sim'ple
Simp'son
—operation
—syndrome
Sims position
sim'tra·zene'
si'mul
sim'u·late', -lat'ed, -lat'ing
sim'u·la'tion
sim'u·la'tor
si'mul·tan·ag'no·si·a
si'mul·ta·ne·ous
si'nal
si·na'pis
sin'a·pism
sin'ca·lide'
sin·cip'i·tal
sin'ci·put pl. -puts or
   sin·cip'i·ta
Sind'bis fever
Sin'ding-Lar'sen-
   Jo·hans'son disease
sin'ew
sine wave
sin'gle
sin'gle-blind'
sin·gul·ta'tion
sin·gul'tus pl. -ti'
sin'is·ter
sin'is·trad'
sin'is·tral
sin'is·tral'i·ty
sin'is·tra'tion
sin'is·trau'ral
sin'is·tro·car'di·a
sin'is·tro·cer'e·bral
sin'is·troc'u·lar
sin'is·troc'u·lar'i·ty
sin'is·tro·gy·ra'tion
sin'is·tro·gy'ric
sin'is·tro·man·u'al
sin'is·trop'e·dal
sin'is·trorse'
sin'is·tro·tor'sion
sin'is·trous
si·no·a'tri·al
si'no·au·ric'u·lar
si'no·bron·chi'tis
si'no·ca·rot'id
si'no·gram'
si·nog'ra·phy

si·no·spi'ral
si'no·vag'i·nal
si'no·ven·tric'u·lar
sin'ter·ing
sin'u·ous
si'nus pl. -nus·es or si'nus
—a'lae' par'vae'
—a·na'lis
—a·or'tae'
—aortae (Val·sal'vae')
—ca·rot'i·cus
—cav'er·no'sus
—cir'cu·lar'is
—co·ro·nar'i·us
—cos'to·me·di·as'ti·na'lis
   pleu'rae'
—du'rae' ma'tris
—ep'i·di·dym'i·dis
—eth'moi·da'lis
—fron·ta'lis
—in'ter·cav'er·no'si'
—in'ter·cav'er·no'sus
   anterior
—intercavernosus posterior
—lac·tif'er·i'
—li·e'nis
—max'il·lar'is
—o·bli'quus per'i·car'di·i'
—oc·cip'i·ta'lis
—of Mor·ga'gni
—of Val·sal'va
—par'a·na·sa'les'
—pe·tro'sus interior
—petrosus superior
—phren'i·co·cos·ta'lis
   pleu'rae'
—pleu'rae'
—poc·u·lar'is
—posterior ca'vi' tym'pa·ni'
—pros·tat'i·cus
—rec·ta'les'
—rec'tus
—re·na'lis
—sag'it·ta'lis inferior
—sagittalis superior
—sig·moi'de·us
—sphe'noi·da'lis
—sphe'no·pa·ri'e·ta'lis
—tar'si'
—ton'sil·lar'is
—trans·ver'sus du'rae'
   ma'tris
—transversus per'i·car'di·i'

—trun'ci' pul'mo·na'lis
—tym'pa·ni'
—un'guis
—u'ro·gen'i·ta'lis
—ve·nar'um ca·var'um
—ve·no'sus
—venosus scle'rae'
—ver'te·bra'les' lon'gi·tu'-
   di·na'les'
si'nus·al
si'nus·i'tis
si'nus·oid'
si'nus·oi'dal
si'nus·oi'dal·i·za'tion
si'nus·ot'o·my
si'phon
si'phon·age
Si'pho·nap'ter·a
Si'phun·cu·la'ta
Si'phun·cu·li'na
Sip'py
—diet
—powder
si·ren'i·form'
si·ren·oid'
si·ren·o·me'li·a
si·ren·om'e·lus pl. -li
si·ri'a·sis pl. -ses'
Sis'ter Mar'y Jo'seph node
Sis'to sign
Sis·tru'rus
site
si·tol'o·gy (dietetics)
   ♦cytology
si'to·ma'ni·a
si'to·pho'bi·a
si'to·stane'
si'to·ther'a·py
si'to·tox'in
si'to·tox'ism
sit·u·a'tion
sit'u·a'tion·al
si'tus pl. si'tus
—in·ver'sus
—inversus vis'cer·um
—mu·ta'tus
—per·ver'sus
—sol'i·tus
—trans·ver'sus
sitz bath
size
Sjö'gren syndrome
ska·tox'yl

skein
ske·lal'gi·a
ske'las·the'ni·a
skel'e·tal
skel'e·ti·za'tion
skel'e·tog'e·nous
skel'e·ton
   —ex·trem'i·ta'tis in·fe'ri·o'-
     ris lib'er·ae'
   —extremitatis su·pe'ri·o'ris
     lib'er·ae'
   —mem'bri' in·fe'ri·o'ris
     lib'er·i
   —membri su·pe'ri·o'ris
     lib'er·i'
skel'e·ton·ize'
Skene
   —duct
   —glands
skene'o·scope'
ske·ni'tis
ske'o·cy·to'sis pl. -ses'
skew
skew'er
skew'foot'
ski'a·gram'
ski·ag'ra·phy
ski·am'e·try
ski'a·po·res'co·py
ski'a·scope'
ski·as'co·py
skid
skill
Skil'lern fracture
skin
Skin'ner box
skin'ny
skip, skipped, skip'ped
Sklow'sky symptom
Skoog method
skull
sky'line'
slake, slaked, slak'ing
slant
sleep, slept, sleep'ing
sleep'less·ness
sleep'walk'er
sleep'walk'ing
sleeve
slice
slide
sling
slip, slipped, slip'ping

slit
slit' lamp' test
slope, sloped, slop'ing
slough
slow
Slu'der
   —method
   —syndrome
sludge
sluice'way'
slum'ber
slur, slurred, slur'ring
slur'ry
small
small'pox'
smear
smeg'ma
   —cli·tor'i·dis
   —em'bry·o'num
   —prae·pu'ti·i'
smeg·mat'ic
smeg'mo·lith'
Smel'lie method
Smith
   —dislocation
   —fracture
   —phenomenon
   —test
Smith'wick' operation
smoke, smoked, smok'ing
smudg'ing
smut
snake
snake'bite'
snake'root'
snap, snapped, snap'ping
snare, snared, snar'ing
sneeze, sneezed, sneez'ing
Snel'len
   —chart
   —reflex
   —test
snore, snored, snor'ing
snow blindness
snuff'box'
snuf'fles
Sny'der test
soap
soap'stone'
sob, sobbed, sob'bing
so·cal'o·in
so'ci·a
   —pa·rot'i·dis

   —pa·ro'tis
so'cial
so'cial·i·za'tion
so'ci·o·cen'tric
so'ci·o·cen'trism
so'ci·o·gen'e·sis pl. -ses'
so'ci·o·log'ic
so'ci·o·log'i·cal
so'ci·ol'o·gy
so'ci·o·med'i·cal
so'ci·om'e·try
so'ci·o·path'
so'ci·o·path'ic
so'ci·op'a·thy
sock
sock'et
so'da
so'da·mide'
Sö'der·bergh' pressure
   reflex
so'di·um
   —an·az'o·lene'
   —an'ti·mo'nyl·glu'co·nate'
   —au'ro·thi'o·mal'ate'
   —eth'a·sul'fate'
   —eth'yl·mer'cu'ri·thi'o·sal'-
     i·cy·late'
   —flu'o·ro·ac'e·tate'
   —flu'o·sil'i·cate'
   —fu'si·date'
   —hy·drox'y·di'one' suc'-
     ci·nate'
   —in'di·go·tin'di·sul'fo·nate'
   —i'o·do·hip'pur·ate'
   —i'o·do·meth'a·mate'
   —i'o·tha·lam'ate
   —ip'o·date'
   —me·thi'o·dal'
   —mor'rhu·ate'
   —ni'tro·fer'ri·cy'a·nide'
   —ric'i·nate'
   —ric'in·o'le·ate'
   —stib'o·glu'co·nate'
   —su'per·ox'ide'
   —tet'ra·bo'rate'
   —tung'state'
so'do·ku
sod'o·mist
sod'o·mite'
sod'o·my
Soem'mer·ing
   —area
   —foramen

—ganglion
—ring
—spot
soft
sol
so'la·na'ceous
so'la·nine'
so·lap'sone'
so'lar
so·lar'i·um *pl.* -i·a
so·lar·i·za'tion
so'lar·ize', -ized', -iz'ing
sol·a'tion
sole
so·le'al
So'le·nog'ly·pha
so'le·no·glyph'ic
so'le·no·nych'i·a
sole'plate'
So'ler·a reaction
so'le·us *pl.* -le·i' *or* -le·us·es
—ac'ces·so'ri·us
sol'id
so·lid'i·fi·ca'tion
so·lid'i·fy', -fied', -fy'ing
sol'i·dus *pl.* -di
sol'ip·sism
sol'i·tar'y
—cells of Mey'nert
sol'-lu'nar
Sol'o·mon rule
Sol·pu'gi·da
sol'u·bil'i·ty
sol'u·bi·li·za'tion
sol'u·bi·lize', -lized', -liz'ing
sol'u·ble
so'lum tym'pa·ni'
so·lute'
so·lu'ti·o'
so·lu'tion
sol'vate'
sol·va'tion
sol'vent
sol·vol'y·sis *pl.* -ses'
so'ma *pl.* -ma·ta *or* -mas
so'mal
so'mas·the'ni·a
so'mat·es·the'si·a
so'mat·es·thet'ic
so·mat'ic
so·mat'i·co·splanch'nic
so·mat'i·co·vis'cer·al
so·ma·tist

so'ma·ti·za'tion
so'ma·tize', -tized', -tiz'ing
so·mat'o·cep'tor
so·mat'o·chrome
so·mat'o·derm'
so·ma·to·did'y·mus
so·ma·to·dym'i·a
so·mat'o·ge·net'ic
so·ma·to·gen'ic
so'ma·tog'e·ny
so'ma·to·log'ic
so'ma·tol'o·gy
so'ma·tome'
so·ma·to·me'din
so·ma·to·meg'a·ly
so·ma·to·met'ric
so·ma·tom'e·try
so·ma·top'a·gus
so·ma·to·path'ic
so·ma·to·phre'ni·a
so·ma·to·plasm
so'ma·to·pleu'ral
so'ma·to·pleure'
so·ma·to·psy'chic
so·ma·to·psy·cho'sis
 pl. -ses'
so·ma·to·sen'so·ry
so·ma·to·splanch'no·pleu'-
 ric
so'ma·to·stat'in
so'ma·to·ther'a·py
so·ma·to·to'ni·a
so·ma·to·ton'ic
so·ma·to·top'ag·no'si·a
so·ma·to·top'ic
so·ma·to·trid'y·mus
so·ma·to·tro'phin
so·ma·to·trop'ic
so·ma·to·tro'pin
so·ma·to·type'
so·ma·to·ty·pol'o·gy
so'ma·trem
so·mat'ro·pin
so·mes·the'si·a
so·mes·thet'ic
so'mite'
som·nam'bu·lance
som·nam'bu·la'tion
som·nam'bu·la·tor
som·nam'bu·lism
som·nam'bu·lisme'
 pro·vo·qué'
som·nam'bu·list

som'ni·al
som'ni·a'tion
som'ni·fa'cient
som·nif'er·ous
som·nif'ic
som·nif'u·gous
som·nil'o·quence
som·nil'o·quism
som·nil'o·quist
som·nil'o·quy
som·nip'a·thist
som·nip'a·thy
som'no·cin'e·mat'o·graph'
som'no·lence
som'no·len·cy
som'no·lent
som·no·len'ti·a
som·no·les'cent
som'no·lism
som'nus
So'mo·gyi
—method
—unit
Son'der·mann canal
sone
Sones
—arteriography
—catheterization
—cineangiography
—technique
son'ic
son'i·cate'
son'i·ca'tion
son'i·tus
Son'ne dysentery
son'o·chem'i·cal
son'o·chem'i·cal·ly
son'o·chem'is·try
son'o·en·ceph'a·lo·gram'
son'o·gram'
son'o·graph'ic
so·nog'ra·phy
son'o·lu'cent
so·nom'e·ter
so·no'rous
so'nus
so·phis'ti·cate'
so·phis'ti·ca'tion
soph'o·ma'ni·a
soph'o·rine'
so'por
so·po'rate', -rat·ed, -rat·ing
sop'o·rif'er·ous

sop'o·rif'ic
so'po·rose'
sor·be·fa'cient
sor'bent
sor'bic
sor'bi·tan'
sor'bite'
sor'bi·tol'
sor'bose'
sor'des' *pl.* sor'des'
sore
sor'ghum
so·ro'ri·a'tion
sorp'tion
sor'rel
so'ta·lol'
so·ter'e·nol'
souf'fle
sound
Souques sign
South'wick osteotomy
soy'bean'
spa
space
—of Burns
—of Dis'se
—of Ret'zi·us
—of Te·non'
spac'er
spaces
—of Lit·tré'
—of Vir'chow-Rob'in
Spal'ding sign
Spal'lan·za'ni law
spal·la'tion
span
spar'ga·no'sis *pl.* -ses'
spare, spared, spar'ing
spar·go'sis *pl.* -ses'
spar'kling
spar'so·my'cin
spar'te·ine'
spasm
spas·mod'ic
spas'mo·gen
spas·mo·gen'ic
spas·mol'o·gy
spas'mo·lyg'mus
spas·mol'y·sis *pl.* -ses'
spas'mo·lyt'ic
spas'mo·phil'i·a
spas'mo·phil'ic
spas'mus

—bron'chi·a'lis
—glot'ti·dis
—mus'cu·lar'is
—nic'ti·tans'
—nu'tans'
—oc'u·li'
spas'tic
spas·tic'i·ty
spa'ti·a
—an'gu·li' i'ri·dis
—anguli i'ri·do·cor'ne·a'lis
—in'ter·cos·ta'li·a
—in'ter·glob'u·lar'i·a
—in'ter·os'se·a met·a·car'pi·
—interossea met·a·tar'si·
—in'ter·vag'i·na'li·a
—zon·u·lar'i·a
spa'tial
spa'tic
spa'ti·um *pl.* -ti·a
—ep'i·scle·ra'le'
—in'ter·cos·ta'le'
—per'i·cho'ri·oi'de·a'le'
—per'i·cho·roi'de·a'le'
—per'i·lym·phat'i·cum
—per'i·ne·i' pro·fun'dum
—perinei su'per·fi'ci·a'le'
—ret'ro·per'i·to·ne·a'le'
—ret'ro·pu'bi·cum
spat'u·la
spat'u·late'
spat'u·la'tion
spe'cial·ist
spe'cial·i·za'tion
spe'cial·ty
spe'cies *pl.* spe'cies'
spe'cies-spe·cif'ic
spe·cif'ic
spec'i·fic'i·ty
spec'i·men
speck'le
spec'ta·cles
spec'ti·no·my'cin
spec'tral
spec'trin
spec'tro·chem'i·cal
spec'tro·chem'is·try
spec'tro·col'o·rim'e·ter
spec'tro·fluo·rom'e·ter
spec'tro·gram'
spec'tro·graph'
spec'tro·graph'ic
spec·trog'ra·phy

spec·trom'e·ter
spec·trom'e·try
spec'tro·mi'cro·scope'
spec'tro·pho·tom'e·ter
spec'tro·pho'to·met'ric
spec'tro·pho·tom'e·try
spec'tro·po'la·rim'e·ter
spec'tro·scope'
spec'tro·scop'ic
spec·tros'co·py
spec'trum *pl.* -tra or -trums
spec'u·lum *pl.* -la or -lums
speech
Spee curve
spe'le·os'to·my
Spen'cer-Par'ker vaccine
Speng'ler fragments
Spens syndrome
sperm *pl.* sperm or sperms
sper'ma·cra'si·a
sper'ma·ta·cra'si·a
sper·mat'ic
sper·mat'i·cid'al
sper·mat'i·cide'
sper'ma·tid
sper'ma·tism
sper'ma·to·blast'
sper'ma·to·blas'tic
sper·mat'o·cele'
sper'ma·to·ce·lec'to·my
sper'ma·to·cid'al
sper'ma·to·cide'
sper'ma·to·cyst'
sper'ma·to·cys·tec'to·my
sper'ma·to·cys'tic
sper'ma·to·cys·ti'tis
sper'ma·to·cys·tot'o·my
sper'ma·to·cy'tal
sper·mat'o·cyte'
sper'ma·to·cy'to·gen'e·sis
sper'ma·to·cy·to'ma
  pl. -mas or -ma·ta
sper'ma·to·gen'e·sis
sper'ma·to·gen'ic
sper'ma·tog'e·nous
sper'ma·tog'e·ny
sper'ma·to·go'ni·um
  pl. -ni·a
sper'ma·toid'
sper'ma·tol'y·sin
sper'ma·tol'y·sis *pl.* -ses'
sper'ma·to·lyt'ic
sper'ma·to·mere'

sper'ma·to·me'rite'
sper'ma·top'a·thy
sper'mat'o·phore'
sper'ma·tor·rhe'a
—dor'mi·en'tum
sper'ma·tos'che·sis
sper'ma·to·tox'in
sper'ma·tox'in
sper'ma·to·zo'a
sper'ma·to·zo'al
sper'ma·to·zo'i·cide'
sper'ma·to·zo'id
sper'ma·to·zo'on' *pl.* -zo'a
sper'ma·tu'ri·a
sper·mec'to·my
sper'mi·a'tion
sper'mi·cid'al
sper'mi·cide'
sper'mi·dine'
sper'mine'
sper'mi·o·gen'e·sis
sper'mi·o·gram'
sper'mi·um *pl.* -mi·a
sper'mo·cy·to'ma *pl.* -mas
or -ma·ta
sper'mo·lith'
sper·mo·lo'ro·pex'y
sper·mol'y·sin
sper·mol'y·sis *pl.* -ses'
sper'mo·neu·ral'gi·a
sper'mo·tox'ic
sper'mo·tox'in
Sper'ry method
spes phthis'i·ca
sphac'e·late', -lat'ed, -lat'ing
sphac'e·la'tion
sphac'e·lism
sphac'e·lo·der'ma
sphac'e·loid
sphac'e·lous
sphac'e·lus
spha'gi·as'mus
spha·gi'tis
sphe'ni·on'
sphe'no·bas'i·lar
sphe'no·ce·phal'ic
sphe'no·ceph'a·lus *pl.* -li'
sphe'no·ceph'a·ly
sphe'no·eth'moid'
sphe'no·fron'tal
sphe'noid'
sphe·noi'dal
sphe'noid·i'tis

sphe'noid·os'to·my
sphe'noid·ot'o·my
sphe'no·ma'lar
sphe'no·man·dib'u·lar
sphe'no·max'il·lar'y
sphe'no-oc·cip'i·tal
sphe'no·pal'a·tine'
sphe'no·pa·ri'e·tal
sphe'no·pe·tro'sal
sphe·no'sis
sphe'no·squa·mo'sal
sphe'no·tem'po·ral
sphe·not'ic
sphe'no·tre'si·a
sphe'no·tribe'
sphe'no·trip'sy
sphe'no·tur'bi·nal
sphe'no·vo'mer·ine
sphe'no·zy'go·mat'ic
sphere
spher'es·the'si·a
spher'ic *or* spher'i·cal
sphe'ro·ceph'a·lus *pl.* -li'
sphe'ro·cyl'in·der
sphe'ro·cyte'
sphe'ro·cyt'ic
sphe'ro·cy·to'sis *pl.* -ses'
sphe'roid'
sphe·roi'dal
sphe·ro'ma *pl.* -mas *or*
-ma·ta
sphe·rom'e·ter
sphe'ro·plast'
spher'ule'
sphinc'ter
—am'pul'lae'
—a'ni' ex·ter'nus
—ani in·ter'nus
—duc'tus cho·led'o·chi'
—of Boy'den
—of Od'di
—pan'cre·at'i·cus
—u're'thrae'
—urethrae mem'bra·na'-
ce·ae'
—ve'si'cae'
sphinc'ter·al
sphinc'ter·al'gi·a
sphinc'ter·ec'to·my
sphinc'ter'ic
sphinc'ter·is'mus
sphinc'ter·i'tis
sphinc'ter·ol'y·sis *pl.* -ses'

sphinc'ter·o·plas'ty
sphinc'ter·o·tome'
sphinc'ter·ot'o·my
sphin'go·lip'id
sphin'go·lip'i·do'sis
pl. -ses'
sphin'go·li'po·dys'tro·phy
sphin'go·my'e·lin
sphin'go·my'e·lin·o'sis
sphin'go·sine'
sphyg'mic *or* sphyg'mi·cal
sphyg'mo·bo·lom'e·ter
sphyg'mo·bo·lom'e·try
sphyg'mo·chron'o·graph'
sphyg'mo·chro·nog'ra·phy
sphyg·mod'ic
sphyg'mo·dy'na·mom'e·
ter
sphyg'mo·gram'
sphyg'mo·graph'
sphyg'mo·graph'ic
sphyg·mog'ra·phy
sphyg'moid'
sphyg'mo·ma·nom'e·ter
sphyg'mo·ma·nom'e·try
sphyg·mom'e·ter
sphyg'mo·os'cil·lom'e·ter
sphyg'mo·pal·pa'tion
sphyg'mo·phone'
sphyg'mo·scope'
sphyg·mos'co·py
sphyg'mo·sys'to·le
sphyg'mo·tech'ny
sphyg'mo·to'no·graph'
sphyg'mo·to·nom'e·ter
sphyg'mus *pl.* -mi'
sphynx'-neck'
sphy·rec'to·my
sphy·rot'o·my
spi'ca *pl.* -cae' *or* -cas
spic'u·la *pl.* -lae'
spic'u·lar
spic'u·late'
spic'ule'
spic'u·lum *pl.* -la
spi'der
Spie'gler
—test
—tumor
Spie'gler-Fendt' sarcoid
spi·ge'li·a
Spi·ge'li·an
—hernia

—lobe
spike
spike'nard'
spill'age
spi·lo'ma *pl.* -mas *or* -ma·ta
spi'lo·pla'ni·a
spi'lus *pl.* -li'
spin, spun, spin'ning
spi'na *pl.* -nae'
 —an'gu·lar'is
 —bif'i·da
 —bifida oc·cul'ta
 —fron·ta'lis
 —hel'i·cis
 —i·li'a·ca anterior inferior
 —iliaca anterior superior
 —iliaca posterior inferior
 —iliaca posterior superior
 —is·chi·ad'i·ca
 —mea'tus
 —men·ta'lis
 —na·sa'lis anterior max·il'-
  lae'
 —nasalis os'sis fron·ta'lis
 —nasalis posterior os'sis
  pal·a·ti'ni'
 —os'sis sphe·noi·da'lis
 —scap'u·lae'
 —su'pra·me·a'tum
 —troch'le·ar'is
 —tym·pan'i·ca major
 —tympanica minor
 —ven·to'sa
spin'a·cene'
spi'nae' pal'a·ti'nae'
spi'nal
spi'nal'gi·a
spi·na'lis
spi'nate'
spin'dle
spine
spi·nif'u·gal
spi·nip'e·tal
spi'no·bul'bar
spi'no·cer'e·bel'lar
spi'no·col·lic'u·lar
spi'no·cor'ti·cal
spi'no·gal'va·ni·za'tion
spi'no·gle'noid'
spi'no·ol'i·var'y
spi·no'sal
spi·no'sus

spi'no·tec'tal
spi'no·tha·lam'ic
spi'no·trans'ver·sar'i·us
spi'nous
spin·thar'i·con'
spin·thar'i·scope'
spin'ther·ism
spi'nu·lose'
spi'ny
spip'er·one'
spi'ra·cle
spi·rad'e·ni'tis sup'pu·ra·
  ti'va
spi·rad'e·no'ma *pl.* -mas *or*
  -ma·ta
spi'ral
spi'ral·i·za'tion
spi'ra·my'cin
spi'reme'
Spi'ril·la·ce·ae'
spi·ril'lar
spi·ril'lar'y
spi·ril'le·mi·a
spi·ril'li·cid'al
spi·ril'lo'sis *pl.* -ses'
spi·ril'lum *pl.* -la
spir'it
spir'i·tous
spir'i·tus
 —fru·men'ti'
Spi'ro·cer'ca
Spi'ro·chae'ta
 —ic'ter·og'e·nes'
 —ic'ter·o·haem'or·rhag'-
  i·ae'
 —mor'sus mu'ris
 —o'ber·mei'er·i'
 —pal'li·da
Spi'ro·chae·ta'ce·ae'
spi'ro·che'tal
spi'ro·chete'
spi'ro·che·te'mi·a
spi'ro·che'ti·cide'
spi'ro·che·tol'y·sis *pl.* -ses'
spi'ro·che·to'sis *pl.* -ses'
spi'ro·che·tot'ic
spi'ro·gram'
spi'ro·graph'
spi'ro·graph'ic
spi·rog'ra·phy
spi·rom'e·ter
spi'ro·met'ric
spi·rom'e·try

spi'ro·no·lac'tone'
Spi·rop'ter·a ne'o·plas'ti·ca
spi'ro·scope'
spi·rox'a·sone'
spis'sat'ed
spis'si·tude'
spit'tle
Spitz nevus
splanch'na·po·phys'e·al
splanch'na·poph'y·sis
  pl. -ses'
splanch'nec·to'pi·a
splanch'nem·phrax'is
splanch'nes·the'si·a
splanch'nic
splanch'ni·cec'to·my
splanch'ni·cot'o·my
splanch'no·blast'
splanch'no·cele' (a hernial
  protrusion)
  ♦ *splanchnocoele*
splanch'no·coele' (part of the
  coelom)
  ♦ *splanchnocele*
splanch'no·cra'ni·um
  pl. -ni·ums *or* -ni·a
splanch'no·di·as'ta·sis
splanch·nog'ra·phy
splanch'no·lith'
splanch'no·li·thi'a·sis
  pl. -ses'
splanch'no·lo'gi·a
splanch·nol'o·gy
splanch'no·meg'a·ly
splanch'no·mi'cri·a
splanch·nop'a·thy
splanch'no·pleu'ral
splanch'no·pleure'
splanch'nop·to'si·a
splanch'nop·to'sis *pl.* -ses'
splanch'no·scle·ro'sis
  pl. -ses'
splanch·nos'co·py
splanch'no·skel'e·ton
splanch'no·so·mat'ic
splanch·not'o·my
splanch'no·tribe'
splash
splay
splay'foot'
spleen
splen'ad·e·no'ma *pl.* -mas
  or -ma·ta

sple·nal′gi·a
sple·nat′ro·phy
sple·nec′ta·sis
sple·nec′to·mize′, -mized′,
 -miz′ing
sple·nec′to·my
splen′ec·to′pi·a
sple·nec′to·py
sple·ne′mi·a
sple·ne′o·lus *pl.* -li
sple·net′ic
sple·ni′al
splen′ic
splen′i·co·pan′cre·at′ic
sple·nic′ter·us
splen′i·fi·ca′tion
splen′i·form′
sple·ni′tis
sple·ni′um *pl.* -ni·a
 —cor′po·ris cal·lo′si′
sple·ni′us *pl.* -ni·i′
 —cer′vi·cis ac′ces·so′ri·us
splen′i·za′tion
sple·no′cele′
sple·no·clei′sis
sple·no′cyte′
sple·no·dyn′i·a
sple·nog′e·nous
sple·no′gram′
sple·no·gran′u·lo′ma·to′sis
 sid′er·ot′i·ca
sple·nog′ra·phy
sple·no·hep′a·to·meg′a·ly
sple′noid′
sple·no·ker′a·to′sis *pl.* -ses′
sple·no·lap′a·rot′o·my
sple·no·lym·phat′ic
sple·nol′y·sis
sple·no′ma *pl.* -mas *or*
 -ma·ta
sple′no·ma·la′ci·a
sple′no·me·ga′li·a
sple′no·meg′a·ly
sple′no·my′e·log′e·nous
sple′no·neph′ric
sple′no·neph′rop·to′sis
sple′no·pan′cre·at′ic
sple·nop′a·thy
sple′no·pex′y
sple′no·phren′ic
sple′no·pneu·mo′ni·a
sple′no·por′to·gram′
sple′no·por·tog′ra·phy

sple′nop·to′sis *pl.* -ses′
sple′no·re′nal
sple′nor·rha′gi·a
sple′nor·rha·phy
sple·no′sis
sple·not′o·my
sple′no·tox′in
sple′no·ty′phoid′
splen′u·lus *pl.* -li′
sple·nun′cu·lus *pl.* -li′
splice, spliced, splic′ing
splint
splint′age
splin′ter
splint′ing
split
split′-thick′ness
split′ting
spo′di·o·my′e·li′tis
spo′do·gram′
spo·dog′ra·phy
spoke
spon′dy·lal′gi·a
spon′dyl·ar·thri′tis
spon′dyl·ar·throc′a·ce′
spon′dyl·ex′ar·thro′sis
 pl. -ses′
spon′dy·lit′ic
spon′dy·li′tis
 —an′ky·lo′poi·et′i·ca
spon′dy·li·ze′ma
spon′dy·lo·ar·thri′tis
spon′dy·loc′a·ce′
spon′dy·lod′e·sis
spon′dy·lo·di·dym′i·a
spon′dy·lod′y·mus
spon′dy·lo·dyn′i·a
spon′dy·lo·lis·the′sis
spon′dy·lo·lis·thet′ic
spon′dy·lol′y·sis
spon′dy·lo·ma·la′ci·a
spon′dy·lop′a·thy
spon′dy·lo·py·o′sis *pl.* -ses′
spon′dy·lo′sis *pl.* -ses′
spon′dy·lo·syn·de′sis
 pl. -ses′
spon′dy·lot′o·my
spon′dy·lous
spon′dy·lus *pl.* -li′
sponge
spon′gi·a
spon′gi·form′
spon′gi·i′tis

spon′gi·o·blast′
spon′gi·o·blas′to·ma
 pl. -mas *or* -ma·ta
 —mul′ti·for′me′
 —po·lar′e′
 —prim′i·ti′vum
 —u′ni·po·lar′e′
spon′gi·o·cyte′
spon′gi·o·cy′to·ma *pl.* -mas
 or -ma·ta
spon′gi·o·form′
spon′gi·oid′
spon′gi·o·neu′ro·blas·to′-
 ma *pl.* -mas *or* -ma·ta
spon′gi·o·plasm
spon′gi·ose′
spon′gi·o′sis
spon′gi·o·si′tis
spon′gi·ot′ic
spon′gy
spon·ta′ne′ous
spon·ta′ne′ous·ly
spoon
spoo′ner·ism
spo·rad′ic
spo·ran′gi·o·phore′
spo·ran′gi·o·spore′
spo·ran′gi·um *pl.* -gi·a
spore
spo′ri·cid′al
spo′ri·cide′
spo·rid′i·um *pl.* -i·a
spo·ro·ag·glu′ti·na′tion
spo′ro·blast′
spo′ro·cyst′
spo′ro·gen′e·sis
spo′ro·gen′ic
spo·rog′e·nous
spo·rog′o·ny
spo′ront′
spo′ro·phyte′
spo′ro·plasm
Spo′ro·thrix′ schenk′i·i′
spo·rot′ri·chin
spo′ro·tri·cho′sis *pl.* -ses′
Spo′ro·zo′a
spo′ro·zo′an
spo′ro·zo′ite′
spo′ro·zo′on′ *pl.* -zo′a
spor·u′lar
spor′u·late′, -lat′ed, -lat′ing
spor′u·la′tion
spor′ule′

spot, spot'ted, spot'ting
spout
sprain
spray
spread, spread, spread'ing
spread'er
Spren'gel deformity
sprue
spud
spur
spu'ri·ous
spu'tum *pl.* -ta *or* -tums
squa'lene'
squa'ma *pl.* -mae'
—fron·ta'lis
—oc·cip'i·ta'lis
—tem'po·ra'lis
squa'mate'
squa'ma·ti·za'tion
squa'mo·bas'al
squa'mo·cel'lu·lar
squa'mo·col'um·nar
squa'mo·fron'tal
squa'moid'
squa'mo·mas'toid'
squa'mo·oc·cip'i·tal
squa'mo·pa·ri'e·tal
squa·mo·pe·tro'sal
squa·mo'sa *pl.* -sae'
squa·mo'sal
squa'mo·sphe'noid'
squa'mo·tem'po·ral
squa'mo·tym·pan'ic
squa'mous
squa'mo·zy'go·mat'ic
square
squar'rose'
squeeze
squill
squint
Ssa·ba'ne·jew-Frank'
  operation
stab, stabbed, stab'bing
sta'bile *(immobile)*
  ♦*stable*
sta·bil'i·ty
sta'bi·lize', -lized', -liz'ing
sta'bi·liz'er
sta'ble *(immutable)*
  ♦*stabile*
stac·ca'to
stach'y·drine'
stach'y·ose'

stacked
stac·tom'e·ter
sta'di·um *pl.* -di·a
—ac'mes'
—am·phib'o·les'
—an·ni'hi·la'ti·o'nis
—aug·men'ti'
—ca·lo'ris
—con·ta'gi·i'
—con·va·les·cen'ti·ae'
—dec·re·men'ti'
—de'crus·ta'ti·o'nis
—des·qua·ma'ti·o·nis
—e·rup'ti·o'nis
—ex'sic·ca'ti·o'nis
—flo·ri'ti·o'nis
—frig'o·ris
—in'cre·men'ti'
—in'cu·ba'ti·o'nis
—ma·ni'a·ca'le'
—ner·vo'sum
—pro'dro·mo'rum
—su·do'ris
—sup'pu·ra'ti·o'nis
—ul'ti·mum
Staeh'li pigment line
staff
stage
stag'nant
stag'nate', -nat'ed, -nat'ing
stag·na'tion
Stahl ear
stain
stain'a·ble
stain'less
stair'step'
stal'a·gom'e·ter
stalk
sta'men *pl.* -mens *or* -mi·na
Sta'mey test
stam'i·na
stam'mer
Stamm gastrostomy
stand
stan'dard
stan'dard·i·za'tion
stan'dard·ize', -ized', -iz'ing
stand'by'
stand'off'
stand'still'
Stan'ford-Bi·net' test
Stan'more' arthroplasty
stan'nate'

stan'nic
stan'nous
stan'num
stan'o·lone'
stan'o·zo'lol'
sta'pe·dec'to·my
sta·pe'di·al
sta·pe'di·o·te·not'o·my
sta·pe'di·o·ves·tib'u·lar
sta·pe'di·us *pl.* -di·i'
sta'pes' *pl.* sta'pes' *or*
  sta·pe'des'
staph'i·sa'gri·a
staph'y·le
staph'y·lec'to·my
staph'yl·e·de'ma
staph'yl·he'ma·to'ma
staph'y·line'
staph'y·li'no·pha·ryn'-
  ge·us
staph'y·li'nus
—ex·ter'nus
—in·ter'nus
—me'di·us
sta·phyl'i·on'
staph'y·li'tis
staph'y·lo·coc'cal
staph'y·lo·coc·ce'mi·a
staph'y·lo·coc'cic
staph'y·lo·coc·co'sis
staph'y·lo·coc'cus *pl.* -ci'
Staph'y·lo·coc'cus
—al'bus
—au're·us
—cit're·us
—ep'i·der'mi·dis
—py·og'e·nes'
staph'y·lo·co'sis *pl.* -ses'
staph'y·lo·der'ma
staph'y·lo·der'ma·ti'tis
staph'y·lo·di·al'y·sis
staph'y·lo·ki'nase'
staph'y·lol'y·sin
staph'y·lo'ma *pl.* -mas *or*
  -ma·ta
—cor'ne·ae'
—u've·a'le'
staph'y·lom'a·tous
staph'y·lon'cus
staph'y·lo·pha·ryn'ge·us
staph'y·lo·phar'yn·gor'-
  rha·phy
staph'y·lo·plas'ty

staph′y·lop·to′sis
staph′y·lor′rha·phy
staph′y·los′chi·sis *pl.* -ses′
staph′y·lot′o·my
staph′y·lo·tox′in
sta′ple
sta′pler
star
starch
Star′gardt′ disease
Star′ling law
start′er
star′tle, -tled, -tling
star·va′tion
starve, starved, starv′ing
sta′sis *pl.* -ses′
state
stat′ic
stat′ics
stat′im
sta′tion
sta′tion·ar′y
sta·tis′tic
sta·tis′ti·cal
sta·tis′tics
stat′o·co′ni·a *sing.* -ni·um
stat′o·cyst′
stat′o·ki·net′ic
stat′o·lith′
sta′to·lon′
sta·tom′e·ter
stat′ur·al
stat′ure
sta′tus
— an′gi·no′sus
— ar·thrit′i·cus
— asth·mat′i·cus
— con′vul·si′vus
— cri·bro′sus
— dys′my′e·li·ni·sa′tus of Vogt
— dys′raph′i·cus
— ep′i·lep′ti·cus
— fi·bro′sus
— lym·phat′i·cus
— mar′mo·ra′tus
— mi·grai′nus
— par′a·thy′re·o·pri′vus
— post
— prae′sens
— rap′tus
— spon′gi·o′sus
— thy′mi·co·lym·phat′i·cus

— thy′mi·cus
— ver′ru·co′sus
— ver·tig′i·no′sus
stat′u·vo′lence
stat′u·vo′lent
Staub′-Trau′gott effect
stau′ri·on′
staves·a′cre
stax′is
stay
stead′y
steal
steam
ste·ap′sin
ste′a·ral′de·hyde′
ste′a·rate′
ste·ar′ic
ste·ar′i·form′
ste′a·rin
ste′a·ro·der′mi·a
ste·ar·rhe′a
— fla·ves′cens
— ni′gri·cans′
— sim′plex
ste′a·ryl
ste′a·ti′tis
ste′a·to·cryp·to′sis *pl.* -ses′
ste′a·to·cys·to′ma mul′-
   ti·plex′
ste′a·tog′e·nous
ste′a·tol′y·sis *pl.* -ses′
ste′a·to·lyt′ic
ste′a·to′ma *pl.* -mas *or* -ma·ta
ste′a·to′ma·to′sis
ste′a·tom′a·tous
ste′a·tom′er·y
ste′a·to·ne·cro′sis
ste′a·to·pyg′i·a
ste′a·top′y·gous
ste′a·tor·rhe′a
ste′a·to′sis *pl.* -ses′
Steele′-Rich′ard·son-
   Ol·szew′ski syndrome
Steell murmur
Steen′bock′ unit
steep
stee′ple
stef′fi·my′cin
ste′ge
steg·no′sis *pl.* -ses′
steg·not′ic
Steg′o·my′ia
Stei′nach′ method

Stein′brock′er class
Steind′ler operation
Stei′nert disease
Stei′ner tumor
Stein′-Lev′en·thal′
   syndrome
Stein test
stel′la *pl.* -lae′
— len′tis hy′a·loi′de·a
— lentis i·rid′i·ca
stel′lar
stel′late′
stel·lec′to·my
stel′lu·la *pl.* -lae′
stel′lu·lae′
— vas′cu·lo′sae′ wins·
   low′i·i′
— ver·hey′en·i·i′
Stell′wag′
— operation
— sign
stem
Sten′der dish
Sten′ger test
sten′i·on′ *pl.* -ni·a
sten′o·car′di·a
sten′o·car′di·ac′
sten′o·ce·phal′ic
sten′o·ceph′a·lous
sten′o·ceph′a·ly
sten′o·cho′ri·a
sten′o·co·ri′a·sis
sten′o·crot′a·phy
sten′o·dont′
sten′o·mer′ic
Ste·no′ni·an duct
sten′o·pe′ic
ste·no′sal
sten·ose′, -nosed′, -nos′ing
ste·no′sis *pl.* -ses′
sten·nos′to·my
sten′o·ther′mal
sten′o·tho′rax′
ste·not′ic
Sten′sen
— duct
— foramen
stent
Sten′ver
— projection
— view
step′down′
ste·pha′ni·al

ste·phan′ic
ste·pha′ni·on′
step′up′
ste·ra′di·an
ster′co·bi′lin
ster′co·bi·lin′o·gen
ster′co·lith′
ster′co·por′phy·rin
ster′co·ra′ceous
ster′co·ral
ster′co·rar′y
ster′co·ro′ma pl. -mas or -ma·ta
ster′co·rous
ster′cus
stere
ster′e·o·ag·no′sis pl. -ses′
ster′e·o·an·es·the′si·a
ster′e·o·ar·throl′y·sis pl. -ses′
ster′e·o·blas′tu·la pl. -las or -lae′
ster′e·o·cam·pim′e·ter
ster′e·o·chem′i·cal
ster′e·o·chem′is·try
ster′e·o·cil′i·a sing. -i·um
ster′e·o·en·ceph′a·lo′tome′
ster′e·o·en·ceph′a·lot′o·my
ster′e·o·fluo·ros′co·py
ster′e·og·no′sis
ster′e·og·nos′tic
ster′e·o·gram′
ster′e·o·graph′
ster′e·og′ra·phy
ster′e·o·i′so·mer
ster′e·o·i·som′er·ism
ster′e·om′e·ter
ster′e·om′e·try
ster′e·o·mon′o·scope′
ster′e·o·oph·thal′mo·scope′
ster′e·o·phan′to·scope
ster′e·o·pho′ro·scope′
ster′e·o·pho′to·mi′cro·graph′
ster′e·o·plasm
ster′e·op′sis
ster′e·op′ter
ster′e·o·ra′di·og′ra·phy
ster′e·o·roent′gen·og′ra·phy
ster′e·o·scope′
ster′e·o·scop′ic

ster′e·os′co·py
ster′e·o·spe·cif′ic
ster′e·o·spec′i·fic′i·ty
ster′e·o·stro′bo·scope′
ster′e·o·tac′tic
ster′e·o·tax′i·a
ster′e·o·tax′ic
ster′e·o·tax′is pl. -tax′es′
ster′e·o·tax′y
ster′e·o·trop′ic
ster′e·ot′ro·pism
ster′e·o·type′
ster′e·o·typ′ic
ster′e·o·ty′py
ster′ic
ster′id
ste·rig′ma pl. -ma·ta or -mas
ster′ig·mat′ic
Ste·rig′ma·to·cys′tis
—cin′na·mo·mi′nus
ster′ile
ster′ile·ly
ste·ril′i·ty
ster′il·i·za′tion
ster′il·ize′, -ized′, -iz′ing
ster′il·iz′er
ster′nad′
ster′nal
ster′nal′gi·a
ster·na′lis
Stern′berg cell
Stern′berg-Reed′ cell
ster′ne·bra pl. -brae′
Stern′heim′er-Mal′bin cells
ster′no·chon′dro·scap′u·lar′is
ster′no·cla·vic′u·lar
ster′no·cla·vic′u·lar′is
ster′no·clei′dal
ster′no·clei′do·mas′toid′
ster′no·cos′tal
ster′no·cos·ta′lis
ster′no·dym′i·a
ster′nod′y·mus
ster′no·dyn′i·a
ster′no·fas·ci·a′lis pl. -les
ster′no·hy′oid′
ster′no·hy·oi′de·us az′y·gos′
ster′no·mas′toid′
ster′no·pa′gi·a
ster·nop′a·gus
ster·nop′a·gy

ster′no·per′i·car′di·al
ster′no·scap′u·lar
ster·nos′chi·sis pl. -ses′
ster′no·thy′roid′
ster·not′o·my
ster′no·tra′che·al
ster′no·ver′te·bral
ster′num pl. -nums or -na
ster′nu·ta′ti·o′
—con′vul′si·va
ster′nu·ta′tion
ster′nu·ta′tor
ster·nu′ta·to′ry
ster′oid′
ste·roi′dal
ste·roid′o·gen′e·sis pl. -ses′
ste·roid′o·gen′ic
ster′ol′
ste′rone′
ster′tor
ster′to·rous
steth·al′gi·a
steth·ar′te·ri′tis
steth′o·gram′
steth′o·graph′
ste·thog′ra·phy
ste·thom′e·ter
steth′o·my·o′si·tis
steth′o·phone′
steth′o·pol′y·scope′
steth′o·scope′
steth′o·scop′ic
ste·thos′co·py
Ste′vens-John′son syndrome
Stew′art-Holmes′ phenomenon
Stew′art-Mo′rel′ syndrome
Stew′art-Treves′ syndrome
sthe′ni·a
sthen′ic
sthe·nom′e·ter
sthen′o·plas′tic
stib′a·mine′
stib′i·ac′ne
stib′i·al·ism
stib′ine′
stib′i·um
sti·bo′ni·um
stib′o·phen′
stich′o·chrome′
stick
Stick′er disease

Stie'da
—disease
—fracture
Stier'lin sign
stiff
stiff'en
stiff'ness
sti'fle, -fled, -fling
stig'ma *pl.* stig·ma'ta *or* -mas
stig'mal
stig·mas'ter·ol'
stig'ma·ta
—ni'gra
—of Ben'e·ke
—ven·tric'u·li'
stig'mat'ic
stig'ma·tism *(an eye condition)*
  ♦*sigmatism*
stig'ma·ti·za'tion
stig'ma·tom'e·ter
stig'mat'o·scope'
stig'ma·tos'co·py
stig'ma·tose'
stil·bam'i·dine'
stil·baz'i·um
stil'bene'
stil·bes'trol'
Stiles'-Craw'ford effect
Still
—disease
—murmur
still'birth'
still'born'
Stil'ler
—disease
—sign
stil'li·cid'i·um
—lac'ri·mar'um
—u'ri'nae'
Stil'ling
—canal
—raphe
—test
Stil'ling-Turk'-Duane'
  syndrome
Still'man cleft
Stim'son method
stim'u·lant
stim'u·late', -lat'ed, -lat'ing
stim'u·la'tion
stim'u·la'tive
stim'u·la'tor
stim'u·la·to'ry

stim'u·lin
stim'u·lus *pl.* -li'
sting
stipe
stip'ple, -pled, -pling
stir'rup
stitch
sto·chas'tic
stock
stock'i·net'
stock'ing
Stock retinal atrophy
Stof'fel operation
stoi'chi·o·met'ric
stoi'chi·om'e·try
Stokes
—expectorant
—law
—operation
Stokes'-Ad'ams syndrome
Stok'vis disease
Stoll
—method
—test
sto'lon'
Stoltz operation
sto'ma *pl.* -ma·ta *or* -mas
sto'ma·ceph'a·lus
stom'ach
stom'ach·ache'
stom'ach·al
sto·mach'ic
sto'mal
sto'ma·tal
sto'ma·tal'gi·a
sto·mat'ic
sto'ma·ti'tis
—ven'e·na'ta
sto'ma·toc'a·ce'
sto'ma·to·ca·thar'sis
sto'ma·to·cyte'
sto'ma·to·dyn'i·a
sto'ma·to·dy·so'di·a
sto'ma·to·gas'tric
sto'ma·to·glos'si'tis
sto'ma·tog·nath'ic
sto'ma·to·log'ic
sto'ma·tol'o·gist
sto'ma·tol'o·gy
sto'ma·to·ma·la'ci·a
sto'ma·to·me'ni·a
sto'ma·to·mi·a
sto·mat'o·my

sto'ma·to·my·co'sis *pl.* -ses'
sto'ma·to·ne·cro'sis
sto'ma·to·no'ma
sto'ma·top'a·thy
sto'ma·to·plas'tic
sto'ma·to·plas'ty
sto'ma·tor·rha'gi·a
sto'ma·tos'chi·sis
sto'ma·to·scope'
sto'ma·to'sis *pl.* -ses'
sto'ma·tot'o·my
sto·men'or·rha'gi·a
sto'mi·on'
sto'mo·de'um *pl.* -de'a *or*
  -de'ums
sto·mos'chi·sis *pl.* -ses'
Sto·mox'ys
stone
Stone operation
Stook'ey reflex
stool
stool'ing
stop'page
sto'rax
store
sto'ri·form'
storm
stra·bis'mal
stra·bis'mic
stra'bis·mom'e·ter
stra'bis·mom'e·try
stra·bis'mus
stra·bom'e·ter
stra·bom'e·try
strab'o·tome'
stra·bot'o·my
strag'u·lum *pl.* -la
strain
strain'er
strait
straight'jack'et
stra·mo'ni·um
strand'y
stran'gle, -gled, -gling
stran'gu·lat'ed
stran'gu·la'tion
stran'gu·ry
strap, strapped, strap'ping
Strass'mann phenomenon
strat'i·fi·ca'tion
strat'i·fied'
strat'i·graph'ic
stra·tig'ra·phy

strat'o·sphere'
stra'tum *pl.* -ta
—al'bum pro·fun'dum cor'-
 po·rum qua'dri·gem'i·
 no'rum
—ba·sa'le'
—basale ep'i·der'mi·dis
—cer'e·bra'le' ret'i·nae'
—ci·ne're·um
—cinereum cer'e·bel'li'
—cir'cu·lar'e' mem·bra'nae'
 tym'pa·ni'
—circulare tu'ni·cae' mus'-
 cu·lar'is col'li'
—circulare tunicae mus-
 cularis in'tes·ti'ni' ten'u·is
—circulare tunicae mus-
 cularis rec'ti'
—circulare tunicae mus-
 cularis tu'bae' u'ter·i'nae'
—circulare tunicae muscularis u·re'thrae' mu'li·e'bris
—circulare tunicae
 muscularis ven·tric'u·li'
—com·pac'tum
—cor'ne·um
—corneum un'guis
—cu·ta'ne·um mem·bra'-
 nae' tym'pa·ni'
—cy·lin'dri·cum
—dis·junc'tum
—ex·ter'num tu'ni·cae'
 mus·cu·lar'is duc'tus
 def'e·ren'tis
—externum tunicae
 muscularis u·re'ter·is
—externum tunicae
 muscularis ve·si'cae'
 u'ri·nar'i·ae'
—fi·bro'sum cap'su·lae'
 ar·tic'u·lar'is
—gan'gli·o·nar'e' ner'vi'
 op'ti·ci'
—ganglionare ret'i·nae'
—gan'gli·o'sum cer'e·bel'li'
—ger'mi·na·ti'vum
—germinativum (Mal·pi'-
 ghi·i')
—germinativum un'guis
—gran'u·lo'sum
—granulosum cer'e·bel'li'
—granulosum ep'i·der'-
 mi·dis

—granulosum fol·lic'u·li'
 o·var'i·ci' ve·sic'u·lo'si
—granulosum o·var'i·i'
—gris'e·um col'lic'u·li'
 su·pe·ri·o'ris
—in·ter'me'di·um
—in·ter'num tu'ni·cae'
 mus'cu·lar'is duc'tus
 def'er·en'tis
—internum tunicae
 muscularis u·re'ter·is
—internum tunicae
 muscularis ve·si'cae'
 u'ri·nar'i·ae'
—in·ter'ol'i·var'e' lem·
 nis'ci'
—lem·nis'ci'
—lon'gi·tu'di·na'le'
 tu'ni·cae' mus'cu·lar'is
 co'li'
—longitudinale tunicae
 muscularis in'tes·ti'ni'
 ten'u·is
—longitudinale tunicae
 muscularis rec'ti'
—longitudinale tunicae
 muscularis tu'bae'
 u'ter·i'nae'
—longitudinale tunicae
 muscularis u·re'thrae
 mu'li·e'bris
—longitudinale tunicae
 muscularis ven·tric'u·li'
—lu'ci·dum
—mal·pi'ghi·i'
—medium tu'ni·cae'
 mus'cu·lar'is duc'tus
 def'er·en'tis
—medium tunicae
 muscularis u·re'ter·is
—medium tunicae
 muscularis ve·si'cae'
 u'ri·nar'i·ae'
—mo·lec'u·lar'e' cer'e·bel'li'
—mu·co'sum
—mucosum mem·bra'nae'
 tym'pa·ni'
—neu'ro·ep'i·the'li·a'le'
 ret'i·nae'
—nu'cle·ar'e' me·dul'lae'
 ob'lon·ga'tae'
—pap'il·lar'e' co'ri·i'
—pig·men'ti' bul'bi' oc'u·li'

—pigmenti cor'po·ris
 cil'i·ar'is
—pigmenti i'ri·dis
—pigmenti ret'i·nae'
—ra'di·a'tum mem·bra'-
 nae' tym'pa·ni'
—re'tic'u·lar'e'
—spi·no'sum ep'i·der'-
 mi·dis
—spon'gi·o'sum
—sub'mu·co'sum
—sub'se·ro'sum
—su'pra·vas'cu·lar'e'
—sy'no·vi·a'le' cap'su·lae'
 ar·tic'u·lar'is
—vas'cu·lar'e'
—zo·na'le' cor'po·rum
 qua'dri·gem'i·no'rum
—zonale thal'a·mi'
Strauss
—phenomenon
—sign
—syndrome
—test
Straus reaction
streak
stream
strem'ma
strength
strep
streph'o·po'di·a
streph'o·sym·bo'li·a
strep'i·tus *pl.* -ti'
—au'ri·um
—u'ter·i'
—u'ter·i'nus
strep'o·gen'in
strep'ti·ce'mi·a
strep'ti·dine'
strep'to·an·gi'na
strep'to·bac'il·lar'y
strep'to·ba·cil'lus *pl.* -li'
Strep'to·ba·cil'lus
—mo·nil'i·for'mis
strep'to·bac·te'ri·a *sing.*
-ri·um
strep'to·bac'ter·in
strep'to·bi·o'sa·mine'
strep'to·coc'cal
Strep'to·coc'ce·ae'
strep'to·coc·ce'mi·a
strep'to·coc'cic
strep'to·coc·co'sis

strep′to·coc′cus *pl.* -ci′
Strep′to·coc′cus
—an′he′mo·lyt′i·cus
—ep′i·dem′i·cus
—fe·ca′lis
—lac′tis
—MG
—py·og′e·nes′
strep′to·dor′nase′
strep′to·gen′in
strep′to·he·mol′y·sin
strep′to·ki′nase′
strep·tol′y·sin
Strep′to·my′ces′
—so·ma′li·en′sis
Strep′to·my′ce·ta·ce·ae′
strep′to·my′cin
strep′to·my·co′sis *pl.* -ses′
strep′to·nic′o·zid
strep′to·ni′grin
strep′tose′
strep′to·sep′ti·ce′mi·a
strep′to·thri′cin
strep′to·tri·cho′sis *pl.* -ses′
strep′to·zo′cin
stress
stretch′er
stri′a *pl.* -ae′
—dis·ten′sa
—in′ter·me′di·a tri·go′ni′
ol′fac·to′ri·i′
—Lan·ci′si·i′
—lon′gi·tu′di·na′lis lat·er·
a′lis cor′po·ris cal·lo′si′
—longitudinalis me′di·a′lis
cor′po·ris cal·lo′si′
—mal′le·ar′is
—mal′le·o·lar′is
—me·di·a′lis tri·go′ni′
ol′fac·to′ri·i′
—med·ul·lar′is thal·a′mi′
—of Gen·na′ri
—of Lang′hans′
—of Ni′ta·buch′
—of Rohr
—ol′fac·to′ri·a
—olfactoria lat′er·a′lis
—sem′i·cir′cu·lar′is
—ter′mi·na′lis
—vas′cu·lar′is duc′tus
coch′le·ar′is
—vascularis of Husch′ke
stri′ae′

—a·cus′ti·cae′
—al′bi·can′tes′ grav′i·
dar′um
—a·tro′phi·cae′
—cer′e·bel·lar′is
—cu′tis dis·ten′sae′
—grav′i·dar′um
—med′ul·lar′es′ fos′sae′
rhom·boi′de·ae′
—medullares ven·tric′u·li′
quar′ti′
—of Bail·lar·ger′
—of Held
—of Mon′a·kov′
—of Pic′co·lo·mi′ni
—of Ret′zi·us
—trans·ver′sae′ cor′po·ris
cal·lo′si′
stri·a′tal
stri′ate′
stri′at′ed
stri·a′tion
stri·a·to·ni′gral
stri·a·to·pal′li·dal
stri·a′tum *pl.* -ta
stric′ture
stri′dent
stri′dor
—den′ti·um
—ser·rat′i·cus
strid′u·lous
string
strin′gent
stri′o·cel′lu·lar
stri′o·cer′e·bel′lar
stri′o·mus′cu·lar
stri′o·ni′gral
stri′o·tha·lam′ic
strip, stripped, strip′ping
stripe
—of Gen·na′ri
stripes of Bail·lar·ger′
strip′per
stro·bi′la *pl.* -lae′
stro′bi·la′tion
stro′bile
stro·bi·loid′
stro·bi′lus *pl.* -li′
stro′bo·scope′
stro′bo·scop′ic
stro′bo·ster′e·o·scope′
Stro′ga·nov′ method
stroke

stro′ma *pl.* -ma·ta
—glan′du·lae′ thy′re·oi′-
de·ae′
—glandulae thy·roi′de·ae′
—i′ri·dis
—o·var′i·i′
—vit′re·um
stro′mal
stro·mat′ic
stro′ma·tin
stro′ma·tog′e·nous
stro′ma·tol′y·sis
stro′ma·to′sis
strom′uhr′
stron′gyle
Stron′gy·loi′des′
—in·tes′ti·na′lis
—ster′co·ra′lis
stron′gy·loi·di·a·sis *pl.* -ses′
stron′gy·loi·do′sis
stron′gy·lo′sis *pl.* -ses′
Stron′gy·lus
stron′ti·a
stron′ti·um
stro·phan′thi·din
stro·phan′thin
stroph′o·ceph′a·lus *pl.* -li′
stroph′o·ceph′a·ly
stroph′u·lus *pl.* -li′
—pru′ri·gi·no′sus
struc′tur·al
struc′ture
stru′ma *pl.* -mae′
—ab′er·ra′ta
—ci·bar′i·a
—con·gen′i·ta
—lin·gua′lis
—lym′pho·ma·to′sa
—ma·lig′na
—med′i·ca·men·to′sa
—o·var′i·i′
—ovarii lu·te′i·no·cel′lu·
lar′e′
—post·bran′chi·a′lis
stru·mec′to·my
Stru′mi·a stain
stru′mi·form′
stru·mi·pri′val
stru·mi·pri′vic
stru′mi·pri′vous
stru·mi′tis
stru′mous
Strüm′pell

—reflex
—sign
Strüm'pell-Ma·rie' disease
Strüm'pell-West'phal
  pseudosclerosis
Strun'sky sign
strut
strych'nine'
strych'nin·ism
strych'nin·i·za'tion
Stu'art factor
stud'y
stump
stunt
stu·pe·fa'cient
stu·pe·fac'tion
stu·pe·fac'tive
stu·pe·fy', -fied', -fy'ing
stu'por
  —mel'an·chol'i·cus
  —vig'i·lans'
stu'por·ous
Sturge'-Web'er disease
Sturm'dorf' operation
stut'ter
stut'ter·er
sty *pl.* sties, *also* stye
sty·co'sis
stye *pl.* styes, *var. of* sty
sty'let
sty'li·form'
sty'lo·glos'sus *pl.* -si'
sty'lo·hy'al
sty'lo·hy'oid'
sty'loid'
sty'lo·man·dib'u·lar
sty'lo·mas'toid'
sty'lo·pha·ryn'ge·us
sty'lus *pl.* -lus·es *or* -li'
sty'ma·to'sis
styp'sis
styp'tic
sty'ra·mate'
Sty'rax
sty'rene'
sty'rol'
sub'ab·dom'i·nal
sub·ac'e·tate'
sub'a·cro'mi·al
sub'a·cute'
sub·al'i·men·ta'tion
sub·an'co·ne'us
sub'a·or'tic

sub·ap'i·cal
sub·ap'o·neu·rot'ic
sub·a'que·ous
sub'a·rach'noid'
sub·ar'cu·ate'
sub'a·re'o·lar
sub·as·trag'a·lar
sub·as·trin'gent
sub'a·tom'ic
sub·au·di'tion
sub·au'ral
sub·au·ric'u·lar
sub·ax'i·al
sub·ax'il·lar'y
sub·bas'al
sub·bra'chi·al
sub·brach'y·ce·phal'ic
sub'cal·car'e·ous
sub'cal·ca·rine'
sub'cal·lo'sal
sub·cap'i·tal
sub·cap'su·lar
sub·car'bon·ate'
sub·car'di·nal
sub·ca·ri'nal
sub·car'ti·lag'i·nous
sub·cel'lu·lar
sub·cer'vi·cal
sub·chlo'ride'
sub·chon'dral
sub·chord'al
sub·cho'ri·al
sub·cho'ri·on'ic
sub·cho·roi'dal
sub·chron'ic
sub·class'
sub·cla'vi·an
sub'cla·vic'u·lar
sub·cla'vi·us *pl.* -vi·i'
sub·clin'i·cal
sub·cli'noid'
sub'col·lat'er·al
sub·con'junc·ti'val
sub·con'scious
sub·con'scious·ness
sub·con·tin'u·ous
sub·cor'a·coid'
sub·cor'ne·al
sub·cor'tex'
sub·cor'ti·cal
sub·cos'tal
sub·cos·tal'gi·a
sub·cra'ni·al

sub·crep'i·tant
sub·crep'i·ta'tion
sub·cru're·us
sub·cul'ture
sub·cu'ra·tive
sub·cu·ta'ne·ous
sub·cu·ta'ne·ous·ly
sub·cu·tic'u·lar
sub·cu'tis
sub·de·lir'i·um
sub·del'toid'
sub·den'tal
sub·der'mal
sub·der'mic
sub·di'a·phrag·mat'ic
sub·dor'sal
sub·duct'
sub·duc'tion
sub·du'ral
sub·en'do·car'di·al
sub·en'do·the'li·al
sub·en'do·the'li·um
sub·e·pen'dy·mal
sub·e·pen'dy·mo'ma
  pl. -mas *or* -ma·ta
sub·ep'i·der'mal
sub·ep'i·glot'tic
sub·ep'i·the'li·al
su'ber·in
su'ber·o'sis
sub·fam'i·ly
sub·fas'ci·al
sub·ga'le·al
sub·gal'late'
sub·ger'mi·nal
sub·gin'gi·val
sub·gle'noid'
sub·glos'sal
sub·glos·si'tis
sub·glot'tic
sub·gran'u·lar
sub'gron·da'tion
sub'he·pat'ic
sub·hu'mer·al
sub·hy'a·loid' *(under the*
  hyaloid membrane)
  ♦*subhyoid*
sub·hy'oid' *(under the hyoid*
  bone)
  ♦*subhyaloid*
sub·ic·ter'ic
su·bic'u·lar
su·bic'u·lum *pl.* -la

—prom'on·to'ri·i'
sub'in·ci'sion
sub'in·fec'tion
sub'in'gui·nal
sub'in·teg'u·men'tal
sub·in'ti·mal
sub·in'vo·lu'tion
sub·i'o·dide'
sub·ja'cent
sub·jec'tive
sub·ju'gal
sub·la'bi·al
sub·la'ti·o'
—ret'i·nae'
sub·la'tion
sub·le'thal
sub'leu·ke'mic
sub'li·mate', -mat'ed,
 -mat'ing
sub'li·ma'tion
sub·lime', -limed', -lim'ing
sub·lim'i·nal
sub·li'mis
sub·line'
sub·lin'gual
sub·lin·gui'tis
sub·lob'u·lar
sub·lux'
sub·lux'at'ed
sub·lux·a'tion
sub'mal·le'o·lar
sub·mam'ma·ry
sub'man·dib'u·lar
sub·mar'gin·al
sub·max'il·lar'y
sub·me'di·al
sub·men'tal
sub'me·sat'i·ce·phal'ic
sub'met·a·cen'tric
sub·mi'cron'
sub·mi'cro·scop'ic
sub·mil'i·ar'y
sub·mor'phous
sub·mu·co'sa pl. -sae' or -sas
sub·mu·co'sal
sub·mu'cous
sub'nar·cot'ic
sub·na'sal
sub·na·sa'le'
sub·na'si·on'
sub·neu'ral
sub·ni'trate'
sub·nor'mal

sub'nor·mal'i·ty
sub'no'to·chord'al
sub·nu'cle·us pl. -cle·i'
sub·nu·tri'tion
sub'oc·cip'i·tal
sub'oc·clu'sal
sub'o·per'cu·lum
sub'op'ti·mal
sub·op'ti·mum pl. -ma
sub·or'bit·al
sub'or'der
sub'or·di·na'tion
sub·ox'ide'
sub·pap'il·lar'y
sub·pap'u·lar
sub·par'a·lyt'ic
sub·pa·ri'e·tal
sub·pa·tel'lar
sub·pec'to·ral
sub'per·i·car'di·al
sub'per·i·os'te·al
sub'per·i·to·ne'al
sub'pha·ryn'ge·al
sub·phren'ic
sub·phy'lum pl. -la
sub·pi'al
sub'pla·cen'ta
sub'pla·cen'tal
sub·pleu'ral
sub·pu'bic
sub·re'nal
sub·ros'tral
sub·sar·to'ri·al
sub·scap'u·lar
sub·scap'u·lar'is
sub·scle'ral
sub·scle·rot'ic
sub·scrip'tion
sub'seg·men'tal
sub·sen·sa'tion
sub'se·ro'sal
sub·se'rous
sub·set'
sub·sib'i·lant
sub·side', -sid'ed, -sid'ing
sub·si'dence
sub·sig'moid'
sub·sis'tence
sub·spe'cies
sub·spi'na'le
sub·spi'nous
sub·stage'
sub·stance

sub·stan'ti·a pl. -ae'
—ad'a·man'ti·na den'tis
—al'ba
—alba me·dul'lae' spi'na·lis
—com·pac'ta
—cor'ti·ca'lis
—corticalis cer'e·bel'li'
—corticalis cer'e·bri'
—corticalis glan'du·lae'
 su'pra·re·na'lis
—corticalis len'tis
—corticalis lym'pho·glan'-
 du·lae'
—corticalis os'sis
—corticalis re'nis
—e·bur'ne·a
—fer'ru·gin'e·a
—ge·lat'i·no'sa
—gelatinosa cen·tra'lis
—gelatinosa Ro·lan'di'
—glan'du·lar'is pros'ta·tae'
—gli·o'sa
—gris'e·a
—grisea cen·tra'lis
 me·dul'lae' spi·na'lis
—grisea centralis mes'en·
 ceph'a·li'
—grisea me·dul'lae' spi'na'-
 lis
—in'ter·me'di·a cen·tra'lis
 me·dul'lae' spi·na'lis
—intermedia lat'er·a'lis
 me·dul'lae' spi·na'lis
—len'tis
—med'ul·lar'is glan'du·lae'
 su'pra·re·na'lis
—medullaris lym'pho·glan'-
 du·lae'
—medullaris re'nis
—mus'cu·lar'is pros'ta·tae'
—ni'gra
—os'se·a den'tis
—per'fo·ra'ta anterior
—perforata posterior
—pro'pri·a cor'ne·ae'
—propria scle'rae'
—re·tic'u·lar'is
—reticularis al'ba
 (Ar·nol'di')
—reticularis alba me·dul'-
 lae' ob'lon·ga'tae'
—reticularis gris'e·a
 me·dul'lae' ob'lon·ga'tae'

—spon'gi•o'sa
sub'stan•tive
sub•ster'nal
sub•ster'no•mas'toid'
sub•stit'u•ent
sub•sti•tute', -tut'ed, -tut'ing
sub'sti•tu'tion
sub'sti•tu'tive
sub'strate'
sub'stra'tum *pl.* -ta
sub'struc'ture
sub•sul'fate'
sub•sul'to•ry
sub•sul'tus
—clo'nus
—ten'di•num
sub'syn•ap'tic
sub•ta'lar
sub•tar'sal
sub•tem'po•ral
sub•te'ni•al
sub•ten'to•ri•al
sub•ter'mi•nal
sub•ter'tian
sub•te•tan'ic
sub•tha•lam'ic
sub•thal'a•mus *pl.* -mi'
sub•thresh'old'
sub•thy'roid•ism
sub'ti•lin
sub•ti•li'sin
sub•to'tal
sub•trac'tion
sub•tra•pe'zi•al
sub•trig'o•nal
sub•tro'chan•ter'ic
sub•trop'i•cal
sub•um•bil'i•cal
sub•un'gual
sub'u•re'thral
sub•vag'i•nal
sub•val'vu•lar
sub•ver'te•bral
sub•vi'ril *(pertaining to virus)*
  ♦*subvirile*
sub•vir'ile *(pertaining to*
  virility)
  ♦*subviril*
sub•vi'ta•min•o'sis
sub•vo•lu'tion
sub•vo'mer•ine'
sub'wak'ing
sub•xiph'oid'

suc'ce•da'ne•ous
suc'ce•da'ne•um *pl.* -ne•a
suc'cen•tu'ri•ate
suc•cif'er•ous
suc'ci•mer
suc'ci•nate'
suc•cin'ic
suc'ci•nyl•cho'line'
suc'ci•nyl•sul'fa•thi'a•zole'
suc•cor•rhe'a
suc•cu•lent
suc•cumb'
suc'cus *(a secretion)*, *pl.* -ci'
  ♦*succus*
—en•ter'i•cus
—gas'tri•cus
—in•tes'ti•na'lis
—pan'cre•at'i•cus
—pro•stat'i•cus
suc•cuss' *(to shake)*
  ♦*succus*
suc•cus'sion
suck
suck'le, -led, -ling
Suc•quet'-Hoy'er canal
su•cral'fate'
su'crase'
su'crate'
su'crose'
su'cro•se'mi•a
su'cro•su'ri•a
suc'tion
Suc•to'ri•a
suc•to'ri•al
su•da'men *pl.* -dam'i•na
su•dam'i•nal
Su'dan'
—stain
su•dan'o•phil'
su•dan'o•phil'i•a
su•dan'o•phil'ic
su•da'tion
sud'den
Su'deck' atrophy
su'do•ker'a•to'sis *pl.* -ses'
su'do•mo'tor
su'dor'
su'do•re'sis
su'do•rif'er•ous
su'do•rif'ic
su'do•rip'a•rous
su•fen'ta•nil
suf'fo•cate', -cat'ed, -cat'ing

suf'fo•ca'tion
suf•fuse', -fused', -fus'ing
suf•fu'sion
sug'ar
sug•gest'i•bil'i•ty
sug•gest'i•ble
sug•ges'tion
sug'gil•la'tion
Su'gi•u'ra procedure
su'i•cid'al
su'i•cide'
su'i•cid•ol'o•gy
su'i•gen'der•ism
Su'ker sign
sul•az'e•pam'
sul•bac'tam
sul'cal
sul'cate'
sul'ci'
—ar•te'ri•o'si'
—cer'e•bel'li'
—cer'e•bri'
—cu'tis
—oc•cip'i•ta'les' lat'er•a'les'
—occipitales su•pe'ri•o'res'
—or'bi•ta'les'
—pal'a•ti'ni' max•il'lae'
—par'a•co'li•ci'
—par'a•gle'noi•da'les'
—tem'po•ra'les' trans•
  ver'si'
—ve'no'si'
sul'ci•form'
sul•con'a•zole'
sul'cus *pl.* -ci'
—am'pul•lar'is
—ant•hel'i•cis trans•ver'sus
—ar•te'ri•ae' oc•cip'i•ta'lis
—arteriae sub•cla'vi•ae'
—arteriae tem'po•ra'lis
  me'di•ae'
—arteriae ver'te•bra'lis
—au'ric'u•lae' posterior
—bas'i•lar'is pon'tis
—bi•cip'i•ta'lis lat'er•a'lis
—bicipitalis me'di•a'lis
—brev'is
—cal'ca•ne'i'
—cal'ca•ri'nus
—can'a•lic'u•li' mas•toi'-
  de•i'
—ca•rot'i•cus
—car'pi'

—cen·tra′lis

—centralis in′su·lae′

—centralis (Ro·lan′di′)

—chi·as′ma·tis

—cin′gu·li′

—cir′cu·lar′is in′su·lae′

—circularis (Rei′li′)

—col·lat′er·a′lis

—co′ro·nar′i·us

—cor′po·ris cal·lo′si′

—cos′tae′

—cru′ris hel′i·cis

—eth′moi·da′lis

—fron·ta′lis inferior

—frontalis superior

—glu·tae′us

—glu·te′us

—ham′u·li′ pter′y·goi′de·i′

—hip′po·cam′pi′

—ho′ri·zon·ta′lis cer′e·bel′li′

—hy′po·tha·lam′i·cus

—hypothalamicus (Mon′ro·i′)

—in′fra·or′bi·ta′lis

—in′fra·pal′pe·bra′lis

—in′ter·me′di·us anterior me·dul′lae′ spi·na′lis

—intermedius posterior me·dul′lae′ spi·na′lis

—in′ter·pa·ri′e·ta′lis

—in′ter·tu·ber′cu·lar′is

—in′ter·ven·tric′u·lar′is anterior

—interventricularis posterior

—in′tra·pa·ri′e·ta′lis

—lac′ri·ma′lis max·il′lae′

—lacrimalis os′sis lac′ri·ma′lis

—lat′er·a′lis anterior me·dul′lae′ ob′lon·ga′tae′

—lateralis anterior me·dul′lae′ spi·na′lis

—lateralis cer′e·bri′

—lateralis mes′en·ceph′a·li′

—lateralis posterior me·dul′lae′ ob′lon·ga′tae′

—lateralis posterior me·dul′lae′ spi·na′lis

—lim′i·tans′

—limitans ven·tric′u·li′ quar′ti′

—limitans ven·tric′u·lo′rum cer′e·bri′

—lon′gi·tu′di·na′lis anterior cor′dis

—longitudinalis posterior

—lu′na′tus

—mal′le·o·lar′is

—ma′tri·cis un′guis cer′e·bri′

—me′di·a′lis cru′ris

—me′di·a′nus lin′guae′

—medianus posterior me·dul′lae′ ob′lon·ga′tae′

—medianus posterior me·dul′lae′ spi·na′lis

—medianus ven·tric′u·li′ quar′ti′

—men′to·la·bi·a′lis

—mus′cu·li′ flex·o′ris hal′lu·cis lon′gi′ cal·ca′ne·i′

—musculi flexoris hallucis longi ta′li′

—musculi per·o·nae′i′ lon′gi′ cal·ca′ne·i′

—musculi peronaei longi os′sis cu·boi′de·i′

—my′lo·hy·oi′de·us

—na′so·la·bi·a′lis

—ner′vi′ oc′u·lo·mo·to′ri·i′

—nervi pe·tro′si′ ma·jo′ris

—nervi petrose mi·no′ris

—nervi petrosi su′per·fi′ci·a′lis ma·jo′ris

—nervi petrosi superficialis mi·no′ris

—nervi ra′di·a′lis

—nervi spi·na′lis

—nervi ul′nar′is

—ob′tu·ra·to′ri·us

—oc·cip′i·ta′lis trans·ver′sus

—oc·cip′i·to·tem′po·ra′lis

—of Mon·ro′

—ol′fac·to′ri·us ca′vi′ na′si′

—olfactorius lo′bi′ fron·ta′lis

—or′bi·ta′lis

—pal′a·ti′nus major max·il′lae′

—palatinus major os′sis pal′a·ti′ni′

—pal′a·to·vag′i·na′lis

—pa·ri′e·to·oc·cip′i·ta′lis

—par·ol·fac′to′ri·us anterior

—parolfactorius posterior

—pe·tro′sus inferior os′sis oc·cip′i·ta′lis

—petrosus inferior os′sis tem′po·ra′lis

—petrosus superior os′sis tem′po·ra′lis

—post′cen·tra′lis

—prae′cen·tra′lis

—pre′cen·tra′lis

—pri·mar′i·us

—prom′on·to′ri·i′

—pter′y·go′pal′a·ti′nus os′sis pal′a·ti′ni′

—pul′mo·na′lis

—rhi′na′lis

—sag′it·ta′lis os′sis fron·ta′lis

—sagittalis ossis oc·cip′i·ta′lis

—sagittalis ossis pa·ri′e·ta′lis

—scle′rae′

—sig′moi′de·us

—si′nus pe·tro′si′ in·fe′ri·o′ris os′sis oc·cip′i·ta′lis

—sinus petrosi inferioris ossis tem′po·ra′lis

—sinus petrosi su·pe′ri·o′ris os′sis tem′po·ra′lis

—sinus sag′it·ta′lis su·pe′ri·o′ris os′sis fron·ta′lis

—sinus sagittalis superioris ossis oc·cip′i·ta′lis

—sinus sagittalis superioris ossis pa·ri′e·ta′lis

—sinus sig·moi′de·i′

—sinus sigmoidei os′sis oc·cip′i·ta′lis

—sinus sigmoidei ossis pa·ri′e·ta′lis

—sinus sigmoidei ossis tem′po·ra′lis

—sinus trans·ver′si′

—spi′ra′lis

—spiralis ex·ter′nus

—spiralis in·ter′nus

—sub·cla′vi·ae′

—sub·cla′vi·us pul′mo′nis

—sub′pa·ri′e·ta′lis

—su′pra·pa·ri′e·ta′lis

—ta'li'
—tem·po·ra'lis inferior
—temporalis me'di·us
—temporalis superior
—ten'di·nis mus'cu·li' fib'u·
lar'is lon'gi' cal·ca'ne·i'
—tendinis musculi flex·o'ris
hal·lu·cis lon'gi'
cal·ca'ne·i'
—tendinis musculi flexoris
hallucis longi ta'li'
—tendinis musculi per'o·
ne'i' lon'gi' cal·ca'ne·i'
—tendinis musculi peronei
longi os'sis cu·boi'de·i'
—ter'mi·na'lis a'tri·i'
dex'tri'
—terminalis lin'guae'
—trans·ver'sus os'sis
oc·cip'i·ta'lis
—transversus ossis pa·ri'e·
ta'lis
—tu'bae' au·di·ti'vae'
—tym·pan'i·cus
—ve'nae' ca'vae'
—venae sub·cla'vi·ae'
—venae um·bil'i·ca'lis
—vo'mer·o·vag'i·na'lis
sul'fa
sul'fa·ben'za·mide'
sul'fa·cet'a·mide'
sulf·ac'id
sul'fa·cy'tine'
sul'fa·di·a'zine'
sul'fa·di'meth·ox'ine'
sul'fa·di'me·tine'
sul'fa·dox'ine'
sul'fa·eth'i·dole'
sul'fa·gua'ni·dine'
sul'fa·lene'
sul'fa·mer'a·zine'
sul'fa·me'ter
sul'fa·meth'a·zine'
sul'fa·meth'i·zole'
sul'fa·meth·ox'a·zole'
sul'fa·me·thox'y·di·a'zine'
sul'fa·me·thox'y·py·rid'a·
zine
sul'fa·mon'o·meth·ox'ine'
sul'fa·mox'ole'
sul'fa·nil'a·mide'
sul·fan'i·late'
sul'fa·nil'ic

sul'fa·pyr'i·dine'
sul'fa·sal'a·zine'
sul'fa·som'i·zole'
sul'fa·tase'
sul'fate'
sul'fa·thi'a·zole'
sul'fa·tide'
sul'fa·ti·do'sis
sul'faz'a·met'
sulf·he'mo·glo'bin
sulf·he'mo·glo'bin·e'mi·a
sulf·hy'drate'
sulf·hy'dryl
sul'fide'
sul'fin·pyr'a·zone
sul'fi·som'i·dine'
sul'fi·sox'a·zole'
sul'fite'
sulf'met·he'mo·glo'bin
sul'fo·bro'mo·phthal'e·in
sul'fo·cy'a·nate'
sul'fo·cy·an'ic
sul'fo·mu'cin
sul·fon'a·mide'
sul'fo·nate'
sul'fone'
sul'fon'ic
sul·fo'ni·um
sul'fon·meth'ane'
sul'fo·nyl
sul'fo·nyl·u're·a
sul'fo·phen'yl·ate'
sul'fo·sal'i·cyl'ic
sul·fox'ide'
sul·fox'one'
sul'fur *also* sulphur
sul'fu·rat'ed
sul'fu·ra'tor
sul'fu·ret'
sul'fu·ric
sul'fur·ous
sul'fur·yl
sul'fy'drate'
sul'in·dac'
su·li'so·ben'zone'
Sul'ko·witch test
sul'lage
Sul'li·van test
sul'pha·fu'ra·zole'
sul'phur *var. of* sulfur
sul·thi'ame'
Sultz·ber'ger-Gar'be
disease

su'mac'
sum·ma'tion
sum'mit
Sum'ner
—method
—sign
sump
sun'burn'
sun'spots'
sun'stroke'
su'per·ab·duc'tion
su'per·ac'id
su'per·a·cid'i·ty
su'per·a·cute'
su'per·al·bu'mi·no'sis
pl. -ses'
su'per·al'i·men·ta'tion
su'per·al'ka·lin'i·ty
su'per·au·ra'le'
su'per·cen'tral
su'per·cer'e·bel'lar
su'per·cil'i·ar'y
su'per·cil'i·um *pl.* -i·a
su'per·con·duct'ing
su'per·di·crot'ic
su'per·dis·ten'tion
su'per·duct'
su'per·duc'tion
su'per·e'go
su'per·e·vac'u·a'tion
su'per·ex·ci'ta'tion
su'per·ex·ten'sion
su'per·fe'cun·da'tion
su'per·fe·cun'di·ty
su'per·fe·ta'tion
su'per·fi'cial
su'per·fi'ci·a'lis
su'per·fi'ci·es'
pl. su'per·fi'ci·es'
su'per·flex'ion
su'per·fu'sion
su'per·gene'
su'per·im·pose', -posed',
-pos'ing
su'per·im'preg·na'tion
su'per·in·duce', -duced',
-duc'ing
su'per·in·fec'tion
su'per·in·vo·lu'tion
su·pe'ri·or
su·pe'ri·or·ly
su'per·lac·ta'tion
su'per·le'thal

su′per·max·il′la
su′per·me′di·al
su′per·na′tant
su′per·nate′
su′per·nor′mal
su′per·nu′mer·ar′y
su′per·nu·tri′tion
su′per·oc·cip′i·tal
su′per·o·in·fe′ri·or
su′per·o·lat′er·al
su′per·o·me′di·al
su′per·o′vu·la′tion
su′per·par′a·mag·net′ic
su′per·par′a·site′
su′per·par′a·sit′ic
su′per·par′a·sit·ism
su′per·phos′phate′
su′per·pig′men·ta′tion
su′per·salt′
su′per·sat′u·rate′, -rat′ed,
  -rat′ing
su′per·scrip′tion
su′per·se·cre′tion
su′per·sen′si·tive
su′per·sen′si·ti·za′tion
su′per·son′ic
su′per·struc′ture
su′per·ten′sion
su′per·ve·nos′i·ty
su′per·ven′tion
su′per·ver′sion
su′per·vi′sor
su′per·vi′so·ry
su′per·volt′age
su′pi·nate′, -nat′ed, -nat′ing
su′pi·na′tion
su′pi·na′tor
su·pine′
sup′ple·ment
sup′ple·men′tal
sup′ple·men′ta·ry
sup·port′
sup·port′er
sup·port′ive
sup·pos′i·to·ry
sup·press′
sup·pres′sant
sup·pres′sion
sup·pres′sive
sup·pres′sor
sup′pu·rant
sup′pu·rate′, -rat′ed, -rat′ing
sup′pu·ra′tion

sup′pu·ra′tive
su′pra·a·or′tic
su′pra·ar·tic′u·lar
su′pra·au·ric′u·lar
su′pra·buc′cal
su′pra·bulge′
su′pra·cal·lo′sal
su′pra·car′di·nal
su′pra·cer′vi·cal
su′pra·chi′as·mat′ic
su′pra·cho′roid′
su′pra·cho·roi′dal
su′pra·cho·roi′de·a
su′pra·cla·vic′u·lar
su′pra·cla·vic′u·lar′is
su′pra·cli′noid′
su′pra·clu′sion
su′pra·con′dy·lar
su′pra·con′dy·loid′
su′pra·cos′tal
su′pra·cos·ta′lis pl. -les′
su′pra·cra′ni·al
su′pra·di′a·phrag·mat′ic
su′pra·ep′i·con′dy·lar
su′pra·ep′i·troch′le·ar
su′pra·ge·nic′u·late′
su′pra·gin′gi·val
su′pra·gle′noid′
su′pra·glot′tal
su′pra·glot′tic
su′pra·gran′u·lar
su′pra·he·pat′ic
su′pra·hy′oid′
su′pra·in′gui·nal
su′pra·le′thal
su′pra·le·va′tor
su′pra·lim′i·nal
su′pra·lum′bar
su′pra·mal·le′o·lar
su′pra·mam′mil·lar′y
su′pra·man·dib′u·lar
su′pra·mar′gin·al
su′pra·mas′toid′
su′pra·max′il·lar′y
su′pra·me·a′tal
su′pra·men′tal
su′pra·na′sal
su′pra·nu′cle·ar
su′pra·oc·cip′i·tal
su′pra·oc·clu′sion
su′pra·oc′u·lar
su′pra·op′tic
su′pra·or′bit·al

su′pra·pa·tel′lar
su′pra·pel′vic
su′pra·pin′e·al
su′pra·pleu′ral
su′pra·pon′tine′
su′pra·pu′bic
su′pra·re′nal
su′pra·re′nal·ec′to·my
su′pra·re·na′lis ab′er·ra′ta
su′pra·re′nal·ism
su′pra·re′nal·op′a·thy
su′pra·scap′u·la
su′pra·scap′u·lar
su′pra·scle′ral
su′pra·sel′lar
su′pra·sep′tal
su′pra·spi′nal
su′pra·spi·na′tus
su′pra·spi′nous
su′pra·sple′ni·al
su′pra·sta·pe′di·al
su′pra·ster′nal
su′pra·ster′ol′
su′pra·tem′po·ral
su′pra·ten·to′ri·al
su′pra·ton′sil·lar
su′pra·tri·gem′i·nal
su′pra·troch′le·ar
su′pra·tym·pan′ic
su′pra·um·bil′i·cal
su′pra·vag′i·nal
su′pra·val′vu·lar
su′pra·ven·tric′u·lar
su′pra·ver′gence
su′pra·ver′sion
su′pra·ves′i·cal
su′pra·vi′tal
su·pro′fen
su′ra pl. -rae′
su′ral
sur·al′i·men·ta′tion
sur′a·min
sur′cin·gle
sur′di·tas
  —ver·ba′lis
sur′di·ty
sur·ex′ci·ta′tion
sur′face
sur′face-ac′tive
sur·fac′tant
sur′geon
sur′ger·y
sur′gi·cal

sur'gi·cal·ly
sur'ro·gate'
sur'sum·duc'tion
sur'sum·ver'gence
sur'sum·ver'gent
sur'sum·ver'sion
sur·veil'lance
sus·cep'ti·bil'i·ty
sus·cep'ti·ble
sus'ci·tate', -tat'ed, -tat'ing
sus'ci·ta'tion
sus·pend'ed
sus·pen'sion
sus·pen'soid'
sus·pen'so'ri·um *pl.* -ri·a
  —hep'a·tis
  —tes'tis
  —ve·si'cae'
sus·pen'so·ry
sus'ten·tac'u·lar
sus'ten·tac'u·lum *pl.* -la
  —ta'li'
su'sur·ra'tion
su·sur'rus
  —au'ri·um
su'ti·lains'
Sut'ton disease
su·tu'ra *pl.* -rae'
  —co'ro·na'lis
  —den·ta'ta
  —eth·moi'de·o·max'il·lar'is
  —eth·moi'do·max'il·lar'is
  —fron·ta'lis
  —fron'to·eth'moi·da'lis
  —fron'to·lac'ri·ma'lis
  —fron'to·max'il·lar'is
  —fron'to·na·sa'lis
  —fron'to·zy'go·mat'i·ca
  —har·mo'ni·a
  —in'ci·si'va
  —in'fra·or'bi·ta'lis
  —in'ter·max'il·lar'is
  —in'ter·na·sa'lis
  —lac'ri·mo·con'cha'lis
  —lac'ri·mo·max'il·lar'is
  —lamb·doi'de·a
  —lim·bo'sa
  —me·top'i·ca
  —na'so·fron·ta'lis
  —na'so·max'il·lar'is
  —no'tha
  —oc·cip'i·to·mas·toi'de·a
  —pal'a·ti'na me·di·a'na

—palatina trans·ver'sa
—pal'a·to·eth'moi·da'lis
—pal'a·to·max'il·lar'is
—pa·ri'e·to·mas·toi'de·a
—pla'na
—sag'it·ta'lis
—ser·ra'ta
—sphe'no·eth'moi·da'lis
—sphe'no·fron·ta'lis
—sphe'no·max'il·lar'is
—sphe'no·or'bi·ta'lis
—sphe'no·pa·ri'e·ta'lis
—sphe'nosqua·mo'sa
—sphe'no·zy'go·mat'i·ca
—squa'mo·mas·toi'de·a
—squa'mo'sa
—squamosa cra'ni·i'
—tem'po·ro·zy'go·mat'i·ca
—ve'ra
—zy'go·mat'i·co·fron·ta'lis
—zy'go·mat'i·co·max'il·lar'is
—zy'go·mat'i·co·tem'po·ra'lis
su·tu'rae' cra'ni·i'
su'tur·al
su'ture, -tured, -tur·ing
Sved'berg' unit
swab, swabbed, swab'bing
swage, swaged, swag'ing
swal'low
Swan'-Ganz' technique
swathe, swathed, swath'ing
sway'back'
sweat
Swe'di·aur' disease
sweep
Sweet syndrome
swell'ing
Swift disease
swine'herd' disease
swing
sy'co·ma *pl.* -mas *or* -ma·ta
sy'co'si·form'
sy·co'sis *(hair-follicle
  inflammation), pl.* -ses'
  ♦*psychosis*
  —bar'bae'
  —cap'il·li·ti·i'
  —con·ta'gi·o'sa
  —fram·boe'si·for'mis
  —men·tag'ra
  —pal'pe·brae' mar'gi·na'lis
  —par'a·sit'i·ca
  —staph'y·log'e·nes'

—vul'gar'is
Syd'en·ham chorea
syl'la·bus *pl.* -bi' *or* -bus·es
syl·lep'sis *pl.* -ses'
syl·vat'ic
Syl'vi·an
  —angle
  —aqueduct
  —fissure
  —ossicle
  —point
  —valve
sym·bal'lo·phone'
sym'bi·o·gen'ic
sym'bi·on'
sym'bi·ont'
sym'bi·o'sis *pl.* -ses'
sym'bi·ote'
sym'bi·ot'ic
sym·bleph'a·ron'
sym·bleph'a·ro'sis
sym'bol
sym·bo'li·a
sym·bol'ic
sym'bol·ism
sym'bol·i·za'tion
sym'bol·o·pho'bi·a
Syme amputation
sym'e·tine'
sym'me·lus *pl.* -li'
sym·met'ric *or*
  sym·met'ri·cal
sym'me·try
sym'pa·ral'y·sis
sym'pa·thec'to·my
sym'pa·thec'to·mize',
  -mized', -miz'ing
sym'pa·thet'ic
sym'pa·thet'i·co·to'ni·a
sym'pa·thet'i·co·ton'ic
sym'pa·thet'o·blast'
sym·path'i·cec'to·my
sym·path'i·co·blast'
sym·path'i·co·blas'to·ma
  pl. -mas *or* -ma·ta
sym·path'i·co·cy·to'ma
  pl. -mas *or* -ma·ta
sym·path'i·co·go·ni'o·ma
  pl. -mas *or* -ma·ta
sym·path'i·co·lyt'ic
sym·path'i·co·mi·met'ic
sym·path'i·co·neu·ri'tis
sym·path'i·cop'a·thy

sym·path′i·co·to′ni·a
sym·path′i·co·ton′ic
sym·path′i·co·trop′ic
sym·path′i·cus
sym′pa·thin
sym′pa·thism
sym′pa·thist
sym′pa·thiz′er
sym·path′o·blast′
sym′pa·tho·blas·to′ma
   pl. -mas or -ma·ta
sym′pa·tho·chro′maf·fin
sym′pa·tho·go′ni·a
sym′pa·tho·go′ni·o′ma
   pl. -mas or -ma·ta
sym′pa·tho·lyt′ic
sym′pa·tho′ma pl. -mas or
   -ma·ta
sym′pa·tho·mi·met′ic
sym′pa·thy
sym·pet′al·ous
sym·pex′is
sym·pha·lan′gi·a
sym·phal′an·gism
sym′phy·o·ceph′a·lus
sym·phys′e·al
sym·phys′i·al
sym·phys′ic
sym·phys′i·ec′to·my
sym·phys′i·ol′y·sis
sym·phys′i·on′
sym′phys·i·or′rha·phy
sym·phys′i·o·tome′
sym·phys′i·ot′o·my
sym′phy·sis pl. -ses′
  —car′ti·lag′i·no′sa
  —lig′a·men·to′sa
  —man·dib′u·lae′
  —os′si·um pu′bis
  —pu′bi·ca
  —pu′bis
  —sa′cro·coc·cyg′e·a
sym′phy·so·dac·tyl′i·a
sym′phys·dac′ty·ly
sym′plasm
sym′plast
sym·po′di·a
sym·po′si·um pl. -si·a
symp′tom
symp′to·mat′ic
symp′to·mat′i·cal·ly
symp′to·mat′o·log′ic
symp′to·ma·tol′o·gy

symp·to′sis
sym′pus
  —a′pus
  —di′pus
  —mon′o·pus
sym·sep′a·lous
syn·a·del′phus
syn·al′gi·a
syn·al′gic
syn·an·the′ma pl. -mas or
  -ma·ta
syn·an′throp·ic
syn·an′throse′
syn·apse′ pl. sy·nap′ses′
syn·ap′sis pl. -ses′
syn·ap′tase′
syn·ap′tene′
syn·ap′tic
syn·ap′to·lem′ma
syn·ap·tol′o·gy
syn·ap′to·some′
syn·ar·thro′di·a
syn·ar·thro′di·al
syn·ar·thro·phy′sis pl. -ses′
syn·ar·thro′sis pl. -ses′
syn·as′to·mo′sis pl. -ses′
syn·can′thus
syn·car′y·on′ var. of
  synkaryon
syn·ceph′a·lus pl. -li
syn·chei′li·a
syn′che·sis var. of synchysis
syn′chon·dro′ses′
  —cra′ni·i′
  —ster·na′les′
syn′chon·dro·si′al
syn′chon·dro′sis pl. -ses′
  —ar′y·cor′nic′u′la·ta
  —ep′i·phys′e·os′
  —in′ter·sphe·noi′da′lis
  —in′tra·oc·cip′i·ta′lis
   anterior
  —intraoccipitalis posterior
  —ma·nu′bri·o·ster·na′lis
  —pet′ro·oc·cip′i·ta′lis
  —sphe′no·oc·cip′i·ta′lis
  —sphe′no·pe·tro′sa
  —ster·na′lis
  —xiph′o·ster·na′lis
syn′chon·drot′o·my
syn′chro·nism
syn′chro·nize′, -nized′,
  -niz′ing

syn′chro·nous
syn′chro·ny
syn′chro·tron′
syn′chy·sis also synchesis
  —scin′til·lans′
syn·ci·ne′sis pl. -ses′
syn·cli′nal
syn·clit′ic
syn·cli·tism
syn·clon′ic
syn·clo′nus pl. -ni′
  —bal′lis′mus
  —tre′mens
syn′co·pal
syn′co·pe′
  —an′gi·no′sa
syn·cop′ic
syn·cy′tial
syn·cy′ti·o′ma pl. -mas or
  -ma·ta
syn·cy′ti·o·tox′in
syn·cy′ti·o·tro′pho·blast′
syn·cy′ti·um pl. -ti·a
syn·dac′tyl
syn·dac′tyl′i·a
syn·dac′tyl·ism
syn·dac′ty·lous
syn·dac′ty·lus
syn·dac′ty·ly
syn·dec′to·my
syn·de·sis
syn·des·mec′to·my
syn·des′mec·to′pi·a
syn·des′mi·tis
syn·des′mo·cho′ri·al
syn·des′mo·di·as′ta·sis
syn·des′mo·lo′gi·a
syn·des′mol′o·gy
syn·des′mo·ma pl. -mas or
  -ma·ta
syn·des′mo·pex′y
syn·des·mor′rha·phy
syn·des·mo′sis pl. -ses′
  —tib′i·o·fib′u·lar′is
  —tym′pa·no·sta·pe′di·a
syn·des·mot′o·my
syn·drome′
syn·drom′ic
syn·ech′i·a pl. -i·ae′
  —vul′vae′
syn·ech′i·al
syn·ech′o·tome′
syn′e·chot′o·my

syn'en·ceph'a·lo·cele'
syn'en·ceph'a·ly
syn·er'e·sis pl. -ses'
syn'er·get'ic
syn·er'gi·a
syn'er·gism
syn'er·gist
syn'er·gis'tic
syn'er·gy
syn'es·the'si·a
syn'es·the'si·al'gi·a
syn·gam'ic
syn'ga·mous
syn'ga·my
syn'ge·ne'ic
syn'ge·ne'si·o·plas'tic
syn'ge·ne'si·o·plas'ty
syn'ge·ne'si·o·trans'plan·
  ta'tion
syn'ge·ne'si·ous
syn·gen·e'sis pl. -ses'
syn'ge·net'ic
syn'hi·dro'sis
syn'i·dro'sis pl. -ses'
syn'i·ze'sis
  —pu·pil'lae'
syn·kar'y·on' also
  syncaryon
syn'ki·ne'si·a
syn'ki·ne'sis pl. -ses'
syn'ki·net'ic
syn'ne·ma'tin
syn'o·don'ti·a
syn·oph'rys
syn'oph·thal'mi·a
syn'oph·thal'mus pl. -mi'
syn·op'si·a
syn·op'to·phore'
syn·or'chi·dism
syn·os'che·os
syn·os'te·o·phyte'
syn·os'tosed'
syn·os·to'sis pl. -ses'
syn·os·tot'ic
syn·o'ti·a
syn·o'tus
syn·o·vec'to·my
syn·o'vi·a
syn·o'vi·al
syn·o'vi·al·o'ma pl. -mas or
  -ma·ta
syn·o'vi·o·en'do·the'li·
  o'ma pl. -mas or -ma·ta

syn·o'vi·o'ma pl. -mas or
  -ma·ta
syn·o'vip'a·rous
syn·o'vi'tis
  —hy'per·plas'ti·ca
syn·tac'tic or syn·tac'ti·cal
syn·tac'tics
syn·tal'i·ty
syn'ta·sis
syn'thase'
syn·tax'is
syn·tec'tic
syn·ther'mal
syn'the·sis pl. -ses'
syn'the·size', -sized', -siz'ing
syn'the·tase'
syn·thet'ic
syn·tho'rax'
syn·ton'ic
syn'to·nin
syn'tro·phism
syn·tro'pho·blast'
syn·tro'phus pl. -phi'
syn·trop'ic
syn'tro·py
syph'i·le'mi·a
syph'i·lid
syph'i·li·on'thus pl. -thi'
syph'i·lis
  —d'em·blée'
  —he·red'i·tar'i·a
  —in'son'ti·um
  —tech'ni·ca
syph'i·lit'ic
syph'i·lo·derm'
syph'i·lo·der'ma
syph'i·lo·der'ma·tous
syph'i·lo·gen'e·sis
syph'i·loid'
syph'i·lol'o·gist
syph'i·lol'o·gy
syph'i·lo'ma pl. -mas or
  -ma·ta
syph'i·lo·nych'i·a
  —ex·ul'cer·ans'
  —sic'ca
syph'i·lop'a·thy
syph'i·lo·pho'bi·a
syph'i·lo·phy'ma pl. -mas or
  -ma·ta
syph'i·lo·psy·cho'sis
  pl. -ses'
syph'i·lous

sy·rig'mo·pho'ni·a
sy·rig'mus
syr'ing·ad'e·no'ma pl.
  -mas or -ma·ta
syr'ing·ad'e·no'sus
sy·ringe'
syr'in·gec'to·my
syr'in·gi'tis
sy·rin'go·bul'bi·a
sy·rin'go·car'ci·no'ma pl.
  -mas or -ma·ta
sy·rin'go·cele' also
  syringocoele
sy·rin'go·coele' var. of
  syringocele
sy·rin'go·coe'li·a
sy·rin'go·cyst'ad·e·no'ma
  pl. -mas or -ma·ta
sy·rin'go·cys·to'ma pl. -mas
  or -ma·ta
sy·rin'go·en·ce·pha'li·a
sy·rin'goid'
syr'in·go'ma pl. -mas or
  -ma·ta
sy·rin'go·me·nin'go·cele'
sy·rin'go·my·e'li·a
sy·rin'go·my·e'li'tis
sy·rin'go·my'e·lo·cele'
sy·rin'go·my'e·lus
sy·rin'go·tome'
syr'in·got'o·my
syr'inx pl. sy·rin'ges' or
  -inx·es
syr'o·sin'go·pine'
syr'up
sys'sar·co'sis pl. -ses'
sys'sar·cot'ic
sys·so'mic
sys·so'mus
sys·tal'tic
sys'tem
sys·te'ma
  —di'ges·to'ri·um
  —lym·phat'i·cum
  —ner'vo'rum cen·tra'le'
  —nervorum per'i·pher'-
    i·cum
  —ner·vo'sum
  —nervosum au'to·nom'-
    i·cum
  —nervosum cen·tra'le'
  —nervosum per'i·pher'-
    i·cum

—nervosum sym·path′-
i·cum
—re·spi′ra·to′ri·um
—u′ro·gen′i·ta′le′
sys′tem·at′ic
sys′tem·a·ti·za′tion
sys′tem·a·tize′, -tized′,
-tiz′ing
sys·tem′ic
sys·tem′i·cal·ly
sys′tem·oid′
sys′to·le
sys·tol′ic
sys·trem′ma *pl.* -ma·ta *or*
-mas
sy·zyg′i·al
syz′y·gy
Sza′bo sign
Szent′-Györ′gyi test
Szy′ma·now′ski operation

T

Taarn′hoj operation
tab′a·co′sis
tab′a·cum
tab′a·gism
tab′a·nid
Ta·ban′i·dae′
Ta·ba′nus
ta′bar·dil′lo
ta·ba·tiére′ a·na·to·mique′
ta·bel′la *pl.* -lae′
ta′bes′
  —cox·ar′i·a
  —do′lo·ro′sa
  —dor·sa′lis
  —er·got′i·ca
  —mes′en·ter′i·ca
ta·bes′cence
ta·bes′cent
ta·bet′ic
ta·bet′i·form′
tab′ic
tab′id
tab′la·ture′
ta′ble
ta′ble·spoon′
tab′let
ta·boo′
ta′bo·pa·ral′y·sis *pl.* -ses′
ta′bo·pa·re′sis *pl.* -ses′
tab′u·la *pl.* -lae′

tab′u·lar
tache
  —bleu·âtre′
  —cé·ré·brale′
  —mé·nin·gé·ale′
  —mo·trice′
  —noire
  —spi·nale
taches
  —blanches
  —du ca·fé′ au lait
  —ro·sées′ len·ti·cu·laires′
ta·chet′ic
ta·chis′to·scope′
ta·chis′to·scop′ic
tach′o·gram′
ta·chog′ra·phy
ta·chom′e·ter
tach′y·al′i·men·ta′tion
tach′y·ar·rhyth′mi·a
tach′y·aux·e′sis *pl.* -ses′
tach′y·car′di·a
  —stru·mo′sa ex′oph·thal′-
mi·ca
tach′y·car′di·ac′
tach′y·car′dic
tach′y·graph′
ta·chyg′ra·phy
tach′y·ki′nin
tach′y·la′li·a
tach′y·lo′gi·a
ta·chym′e·ter
tach′y·pha′gi·a
tach′y·pha′si·a
tach′y·phe′mi·a
tach′y·phra′si·a
tach′y·phy·lax′is *pl.* -lax′es′
tach′yp·ne′a
tach′yp·ne′ic
tach′y·rhyth′mi·a
ta·chys′ter·ol′
tach′y·sys′to·le
tac′rine′
tac′tile
tac′tion
tac·tom′e·ter
tac′tor
tac′tu·al
tae′di·um vi′tae′
tae′ni·a
  —cho·roi′de·a
  —for′ni·cis
  —hip′po·cam′pi′

  —li′ber·a
  —mes′o·co′li·ca
  —o′men·ta′lis
  —pon′tis
  —tec′tae′
  —te′lae′
  —ter′mi·na′lis
  —thal′a·mi′
  —tu′bae′
  —ven·tric′u·li quar′ti
Tae′ni·a
  —e·chi′no·coc′cus
  —na′na
  —sag′i·na′ta
  —so′li·um
tae′ni·a·cide′ *also* teniacide
tae′ni·ae′
  —a·cus′ti·cae′
  —co′li
  —of Val·sal′va
  —py·lo′ri
  —te·lar′um
tae′ni·a·fuge′ *also* teniafuge
Tae′ni·a·rhyn′chus
tae·ni′a·sis *also* teniasis
tae′ni·form′ *also* teniform
tae′ni·oid′ *also* tenioid
tae·ni′o·la *var. of* teniola
tag
tag′ma
tail
  —of Spence
tai′pan
Ta·ka′ta-A′ra test
Ta′ka·ya′su
  —arteritis
  —disease
  —syndrome
take′down′
take′off′
ta·lal′gi·a
ta′lar
tal′bu·tal′
talc
tal·co′sis *pl.* -ses′
tal′cum
tal′i·pes′
  —ar′cu·a′tus
  —cal·ca′ne·o·ca′vus
  —cal·ca′ne·o·val′gus
  —cal·ca′ne·us
  —ca′vo·val′gus
  —ca′vus

—e·qui'no·ca'vus
—e·qui'no·val'gus
—e·qui'no·var'us
—e·qui'nus
—per·ca'vus
—pla'nus
—spas·mod'i·ca
—val'gus
—var'us
tal'i·pom'a·nus
Tal'ler·man treatment
tal'low
Tall'quist method
Tal'ma operation
ta'lo·cal·ca'ne·al
ta'lo·cal·ca'ne·o·na·vic'u·lar
ta'lo·cru'ral
ta'lo·fib'u·lar
ta'lo·mal·le'o·lar
tal'on
ta'lo·na·vic'u·lar
tal'o·nid
tal'ose'
ta'lo·tib'i·al
ta'lus *pl.* -li'
ta'ma
tam'a·rind
tam·bour'
Tamm'-Hors'fall' protein
ta·mox'i·fen
tam'pon'
tam'pon·ade'
tam'pon·age'
tam'pon·ing
tam·pon'ment
ta'na·pox'
tan'dem
tan'gent
tan·gen'tial
Tan·gier' disease
tan'gle
tank
tan'nase'
tan'nate'
Tan'ner operation
tan'nic
tan'nin
Tan·ret' reagent
tan'ta·lum
tan'trum
tap, tapped, tap'ping
tape

ta·pei'no·ceph'a·ly
ta·pe'tal
ta·pe'to·ret'i·nal
ta·pe'tum *pl.* -ta
—al·ve'o·li'
—lu'ci·dum
tape'worm'
taph'e·pho'bi·a
Ta'pi·a syndrome
tap'i·no·ce·phal'ic
tap'i·no·ceph'a·ly
ta'pir·oid'
ta·pote'ment
tar
ta·ran'tu·la *pl.* -las *or* -lae'
ta·rax'a·cum
Tar·dieu' ecchymoses
tar'di·grade'
tar'dive
tare
tar'get
Tar'lov cyst
Tar·nier' sign
ta'ro
tar'ry
tars·ad'e·ni'tis
tar'sal
tar·sa'le *pl.* -li·a
tar'sal'gi·a
tar'sa'lis
tar·sec'to·my
tar·si'tis
tar'so·chei'lo·plas'ty
tar'so·cla'si·a
tar·soc'la·sis
tar'so·ma·la'ci·a
tar'so·met'a·tar'sal
tar'so·pha·lan'ge·al
tar'so·phy'ma *pl.* -mas *or* -ma·ta
tar'so·pla'si·a
tar'so·plas'ty
tar'sop·to'si·a
tar'sop·to'sis *pl.* -ses'
tar·sor'rha·phy
tar'so·tar'sal
tar'so·tib'i·al
tar·sot'o·my
tar'sus *pl.* -si'
—inferior pal'pe·brae'
—superior palpebrae
tar'tar
tar·tar'ic

tar'trate'
tar'tra·zine'
tar·tron'ic
Tash'kent' ulcer
taste', tast'ed, tast'ing
tat·too'
tat·too'ing
Tau'ber test
tau'rine'
tau'ro·cho·lan'o·poi·e'sis
  pl. -ses'
tau'ro·cho'late'
tau'ro·cho'lic
tau'ro·dont'
tau'ro·don'ti·a
Taus'sig-Bing'
—anomaly
—complex
—malformation
—syndrome
Taus'sig-Bla'lock'
  operation
tau'to·me'ni·al
tau'to·mer
tau·tom'er·al
tau·tom'er·ase'
tau'to·mer'ic
tau·tom'er·ism
Ta·wa'ra node
tax'is *pl.* tax'es'
tax·o'di·um
tax'ol'
tax'on' *pl.* tax'a
tax·o·nom'ic
tax·on'o·mist
tax·on'o·my
Tay choroiditis
Tay'-Sachs' disease
tear, teared, tear'ing
tease, teased, teas'ing
tea'spoon'
teat
tech·ne'ti·um
tech'nic
tech'ni·cal
tech·ni'cian
tech'nics
tech·nique'
tech·nol'o·gist
tech·nol'o·gy
tec'lo·zan'
tec'tal
tec'ti·form'

tec'to·bul'bar
tec'to·ceph'a·ly
tec'to·cer'e·bel'lar
tec·ton'ic
tec'to·ri'al
tec'to·ri·um
tec'to·ru'bral
tec'to·spi'nal
tec'tum *pl.* -ta
—mes'en·ceph'a·li'
te'di·ous
teethe, teethed, teeth'ing
Tee'van law
tef'lu·rane'
teg'men *pl.* -mi·na
—mas·toi'de·um
—tym'pa·ni'
—ven·tric'u·li' quar'ti'
teg·men'tal
teg·men'tum *pl.* -ta
—rhom'ben·ceph'a·li'
teg'u·ment
teg'u·men'tal
teg'u·men'ta·ry
Teich'mann
—crystals
—test
tei·cho'ic
tei·chop'si·a
tek'no·cyte'
te'la *pl.* -lae'
—ad'i·po'sa
—cho'ri·oi'de·a ven·tric'-
u·li' quar'ti'
—chorioidea ventriculi
ter'ti·i'
—cho·roi'de·a ven·tric'u·li'
quar'ti'
—choroidea ventriculi
ter'ti·i'
—sub'cu·ta'ne·a
—sub'mu·co'sa
—submucosa co'li'
—submucosa e·soph'a·gi'
—submucosa in'tes·ti'ni'
rec'ti'
—submucosa intestini
ten'u·is
—submucosa oe·soph'a·gi'
—submucosa pha·ryn'gis
—submucosa rec'ti'
—submucosa tra'che·ae' et
bron·cho'rum

—submucosa tu'bae'
u'ter·i'nae'
—submucosa ven·tric'u·li'
—submucosa ves'i·cae'
u'ri·nar'i·ae'
—sub'se·ro'sa
—subserosa co'li'
—subserosa hep'a·tis
—subserosa in'tes·ti'ni'
ten'u·is
—subserosa per'i·to·nae'i'
—subserosa per'i·to·ne'i'
pa·ri'e·ta'lis
—subserosa peritonei
vis'ce·ra'lis
—subserosa tu'bae'
u'ter·i'nae'
—subserosa u'ter·i'
—subserosa ven·tric'u·li'
—subserosa ves'i·cae'
fel'le·ae'
—subserosa vesicae
u'ri·nar'i·ae'
tel·al'gi·a
tel·an'gi·ec·ta'si·a
tel·an'gi·ec·ta'sis *pl.* -ses'
—fa'ci·e'i'
—lym·phat'i·ca
tel·an'gi·ec·tat'ic
tel·an'gi·ec·to'des'
tel·an'gi·o'ma *pl.* -mas *or*
-ma·ta
tel·an'gi·on'
tel·an'gi·o'sis *pl.* -ses'
tel·an'gi·tis
te'lar
tel·au'gic
tel'e·an·gi·ec·ta'sis *pl.* -ses'
tel'e·car'di·o·gram'
tel'e·car'di·og'ra·phy
tel'e·car'di·o·phone'
tel'e·cep'tor
tel'e·ci·ne'si·a
tel'e·ci·ne'sis *pl.* -ses'
tel'e·co'balt
tel'e·cu'rie·ther'a·py
tel'e·den'drite'
tel'e·den'dron
tel'e·di'ag·no'sis
tel'e·fluo·ros'co·py
tel'e·ki·ne'sis *pl.* -ses'
tel'e·lec'tro·car'di·o·gram'
te·lem'e·ter

te·lem'e·try
tel'en·ce·phal'ic
tel'en·ceph'a·lon'
tel'e·neu'rite'
tel'e·neu'ron'
tel'e·o·log'ic *or*
te'le·o·log'i·cal
tel'e·ol'o·gy
tel'e·o·mi·to'sis
tel'e·o·morph'
tel'e·or·gan'ic
tel'e·o·ther'a·peu'tics
te·lep'a·thy
tel'e·phone'
tel'e·ra'di·og'ra·phy
tel'e·ra'di·um
tel'er·gy
tel'e·roent'gen·o·gram'
tel'e·roent'ge·nog'ra·phy
tel'e·scope'
tel'es·the'si·a
tel'e·sys·tol'ic
tel'e·ther'a·py
tel·lu'ric
tel·lu'ri·um
tel'o·cen'tric
tel'o·coele'
tel'o·den'dri·a
tel'o·den'dron
tel'o·gen
tel'og·no'sis
tel'o·lec'i·thal
tel'o·lem'ma
tel'o·mer
tel'o·mere'
te·lom'er·i·za'tion
te·lom'er·ize', -ized', -iz'ing
tel'o·phase'
Tel'o·spo·rid'i·a
tel'o·syn·ap'sis
te·maz'e·pam
tem'per
tem'per·a·ment
tem'per·ance
tem'per·ate
tem'per·a·ture
tem'plate
tem'ple
tem'po·la'bile
tem'po·ra
tem'po·ral
tem'po·ra'lis
—su'per·fi'ci·a'lis

tem'po·rar'y
tem'po·ro·au·ric'u·lar
tem'po·ro·fa'cial
tem'po·ro·fron'tal
tem'po·ro·hy'oid'
tem'po·ro·ma'lar
tem'po·ro·man·dib'u·lar
tem'po·ro·max'il·lar'y
tem'po·ro·oc·cip'i·tal
tem'po·ro·pa·ri'e·tal
tem'po·ro·pon'tine'
tem'po·ro·spa'tial
tem'po·ro·sphe'noid'
tem'po·sta'bile
tem'po·ro·zy'go·mat'ic
tem'u·lence
tem'u·len'ti·a
te·na'cious
te·nac'i·ty
te·nac'u·lum *pl.* -la *or* -lums
ten·al'gi·a
　—crep'i·tans'
ten'den·cy
ten'der
ten'der·ness
ten'di·ni'tis
ten'di·no·plas'ty
ten'di·no·su'ture
ten'di·nous
ten'do *pl.* -di·nes'
　—A·chil'lis
　—cal·ca'ne·us
　—con'junc·ti'vus
　—cri'co·e·soph'a·ge'us
ten'dol'y·sis
ten'do·mu'cin
ten'don
　—of Zinn
　—organ of Gol'gi
ten'do·ni'tis
ten'do·plas'ty
ten'do·syn'o·vi'tis
ten'do·vag'i·nal
ten'do·vag'i·ni'tis
　—crep'i·tans'
　—gran'u·lo'sa
　—ste'no'sans'
te·neb'ric
Te·neb'ri·o
te·nec'to·my
te·nes'mic
te·nes'mus
te·ni'a *pl.* -ni·ae', *also* taenia

te'ni·a·cide' *var. of* taeniacide
te'ni·a·fuge' *var. of*
　taeniafuge
te'ni·al
te·ni'a·sis *var. of* taeniasis
te'ni·form' *var. of* taeniform
te'ni·oid' *var. of* taenioid
te·ni'o·la *also* taeniola
　—ci·ne're·a
ten'i·po'side'
ten'o·de'sis *pl.* -ses'
ten'o·dyn'i·a
ten'o·fi'bril
te·nol'y·sis
te·nom'e·ter
ten'o·my'o·plas'ty
ten'o·my·ot'o·my
Te·non' capsule
ten'o·nec'to·my
ten'o·ni'tis
te·non'to·dyn'i·a
ten'on·tog'ra·phy
te·non'to·my'o·plas'ty
te·non'to·my·ot'o·my
te·non'to·phy'ma
te·non'to·the·ci'tis
　—pro·lif'er·a cal·car'e·a
ten'o·phyte'
ten'o·plas'tic
ten'o·plas'ty
ten'o·re·cep'tor
te·nor'rha·phy
ten'o·si'tis
ten'os·to'sis *pl.* -ses'
ten'o·sus·pen'sion
ten'o·su'ture
ten'o·syn'o·vec'to·my
ten'o·syn'o·vi·al
ten'o·syn'o·vi·o'ma *pl.*
　-mas *or* -ma·ta
ten'o·syn'o·vi'tis
　—crep'i·tans'
ten'o·tome'
te·not'o·mize', -mized',
　-miz'ing
te·not'o·my
ten'o·vag'i·ni'tis
ten'sion
ten'si·ty
ten'sive
ten'sor
　—cap'su·lar'is ar·tic'u·la'-
　ti·o'nis met'a·car'po·pha·

lan'ge·i' dig'i·ti'
　—fas'ci·ae' la'tae' reflex
　—lam'i·nae' pos·te'ri·o'ris
　va·gi'nae' mus'cu·lae'
　rec'ti' ab·dom'i·nis
　—lig'a·men'ti' an'nu·lar'is
　—pa·la'ti' muscle
　—ve'li' pal·a·ti'ni' muscle
tent
ten'ta·tive
ten·tig'i·nous
ten·ti'go
　—ve·ne're·a
ten·to'ri·al
ten·to'ri·um *pl.* -ri·a
　—cer'e·bel'li'
ten'u·ate', -at'ed, -at'ing
ten'u·ous
teph'ro·my'e·li'tis
tep'id
ter'a·mor'phous
ter'as *pl.* ter'a·ta
ter·at'ic
ter'a·tism
ter'a·to·blas·to'ma *pl.* -mas
　or -ma·ta
ter'a·to·car'ci·no'ma
　pl. -mas *or* -ma·ta
ter'a·to·gen
ter'a·to·gen'e·sis *pl.* -ses'
ter'a·to·ge·net'ic
ter'a·to·gen'ic
ter'a·to·ge·nic'i·ty
ter'a·tog'e·nous
ter'a·tog'e·ny
ter'a·toid'
ter'a·to·log'ic *or*
　ter'a·to·log'i·cal
ter'a·tol'o·gy
ter'a·to'ma *pl.* -mas *or* -ma·ta
ter'a·to·pho'bi·a
ter'a·to'sis *pl.* -ses'
ter'a·to·sper'mi·a
te·ra'zo·sin
ter'bi·um
ter·bu'ta·line'
ter·con'a·zole'
te're'
ter'e·bene'
ter'e·bin'thi·nate'
ter'e·bin'thine'
ter'e·bin'thism
ter'e·bra·che'sis *pl.* -ses'

ter'e·brat'ing
ter'e·bra'tion
te'res' *pl.* ter'e·es'
ter·fen'a·dine'
ter'gal
ter in di'e
term
ter'mi·nad'
ter'mi·nal
ter'mi·nal·i·za'tion
ter'mi·nal·ly
ter'mi·na'ti·o'
   pl. -na'ti·o'nes'
ter'mi·na'tion
ter'mi·na'ti·o'nes'
   ner·vo'rum li'ber·ae'
ter'mi·ni'
   —ad mem'bra spec·tan'tes'
   —gen'e·ra'les'
   —on'to·ge·net'i·ci'
   —si'tum et di·rec'ti·o'nem
     par'ti·um cor'po·ris
     in'di·can'tes'
ter'mi·nol'o·gy
ter'mi·nus *pl.* -ni'
ter'na·ry
ter·o'·di'line'
ter·ox'a·lene'
ter'pe·nism
ter'pin
ter·pin'e·ol'
ter'pi·nol'
ter'ra *pl.* -rae'
   —al'ba
   —sig'il·la'ta
Ter'ry
   —method
   —stain
ter'tian
ter'ti·a·rism
ter'ti·ar'y
ter'ti·grav'i·da
ter·tip'a·ra
tes'la
Tes'la current
tes'sel·lat'ed
test
tes·ta'ceous
tes·tal'gi·a
test'cross'
tes·tec'to·my
test'er
tes'ti·cle

tes·tic'u·lar
tes'tis *pl.* -tes'
tes·ti'tis
tes'toid'
tes'to·lac'tone'
tes·tos'ter·one'
tet'a·nal
te·ta'ni·a
te·tan'ic
te·tan'i·form'
tet'a·nig'e·ous
tet'a·nil'la
tet'a·nin
tet'a·nism
tet'a·ni·za'tion
tet'a·nize', -nized', -niz'ing
tet'a·no·can'na·bin
tet'a·node'
tet'a·noid'
tet'a·nol'y·sin
tet'a·nol'y·sis *pl.* -ses'
tet'a·nom'e·ter
tet'a·no·mo'tor
tet'a·no·spas'min
tet'a·nus
   —in'fan'tum
   —ne'o·na·to'rum
tet'a·ny
te·tar'ta·no'pi·a
te·tar'ta·nop'si·a
te·tar'to·cone'
te·tar'to·co'nid
tet'ra·ba'sic
tet'ra·ben'zine'
tet'ra·bra'chi·us
tet'ra·caine'
tet'ra·chei'rus
tet'ra·chlor·eth'ane'
tet'ra·chlo'ride'
tet'ra·chlo'ro·eth'ane'
tet'ra·chlo'ro·eth'yl·ene'
tet'ra·chlo'ro·meth'ane'
tet'ra·chlo'ro·sal'i·cyl·an'i·
   lide'
tet'ra·coc'cus *pl.* -ci
tet'ra·cy'cline'
tet'rad'
tet'ra·dac'tyl
tet'ra·dac'ty·ly
tet'ra·eth'yl
tet'ra·eth'yl·am·mo'ni·um
tet'ra·eth'yl·thi'u·ram
tet'ra·gen'ic

te·trag'e·nous
tet'ra·hy'dric
tet'ra·hy'dro·a·mi'no·ac'ri·
   dine'
tet'ra·hy'dro·can·nab'i·nol'
tet'ra·hy'dro·cor'ti·sol'
tet'ra·hy'dro·zo'line'
Tet'ra·hy'me·na
tet'ra·i·o'do·phe'nol·
   phthal'e·in
tet'ra·i·o'do·phthal'e·in
te·tral'o·gy
   —of Fal'lot'
tet'ra·mas'ti·a
tet'ra·mas'ti·gote'
tet'ra·ma'zi·a
te·tram'e·lus
tet'ra·mer
tet'ra·mer'ic
te·tram'er·ism
te·tram'er·ous
tet'ra·meth'yl·am·mo'-
   ni·um
tet'ra·meth'yl·ene·di'a·
   mine'
tet'ra·ni'trol'
tet'ra·nop'si·a
tet'ra·o'tus
tet'ra·pa·re'sis
tet'ra·pep'tide'
Tet'ra·pet'a·lo·ne'ma
   per'stans'
tet'ra·pho'co·me'li·a
tet'ra·ple'gi·a
tet'ra·ploid'
tet'ra·ploi'dy
tet'ra·pod'
tet'ra·pus
tet'ra·pyr'role'
tet'ra·sac'cha·ride'
te·tras'ce·lus
tet'ra·so'mic
tet'ra·so'my
tet'ras'ter
tet'ra·sti·chi'a·sis
tet'ra·thi'o·nate'
tet'ra·tom'ic
tet'ra·vac'cine'
tet'ra·va'lent
tet'ra·zole'
tet'ra·zo'li·um
tet'ro·do·tox'i·ca'tion
tet'ro·do·tox'ism

tet'ro·nal
tet'roph·thal'mus
tet'ro·quin'one'
tet'rose'
te·tro'tus
te·trox'ide'
te·tryd'a·mine'
tex'is
tex'ti·form'
tex'to·blas'tic
tex'tur·al
tex'ture
tex'tus   *pl.* tex'tus
thal'a·mec'to·my
thal'a·men·ce·phal'ic
thal'a·men·ceph'a·lon'
tha·lam'ic
thal'a·mo·coele'
thal'a·mo·cor'ti·cal
thal'a·mo·ge·nic'u·late
thal'a·mo·len·tic'u·lar
thal'a·mo·mam'mil·lar'y
thal'a·mo·pa·ri'e·tal
thal'a·mo·teg·men'tal
thal'a·mot'o·my
thal'a·mus   *pl.* -mi'
thal'as·se'mi·a
thal'as·se'mic
thal'as·so·pho'bi·a
thal'as·so·po'si·a
thal'as·so·ther'a·py
tha·lid'o·mide'
thal'li·um
thal'lo·phyte'
thal'lo·spore'
thal'lous chlo'ride'
thal'lus   *pl.* -li
Thal procedure
tha·mu'ri·a
than'a·to·bi'o·log'ic
than'a·to·gno·mon'ic
than'a·toid'
than'a·tol'o·gy
than'a·to·ma'ni·a
than'a·to·pho'bi·a
than'a·to·phor'ic
than'a·top'sy
than'a·tos
thau·mat'ro·py
Thay'er-Doi'sy unit
thea'ism
the·ba'ic
the·ba'ine'

the·be'si·an
the·ca   *pl.* -cae'
—ex·ter'na
—fol·lic'u·li'
—in·ter'na
the'cal
the'cate
the·ci'tis
the'co·dont'
the·co'ma   *pl.* -mas or -ma·ta
the'co·ma·to'sis
the'co·steg·no'sis
The'den method
Thei·le'ri·a
Thei'ler virus
the'in
the'ine'
the'in·ism
the·lal'gi·a
the·lar'che
the·las'is
The·la'zi·a
the·la·zi'a·sis
the'le·plas'ty
the·ler'e·thism
the·li·o'ma   *pl.* -mas or -ma·ta
the·li'tis
the'li·um   *pl.* -li·a
the·lon'cus   *pl.* -ci'
the'lor·rha'gi·a
the'lo·thism
thel'y·gen'ic
thel'y·to'ci·a
the·lyt'o·ky
The·mat'ic Ap'per·cep'-
    tion Test
the'nad'
the'nal
the'nar'
then'yl·di'a·mine'
then'yl·pyr'a·mine'
the'o·bro'mine'
the'o·ma'ni·a
the'o·pho'bi·a
the'o·phyl'line'
the'o·ple'gi·a
the'o·ret'ic   *or* the'o·ret'i·cal
the'o·ry
the'o·ther'a·py
thèque
ther'a·peu'sis   *pl.* -ses'
ther'a·peu'tic   *or*
    ther'a·peu'ti·cal

ther'a·peu'tics
ther'a·peu'tist
ther'a·pi'a ster'i·li'sans'
    mag'na
ther'a·pist
ther'a·py
ther'en·ceph'a·lous
Ther'i·di·i·dae'
the'ri·od'ic
the'ri·o·gen'o·log'ic
the'ri·o·ge·nol'o·gy
the'ri·o'ma   *pl.* -mas or
    -ma·ta
therm
therm·aer'o·ther'a·py
ther'mal
therm'al·ge'si·a
ther·mal'gi·a
therm'an·al·ge'si·a
therm'an·es·the'si·a
ther'ma·to·log'ic
ther'ma·tol'o·gy
ther·me·lom'e·ter
therm·es·the'si·a
therm·es·the'si·om'e·ter
therm·hy'per·es·the'si·a
therm·hyp·es·the'si·a
ther'mic
ther'mis·tor
ther'mo·an·al·ge'si·a
ther'mo·an·es·the'si·a
ther·mo·cau'ter·y
ther'mo·chem'is·try
ther·moch'ro·ism
ther'mo·co·ag'u·la'tion
ther'mo·cou'ple
ther'mo·cur'rent
ther'mo·dif·fu'sion
ther'mo·di·lu'tion
ther'mo·du'ric
ther'mo·dy·nam'ics
ther'mo·e·lec'tric
ther'mo·e·lec·tric'i·ty
ther'mo·ex·ci'to·ry
ther'mo·gen'e·sis
ther'mo·gen'ic
ther'mo·gen'ics
ther·mog'e·nous
ther'mo·gram'
ther'mo·graph'
ther'mo·graph'ic
ther·mog'ra·phy
ther·mo·hy'per·al·ge'si·a

ther'mo·hy'per·es·the'si·a

ther'mo·hyp'es·the'si·a

ther'mo·in·hib'i·to'ry

ther'mo·ker'a·to·plas'ty

ther'mo·la'bile

ther·mol'o·gy

ther'mo·lu'mi·nes'cence

ther'mo·lu'mi·nes'cent

ther·mol'y·sis

ther'mo·lyt'ic

ther'mo·mas·sage'

ther'mo·mas·tog'ra·phy

ther·mom'e·ter

ther'mo·met'ric

ther·mom'e·try

ther'mo·neu·ro'sis

ther'mo·phile'

ther'mo·phil'ic

ther'mo·pho'bi·a

ther'mo·phore'

ther'mo·pile'

ther'mo·pla·cen·tog'ra·phy

ther'mo·plas'tic

ther'mo·ple'gi·a

ther'mo·pol'yp·ne'a

ther'mo·re·cep'tor

ther'mo·scope'

ther'mo·set'

ther'mo·sta'ble

ther'mo·sta'sis

ther'mo·ste·re·o'sis

ther'mo·stro'muhr' of Rein

ther'mo·sys'tal'tic

ther'mo·sys'tal·tism

ther'mo·tac'tic

ther'mo·tax'ic

ther'mo·tax'is

ther'mo·ther'a·py

ther·mot'ics

ther'mo·to·nom'e·ter

ther'mo·tra'che·ot'o·my

ther'mo·trop'ic

ther·mot'ro·pism

the'ro·mor'phi·a

the'ro·mor'phism

the·sau'ris·mo'sis *pl.* -ses'

the'sis *pl.* -ses'

the'ta

the'tin

thev'e·tin

thi'a·ben'da·zole'

thi'a·cet'a·zone'

thi·am'i·nase'

thi'a·mine'

thi·am'i·prine'

thi·am'phen'i·col'

thi·am'y·lal'

thi·az'e·sim

thi'a·zine'

thi'a·zole'

thi'a·zol·sul'fone'

thick'en

thick'ness

Thie'mann disease

Thiersch

—graft

—operation

thi·eth'yl·per'a·zine'

thigh

thigh'bone'

thig·man'es·the'si·a

thig'mes·the'si·a

thig'mo·tax'is *pl.* -tax'es'

thig'mo·trop'ic

thig·mot'ro·pism

thi·hex'i·nol'

thi·mer'o·sal'

thi'o·ac'e·tal

thi'o·al'de·hyde'

thi'o·bar·bit'u·rate'

thi'o·bar'bi·tu'ric

thi'o·car'ba·mide'

thi'o·chrome'

thi·oc'tic

thi'o·cy'a·nate'

thi'o·cy·an'ic

thi'o·di·phen'yl·am'ine

thi'o·gua'nine'

thi'ol'

thi'o·mer'sa·late'

thi'o·ne'ine

thi·on'ic

thi'o·pen'tal'

thi'o·pen'tone'

thi'o·phene'

thi'o·pro'pa·zate'

thi'o·rid'a·zine'

thi'o·sem'i·car'ba·zone'

thi'o·sul'fate'

thi'o·sul·fu'ric

thi'o·tep'a

thi'o·thix'ene'

thi'o·u'ra·cil

thi'o·u·re'a

thi·phen'a·mil

thi'ram'

third'-de·gree'

—burn

—heart block

thirst

Thi'ry fistula

thix'o·trop'ic

thix·ot'ro·pism

thix·ot'ro·py

thlip'sen·ceph'a·lus *pl.* -li'

Tho'ma ampulla

Thom'as

—method

—sign

—test

Thom'as-La'vol·lay' method

Tho'minx' aer'o·phil'a

Thom'sen disease

thon·zo'ni·um

thon·zyl'a·mine'

tho'ra·cal'gi·a

tho'ra·cec'to·my

tho'ra·cen·te'sis *pl.* -ses'

tho·rac'ic

tho·rac'i·co·hu'mer·al

tho·rac'i·co·lum'bar

tho'ra·co·ab·dom'i·nal

tho'ra·co·a·cro'mi·al

tho'ra·co·bron·chot'o·my

tho'ra·co·ce'li·ot'o·my

tho'ra·co·ce·los'chi·sis *pl.* -ses'

tho'ra·co·cen·te'sis *pl.* -ses'

tho'ra·co·cyl·lo'sis *pl.* -ses'

tho'ra·co·cyr·to'sis

tho'ra·co·del'phus

tho'ra·co·did'y·mus

tho'ra·co·dyn'i·a

tho'ra·co·gas'tro·did'y·mus

tho'ra·co·gas'tros'chi·sis *pl.* -ses'

tho'ra·co·lap'a·rot'o·my

tho'ra·co·lum'bar

tho'ra·col'y·sis *pl.* -ses'

tho'ra·com'e·lus

tho'ra·com'e·ter

tho'ra·com'e·try

tho'ra·co·my'o·dyn'i·a

tho'ra·cop'a·gus *pl.* -gus·es *or* -gi'

—par'a·sit'i·cus

—tri·bra'chi·us

—tri′pus
tho′ra·co·par′a·ceph′a·lus
  pl. -li′
  —pseu′do·a·cor′mus
tho′ra·cop′a·thy
tho′ra·co·plas′ty
tho′ra·co·pneu′mo·plas′ty
tho′ra·cos′chi·sis *pl.* -ses′
tho·ra′co·scope′
tho′ra·co·scop′ic
tho′ra·cos′co·py
tho′ra·co·ste·no′sis
tho′ra·cos′to·my
tho′ra·cot′o·my
tho′ra·del′phus
tho′rax′ *pl.* -rax′es *or* -ra′ces′
Tho′rel bundle
tho′ri·um
Thorn test
tho′ron′
thought
tho·zal′i·none′
thread
thread′worm′
thre′o·nine′
thre′ose′
threp·sol′o·gy
thresh′old′
thrill
thrix an′nu·la′ta
throat
throb, throbbed, throb′bing
Throck′mor′ton reflex
throe
throm′bal·lo′sis
throm′base′
throm′bas·the′ni·a
throm·bec′to·my
throm′bin
throm·bin′o·gen
throm′bo·an′gi·i′tis
  —cu·ta′ne·o·in·tes′ti·na′lis
    dis·sem′i·na′ta
  —o·blit′er·ans′
throm′bo·ar·ter·i′tis
throm′bo·as·the′ni·a
throm′bo·blast′
throm′bo·cav′er·no·si′tis
throm·boc′la·sis
throm′bo·clas′tic
throm′bo·cyst′
throm′bo·cys′tis
throm′bo·cyte′

throm′bo·cy·the′mi·a
throm′bo·cyt′ic
throm′bo·cy′to·crit
throm′bo·cy′tol′y·sin
throm′bo·cy′tol′y·sis
throm′bo·cy′to·lyt′ic
throm′bo·cy′to·path′i·a
throm′bo·cy′to·path′ic
throm′bo·cy′top′a·thy
throm′bo·cy′to·pe′ni·a
throm′bo·cy′to·pe′nic
throm′bo·cy′to·pher′e·sis
throm′bo·cy′to·poi·e′sis
  pl. -ses′
throm′bo·cy′to·poi·et′ic
throm′bo·cy′to·sis *pl.* -ses′
throm′bo·em′bo·lec′to·my
throm′bo·em·bol′ic
throm′bo·em′bo·lism
throm′bo·em′bo·li·za′tion
throm′bo·em′bo·lus *pl.* -li′
throm′bo·en·dar′ter·ec′-
  to·my
throm′bo·end′ar·te·ri′tis
throm′bo·en′do·car·di′tis
throm′bo·gen
throm′bo·gen′e·sis *pl.* -ses′
throm′bo·gen′ic
throm′boid′
throm′bo·ki′nase′
throm′bo·ki·ne′sis *pl.* -ses′
throm′bo·lym′phan·gi′tis
throm·bol′y·sis *pl.* -ses′
throm′bo·lyt′ic
throm′bo·neu·ro′sis *pl.* -ses′
throm′bo·path′i·a
throm·bop′a·thy
throm′bo·pe′ni·a
throm′bo·pe′nic
throm′bo·phil′i·a
throm′bo·phle·bi′tis
throm′bo·plas′tic
throm′bo·plas′tid
throm′bo·plas′tin
throm′bo·plas′tin′o·gen
throm′bo·poi·e′sis
throm′bo·poi·et′ic
throm·bose′, -bosed′,
  -bos′ing
throm·bo′sis *pl.* -ses′
throm′bo·sta′sis *pl.* -ses′
throm′bo·sthe′nin
throm·bot′ic

throm·box′ane′
throm′bus *pl.* -bi′
  —ne′o·na·to′rum
  —vul′vae′
throt′tle, -tled, -tling
throw′back′
thrush
thryp′sis
thu′ja
thu′jone′
thu′li·um
thumb
thyme
thy·mec′to·mize′, -mized′,
  -miz′ing
thy·mec′to·my
thy′mer·ga′si·a
thy′mer·ga′sic
thy′mic
thy′mi·co·lym·phat′ic
thy·mi·dine′
thy′mine′
thy′mi·on′
thy·mi′tis
thy′mo·cyte′
thy′mo·gen′ic
thy·mo·ke′sis
thy·mo·ki·net′ic
thy′mol′
thy′mo·lep′tic
thy·mol·phthal′e·in
thy·mol′y·sis
thy·mo·lyt′ic
thy·mo′ma *pl.* -mas *or*
  -ma·ta
thy′mo·me·tas′ta·sis
  pl. -ses′
thy′mo·no′ic
thy·mo·nu·cle′ic
thy′mo·path′ic
thy·mop′a·thy
thy′mo·pha·ryn′ge·al
thy′mo·priv′ic
thy·mop′ri·vous
thy′mo·tox′ic
thy′mo·tox′in
thy·mox′a·mine′
thy′mus *pl.* -mus·es *or* -mi′
thy·mus·ec′to·my
thy′ro·ad′e·ni′tis
thy′ro·a·pla′si·a
thy′ro·ar′y·te′noid′
thy′ro·cal′ci·to′nin

thy′ro·car′di·ac′
thy′ro·car·di′tis
thy′ro·cele′
thy′ro·cer′vi·cal
thy′ro·chon·drot′o·my
thy′ro·cri·cot′o·my
thy′ro·ep′i·glot′tic
thy′ro·gen′ic
thy·rog′e·nous
thy′ro·glob′u·lin
thy′ro·glos′sal
thy′ro·hy′al
thy′ro·hy′oid′
thy′roid′
thy·roi′dal
thy·roi′de·a
thy′roid·ec′to·mize′,
 -mized′, -miz′ing
thy′roid·ec′to·my
thy′roid·ism
thy′roid·i′tis
thy′roid·i·za′tion
thy′roid·ot′o·my
thy·roi′do·tox′in
thy′ro·me·dan′
thy′ro·meg′a·ly
thy′ro·mi·met′ic
thy·ron′cus
thy′ro·nine′
thy′ro·nyl
thy′ro·par′a·thy′roid·ec′-
 to·my
thy′ro·pe′ni·a
thy′ro·pha·ryn′ge·al
thy′ro·pha·ryn′ge·us
thy′ro·pri′val
thy′ro·priv′ic
thy′ro·pro′tein′
thy′rop·to′sis
thy·ro′sis pl. -ses′
thy′ro·ther′a·py
thy′ro·tome′
thy·rot′o·my
thy′ro·tox·e′mi·a
thy′ro·tox′ic
thy′ro·tox′i·co′sis pl. -ses′
thy′ro·tox′in
thy′ro·trop′ic
thy·rot′ro·pin
thy·rot′ro·pism
thy·rox′ine′
thy·rox′i·ne′mi·a
tib′i·a pl. -ae′ or -as

tib′i·ad′
tib′i·al
tib′i·a′le
 —ex·ter′num
 —pos·ti′cum
tib′i·al′gi·a
tib′i·a′lis
 —se·cun′dus
tib′i·o·fem′o·ral
tib′i·o·fib′u·lar
tib′i·o·na·vic′u·lar
tib′i·o·scaph′oid′
tib′i·o·tar′sal
ti′bro·fan′
tic (spasm)
 ♦tick
 —con′vul·sif′
 —de sa·laam′
 —dou·lou·reux′
 —of Gilles de la Tou·rette′
 —ro·ta·toire′
ti′car·cil′lin
tick (insect)
 ♦tic
ti·clo′pi·dine′
tic′po·lon′ga
tic·tol′o·gy
tid′al
tide
tie
Tie′de·mann
 —gland
 —nerve
Tiet′ze
 —disease
 —syndrome
ti·ges′tol′
tight
tight′ness
ti·gog′e·nin
tig′o·nin
ti′groid′
ti·grol′y·sis
Til·laux′ disease
tilt
tim′bre
ti′mo·lol′
tin
tinc′tion
tinc·to′ri·al
tinc·tu′ra
tinc′ture
tine

tin′e·a
 —am′i·an·ta′ce·a
 —bar′bae′
 —cap′i·tis
 —cir′ci·na′ta
 —cor′po·ris
 —cru′ris
 —de·cal′vans′
 —fa′ci·a′le′
 —fa′ci·e′i′
 —fa·vo′sa
 —gla·bro′sa
 —im′bri·ca′ta
 —ni′gra
 —no·do′sa
 —ton′su·rans′
 —un′gui·um
 —ver′si·co′lor
Ti·nel′ sign
Tine test
tin′gi·ble
tin′gle, -gled, -gling
tin·ni′tus
 —au′ri·um
 —cra′ni·i′
tin·tom′e·ter
ti′o·con′a·zole′
tip′ping
ti′queur′
tire, tired, tir′ing
Ti·se′li·us apparatus
tis′sue
tis′su·lar
ti·ta′ni·um
ti′ter also titre
tit′il·la′tion
ti′trate′, -trat′ed, -trat′ing
ti·tra′tion
ti′tre var. of titer
ti·trim′e·ter
ti·tri·met′ric
ti·trim′e·try
tit′u·ba′tion
Tit′y·us
to·bac′co
To′bey-Ay′er test
to′bra·my′cin
to·cai′nide′
to·co·al·gog′ra·phy
to′co·graph′
to·cog′ra·phy
to·col′o·gy
to·com′e·ter

to·com′e·try
to·coph′er·ol′
to·coph′er·so′lan′
to·co·pho′bi·a
to′cus
Todd
—cirrhosis
—palsy
—paralysis
—process
toe
toe′ing
toe′nail′
to′ga·vi′rus
tog′gle
toi′let
Toi·son′ solution
to·ko·dy′na·mom′e·ter
to·laz′a·mide′
to·laz′o·line′
tol·bu′ta·mide′
tol′er·ance
tol′er·ant
tol′er·ate′, -at′ed, -at′ing
tol′er·a′tion
tol′er·o·gen
Tol′lens test
tol′me·tin
tol·naf′tate′
to·lo′ni·um
To·lo′sa-Hunt′ syndrome
tol·pyr′ra·mide′
tol′u·ene′
to·lu′ic
to·lu′i·dine′
tol′u·yl·ene′
tol′yl
to′ma·tine′
Tomes
—fibers
—granular layer
—process
Tom′ma·sel′li syndrome
to′mo·gram′
to′mo·graph′
to′mo·graph′ic
to·mog′ra·phy
to·mo·ma′ni·a
ton′al
ton′a·pha′si·a
tone
tongs
tongue

tongue′-tie′
ton′ic
ton′ic-clon′ic
to·nic′i·ty
To′ni-Fan·co′ni syndrome
to·ni·tro·pho′bi·a
ton′o·clon′ic
to·no·fi′bril
to·no·gram′
to·no·graph′
to·nog′ra·phy
to·nom′e·ter
to·nom′e·try
to·no·plast′
to·no·scil·log′ra·phy
to·no·scope′
ton′sil
ton·sil′la *pl.* -lae′
—cer′e·bel′li′
—lin·gua′lis
—pal′a·ti′na
—pha·ryn′ge·a
—tu·bar′i·a
ton′sil·lar
ton′sil·lar′y
ton′sil·lec′tome′
ton′sil·lec′to·my
ton′sil·lit′ic
ton′sil·li′tis
ton′sil·lo·lith′
ton′sil·lo·phar′yn·gi′tis
ton′sil·lo·tome′
ton′sil·lot′o·my
ton′sil·lo·ty′phoid′
ton′sil·sec′tor
ton′sure
to′nus
tooth *pl.* teeth
tooth′ache′
toothed
Tooth muscular atrophy
top′ag·no′sis
to·pal′gi·a
to·pec′to·my
top′es·the′si·a
Töp′fer
—reagent
—test
to·pha′ceous
to′phus *pl.* -phi′
top′ic *or* top′i·cal
top′i·cal·ly
To·pi·nard′ angle

top′o·al′gi·a
top′o·an·es·the′si·a
top′o·gen′e·sis
top′og·no′si·a
top′og·no′sis
top′og·nos′tic
top′o·graph′ic
to·pog′ra·phy
top′o·i·som′er·ase′
to·pol′o·gy
top′o·nar·co′sis *pl.* -ses′
top′o·neu·ro′sis *pl.* -ses′
top′o·nym
top′o·pho′bi·a
top′o·phone′
tor′cu·lar He·roph′i·li′
To·rek′ operation
tor′ic
Tor′kild·sen
—procedure
—shunt operation
tor′mi·na
—al′vi′
tor′mi·nal
Torn′waldt′
—bursitis
—disease
to′rose′
tor·pes′cence
tor′pid
tor·pid′i·ty
tor′por
—in·tes′ti·no′rum
torque
torr
tor′re·fac′tion
tor′re·fy
tor·sade′ de pointes′
tor′si·oc·clu′sion
tor′si·om′e·ter
tor′sion
tor′sive
tor′si·ver′sion
tor′so *pl.* -sos, -si′, *or* -soes
tor′soc·clu′sion
tort
tor′ti·col′lar
tor′ti·col′lis
—spas′ti·ca
tor′ti·pel′vis
tor′tu·os′i·ty
tor′tu·ous
tor′u·li tac′ti·les′

tor'u·lo'ma *pl.* -mas *or*
-ma·ta
Tor'u·lop'sis ne'o·for'-
mans'
tor'u·lo'sis
tor'u·lus *pl.* -li'
to'rus *pl.* -ri'
—gen'i·ta'lis
—lev'a·to'ri·us
—oc·cip'i·ta'lis
—pal'a·ti'nus
—pu'bi·cus
—tu·bar'i·us
—u're·ter'i·cus
—u'ter·i'nus
to'sy·late'
to'tal
To'ti operation
to·tip'o·tence
to'ti·po·ten·cy
to·tip'o·tent
to'ti·po·ten'tial
to'ti·po·ten'ti·al'i·ty
touch
Tou·raine' aphthosis
tour de maî'tre
Tou·rette'
—disease
—syndrome
Tour·nay' sign
tour'ni·quet
Tou'ton cells
tow
tow'el
Towne
—projection
—view
Town'send operation
tox'al·bu'min
tox'a·phene'
Tox·as'ca·ris
tox·e'mi·a
tox·e'mic
tox·en'zyme'
tox'ic
tox'i·cant
tox'i·ce'mi·a
tox'i·cide'
tox·ic'i·ty
tox'i·co·den'drol'
Tox'i·co·den'dron
tox'i·co·der'ma·ti'tis
tox'i·co·der'ma·to'sis

tox'i·co·gen'ic
tox'i·coid'
tox'i·co·log'ic *or*
tox'i·co·log'i·cal
tox'i·col'o·gist
tox'i·col'o·gy
tox'i·co·ma'ni·a
tox'i·co·ma'ni·ac'
tox'i·co·path'ic
tox'i·cop'a·thy
tox'i·co·pex'is
tox'i·co·phid'i·a
tox'i·co·pho'bi·a
tox'i·co'sis *pl.* -ses'
tox'i·der'ma·to'sis *pl.* -ses'
tox'i·der·mi'tis
tox·if'er·ine'
tox·if'er·ous
tox'i·gen'ic
tox'i·ge·nic'i·ty
tox·ig'e·nous
tox'ig·nom'ic
tox'in
tox'in-an'ti·tox'in
tox'in·e'mi·a
tox'in·fec'tion
tox'i·no'sis *pl.* -ses'
tox·ip'a·thy
tox'i·phre'ni·a
tox·is'ter·ol'
tox'i·ther'a·py
tox'i·tu·ber'cu·lide'
Tox'o·car'a
tox'o·ca·ri'a·sis
tox'oid'
tox'o·lec'i·thin
tox'o·no'sis *pl.* -ses'
tox'o·phil'
tox'o·phil'ic
tox'o·phore'
tox·oph'o·rous
Tox'o·plas'ma
—gon'di·i'
tox'o·plas·mat'ic
tox'o·plas'mic
tox'o·plas'min
tox'o·plas·mo'sis *pl.* -ses'
Toyn'bee
—corpuscle
—ligament
tra·bec'u·la *pl.* -lae'
—sep'to·mar'gi·na'lis
tra·bec'u·lae'

—car'ne·ae'
—cor'dis
—cor'po·ris spon'gi·o'si'
—cor'po·rum cav'er·no·so'-
rum
—li·e'nis
tra·bec'u·lar
tra·bec'u·late'
tra·bec'u·la'tion
tra·bec'u·lec'to·my
tra·bec'u·lo·plas'ty
tra·bec'u·lot'o·my
trabs *pl.* tra'bes'
trace
trac'er
tra'che·a *pl.* -ae' *or* -as
tra'che·a·ec'ta·sy
tra'che·al
tra'che·al'gi·a
tra'che·i'tis
tra'che·lec'to·my
tra'che·le'ma·to'ma *pl.*
-mas *or* -ma·ta
tra'che·lism
tra'che·lis'mus
tra'che·li'tis
tra'che·lo·cyl'lo'sis
tra'che·lo·cys·ti'tis
tra'che·lo·dyn'i·a
tra'che·lo·ky·pho'sis
tra'che·lo·mas'toid'
tra'che·lo·par'a·si'tus
tra'che·lo·pex'i·a
tra'che·lo·plas'ty
tra'che·lor·rha·phy
tra'che·lor·rhec'tes'
tra'che·los'chi·sis *pl.* -ses'
tra'che·lo·syr'in·gor'rha·
phy
tra'che·lot'o·my
tra'che·o·blen'nor·rhe·a
tra'che·o·bron'chi·al
tra'che·o·bron·chi'tis
tra'che·o·bron·chos'co·py
tra'che·o·cele'
tra'che·o·e·soph'a·ge'al
tra'che·o·fis'sure
tra'che·o·gen'ic
tra'che·o·gram'
tra'che·og'ra·phy
tra'che·o·la·ryn'ge·al
tra'che·o·lar'yn·got'o·my
tra'che·o·ma·la'ci·a

tra′che·o·path′i·a
  os′te·o·plas′ti·ca
tra′che·op′a·thy
tra′che·o·pha·ryn′ge·al
tra′che·oph′o·ny
tra′che·o·plas′ty
tra′che·o·py·o′sis
tra′che·or·rha′gi·a
tra′che·or′rha·phy
tra′che·os′chi·sis *pl.* -ses′
tra′che·o·scop′ic
tra′che·os′co·py
tra′che·o·ste·no′sis *pl.* -ses′
tra′che·os′to·ma *pl.* -ma·ta
  or -mas
tra′che·os′to·my
tra′che·o·tome′
tra′che·ot′o·mist
tra′che·ot′o·mize′, -mized′,
  -miz′ing
tra′che·ot′o·my
tra·chi′tis
tra·cho′ma
tra·cho′ma·tous
tra′chy·chro·mat′ic
tra′chy·o·nych′i·a
tra′chy·pho′ni·a
trac′ing
track
tract
  —of Al′len
  —of Schütz
trac′tion
trac′tor
trac·tot′o·my
trac′tus *pl.* trac′tus
  —cen·tra′lis thy′mi′
  —cer′e·bel′lo·ru·bra′lis
  —cer′e·bel′lo·tha·lam′i·cus
  —cor′ti·co·hy′po·tha·lam′i·ci′
  —cor′ti·co·pon·ti′ni′
  —cor′ti·co·pon·ti′nus
  —corticopontinus mes′en·
    ce·phal′i·cus
  —corticopontinus pon′tis
  —cor′ti·co·spi·na′lis
    anterior
  —corticospinalis lat′er·a′lis
  —dor′so·lat′er·a′lis
  —fron′to·pon·ti′nus
  —gen′i·ta′lis
  —il′i·o·tib′i·a′lis
  —iliotibialis (Mais·si·a′ti′)

  —mes′en·ce·phal′i·cus
    ner′vi′ tri·gem′i·ni′
  —ner·vo′si′ as·so′ci·a′-
    ti·o′nis
  —nervosi com·mis′su·
    ra′les′
  —nervosi pro·jec′ti·o′nis
  —oc·cip′i·to·pon·ti′nus
  —ol′fac·to′ri·us
  —o·li′vo·cer′e·bel·lar′is
  —op′ti·cus
  —pa·ri′e·to·pon·ti′nus
  —py·ram′i·da′les′
  —py·ram′i·da′lis anterior
  —pyramidalis lat′er·a′lis
  —pyramidalis me·dul′lae′
    ob′lon·ga′tae′
  —pyramidalis mes′en·ce·
    phal′i·cus
  —pyramidalis pon′tis
  —re·tic′u·lo·spi·na′lis
  —ru′bro·spi·na′lis
  —sol′i·tar′i·us
  —spi·na′lis ner′vi′ tri·gem′-
    i·ni′
  —spi′no·cer′e·bel·lar′is
    anterior
  —spinocerebellaris posterior
  —spi′no·tec′ta·lis
  —spi′no·tha·lam′i·cus
    anterior
  —spinothalamicus
    lat′er·a′lis
  —spi·ra′lis fo·ram′i·no′sus
  —su′pra·op′ti·co·hy′po·phys′i·a′lis
  —sys·te′ma·tis ner·vo′si′
    cen·tra′lis
  —tec′to·spi·na′lis
  —teg′men·ta′lis cen·tra′lis
  —tem′po·ro·pon·ti′nus
  —ves·tib′u·lo·spi·na′lis
Tra′cy method
trade′mark′
trag′a·canth′
tra′gal
Tra′gi·a
trag′i·on′
trag′o·mas·chal′i·a
trag′o·pho′ni·a
tra·goph′o·ny
trag′o·po′di·a
tra′gus *pl.* -gi′
trail′er

train′a·ble
trait
tram′a·dol′
tra·maz′o·line′
trance
tran′ex·am′ic
tran′quil·ize′, -ized′, -iz′ing
tran′quil·iz′er
trans′ab·dom′i·nal
trans·a·cet′y·lase′
trans·ac′tion
trans·ac′tion·al
trans·ac′y·la′tion
trans·am′i·nase′
trans·an′i·ma′tion
trans·a·or′tic
trans·a′tri·al
trans·au′di·ent
trans·ax′o·nal
trans·cav′i·tar′y
trans·cer′vi·cal
trans·con′dy·lar
trans·cor′ti·cal
trans·cor′tin
trans·cra′ni·al
tran·scrip′tase′
tran·scrip′tion
tran·scrip′tion·ist
trans·cu′ta·ne·ous
trans·der′mal
trans·duce′
trans·duc′er
trans·duc′tion
trans·du′o·de′nal
tran·sect′
tran·sec′tion
trans·fer′, -ferred′, -fer′ring
trans′fer·ase′
trans′fer·ence
trans′fer·rin
trans·fix′
trans·fix′ion
trans′fo·rate′, -rat′ed, -rat′ing
trans·fo·ra′tion
trans·fo·ra′tor
trans·form′
trans·for·ma′tion
trans·form′er
trans·fuse′, -fused′, -fus′ing
trans·fu′sion
trans·fu′sion·al
trans·he·pat′ic
trans·hi·a′tal

tran'sient
trans·il'i·ac'
trans·il·lu'mi·nate'
trans·il·lu'mi·na'tion
trans·isth'mi·an
tran·sis'tor
tran·si'tion·al
tran·si'tiv·ism
tran'si·to'ry
tran'si·to·zo'o·no'sis
trans'late'
trans·la'tion
trans·lin'gual
trans·lo·ca'tion
trans·lu'cent
trans·lu'mi·nal
trans·mal'le·o·lar
trans·max'il·lar'y
trans·mem'brane'
trans·meth'yl·ase'
trans'meth·yl·a'tion
trans·mi·gra'tion
trans·mis·si·bil'i·ty
trans·mis'si·ble
trans·mis'sion
trans·mit', -mit'ted, -mit'ting
trans·mit'ta·ble
trans·mit'tance
trans·mit'ter
trans·mu'ral
trans'mu·ta'tion
trans·oc'u·lar
tran'so·nance
trans·or'bi·tal
trans·os'se·ous
trans·os'te·al
trans·pal'a·tal
trans·par'en·cy
trans·par'ent
trans·pep'ti·dase'
trans·pep'ti·da'tion
trans·per'i·to·ne'al
trans'phos·pho'ryl·ase'
trans'phos·pho'ry·la'tion
tran·spir'a·ble
tran'spi·ra'tion
tran·spire'
trans·pla·cen'tal
trans·plant' *n.*
trans·plant' *v.*
trans'plan·ta'tion
trans·pleu'ral
trans'port'

trans·pose', -posed', -pos'ing
trans'po·si'tion
trans'py·lor'ic
trans·ra'di·al
trans·ra'di·ant
trans·sa'cral
trans·scaph'oid'
trans·sec'tion
trans·seg·men'tal
trans·sep'tal
trans·sex'u·al
trans·sex'u·al·ism
trans'ten·to'ri·al
trans'tha·lam'ic
trans'tho·rac'ic
trans·tra'che·al
trans·tri·que'tral
trans'tym·pan'ic
tran'sub·stan'ti·a'tion
tran·su'date'
tran'su·da'tion
tran·sude', -sud'ed, -sud'ing
trans·u'ran'ic
trans·u·re'thral
trans·vag'i·nal
trans·ve'nous
trans'ver·sa'lis
trans·verse'
trans'ver·sec'to·my
trans·ver'sion
trans·ver·sot'o·my
trans·ver'sus
—nu'chae'
trans·ves'i·cal
trans·ves'tism
trans·ves'tite'
trans·ves'ti·tism
tran'yl·cy'pro·mine'
tra·pe'zi·al
tra·pe'zi·form'
tra·pe'zi·o·met'a·car'pal
tra·pe'zi·um *pl.* -zi·ums *or* -zi·a
tra·pe'zi·us
trap'e·zoid'
trap'e·zoi'dal
Trapp formula
trap'ping
Trau'be
—membrane
—murmur
—sign
—space

—waves
Trau'be-Her'ing waves
trau'ma *pl.* -ma·ta *or* -mas
trau·mat'ic
trau'ma·tism
trau'ma·tize', -tized', -tiz'ing
trau'ma·tol'o·gy
trau'ma·top'a·thy
trau'ma·top·ne'a
trau'ma·to'sis *pl.* -ses'
Traut'mann triangle
tra·vail'
tray
traz'o·done'
Trea'cher Col'lins syndrome
trea'cle
tread'mill'
treat
treat'a·ble
treat'ment
tre·ha'la
tre·ha'lose'
Treitz
—fossa
—hernia
—muscle
tre'ma
tre·mat'ic
Trem'a·to'da
trem'a·tode'
trem'a·to·di'a·sis *pl.* -ses'
trem'ble, -bled, -bling
trem'el·loid'
trem'el·lose'
trem'e·tol'
trem'o·gram'
trem'o·graph'
trem'o·la'bile'
trem'o·pho'bia
trem'or
—ar'tu·um
—cap'i·tis
—cor'dis
—me·tal'li·cus
—po·ta'to·rum
—sat'ur·ni'nus
—ten'di·num
trem'u·lous
Tren·del'en·burg'
—position
—test
tre·pan', -panned', -pan'ning

trep'a·na'tion
trep'a·nize', -nized', -niz'ing
treph'i·na'tion
tre·phine', -phined',
   -phin'ing
treph'o·cyte'
trep'i·dant
tre·pi'da'ti·o'
  —cor'dis
trep'i·da'tion
trep'o·ne'ma *pl.* -ma·ta *or*
  -mas
Trep'o·ne'ma
  —a·mer'i·ca'num
  —ca·ra'te·um
  —cu·nic'u·li'
  —her're·jo'ni'
  —pal'li·dum
  —per·ten'u·e'
  —pic'tor'
  —pin'tae'
trep'o·ne'mal
trep'o·ne'ma·to'sis *pl.* -ses'
trep'o·neme'
trep'o·ne·mi'a·sis *pl.* -ses'
trep'o·ne'mi·cid'al
trep'o·ne'min
tre·pop'ne·a
trep'pe
Tre·sil'i·an sign
tret'i·noin'
tri·ac'e·tate'
tri·ac'e·tin
tri·ac'e·tyl·o'le·an'do·my'-
  cin
tri'ad'
  —of Whip'ple
tri'ad·i'tis
tri·age'
tri'al
tri·am·cin'o·lone'
tri·am'py·zine'
tri·am'ter·ene'
tri'an·gle
  —of Ca·lot'
  —of Gom·bault'-Phi·lippe'
tri·an'gu·lar
tri·an'gu·lar'is
tri·an'gu·la'tion
Tri·at'o·ma
Tri'a·to'mi·nae'
tri·a'tri·al
tri·ax'i·al

tri·a'zo·lam
trib'a·dy
tri·ba'sic
tri·bas'i·lar
tribe
trib'o·lu·mi·nes'cence
tri·bra'chi·us
tri·bro'mo·eth'a·nol'
tri·bro'mo·meth'ane'
tri·brom'sa·lan'
trib'u·tar'y
tri·bu'ty·rin
tri·car'box·yl'ic
tri·cel'lu·lar
tri'ceps'
  —ex·ten'sor cu'bi·ti'
tri·cet'a·mide'
trich·a·tro'phi·a
trich·es·the'si·a
tri·chi'a·sis
tri·chi'na *pl.* -nae'
Trich·i'nel'la
  —spi·ra'lis
trich'i·nel·lo'sis *pl.* -ses'
trich'i·ni'a·sis *pl.* -ses'
trich'i·no·scope'
trich'i·no·scop'ic
trich'i·no'sis *pl.* -ses'
trich'i·nous
trich'i·on'
tri·chi'tis
tri'chlor·eth'yl·ene'
tri·chlor'fon
tri'chlor·meth'ane'
tri'chlor·me·thi'a·zide'
tri·chlo'ro·ac'et·al'de·hyde'
tri·chlo'ro·a·ce'tic
tri·chlo'ro·bu'tyl
tri·chlo'ro·eth'yl·ene'
tri·chlo'ro·meth'ane'
tri·chlo'ro·mo'no·fluor'o·
  meth'ane'
trich'o·an'es·the'si·a
trich'o·be'zoar'
Trich'o·bil·har'zi·a
  —el'vae'
  —o'cel·la'ta
  —phy·sel'lae'
  —stag'ni·co'lae'
  —szi·da'ti
trich'o·car'di·a
trich'o·ceph'a·li'a·sis
  pl. -ses'

trich'o·cla'si·a
tri·choc'la·sis
trich'o·clas·ma'ni·a
trich'o·cryp·to'sis *pl.* -ses'
trich'o·cyst'
Trich'o·dec'tes'
Trich'o·der'ma
trich'o·ep'i·the'li·o'ma
  pl. -mas *or* -ma·ta
  —pap'u·lo'sum mul'ti·plex'
trich'o·es·the'si·a
trich'o·es·the'si·om'e·ter
trich'o·gen
trich'o·gen'ic
tri·cog'e·nous
trich'o·glos'si·a
trich'o·hy'a·lin
trich'oid'
trich'o·lith'
trich'o·lo'gi·a
tri·chol'o·gy
tri·cho'ma *pl.* -mas *or* -ma·ta
trich'o·ma·de'sis
trich'o·ma'ni·a
tri·cho'ma·tose'
tri·cho'ma·to'sis
trich'ome'
trich'o·mo'na·cid'al
trich'o·mo'na·cide'
trich'o·mo'nad'
tri·chom'o·nal
Trich'o·mo'nas
  —hom'i·nis
  —vag'i·na'lis
  —vag'i·ni'tis
trich'o·mo·ni'a·sis *pl.* -ses'
trich'o·mo'ni·cide'
Trich'o·my·ce'tes'
trich'o·my·co'sis *pl.* -ses'
  —ax'il·lar'is
  —bar'bae'
  —cap'il·li'ti·i'
  —cir'ci·na'ta
  —fa·vo'sa
  —fla'va ni'gra
  —no·do'sa
  —pal'mel·li'na
  —pus'tu·lo'sa
  —ru'bra
tri'chon'
trich'o·no·car'di·o'sis
trich'o·no·do'sis
trich'o·no'sis *pl.* -ses'

trich'o·path'ic
trich'o·path'o·pho'bi·a
tri·chop'a·thy
trich'o·pha'gi·a
tri·choph'a·gy
trich'o·pho'bi·a
trich'o·phyte'
trich'o·phy'tid
trich'o·phy'tin
trich'o·phy'to·be'zoar'
trich'o·phy'ton' *pl.* -ta *or*
　-tons'
trich'o·phy·to'sis *pl.* -ses'
trich'o·pti·lo'sis
trich'or·rhe'a
trich'or·rhex'is
　—no'do'sa
tri·chos'chi·sis
tri·chos'co·py
trich'o·sid'er·in
tri·cho'sis *pl.* -ses'
Tri·chos'po·ron' bei·gel'i·i'
trich'o·spo·ro'sis *pl.* -ses'
trich'o·sta'sis spi'nu·lo'sa
trich'o·stron'gy·li'a·sis
trich'o·stron'gy·lo'sis
Trich'o·stron'gy·lus
trich'o·the'cin
trich'o·til'lo·ma'ni·a
trich'o·til'lo·man'ic
tri·chot'o·my
tri'chro'ic
tri·chro·ism
tri'chro·mat'
tri'chro·mat'ic
tri'chro·ma·tism
tri'chro·ma·top'si·a
tri'chrome'
tri'chro'mic
trich'ter·brust'
trich'u·ri'a·sis *pl.* -ses'
Trich·u'ris
　—trich'i·u'ra
tri·cip'i·tal
tri'clo·bi·so'ni·um
tri'clo·car'ban'
tri·clo·fen·ol'
tric'lo·fos'
tri'corn'
tri·cor'nute'
tri·cre'sol'
tri·crot'ic
tri'cro·tism

tri·cus'pid
tri·cus'pi·date'
tri·cy'cla·mol'
tri·cy'clic
tri·dac'tyl
tri·dac'tyl·ism
tri·dac'ty·lous
tri'dent'
tri·den'tate'
tri·der'mic
tri·der·mo'ma *pl.* -mas *or*
　-ma·ta
tri·di·hex·eth'yl
trid'y·mite'
trid'y·mus
tri'en·ceph'a·lus *pl.* -li'
tri'en·tine'
tri·eth'a·nol'a·mine'
tri·eth'yl·am'ine'
tri·eth'yl·ene·mel'a·mine'
tri·eth'yl·ene·thi'o·phos·
　pho'ra·mide'
tri·fa'cial
tri'fid
tri·flu'mi·date'
tri·flu'o·per'a·zine'
tri·flu·per'i·dol'
tri·flu·pro'ma·zine'
tri·flu'ri·dine'
tri·fo'cal
tri'fur·cate', -cat'ed, -cat'ing
tri'fur·ca'tion
tri·gas'tric
tri·gas'tri·cus
tri·gem'i·nal
tri·gem'i·no·tha·lam'ic
tri·gem'i·nus *pl.* -ni'
tri·gem'i·ny
tri·gen'ic
tri·glyc'er·ide'
tri·go'na fi·bro'sa cor'dis
trig'o·nal
tri'gone'
　—of Lieu·taud'
tri'gon·ec'to·my
Trig'o·nel'la
trig'o·nel'line'
tri·gon'id
tri'go·ni'tis
trig'o·no·ce·phal'ic
trig'o·no·ceph'a·lus *pl.* -li'
trig'o·no·ceph'a·ly
tri·go'no·tome'

tri·go'num *pl.* -nums *or* -na
　—a·cus'ti·ci'
　—ca·rot'i·cum
　—col·lat'er·a'le'
　—del·toi'de·o·pec'to·ra'le'
　—fem'o·ra'le'
　—fi·bro'sum cor'dis
　　(dex'trum et si·nis'trum)
　—ha·ben'u·lae'
　—in'gui·na'le'
　—in'ter·pe·dun'cu·lar'e'
　—lem·nis'ci'
　—lum·ba'le'
　—lumbale (Pet'i·ti')
　—ner'vi' hy'po·glos'si'
　—nervi va'gi'
　—ol'fac·to'ri·um
　—o'mo·cla·vic'u·lar'e'
　—sub·man·dib'u·lar'e'
　—u'ro·gen'i·ta'le'
　—ve·si'cae'
　—vesicae (Lieu·tau'di')
tri'hex·y·phen'i·dyl
tri·hy'brid
tri·hy'dric
tri'hy·drox'y·ben·zo'ic
tri'hy·drox'y·pro'pane'
tri·i'o·do·eth'i·on'ic
tri·i'o·do·meth'ane'
tri·i'o·do·thy'ro·nine'
tri·ke'to·hy'drin·dene'
tri·ke'to·pu'rine'
tri'labe'
tri·lam'i·nar
tri·lat'er·al
tri·li'no·le'in
tri·lo'bate'
tri·lo·bec'to·my
tri·loc'u·lar
tril'o·gy of Fal'lot
tri·lo'stane'
tri·mal'le·o·lar
tri·man'u·al
tri·mas'ti·gote'
tri·men'su·al
tri·mep'ra·zine'
Trim'e·re·su'rus
tri·mes'ter
tri·meth'a·di'one'
tri·meth'a·phan' cam'syl·
　ate'
tri·meth'i·din'i·um meth'o·
　sul'fate'

tri·meth'o·benz'a·mide'
tri·meth'o·prim
tri'meth·yl·am'ine'
tri·meth'yl·ene'
tri·meth'yl·gly'cine'
tri·meth'yl·xan'thine'
tri·met'o·zine
tri'me·trex'ate' glu·cu'-
 ro·nate'
tri·mip'ra·mine'
tri'mix'
trim'mer
tri·mor'phic
tri·mor'phism
tri·mor'phous
tri·mox'a·mine'
tri·neu'ral
tri·ni'tro·glyc'er·in
tri·ni'tro·phe'nol'
tri·ni·tro·tol'u·ene'
tri·no'mi·al
tri·nu'cle·ate'
tri·nu'cle·o·tide'
tri·o·ceph'a·lus
tri·o'le·in
tri·o·lism
tri'oph·thal'mos
tri·o'pod'y·mus
tri·or'chid
tri·or'chid·ism
tri·o'tus
tri·ox'ide'
tri·ox'sa·len
tri·ox'y·meth'yl·ene'
tri·ox'y·pu'rine'
tri·pal'mi·tin
trip'a·ra
tri·par'tite'
tri·pe·len'na·mine'
tri·pep'tide'
tri·pha·lan'gism
tri·pha·lan'gy
tri·phar'ma·con
tri·pha'sic
tri·phos'pha·tase'
tri'ple
tri·ple'gi·a
trip'let
trip'lex'
trip'lo·blas'tic
trip'loid'
trip'loi'dy
trip'lo·ko'ri·a

trip·lo'pi·a
tri'pod'
tri'pod·ing
tri·pro'li·dine'
tri'pro·so'pus
trip'sis
tri'pus
tri·que'tral
tri·que'trous
tri·que'trum *pl.* -tra
tri·ra'di·al
tri·ra'di·ate
tri·ra'di·us *pl.* -di·i'
tri·sac'cha·ride'
tri'sect'
tris'kai·dek'a·pho'bi·a
tris'mus
tri·so'mic
tri·so'mus
tri'so·my
tri·splanch'nic
tri·ste'a·rin
tri·stich'i·a
tris'ti·chi'a·sis
tris'ti·ma·ni·a
tris'tis
tri·sul'cate'
tri·sul'fam
tri·sul'fa·py·rim'i·dines'
tri'ta·nope'
tri'ta·no'pi·a
tri·ter'pene'
trit'i·ate'
tri·ti'ce·o·glos'sus
tri·ti'ceous
tri·ti'ce·um *pl.* -ce·i'
trit'i·co·nu·cle'ic
trit'i·um
trit'o·cone'
trit'o·co'nid
tri'ton
tri·tu'ber·cu·lar
trit'u·ra·ble
trit'u·rate', -rat'ed, -rat'ing
trit'u·ra'tion
trit'u·ra'tor
tri·va'lence
tri·va'len·cy
tri·va'lent
tri'valve'
tri·val'vu·lar
triv'i·al
tro'car' *also* trochar

tro·chan'ter
tro'chan·ter'ic
tro·chan'tin
tro·chan·tin'i·an
tro'char' *var. of* trocar
tro'che
tro'chin
tro·chis·ca'tion
tro·chis'cus *pl.* -ci'
troch'i·ter
troch'le·a *pl.* -ae'
 —fib'u·lar'is
 —hu'mer·i'
 —mus'cu·lar'is
 —mus'cu·li' ob·li'qui'
  oc'u·li' su·pe'ri·o'ris
 —musculi obliqui superioris
 —per'o·ne·a'lis
 —pha·lan'gis
 —ta'li
troch'le·ar
troch'le·ar'i·form'
troch'le·ar'is
troch'o·car'di·a
troch'o·ce·pha'li·a
tro'cho·ceph'a·lus
tro'cho·ceph'a·ly
tro'choid'
tro·choi'des'
tro'cho·ri'zo·car'di·a
Trog'lo·tre'ma
 —sal·min'co·la
Trog'lo·tre·mat'i·dae'
Troi·sier'
 —sign
 —syndrome
trol'a·mine'
tro'land
tro'le·an'do·my'cin
trol·ni'trate'
Tröltsch
 —corpuscles
 —recesses
Trom·bic'u·la
 —al'fred·du'ge·si'
 —ir'ri·tans'
trom·bic'u·lo'sis *pl.* -ses'
tro·meth'a·mine'
Trom'mer test
Tröm'ner sign
trom'o·ma'ni·a
tro'na
tro'pa·co'caine'

tro'pane'
tro'pate'
tro·pe'o·lin
troph·ec'to·derm'
troph'e·de'ma
tro·phe'si·al
tro·phe'sic
troph'e·sy
troph'ic
tro·phic'i·ty
troph'ism
troph'o·blast'
troph'o·blas'tic
troph'o·blas·to'ma *pl.* -mas
  or -ma·ta
troph'o·chrome'
troph'o·chro·mid'i·a
troph'o·cyte'
troph'o·derm'
troph'o·der'mal
troph'o·der'ma·to·neu·ro'-
  sis *pl.* -ses'
troph'o·dy·nam'ics
tro·phol'o·gy
troph'o·neu·ro'sis *pl.* -ses'
troph'o·neu·rot'ic
troph'o·no'sis *pl.* -ses'
troph'o·nu'cle·us *pl.* -cle·i'
tro·phop'a·thy
troph'o·plast'
troph'o·spon'gi·a
troph'o·spon'gi·um
troph'o·tax'is *pl.* -tax'es'
troph'o·ther'a·py
troph'o·trop'ic
tro·phot'ro·pism
troph'o·zo'ite'
tro'pi·a
trop'ic
trop'i·cal
tro·pic'a·mide'
tro'pine'
tro'pism
tro'po·chrome'
tro'po·col'la·gen
tro·pom'e·ter
tro'po·my'o·sin
tro'po·nin
tro'po·pause'
tro'po·sphere'
trou'sers
Trous·seau'
  —disease

—mark
—sign
trox'i·done'
troy
Tru·e'ta shunt
trun'cal
trun'cate', -cat'ed, -cat'ing
trun'ci'
  —in·tes'ti·na'les'
  —lum·ba'les'
  —lumbales (dex'ter et
   si·nis'ter)
  —plex'us bra·chi·a'lis
trun'co·co'nal
trun'cus *pl.* -ci'
  —ar·te'ri·o'sus
  —bra·chi·o·ce·phal'i·cus
  —bron·cho·me·di·as·ti·na'lis
  —bronchomediastinalis
   dex'ter
  —ce·li'a·cus
  —cor'po·ris cal·lo'si'
  —cos'to·cer'vi·ca'lis
  —fas·cic'u·li' a'tri·o·ven·
   tric'u·lar'is
  —inferior plex'us bra·chi·a'lis
  —in·tes'ti·na'lis
  —jug'u·lar'is
  —lin'guo·fa'ci·a'lis
  —lum'bo·sa·cra'lis
  —me'di·us plex'us
   bra·chi·a'lis
  —pul'mo·na'lis
  —sub·cla'vi·us
  —superior plex'us
   bra·chi·a'lis
  —sym·path'i·cus
  —thy're·o·cer'vi·ca'lis
  —thy'ro·cer'vi·ca'lis
  —trans·ver'sus
  —va·ga'lis anterior
  —vagalis posterior
trunk
truss
try'pan
try·pan'o·cid'al
try·pan'o·cide'
try·pan·ol'y·sis
Try·pan'o·so'ma
  —bru'ce·i'
  —cru'zi'
  —eq'ui·per'dum
  —ev'an·si'

  —gam'bi·en'se'
  —hip'pi·cum
  —lew'i·si'
  —rho·de'si·en'se'
  —vi'vax'
try·pan'o·so'mal
Try·pan'o·so·mat'i·dae'
try·pan'o·some'
try·pan'o·so·mi'a·sis *pl.* -ses'
try·pan'o·som'ic
try·pan'o·so'mi·cid'al
tri·pan'o·so'mi·cide'
try·pan'o·so·mid'
tryp·ar'sa·mide'
tryp'sin
tryp·sin'o·gen
tryp'ta·mine'
tryp'tase'
tryp'tic
tryp·to·lyt'ic
tryp'to·phan
tryp'to·phan·ase'
tryp'to·phan·e'mi·a
tryp'to·phan·u'ri·a
tryp'to·phyl
tset'se
Tsu·chi'ya reagent
tsu'tsu·ga·mu'shi
tu'a·mi'no·hep'tane'
tu'ba *pl.* -bae'
  —au'di·ti'va
  —auditiva (Eu·sta'chi·i')
  —u'ter·i'na
  —uterina (Fal·lop'pi·i')
tu'bal
tube
tu·bec'to·my
tu'ber *pl.* -bers *or* -ber·a
  —cal·ca'ne·i'
  —ci·ne're·um
  —fron·ta'le'
  —is'chi·ad'i·cum
  —max·il'lae
  —max·il·lar'e'
  —o'men·ta'le' hep'a·tis
  —omentale pan·cre'a·tis
  —pa·ri'e·ta'le'
  —ver'mis
tu'ber·al
tu'ber·cle
tu·ber'cu·la co·ro'nae'
  den'tis
tu·ber'cu·lar

tu·ber′cu·late′
tu·ber′cu·la′tion
tu·ber′cu·lid
tu·ber′cu·lig′e·nous
tu·ber′cu·lin
tu·ber′cu·lin·i·za′tion
tu·ber′cu·li′tis
tu·ber′cu·li·za′tion
tu·ber′cu·lo·cele′
tu·ber′cu·lo·cid′al
tu·ber′cu·lo·ci′din
tu·ber′cu·lo·derm′
tu·ber′cu·lo·der′ma
tu·ber′cu·lo·fi′broid′
tu·ber′cu·lo·fi·bro′sis
  pl. -ses′
tu·ber′cu·loid′
tu·ber′cu·lo′ma *pl.* -mas *or*
  -ma·ta
 —en plaque
tu·ber′cu·lo·pro′tein′
tu·ber′cu·lose′
tu·ber′cu·lo·sil′i·co′sis
tu·ber′cu·lo′sis
 —cu′tis
 —cutis in·du′ra·ti′va
 —cutis o′ri·fi′ci·a′lis
 —li′che·noi′des′
 —lu·po′sa
 —ver′ru·co′sa
tu·ber′cu·lo·stat′ic
tu·ber′cu·lo·ste′ar·ic
tu·ber′cu·lot′ic
tu·ber′cu·lous
tu·ber′cu·lum *pl.* -la
 —a·cus′ti·cum
 —ad·duc·to′ri·um
 —an·te′ri·us at·lan′tis
 —anterius thal·a′mi′
 —anterius ver′te·brar′um
  cer′vi·ca′li·um
 —ar·tic′u·lar′e′ os′sis
  tem′po·ra′lis
 —au·ric′u·lae′
 —auriculae (Dar′wi·ni′)
 —ca·rot′i·cum ver′te·brae′
  cer′vi·ca′lis VI
 —cau·da′tum
 —ci·ne′re·um
 —co·noi′de·um
 —cor·nic′u·la′tum
  (San′to·ri′ni′)

—co·ro′nae′ den′tis
—cos′tae′
—cu′ne·i·for′me′
—cuneiforme (Wris·ber′gi′)
—ep′i·glot′ti·cum
—gen′i·ta′le′
—im′par′
—in·fra·gle′noi·da′le′
—in·ter·con·dy·lar′e′
  lat′er·a′le′
—intercondylare me·di·a′le′
—in′ter·con′dy·loi·de·um
  lat′er·a′le′
—intercondyloideum
  me·di·a′le′
—in′ter·ve·no′sum
—intervenosum (Low′e·ri′)
—jug′u·lar′e′ os′sis
  oc·cip′i·ta′lis
—la′bi·i′ su·pe′ri·o′ris
—lat′er·a′le′ pro·ces′sus
  pos·te′ri·o′ris ta′li′
—lin′gua′le′ lat′er·a′le′
—linguale me·di·a′le′
—ma′jus hu′mer·i′
—mar′gi·na′le′ os′sis
  zy′go·mat′i·ci′
—me′di·a′le′ pro·ces′sus
  pos·te′ri·o′ris ta′li′
—men·ta′le′ man·dib′u·lae′
—mi′nus hu′mer·i′
—mus′cu·li′ sca·le′ni′
  an·te′ri·o′ris
—nu′cle·i′ cu′ne·a′ti′
—nuclei grac′i·lis
—ob·tu·ra·to′ri·um
  an·te′ri·us
—obturatorium pos·te′ri·us
—of San′to·ri′ni
—os′sis mul·tan′gu·li′
  ma·jo′ris
—ossis na·vic′u·lar′is
—ossis sca·phoi′de·i′
—ossis tra·pe′zi·i′
—pha·ryn′ge·um
—pos·te′ri·us at·lan′tis
—posterius ver′te·brar′um
  cer′vi·ca′li·um
—pu′bi·cum os′sis pu′bis
—sca·le′ni′ (Lis·fran′ci′)
—sel′lae′ tur′ci·cae′
—su′pra·gle′noi·da′le′
—su′pra·tra′gi·cum

—thy′re·oi′de·um in·fe′ri·us
—thyreoideum su·pe′ri·us
—thy′roi′de·um in·fe′ri·us
—thyroideum su·pe′ri·us
tu′ber·o·hy′po·phys′e·al
tu′ber·o′sis
tu′ber·os′i·tas′ *pl.* -os·i′ta′tes′
 —co′ra·coi′de·a cla·vic′-
  u′lae′
 —cos′tae′ II
 —cos′ta′lis cla·vic′u·lae′
 —del·toi′de·a
 —glu′tae·a
 —glu′te·a
 —i·li′a·ca
 —in·fra·gle′noi·da′lis
 —mas′se·ter′i·ca
 —mus′cu·li′ ser·ra′ti′
  an·te·ri·o′ris
 —os′sis cu·boi′de·i′
 —ossis met·a·tar·sa′lis I
 —ossis metatarsalis V
 —ossis na·vic′u·lar′is
 —pha·lan′gis dis·ta′lis
 —pter′y·goi′de·a
 —ra′di·i′
 —sa′cra′lis
 —su′pra·gle′noi·da′lis
 —tib′i·ae′
 —ul′nae′
 —un·guic′u·lar′is
tu′ber·os′i·ty
tu′ber·ous
tub′ing
tu′bo·ab·dom′i·nal
tu′bo·ad·nex′o·pex′y
tu′bo·cu·ra′re
tu′bo·cu·ra′rine′
tu′bo·lig′a·men′ta·ry
tu′bo·lig′a·men′tous
tu′bo·o·var′i·an
tu′bo·o·var′i·ot′o·my
tu′bo·per′i·to·ne′al
tu′bo·plas′ty
tu′bo·tym′pa·nal
tu′bo·tym·pan′ic
tu′bo·u′ter·ine
tu′bo·vag′i·nal
tu′bu·lar
tu′bule
tu′bu·li′
 —lac·tif′er·i′
 —re·na′les′

—renales con·tor′ti′
—renales rec′ti′
—sem′i·nif′er·i′ con·tor′ti′
—seminiferi rec′ti′
tu′bu·lin
tu′bu·li·za′tion
tu′bu·lize′, -lized′, -liz′ing
tu′bu·lo·ac′i·nar
tu′bu·lo·ac′i·nous
tu′bu·lo·al·ve′o·lar
tu′bu·lo·cyst′
tu′bu·lo·in′ter·sti′tial
tu′bu·lo·rac′e·mose′
tu′bu·lor·rhex′is
tu′bu·lus *pl.* -li′
tu′bus *pl.* -bi′
  —di′ges·to′ri·us
  —med′ul·lar′is
  —ver′te·bra′lis
Tuf·fier′
  —ligament
  —test
tuft
tu·la·re′mi·a
tu′me·fa′cient
tu′me·fac′tion
tu′me·fy′, -fied′, -fy′ing
tu·men′ti·a
tu·mes′cence
tu·mes′cent
tu′mid
tu·mid′i·ty
tu′mor
tu′mor·af′fin
tu′mor·al
tu′mor·i·cid′al
tu′mor·i·gen′ic
tu′mor·let
tu′mor·ous
tu·mul′tus
  —cor′dis
  —ser·mo′nis
Tun′ga
  —pen′e·trans′
tun·gi·a′sis *pl.* -ses′
tung′sten
tu′nic
tu′ni·ca *pl.* -cae′
  —ad·ven·ti′ti·a
  —adventitia duc′tus
    def′e·ren′tis
  —adventitia e·soph′a·gi′
  —adventitia oe·soph′a·gi′

—adventitia tu′bae′
  u′ter·i′nae′
—adventitia u·re′ter·is
—adventitia ve·si′cae′
  sem′i·na′lis
—adventitia ve·sic′u·lae′
  sem′i·na′lis
—al′bu·gin′e·a
—albuginea cor′po·ris
  spon′gi·o′si′
—albuginea cor′po·rum
  cav′er·no·so′rum
—albuginea li·e′nis
—albuginea oc′u·li′
—albuginea o·var′i·i′
—albuginea pe′nis
—albuginea tes′tis
—con′junc·ti′va
—conjunctiva bul′bi′
—conjunctiva pal′pe·
  brar′um
—dar′tos′
—de·cid′u·a
—e′las′ti·ca
—ex·ter′na
—externa the′cae′
  fol·lic′u·li′
—externa va·so′rum
—fi·bro′sa
—fibrosa bul′bi′
—fibrosa hep′a·tis
—fibrosa li·e′nis
—fibrosa oc′u·li′
—fibrosa re′nis
—in·ter′na
—interna bul′bi′
—interna the′cae′ fol·lic′u·li′
—in′ti·ma
—me′di·a
—mu·co′sa
—mucosa ca′vi′ tym′pa·ni′
—mucosa co′li′
—mucosa duc′tus
  def′e·ren′tis
—mucosa e·soph′a·gi′
—mucosa in′tes·ti′ni′
  cras′si′
—mucosa intestini rec′ti′
—mucosa intestini ten′u·is
—mucosa la·ryn′gis
—mucosa lin′guae′
—mucosa na′si′
—mucosa oe·soph′a·gi′

—mucosa o′ris
—mucosa pha·ryn′gis
—mucosa rec′ti′
—mucosa tra′che·ae′ et
  bron·cho′rum
—mucosa tu′bae′ au′di·ti′-
  vae′
—mucosa tubae u′ter·i′nae′
—mucosa tym·pan′i·ca
—mucosa u·re′ter·is
—mucosa u·re′thrae′
  fem′i·ni′nae′
—mucosa urethrae
  mu′li·e′bris
—mucosa u′ter·i′
—mucosa va·gi′nae′
—mucosa ven·tric′u·li′
—mucosa ve·si′cae′ fel′-
  le·ae′
—mucosa vesicae u·ri·nar′-
  i·ae′
—mucosa ve·sic′u·lae′
  sem′i·na′lis
—mus′cu·lar′is
—muscularis bron·cho′rum
—muscularis cer′vi·cis
  u′ter·i′
—muscularis co′li′
—muscularis duc′tus
  def′e·ren′tis
—muscularis e·soph′a·gi′
—muscularis in′tes·ti′ni′
  cras′si′
—muscularis intestini rec′ti′
—muscularis intestini
  ten′u·is
—muscularis oe·soph′a·gi′
—muscularis pha·ryn′gis
—muscularis rec′ti′
—muscularis tra′che·ae′ et
  bron·cho′rum
—muscularis tu′bae′
  u′ter·i′nae′
—muscularis u·re′ter·is
—muscularis u·re′thrae′
  fem′i·ni′nae′
—muscularis urethrae
  mu′li·e′bris
—muscularis u′ter·i′
—muscularis va·gi′nae′
—muscularis ven·tric′u·li′
—muscularis ve·si′cae′
  fel′le·ae′

—muscularis vesicae
u′ri·nar′i·ae′
—muscularis ve·sic′u·lae′
sem′i·na′lis
—pro′pri·a co′ri·i′
—propria mu·co′sa
—propria tu′bu·li′ sem′i·
nif′er·i′
—se·ro′sa
—serosa co′li′
—serosa hep′a·tis
—serosa in′tes·ti′ni′ cras′si′
—serosa intestini ten′u·is
—serosa li·e′nis
—serosa per′i·to′nae′i′
—serosa per′i·to·ne′i′ pa·ri′-
e·ta′lis
—serosa peritonei vis′cer·a′-
lis
—serosa tu′bae′ u′ter·i′nae′
—serosa u′tre·i′
—serosa ven·tric′u·li′
—serosa ve·si′cae′ fel′le·ae′
—serosa vesicae u′ri·nar′-
i·ae′
—sub′mu·co′sa
—submucosa u·re′thrae′
mu′li·e′bris
—tes′tis
—u′ve·a
—vag′i·na′lis com·mu′nis
—vaginalis pro′pri·a tes′tis
—vaginalis tes′tis
—vas′cu·lo′sa bul′bi′
—vasculosa len′tis
—vasculosa oc′u·li′
—vasculosa tes′tis
tu′ni·cae′
—fu·nic′u·li′ sper·mat′i·ci′
—funiculi spermatici et
tes′tis
tun′nel
—of Cor′ti′
tu′ran·ose′
tur′bid
tur′bi·dim′e·ter
tur′bi·di·met′ric
tur′bi·dim′e·try
tur·bid′i·ty
tur′bi·nal
tur′bi·nate′
tur′bi·nat′ed
tur′bi·nec′to·my

tur′bi·no·tome′
tur′bi·not′o·my
tur′bu·lence
tur′bu·lent
Türck
—bundle
—column
—trachoma
Tur·cot′ syndrome
tur·ges′cence
tur·ges′cent
tur′gid
tur·gid′i·ty
tur′gor
tu·ris′ta
Türk
—cell
—leukocyte
Tur′ling·ton balsam
tur′mer·ic
turn
Tur′ner
—sign
—syndrome
tur′pen·tine′
tur′ri·ceph′a·ly
Tu′ryn sign
tusk
tus′sal
tus·se′do
tus·sic′u·la
tus·sic′u·lar
tus·sic′u·la′tion
Tus′si·la′go
tus′sis
—con′vul·si′va
tus′sive
tu·ta′men pl. -tam′i·na
Tut′hill method
Tut′tle operation
twang
tweez′ers
twig
twin
twinge, twinged, twing′ing
Twi′ning
—kink
—line
twin′ning
twist
twitch
ty·bam′ate′
tyl′i·on′ pl. -i·a

ty·lo′ma pl. -mas or -ma·ta
ty·lo′sis pl. -ses′
—pal·mar′is et plan·tar′is
ty·lot′ic
ty·lox′a·pol′
tym′pa·nal
tym′pa·nec′to·my
tym·pan′i·a
tym·pan′ic
tym·pan′i·on
tym′pa·nism
tym′pa·ni′tes′ (abdominal
distention)
♦ tympanitis
tym′pa·nit′ic
tym′pa·ni′tis (inflammation of
the tympanum)
♦ tympanites
tym′pa·no·eu·sta′chi·an
tym′pa·no·man·dib′u·lar
tym′pa·no·mas′toid′
tym′pa·no·mas·toi·di′tis
tym′pa·no·plas′ty
tym′pa·no·scle·ro′sis
pl. -ses′
tym′pa·no·sis pl. -ses′
tym′pa·no·squa·mo′sal
tym′pa·no·squa′mous
tym′pa·no·sta·pe′di·al
tym′pa·no·sym′pa·thec′-
to·my
tym′pa·no·tem′po·ral
tym′pa·not′o·my
tym′pa·nous
tym′pa·num pl. -na or -nums
tym′pa·ny
Tyn′dall
—effect
—phenomenon
tyn′dal·li·za′tion
type, typed, typ′ing
typh′lec′ta·si·a
typh·lec′ta·sis
typh·lec′to·my
typh·len·ter′i·tis
typh·li′tis
typh′lo·cele′
typh′lo·co·li′tis
typh′lo·dic′li·di′tis
typh′lo·em·py·e′ma
typh′lo·en·ter′i·tis
typh′loid′
typh′lo·lex′i·a

typh'lo·li·thi'a·sis
typh'lo·meg'a·ly
typh'lo·pex'y
typh'lo·pto'sis
typh·lo'sis
typh'lo·sole'
typh'lo·spasm
typh'lo·ste·no'sis *pl.* -ses'
typh'los'to·my
typh·lot'o·my
typh'lo·u·re'ter·os'to·my
ty'pho·bac'il·lo'sis of
　　Lan'dou·zy'
ty'pho·bac'ter·in
ty'phoid'
ty·phoi'dal
ty'pho·ma·lar'i·al
ty'pho·ma'ni·a
ty'pho·pneu·mo'ni·a
ty'phous
ty'phus
　—ex·an·thé·ma·tique'
typ'i·cal
ty'po·scope'
ty'pus de·gen'er·a·ti'vus
　am'ste·lo'da·men'sis
ty'ra·mine'
tyr'an·nism
ty·rem'e·sis
ty'ro·ci'dine'
Ty'rode' solution
ty·rog'e·nous
ty'roid'
ty'ro·pa·no'ate'
ty'ros'a·mine'
ty'ro·si·nase'
ty'ro·sine'
ty'ro·si·ne'mi·a
ty'ro·si·no'sis
ty'ro·si·nu'ri·a
ty'ro·sy·lu'ri·a
ty'ro·thri'cin
ty'ro·tox'ism
Ty'son glands
ty've·lose'
Tyz'zer disease
Tzanck test

U

u'ber·ous
u'ber·ty
u'bi·qui'nol'

u'bi·qui·none'
ud'der
Uf'fel·mann test
Uhl anomaly
Uht'hoff sign
ul'cer
ul'cer·ate', -at'ed, -at'ing
ul'cer·a'tion
ul'cer·a·tive
ul'cer·o·gan'gre·nous
ul'cer·o·gen'ic
ul'cer·o·glan'du·lar
ul'cer·o·gran'u·lo'ma
　pl. -mas *or* -ma·ta
ul'cer·o·mem'bra·nous
ul'cer·ous
ul'cus *pl.*
　—am'bu·lans
　—can·cro'sum
　—cru'ris
　—in'du·ra'tus
　—mol'le'
　—ser'pens
　—tu·ber'cu·lo'sum
　—ve·ne're·um
　—ven·tric'u·li'
　—vul'vae' a·cu'tum
u·lec'to·my
u·le·gy'ri·a
u·ler'y·the'ma
　—cen·trif'u·gum
　—oph'ry·og'e·nes'
　—sy'co·si·for'me'
u·let'ic
u·lex'ine'
u·li'tis
Ull'rich-Tur'ner syndrome
ul'na *pl.* -nae' *or* -nas
ul'nad'
ul'nar
ul·nar'is
ul'no·car'pe·us
ul'no·ra'di·al
u·loc'a·ce
u·lo·der'ma·ti'tis
u·lo·glos·si'tis
u'loid'
u·lon'cus
u·lor·rha'gi·a
u·lor·rhe'a
u·lo'sis
U'lo·so'ni·a par'vi·cor'nis
u·lot'ic

u·lot'o·my
Ul'rich test
ul'ti·mate
ul'ti·mum mo'ri·ens
ul'tra·brach'y·ce·phal'ic
ul'tra·brach'y·cra'ni·al
ul'tra·cen·trif'u·gal
ul'tra·cen·trif'u·ga'tion
ul'tra·cen·trif'u·fuge'
ul'tra·dol'i·cho·cra'ni·al
ul'tra·fast'
ul'tra·fil'ter
ul'tra·fil·tra'tion
ul'tra·len'te
ul'tra·mi'cro·scope'
ul'tra·mi'cro·scop'ic *or*
　ul'tra·mi'cro·scop'i·cal
ul'tra·mi·cros'co·py
ul'tra·mi'cro·tome'
ul'tra·phag'o·cy·to'sis
　pl. -ses'
ul'tra·red'
ul'tra·son'ic
ul'tra·son'o·gram'
ul'tra·son'o·graph'ic
ul'tra·so·nog'ra·phy
ul'tra·son'o·scope'
ul'tra·sound'
ul'tra·struc'ture
ul'tra·vi'o·let
ul'tra·vi'rus
ul'u·la'tion
um·bel'li·fer
um'bel·lif'er·ous
um'ber
Um'ber test
um·bi·lec'to·my
um·bil'i·cal
um·bil'i·cate
um·bil'i·cat'ed
um·bil'i·ca'tion
um·bil'i·cus *pl.* -ci' *or*
　-cus·es
um·bo' *pl.* -bos' *or* um·bo'-
nes'
　—mem·bra'nae' tym'pa·ni'
um'bo·nate'
um·bras'co·py
um·brel'la
un·bal'ance, -anced, -anc'ing
un'cal
un'ci·a *pl.* -ae'
un'ci·form'

un'ci·nal
un'ci·na·ri'a·sis *pl.* -ses'
un'ci·nate'
un'ci·pi'si·for'mis
un·com'pen·sat·ed
un·com'pli·cat'ed
un·con·di'tion·al
un·con·di'tioned
un·con'ju·gat'ed
un·con'scious
un·con'scious·ness
un·co·ver'te·bral
unc'tion
unc'tu·ous
un'cus *pl.* -ci'
  —gy'ri' hip'po·cam'pi'
un'de·cy·len'ic
un'der·a·chieve', -chieved',
  -chiev'ing
un'der·a·chiev'er
un'der·arm'
un'der·cut'
un'der·de·vel'oped
un'der·nour'ished
un'der·nu·tri'tion
un'der·sur'face
un'der·toe'
un'der·weight'
Un'der·wood' disease
un'de·scend'ed
un·dif'fer·en'ti·at·ed
un·dine'
un'din·ism
un'dis·placed'
un·do'ing
un'du·lant
un'du·late'
un'du·la'tion
un'du·la·to'ry
un'en·cap'su·lat·ed
un'en·hanced'
un·e'qual
un'e·rupt'ed
un'gual
un'guent
un·guen'tum
un'gui·nal
un'guis *pl.* -gues'
  —in'car·na'tus
un·health'y
u'ni·ar·tic'u·lar
u'ni·ax'i·al
u'ni·cam'er·al

u'ni·cel'lu·lar
u'ni·cen'tral
u'ni·cen'tric
u'ni·ceps'
u'ni·cep'tor
u'ni·cor'nous
u'ni·cus'pid
u'ni·cus'pi·date'
u'ni·di·rec'tion·al
u'ni·fa·mil'ial
u'ni·fo'cal
u'ni·glan'du·lar
u'ni·grav'i·da
u'ni·lat'er·al
u'ni·lat'er·al·ly
u'ni·lo'bar
u'ni·loc'u·lar
un'in·cised'
un'in·hib'it·ed
u'ni·nu'cle·ar
u'ni·nu'cle·ate'
u'ni·oc'u·lar
un'ion
u'ni·o'val
u'ni·o'vu·lar
u·nip'ar·a
u'ni·par'i·ens
u·nip'a·rous
u'ni·pen'nate'
u'ni·po'lar
u'ni·po'ten·cy
u·nip'o·tent
u'ni·po·ten'tial
u'ni·sep'tate'
u'ni·sex'u·al
u'nit
u'ni·tar'y
u'ni·va'lent
u'ni·ver'sal
un·load'ing
un·mod'i·fied'
un·my'e·li·nat·ed
Un'na
  —bodies
  —boot
  —stain
Un'na-Pap'pen·heim'
  stain
Un'na-Thost' syndrome
un·of·fi'cial
un·or'ga·nized'
un'phys·i·o·log'ic
un're·al'it·y

un're·sect'a·ble
un're·solved'
un're·spon'sive
un·rest'
un·sat'u·rat'ed
un·sex'
un·sound'
un·sound'ness
un·spec'i·fied'
un·sta'ble
un·stri'at·ed
Un'ver·richt
  —disease
  —myoclonus
un·well'
up·go'ing
up'per
up'right'ing
up'stroke'
up'take'
up'time'
u'ra·chal
u'ra·chus
u'ra·cil
u'ra·cra'si·a
u'ra·cra'ti·a
u'ra·gogue'
u'ra·mil
u'ra·nal
u·ra·nal'y·sis *pl.* -ses'
u'ra·nin
u·ran'i·nite'
u·ra·nis'co·la'li·a
u·ra·nis'co·plas'ty
u·ra·nis·cor'rha·phy
u·ra·nis'cus
u·ra'ni·um
u·ra·no·pho'bi·a
u·ra·no·plas'tic
u·ra·no·plas'ty
u·ra·no·ple'gi·a
u·ra·nor'rha·phy
u·ra·nos·chi·sis *pl.* -ses'
u·ran'o·schism
u'ra·no·schis'ma
u·ra·no·staph'y·lo·plas'ty
u·ra·no·staph'y·lor'rha·phy
u·ra·no·staph'y·los'chi·tis
u'ra·nyl
u·ra·ro'ma
u'rase'
u'ra·sin
u'rate'

u·ra·te′mi·a
u·rat′ic
u·ra·to′ma *pl.* -mas *or*
  -ma·ta
u·ra·to′sis
u·ra·tu′ri·a
u·re′a
u·re·am′e·ter
u·re·am′e·try
U·re′a·plas′ma u·re′a·lyt′-
  i·cum
u′re·ase′
u·rec′chy·sis
u·re·de′ma
u·re·dep′a
u·re·he·pat′ic
u′re·ide′
u·re′mi·a
u·re′mic
u·re′mi·gen′ic
u′re·o·tel′ic
u′re·o·tel′ism
u·re′si·es·the′si·a
u·re′si·es·the′sis
u·re′sis
u·re′tal
u·re′ter
u·re′ter·al
u·re′ter·al′gi·a
u·re′ter·ec·ta′si·a
u·re′ter·ec·ta·sis *pl.* -ses′
u·re′ter·ec′to·my
u·re′ter·ic
u·re·ter·i′tis
  —cys′ti·ca
u·re′ter·o·cele′
u·re′ter·o·ce·lec′to·my
u·re′ter·o·cer′vi·cal
u·re′ter·o·co·los′to·my
u·re′ter·o·cu·ta′ne·os′-
  to·my
u·re′ter·o·cys′ta·nas′to·
  mo′sis *pl.* -ses′
u·re′ter·o·cys′tic
u·re′ter·o·cys′to·scope′
u·re′ter·o·cys·tos′to·my
u·re′ter·o·di·al′y·sis *pl.* -ses′
u·re′ter·o·en·ter′ic
u·re′ter·o·en′ter·os′to·my
u·re′ter·o·gram′
u·re′ter·og′ra·phy
u·re′ter·o·hem′i·ne·phrec′-
  to·my

u·re′ter·o·hy′dro·ne·phro′-
  sis *pl.* -ses′
u·re′ter·o·il′e·al
u·re′ter·o·il′e·os′to·my
u·re′ter·o·in·tes′ti·nal
u·re′ter·o·lith′
u·re′ter·o·li·thi′a·sis *pl.* -ses′
u·re′ter·o·li·thot′o·my
u·re′ter·ol′y·sis *pl.* -ses′
u·re′ter·o·me′a·tot′o·my
u·re′ter·o·meg′a·ly
u·re′ter·o·ne′o·cys·tos′-
  to·my
u·re′ter·o·ne′o·py′e·los′-
  to·my
u·re′ter·o·ne·phrec′to·my
u·re′ter·op′a·thy
u·re′ter·o·pel′vic
u·re′ter·o·pel′vi·o·plas′ty
u·re′ter·o·phleg′ma
u·re′ter·o·plas′ty
u·re′ter·o·proc·tos′to·my
u·re′ter·o·py′e·li′tis
u·re′ter·o·py′e·log′ra·phy
u·re′ter·o·py′e·lo·ne·os′-
  to·my
u·re′ter·o·py′e·lo·ne·phri′-
  tis
u·re′ter·o·py′e·lo·ne·
  phros′to·my
u·re′ter·o·py′e·lo·plas′ty
u·re′ter·o·py′e·los′to·my
u·re′ter·o·py·o′sis
u·re′ter·o·rec′tal
u·re′ter·or·rha′gi·a
u·re′ter·or′rha·phy
u·re′ter·o·sig′moid·os′-
  to·my
u·re′ter·o·ste·no′sis *pl.* -ses′
u·re′ter·os′to·ma *pl.* -mas *or*
  -ma·ta
u·re′ter·os′to·my
u·re′ter·o·the′cal
u·re′ter·ot′o·my
u·re′ter·o·u·re′ter·al
u·re′ter·o·u·re′ter·os′to·my
u·re′ter·o·u′ter·ine′
u·re′ter·o·vag′i·nal
u·re′ter·o·ves′i·cal
u·re′ter·o·ves′i·co·plas′ty
u·re′ter·o·ves′i·cos′to·my
u′re·thane′
u·re′thra *pl.* -thras *or* -thrae′

—fem′i·ni′na
—mas′cu·li′na
—mu′li·e′bris
—vi·ri′lis
u·re′thral
u′re·thral′gi·a
u·re′thra·tre′si·a
u·re′threc′to·my
u·re′threm·phrax′is
u′re·thrism
u′re·thri′tis
  —cys′ti·ca
  —o′ri·fi′ci·i′ ex·ter′ni′
  —ve·ne′re·a
u·re′thro·blen′nor·rhe′a
u·re′thro·bul′bar
u·re′thro·cele′
u·re′thro·cu·ta′ne·ous
u·re′thro·cys·ti′tis
u·re′thro·cys′to·cele′
u·re′thro·dyn′i·a
u·re′thro·gram′
u·re′thro·graph′
u·re·throg′ra·phy
u·re′throm·e′ter
u·re′throm′e·try
u·re′thro·pe′nile′
u·re′thro·per′i·ne′al
u·re′thro·per′i·ne′o·scro′tal
u·re′thro·phy′ma
u·re′thro·plas′ty
u·re′thro·pros·tat′ic
u·re′thro·rec′tal
u·re′thror·rha′gi·a
u·re′thror′rha·phy
u·re′thror·rhe′a
  —ex li·bid′i·ne′
u·re′thro·scope′
u·re′thro·scop′ic
u·re·thros′co·py
u·re′thro·spasm
u·re′thro·stax′is
u·re′thro·ste·no′sis *pl.* -ses′
u·re·thros′to·my
u·re′thro·tome′
u·re·throt′o·my
u·re′thro·tri·go·ni′tis
u·re′thro·vag′i·nal
u·re′thro·ves′i·cal
u·re′thro·ves′i·co·vag′i·nal
u·ret′ic
urge
ur′gen·cy

ur'hi·dro'sis *pl.* -ses'
u'ric
u'ric·ac'i·de'mi·a
u'ric·ac'i·du'ri·a
u'ri·case'
u'ri·ce'mi·a
u'ri·col'y·sis
u'ri·co·lyt'ic
u'ri·co·su'ri·a
u'ri·co·su'ric
u'ri·co·tel'ic
u'ri·co·tel'ism
u'ri·dine'
u'ri·dro'sis *pl.* -ses'
u'ri·dyl
u'ri·dyl'ic
u'ri·es'the·sis
u·ri'na
  —chy'li'
  —ju'men·to'sa
  —po'tus
  —san'gui·nis
u'ri·nal
u'ri·nal'y·sis *pl.* -ses'
u'ri·nar'y
u'ri·nate', -nat'ed, -nat'ing
u'ri·na'tion
u'ri·na'tive
u'rine
u'ri·nif'er·ous
u'ri·nif'ic
u'ri·nip'a·rous
u'ri·no·cry·os'co·py
u'ri·no·gen'i·tal
u'ri·nog'e·nous
u'ri·nol'o·gy
u'ri·no·ma *pl.* -mas *or* -ma·ta
u'ri·nom'e·ter
u'ri·nom'e·try
u'ri·no·scop'ic
u'ri·nos'co·py
u'ri·nous
u'ri·po'si·a
u·ri'tis
u'ro·ac'i·dim'e·ter
u'ro·am·mo'ni·ac'
u'ro·an'the·lone'
u'ro·az'o·tom'e·ter
u'ro·ben·zo'ic
u'ro·bi'lin
u'ro·bi'lin·e'mi·a
u'ro·bi'li·nic'ter·us
u'ro·bi·lin'o·gen

u'ro·bi·lin'o·ge·nu'ri·a
u'ro·bi'li·noi'din
u'ro·bi'li·nu'ri·a
u'ro·can'ic
u'ro·cele'
u·roch'er·as
u'ro·che'zi·a
u'ro·chlo'ral'ic
u'ro·chrome'
u'ro·chro'mo·gen
u'ro·clep'si·a
u'ro·cris'i·a
u'ro·cri'sis *pl.* -ses'
u'ro·cy'a·nin
u'ro·cy·an'o·gen
u'ro·cy'a·nose'
u'ro·cy'a·no'sis
u'ro·cys'tis
u'ro·cys·ti'tis
u'ro·de'um
u'ro·dy·nam'ics
u'ro·dyn'i·a
u'ro·e·de'ma
u'ro·en'ter·one'
u'ro·er'y·thrin
u'ro·fla'vin
u'ro·fol'li·tro'pin
u'ro·fus'cin
u'ro·fus'co·he'ma·tin
u'ro·gas'trone'
u'ro·gen'i·tal
u·rog'e·nous
u'ro·glau'cin
u'ro·gram'
u·rog'ra·phy
u'ro·gra·vim'·ter
u'ro·he'ma·tin
u'ro·he'ma·to·ne·phro'sis
u'ro·he'ma·to·por'phy·rin
u'ro·hy'per·ten'sin
u'ro·ki'nase'
u'ro·ky·mog'ra·phy
u'ro·leu·kin'ic
u'ro·lith'
u'ro·li·thi'a·sis
u'ro·lith'ic
u'ro·li·thot'o·my
u'ro·log'ic *or* u'ro·log'i·cal
u·rol'o·gist
u·rol'o·gy
u'ro·lu'te·in
u'ro·man'cy

u'ro·man'ti·a
u'ro·mel'a·nin
u·rom'e·lus
u·rom'e·ter
u·ron'cus
u'ro·ne·phro'sis
u·ron'ic
u'ro·nol'o·gy
u'ro·non·com'e·try
u'ro·nos'co·py
u·rop'a·thy
u'ro·pe'ni·a
u'ro·pep'sin
u'ro·phan'ic
u'ro·phe'in
u'ro·phil'i·a
u'ro·pla'ni·a
u'ro·poi·e'sis
u'ro·poi·et'ic
u'ro·por'phy·rin
u'ro·por'phy·rin'o·gen
u'ro·psam'mus
u'ro·ra'di·ol'o·gy
u'ro·rec'tal
u'ro·ro'se·in
u·ror·rha'gi·a
u·ror·rhe'a
u·ror·rho'din
u·ror·rho·din'o·gen
u'ro·ru'bin
u'ro·ru·bin'o·gen
u·ros'che·sis
u·ro'sa·cin
u·ros'che·o·cele'
u'ro·scop'ic
u·ros'co·py
u'ro·sem'i·ol'o·gy
u'ro·sep'sis
u'ro·sep'tic
u'ro·spec'trin
u'ro·ste'a·lith'
u'ro·the'li·al
u'ro·the'li·um
u'ro·tox'i·a
u'ro·tox'ic
u'ro·tox·ic'i·ty
u'ro·tox'in
u'ro·tox'y
u'ro·u·re'ter
u'ro·xan'thin
ur'so·de·ox'y·cho'lic
ur'so·di'ol'
ur·ti'ca

ur'ti·cant
ur'ti·car'i·a
— bul·lo'sa
— fac·ti'ti·a
— hem'or·rhag'i·ca
— med'i·ca·men·to'sa
— pap'u·lo'sa
— pig'men·to'sa
— so·lar'is
ur'ti·car'i·al
ur'ti·car'i·o·gen'ic
ur'ti·cate'
ur'ti·ca'tion
u·ru'shi·ol'
us'ne·in
us'nic
us'ti·lag'i·nism
Us'ti·la'go
— may'dis
— ze'ae'
us'tion
us·tu·la'tion
U·su'tu fever
u'ta
u·ter·al'gi·a
u'ter·ine
u'ter·is'mus
u·ter·i'tis
u'ter·o·ab·dom'i·nal
u'ter·o·ad·nex'al
u'ter·o·cer'vi·cal
u'ter·o·col'ic
u'ter·o·dyn'i·a
u'ter·o·en·ter'ic
u'ter·o·fix·a'tion
u'ter·o·ges·ta'tion
u'ter·og'ra·phy
u'ter·o·in·tes'ti·nal
u'ter·o·lith'
u'ter·om'e·ter
u'ter·o·o·var'i·an
u'ter·o·pa·ri'e·tal
u'ter·o·pel'vic
u'ter·o·pex'i·a
u'ter·o·pex'y
u'ter·o·pla·cen'tal
u'ter·o·plas'ty
u'ter·o·rec'tal
u'ter·o·sa'cral
u'ter·o·sal'pin·gog'ra·phy
u'ter·o·scope'
u'ter·ot'o·my

u'ter·o·ton'ic
u'ter·o·trac'tor
u'ter·o·trop'ic
u'ter·o·tu'bal
u'ter·o·tu·bog'ra·phy
u'ter·o·vag'i·nal
u'ter·o·ven'tral
u'ter·o·ves'i·cal
u'ter·us pl. u'ter·i'
— a·col'lis
— ar'cu·a'tus
— bi·cor'nis
— bi·loc'u·lar'is
— di·del'phys
— du'plex'
— mas'cu·li'nus
— par'vi·col'lis
— sep'tus
— u·ni·cor'nis
u'tri·cle
u·tric'u·lar
u·tric'u·li'tis
u·tric'u·lo·sac'cu·lar
u·tric'u·lus pl. -li'
— mas'cu·li'nus
— pros·tat'i·cus
u'va-ur'si'
u've·a
u've·al
u've·it'ic
u've·i'tis
u've·o·en·ceph'a·li'tis
u've·o·lab'y·rin·thi'tis
u've·o·men·in·gi'tis
u've·o·me·nin'go·en·ceph'a·li'tis
u've·o·neu'rax·i'tis
u've·o·pa·rot'id
u've·o·par'o·ti'tis
u've·o·scle·ri'tis
u'vi·form'
u'vi·o·fast'
u'vi·om'e·ter
u'vi·o·re·sis'tant
u'vi·o·sen'si·tive
u'vu·la pl. -las or -lae'
— cer'e·bel'li'
— fis'sa
— pal·a·ti'na
— ver'mis
— ve·si'cae'
u'vu·lap·to'sis
u'vu·lar

u'vu·la·tome' var. of
uvulotome
u'vu·lec'to·my
u'vu·li'tis
u'vu·lo·nod'u·lar
u'vu·lop·to'sis
u'vu·lo·tome' also
uvulatome
u'vu·lot'o·my

V

vac'cin
vac'ci·na·ble
vac'ci·nal
vac'ci·nate', -nat·ed, -nat·ing
vac'ci·na'tion
vac'ci·na·tor
vac·cine'
vac·cin'i·a
— gan'gre·no'sa
— ne·cro'sum
vac·cin'i·al
vac·cin'i·form'
vac·ci·ni·o'la
vac'ci·noid'
vac·cin'o·style'
vac'ci·no·ther'a·py
vac'u·o'lar
vac'u·o·late'
vac'u·o·lat'ed
vac'u·o·la'tion
vac'u·ole'
vac'u·o·li·za'tion
vac'u·ome'
vac'u·um pl. -u·ums or -u·a
va'gal
va·gi'na pl. -nas or -nae'
— bul'bi'
— ca·rot'i·ca fas'ci·ae'
cer'vi·ca'lis
— den'tis
— ex·ter'na ner'vi op'ti·ci'
— fi·bro'sa ten'di·nis
— in·ter'na ner'vi op'ti·ci'
— mas'cu·li'na
— mu·co'sa in·ter·tu·ber'cu·lar'is
— mus'cu·li' rec'ti' ab·dom'i·nis
— pro·ces'sus sty·loi'de·i'
— sy·no'vi·a'lis com·mu'nis mus'cu·lo'rum flex·o'rum

—synovialis in'ter·tu·ber'-
cu·lar'is
—synovialis mus'cu·li'
ob·li'qui' su·pe'ri·o'ris
—synovialis mus'cu·lo'rum
fib'u·lar'i·um com·mu'nis
—synovialis musculorum
per'o·ne·o'rum
com·mu'nis
—synovialis ten'di·nis
—synovialis tendinis
mus'cu·li' flex·o'ris car'pi'
ra'di·a'lis
—synovialis tendinis mus-
culi flexoris hal'lu·cis
lon'gi'
—synovialis tendinis mus-
culi tib'i·a'lis pos·te'ri·o'ris
—ten'di·nis mus'cu·li'
ex'ten·so'ris car'pi'
ul·nar'is
—tendinis musculi extenso-
ris dig'i·ti' min'i·mi'
—tendinis musculi extenso-
ris hal'lu·cis lon'gi'
—tendinis musculi extenso-
ris pol'li·cis lon'gi'
—tendinis musculi fib'u·
lar'is lon'gi'
—tendinis musculi flex·o'ris
hal'lu·cis lon'gi'
—tendinis musculi flexoris
pol'li·cis lon'gi'
—tendinis musculi per'o·
nae'i' lon'gi'
—tendinis musculi per'o·
ne'i' lon'gi'
—tendinis musculi tib'i·a'lis
an·te'ri·o'ris
—tendinis musculi tibialis
pos·te'ri·o'ris
—ten'di·num mus'cu·li'
ex'ten·so'ris dig'i·to'rum
pe'dis lon'gi'
—tendinum musculi flex·o'-
ris dig'i·to'rum pe'dis
lon'gi'
—tendinum mus'cu·lo'rum
ab'duc·to'ris lon'gi' et ex'-
ten·so'ris brev'is pol'li·cis
—tendinum musculorum
ex'ten·so'ris dig'i·to'rum
et ex'ten·so'ris in'di·cis

—tendinum musculorum
ex'ten·so'rum car'pi'
ra'di·a'li·um
—tendinum musculorum
flex·o'rum com·mu'ni·um
—tendinum musculorum
per'o·nae·o'rum com·
mu'nis
—va·so'rum
va·gi'nae'
—fi·bro'sae' dig'i·to'rum
ma'nus
—fibrosae digitorum pe'dis
—mu·co'sae' dig'i·to'rum
ma'nus
—mucosae digitorum pe'dis
—ner'vi' op'ti·ci'
—sy'no·vi·a'les' dig'i·to'-
rum ma'nus
—synoviales digitorum
pe'dis
—synoviales ten'di·num
dig'i·to'rum ma'nus
—synoviales tendinum
digitorum pe'dis
—ten'di·num dig'i·ta'les'
ma'nus
—tendinum digitales pe'dis
vag'i·nal
vag'i·nal·ec'to·my
vag'i·na·li'tis
va·gi'na·pex'y
vag'i·nate'
vag'i·nec'to·my
vag'i·nif'er·ous
vag'i·nis'mus
vag'i·ni'tis
vag'i·no·ab·dom'i·nal
vag'i·no·cele'
vag'i·no·cu·ta'ne·ous
vag'i·no·dyn'i·a
vag'i·no·fix·a'tion
vag'i·no·la'bi·al
vag'i·no·my·co'sis *pl.* -ses'
vag'i·nop'a·thy
vag'i·no·per'i·ne'al
vag'i·no·per'i·ne·or·rha·
phy
vag'i·no·per'i·ne·ot'o·my
vag'i·no·per'i·to·ne'al
vag'i·no·pex'y
vag'i·no·plas'ty
vag'i·no·scope'

vag'i·nos'co·py
vag'i·not'o·my
vag'i·no·ves'i·cal
vag'i·no·vul'var
va·gi'tus
—u'ter·i'nus
—vag'i·na'lis
va'go·ac·ces'so·ry
va'go·gram'
va'go·hy'po·glos'sal
va·gol'y·sis
va'go·lyt'ic
va'go·mi·met'ic
va'go·pres'sor
va·got'o·mize'
va·got'o·my
va'go·to'ni·a
va'go·ton'ic
va·got'o·nin
va'go·trop'ic
va'go·va'gal
va'grant
va'gus *pl.* -gi'
va'gus·stoff'
va'lence
va'len·cy
va'lent
Va·len'tin'
—corpuscles
—ganglion
val'er·ate'
va·ler'ic
val'e·tham'ate'
val'e·tu'di·nar'i·an
val'e·tu'di·nar'i·an·ism
val'gus
val'id
val'i·da'tion
va·lid'i·ty
val'ine'
val'i·ne'mi·a
val'late'
val·lec'u·la *pl.* -lae'
—cer'e·bel'li'
—ep'i·glot'ti·ca
—lin'guae'
—un'guis
val·lec'u·lar
Val·leix' points
Val·let' mass
val'lum *pl.* -la *or* -lums
—un'guis
val·noc'ta·mide'

val·pro'ate'
val·pro'ic
Val·sal'va
—maneuver
—sinus
—test
Val'su·a'ni disease
val'va *pl.* -vae'
—a·or'tae'
—a'tri·o·ven·tric'u·lar'is
   dex'tra
—atrioventricularis si·nis'-
   tra
—il'e·o·ce·ca'lis
—mi·tra'lis
—tri·cus'pi·da'lis
—trun'ci' pul'mo·na'lis
val'ue
valve
val'vi·form'
val'vo·tome'
val·vot'o·my
val'vu·la *pl.* -lae'
—bi·cus'pi·da'lis
—co'li'
—fo·ram'i·nis o·va'lis
—fos'sae' na·vic'u·lar'is
—lym·phat'i·ca
—pro·ces'sus ver'mi·for'-
   mis
—py·lo'ri'
—sem'i·lu·nar'is anterior
   ar·te'ri·ae' pul'mo·na'lis
—semilunaris anterior
   trun'ci' pul'mo·na'lis
—semilunaris dex'tra
   a·or'tae'
—semilunaris dextra
   ar·te'ri·ae' pul'mo·na'lis
—semilunaris dextra
   val'vae' a·or'tae'
—semilunaris dextra valvae
   trun'ci' pul'mo·na'lis
—semilunaris posterior
   a·or'tae'
—semilunaris posterior
   val'vae a·or'tae'
—semilunaris si·nis'tra
   a·or'tae'
—semilunaris sinistra
   ar·te'ri·ae' pul'mo·na'lis
—semilunaris sinistra
   val'vae' a·or'tae'

—semilunaris sinistra
   valvae trun'ci'
   pul'mo·na'lis
—si'nus co'ro·nar'i·i'
—sinus coronarii
   (The·be'si·i')
—spi'ra'lis (Heis'ter·i')
—tri·cus'pi·da'lis
—ve'nae' ca'vae' in·fe'ri·o'-
   ris
—venae cavae inferioris
   (Eu·sta'chi·i')
—ve·no'sa
val'vu·lae'
—a·na'les'
—con'ni·ven'tes'
—sem'i·lu·nar'es' a·or'tae'
—semilunares ar·te'ri·ae'
   pul'mo·na'lis
val'vu·lar
val'vu·lec'to·my
val'vu·li'tis
val'vu·lo·plas'ty
val'vu·lo·tome'
val'vu·lot'o·my
van'a·date'
va·na'di·um
va·na'di·um·ism
van Bo'gaert
   leukoencephalitis
van'co·my'cin
van Deen test
van den Bergh
—disease
—test
van der Hoeve syndrome
van Ge·huch'ten cell
Van Gie'son stain
van Han'se·mann cells
Van Hoorne canal
va·nil'la
va·nil'lic
va·nil'lin
va·nil'lism
van'il·lyl·man·del'ic
Van Slyke
—apparatus
—method
van't Hoff law
va'po·cau'ter·i·za'tion
va'por
va·po'res' u'ter·i'ni'
va·por·i·za'tion

va'por·ize', -ized', -iz'ing
va'por·iz'er
va'po·ther'a·py
Va·quez' disease
var'i·a·bil'i·ty
var'i·a·ble
var'i·ance
var'i·ant
var'i·a'tion
var'i·ca'tion
var'i·ce'al
var'i·cec'to·my
var'i·cel'la
—gan'gre·no'sa
—in·oc'u·la'ta
var'i·cel·la'tion
var'i·cel'li·form'
var'i·cel'loid'
var·ic'i·form'
var'i·co·bleph'a·ron'
var'i·co·cele'
var'i·co·ce·lec'to·my
var'i·cog'ra·phy
var'i·coid'
var'i·com'pha·lus *pl.* -li'
var'i·co·phle·bi'tis
var'i·cose'
var'i·co'sis *pl.* -ses'
var'i·cos'i·ty
var'i·cot'o·my
va·ric'u·la *pl.* -las *or* -lae'
var'i·e·gate'
va·ri'e·ty
var'i·form'
va·ri'o·la
—vac·cin'i·a
—ve'ra
va·ri'o·lar
var'i·o·late', -lat'ed, -lat'ing
var'i·o·la'tion
var'i·ol'ic
var'i·ol'i·form'
var'i·o·li·za'tion
var'i·o·loid'
va·ri'o·lous
va·ri'o·lo·vac·cine'
va·ri'o·lo·vac·cin'i·a
var'ix *pl.* -i·ces'
—lym·phat'i·cus
var'us
vas *pl.* va'sa
—af'fer·ens ar·te'ri·ae'
   in'ter·lob·u·lar'is

—afferens glo·mer′u·li′
re·na′lis
—a·nas′to·mot′i·cum
—cap′il·lar′e′
—col·lat′er·a′le′
—def′er·ens
—ef′fer·ens ar·te′ri·ae′
in′ter·lob′u·lar′is
—efferens glo·mer′u·li′
re·na′lis
—lym·phat′i·cum
—prom′i·nens
—spi·ra′le′
va′sa
—ab′er·ran′ti·a hep′a·tis
—af′fe·ren′ti·a lym′pho·
glan′du·lae′
—afferentia no′di′
lym·phat′i·ci′
—au′ris in·ter′nae′
—brev′is
—def′e·ren′ti·a
—ef′fe·ren′ti·a
lym′pho·glan′du·lae′
—efferentia no′di′
lym·phat′i·ci′
—lym·phat′i·ca
—lymphatica pro·fun′da
—lymphatica su·per·fi′ci·a′-
li·a
—prae′vi·a
—rec′ta
—san·guin′e·a ret′i·nae′
—va·so′rum
va′sal
vas′cu·lar
vas′cu·lar′i·ty
vas′cu·lar·i·za′tion
vas′cu·lar·ize′, -ized′, -iz′ing
vas′cu·la·ture
vas′cu·li′tis
vas′cu·lo·gen′e·sis
vas′cu·lo·lym·phat′ic
vas′cu·lop′a·thy
vas′cu·lum pl. -la
va·sec′to·mize′, -mized′,
-miz′ing
va·sec′to·my
vas′i·cine′
vas′i·fac′tion
vas′i·fac′tive
va·si′tis
va·so·ac′tive

va·so·con·stric′tion
va′so·con·stric′tive
va′so·con·stric′tor
va′so·den′tin
vas·o·de·pres′sion
va′so·de·pres′sor
va′so·dil′a·ta′tion
va′so·di·la′tion
va′so·di·la′tive
va′so·di·la′tor
va′so·ep′i·did′y·mos′to·my
va′so·for·ma′tion
va′so·for′ma·tive
va′so·gan′gli·on pl. -gli·ons
or -gli·a
va′so·gen′ic
va·sog′ra·phy
va′so·hy′per·ton′ic
va′so·hy′po·ton′ic
va′so·in·hib′i·tor
va′so·in·hib′i·to′ry
va′so·li·ga′tion
va′so·mo′tion
va′so·mo′tor
vas·o·mo·to′ri·al
va′so·mo·tric′i·ty
vas·o·neu·rop′a·thy
va′so·neu·ro′sis pl. -ses′
va′so·or′chid·os′to·my
va′so·pa·ral′y·sis pl. -ses′
va′so·pa·re′sis pl. -ses′
va′so·pres′sin
va′so·pres′sor
va′so·punc′ture
va′so·re′flex
va′so·re·lax·a′tion
va·sor′rha·phy
va′so·sec′tion
va′so·sen′so·ry
va′so·spasm
va′so·spas′tic
va′so·stim′u·lant
va·sos′to·my
va′so·to′cin
va·sot′o·my
va′so·to′ni·a
va′so·ton′ic
va′so·to′nin
va′so·tribe′
va′so·troph′ic
va·so·trop′ic
va·so·va′gal
va′so·va·sos′to·my

va′so·va·sot′o·my
va′so·ve·sic′u·lec′to·my
va′so·ve·sic′u·li′tis
vas′tus pl. -ti′
Va′ter
—ampulla
—corpuscle
Va′ter-Pa·ci′ni corpuscle
vault
Veau operation
vec′tion
vec′tis
vec′tor
vec′tor·car′di·o·gram′
vec′tor·car′di·o·graph′
vec′tor·car′di·og′ra·phy
vec·to′ri·al
ve′cu·ro′ni·um
Ved′der sign
veg′an′
veg′an·ism
veg′e·ta·ble
veg′e·tar′i·an
veg′e·tar′i·an·ism
veg′e·ta′tion
veg′e·ta′tive
veg′e·to·an′i·mal
ve′hi·cle
veil
Veil′lo·nel′la
—al′ca·les′cens
—dis·coi′des′
—or·bic′u·lus
—par′vu·la
—ren′i·for′mis
Veil·lon′ tube
vein
—of Lab·bé′
—of Tro′lard′
ve·la′men pl. -lam′i·na
—vul′vae′
vel′a·men′tous
vel′a·men′tum pl. -ta
ve′lar
vel′li·cate′, -cat′ed, -cat′ing
vel′li·ca′tion
vel′lus
ve·loc′i·ty
ve′lo·pha·ryn′ge·al
Vel·peau′ deformity
ve′lum pl. -la
—in′ter·pos′i·tum rhom′-
ben·ceph′a·li′

—med'ul·lar'e' an·te'ri·us
—medulllare in·fe'ri·us
—medullare pos·te'ri·us
—medullare su·pe'ri·us
—pa·la'ti'
—pal'a·ti'num
—pen'du·lum pa·la'ti'
—ter'mi·na'le'

ve'na *pl.* -nae'
—a·nas'to·mot'i·ca inferior
—anastomotica superior
—an'gu·lar'is
—ap'pen·dic'u·lar'is
—aq'ue·duc'tus coch'le·ae'
—aqueductus ves·tib'u·li'
—au·ric'u·lar'is posterior
—ax'il·lar'is
—az'y·gos'
—ba·sa'lis
—basalis com·mu'nis
—basalis inferior
—basalis (Ro'sen·tha'li')
—basalis superior
—ba·sil'i·ca
—bron'chi·a'les' an·te'ri·o'res'
—bul'bi' pe'nis
—bulbi ves·tib'u·li'
—can'a·lic'u·li' coch'le·ae'
—ca'na·lis pter'y·goi'de·i'
—canalis pterygoidei (Vi'di·i')
—ca'va
—cava inferior
—cava superior
—cen'tra'lis glan'du·lae' sup'pra·re·na'lis
—centralis ret'i·nae'
—ce·phal'i·ca
—cephalica ac'ces·so'ri·a
—cer'e·bri' anterior
—cerebri mag'na
—cerebri magna (Ga·le'ni')
—cerebri me'di·a
—cerebri media pro·fun'da
—cerebri media su·per·fi'ci·a'lis
—cer'vi·ca'lis pro·fun'da
—cho'ri·oi'de·a
—cho'roi'de·a
—cir'cum·flex'a il'i·i' pro·fun'da
—circumflexa ilii su'per·fi'ci·a'lis

—col'i·ca dex'tra
—colica me'di·a
—colica si·nis'tra
—com'i·tans'
—comitans ner'vi' hy'po· glos'si'
—cor'dis mag'na
—cordis me'di·a
—cordis par'va
—co'ro·nar'i·a ven·tric'u·li'
—cu·ta'ne·a
—cys'ti·ca
—di·plo'i·ca fron·ta'lis
—diploica oc·cip'i·ta'lis
—diploica tem·po·ra'lis anterior
—diploica temporalis posterior
—dor·sa'lis cli·to'ri·dis
—dorsalis clitoridis pro· fun'da
—dorsalis pe'nis
—dorsalis penis pro·fun'da
—em'is·sar'i·a
—emissaria con'dy·lar'is
—emissaria mas·toi'de·a
—emissaria oc·cip'i·ta'lis
—emissaria pa·ri'e·ta'lis
—ep'i·gas'tri·ca inferior
—epigastrica su'per·fi'- ci·a'lis
—epigastrica superior
—eth'moi·da'lis
—ethmoidalis anterior
—ethmoidalis posterior
—fa'ci·a'lis
—facialis anterior
—facialis com·mu'nis
—fascialis posterior
—fa'ci·e'i' pro·fun'da
—fem'o·ra'lis
—fem'o·ro·pop·lit'e·a
—Ga·le'ni'
—gas'tri·ca dex'tra
—gastrica si·nis'tra
—gas'tro·ep'i·plo'i·ca dex'tra
—gastroepiploica si·nis'tra
—haem'or·rhoi·da'lis me'di·a
—haemorrhoidalis superior
—hem'i·az'y·gos'
—hemiazygos ac'ces·so'ri·a

—hy'po·gas'tri·ca
—il'e·o·col'i·ca
—i·li'a·ca com·mu'nis
—iliaca ex·ter'na
—iliaca in·ter'na
—il'e·o·lum·ba'lis
—in'ter·cos·ta'lis superior dex'tra
—intercostalis superior si·nis'tra
—intercostalis su·pre'ma
—in'ter·ver'te·bra'lis
—jug'u·lar'is anterior
—jugularis ex·ter'na
—jugularis in·ter'na
—la·bi·a'lis inferior
—labialis superior
—lac'ri·ma'lis
—la·ryn'ge·a inferior
—laryngea superior
—li'e·na'lis
—lin·gua'lis
—lum·ba'lis as·cen'dens
—mam·mar'i·a in·ter'na
—me'di·a'na an'te·bra'chi·i'
—mediana an'ti·bra'chi·i'
—mediana ba·sil'i·ca
—mediana ce·phal'i·ca
—mediana col'li'
—mediana cu'bi·ti'
—mes'en·ter'i·ca inferior
—mesenterica superior
—na'so·fron·ta'lis
—ob·li'qua a'tri·i' si·nis·tri'
—obliqua atrii sinistri (Mar·shal'li')
—oc·cip'i·ta'lis
—oph·thal'mi·ca inferior
—ophthalmica superior
—oph·thal'mo·me·nin'ge·a
—o·var'i·ca
—ovarica dex'tra
—ovarica si·nis'tra
—pal'a·ti'na
—palatina ex·ter'na
—phren'i·ca inferior
—pop·lit'e·a
—por'tae'
—posterior ven·tric'u·li' si·nis'tri'
—pre'py·lo'ri·ca
—pro·fun'da fem'o·ris
—profunda lin'guae'

—pu·den'da in·ter'na
—pul·mo·na'lis inferior
dex'tra
—pulmonalis inferior
si·nis'tra
—pulmonalis superior
dex'tra
—pulmonalis superior
si·nis'tra
—rec·ta'lis me'di·a
—rectalis superior
—ret'ro·man·dib'u·lar'is
—sa·cra'lis me'di·a
—sacralis me·di·a'na
—sa·phe'na ac'ces·so'ri·a
—saphena mag'na
—saphena par'va
—scap'u·lar'is dor·sa'lis
—sep'ti' pel·lu'ci·di'
—sper·mat'i·ca
—spi·ra'lis mo·di'o·li'
—ster'no·clei'do·mas·toi'de·a
—stri·a'ta
—sty'lo·mas·toi'de·a
—sub·cla'vi·a
—sub·cos·ta'lis
—sub·lin·gua'lis
—sub·men·ta'lis
—su'pra·or'bi·ta'lis
—su'pra·re·na'lis dex'tra
—suprarenalis si·nis'tra
—su'pra·scap'u·lar'is
—tem'po·ra'lis me'di·a
—ter'mi·na'lis
—tes·tic'u·lar'is
—testicularis dex'tra
—testicularis si·nis'tra
—thal'a·mo·stri·a'ta
—tho·ra·ca'lis lat'er·a'lis
—tho'rac'i·ca in·ter'na
—thoracica lat'er·a'lis
—tho'ra·co·a·cro'mi·a'lis
—thy're·oi'de·a i'ma
—thyreoidea superior
—thy'roi'de·a inferior
—thyroidea superior
—trans·ver'sa fa'ci·e'i'
—transversa scap'u·lae'
—um·bil'i·ca'lis
—umbilicalis si·nis'tra
—ver'te·bra'lis
—vertebralis ac'ces·so'ri·a
—vertebralis anterior

ve'na·ca'vo·gram'
ve'na·ca·vog'ra·phy
ve'nae'
—a·non'y·mae' dex'tra et
si·nis'tra
—ar'ci·for'mes' re'nis
—ar·cu·a'tae' re'nis
—ar·tic'u·lar'es' man·dib'-
u·lae'
—articulares tem'po·ro·
man·dib'u·lar'es'
—au·di·ti'vae' in·ter'nae'
—au·ric'u·lar'es' an·te'ri·o'-
res'
—ba'si·ver'te·bra'les'
—bra'chi·a'les'
—bra·chi·o·ce·phal'i·cae'
dex'tra et si·nis'tra
—bron'chi·a'les'
—bronchiales pos·te'ri·o'-
res'
—cav'er·no'sae' pe'nis
—cen·tra'les' hep'a·tis
—cer'e·bel'li' in·fe'ri·o'res'
—cerebelli su·pe'ri·o'res'
—cer'e·bri'
—cerebri in·fe'ri·o'res'
—cerebri in·ter'nae'
—cerebri su·pe'ri·o'res'
—cho·roi'de·ae' oc'u·li'
—cil'i·ar'es'
—ciliares an·te'ri·o'res'
—ciliares pos·te'ri·o'res'
—cir'cum·flex'ae' fem'o·ris
lat'er·a'les'
—circumflexae femoris
me'di·a'les'
—col'i·cae' dex'trae'
—com'i·tan'tes'
—con·junc'ti·va'les'
—conjunctivales an·te'ri·o'-
res'
—conjunctivales pos·te'ri·
o'res'
—cor'dis
—cordis an·te'ri·o'res'
—cordis min'i·mae'
—cos'to·ax'il·lar'es'
—dig'i·ta'les' com·mu'nes'
pe'dis
—digitales dor·sa'les' pe'dis
—digitales pal·mar'es'
—digitales pe'dis dor·sa'les'

—digitales plan·tar'es'
—digitales vo·lar'es' com·
mu'nes'
—digitales volares pro'-
pri·ae'
—di·plo'i·cae'
—dor·sa'les' cli·to'ri·dis
su'per·fi'ci·a'les'
—dorsales lin'guae'
—dorsales pe'nis sub'cu·ta'-
ne·ae'
—dorsales penis su'per·fi'ci·
a'les'
—du'o·de·na'les'
—em'is·sar'i·ae'
—ep'i·gas'tri·cae' su·pe'ri·
o'res'
—ep'i·scle·ra'les'
—e'so·phag'e·ae'
—eth'moi·da'les'
—fib'u·lar'es'
—fron·ta'les'
—gas'tri·cae' brev'es'
—ge'nus
—glu'tae·ae' in·fe'ri·o'res'
—glutaeae su·pe'ri·o'res'
—glu'te·ae' in·fe'ri·o'res'
—gluteae su·pe'ri·o'res'
—haem'or·rhoi·da'les'
in·fe'ri·o'res'
—he·pat'i·cae'
—hepaticae dex'trae'
—hepaticae me'di·ae'
—hepaticae si·nis'trae'
—in'ter·cap'i·ta'les'
—in'ter·ca·pit'u·lar'es'
ma'nus
—intercapitulares pe'dis
—in'ter·cos·ta'les'
—intercostales an·te'ri·o'-
res'
—intercostales pos·te'ri·o'-
res' (IV-XI)
—in'ter·lo·bar'es' re'nis
—in'ter·lob'u·lar'es'
hep'a·tis
—interlobulares re'nis
—in'ter·ver'te·bra'les'
—in·tes'ti·na'les'
—je·ju'na'les' et il'e·i'
—la'bi·a'les' an·te'ri·o'res'
—labiales in·fe'ri·o'res'
—labiales pos·te'ri·o'res'

—lab'y·rin'thi'
—lum·ba'les'
—lumbales (I et II)
—lumbales (III et IV)
—mas'se·ter'i·cae'
—max'il·lar'es'
—me'di·as'ti·na'les'
—mediastinales an·te'ri·o'-res'
—me·nin'ge·ae'
—meningeae me'di·ae'
—met'a·car'pe·ae' dor·sa'les'
—metacarpeae pal·mar'es'
—metacarpeae vo·lar'es'
—met'a·tar'se·ae' dor·sa'-les' pe'dis
—metatarseae plan·tar'es'
—mus'cu·lar'es'
—mus'cu·lo·phren'i·cae'
—na·sa'les' ex·ter'nae'
—ob·tu·ra·to'ri·ae'
—oe'so·phag'e·ae'
—pal'pe·bra'les'
—palpebrales in·fe'ri·o'res'
—palpebrales su·pe'ri·o'res'
—pan·cre·at'i·cae'
—pan·cre·at'i·co·du'o·de·na'les'
—par'a·um·bil'i·ca'les'
—pa·rot'i·de·ae'
—parotideae an·te'ri·o'res'
—parotideae pos·te'ri·o'res'
—par'um·bil'i·ca'les' (Sap·pey'i')
—pec'to·ra'les'
—per'fo·ran'tes'
—per'i·car·di·a'cae'
—per'i·car·di·a·co·phren'i·cae'
—per'o·nae'ae'
—per'o·ne'ae'
—pha·ryn'ge·ae'
—phren'i·cae' in·fe'ri·o'res'
—phrenicae su·pe'ri·o'res'
—pop·lit'e·ae'
—pro·fun'dae' cli·to'ri·dis
—profundae fem'o·ris
—profundae pe'nis
—pu·den'dae' ex·ter'nae'
—pul'mo·na'les'
—pulmonales dex'trae'
—pulmonales si·nis'trae'
—ra'di·a'les'
—rec·ta'les' in·fe'ri·o'res'

—rectales me'di·ae'
—re·na'les'
—re'nis
—sa·cra'les' lat·er·a'les'
—scro·ta'les' an·te'ri·o'res'
—scrotales pos·te'ri·o'res'
—sig'moi'de·ae'
—spi'na'les'
—spinales ex·ter'nae' an·te'ri·o'res'
—spinales externae pos·te'ri·o'res'
—spinales in·ter'nae'
—stel'la'tae'
—sub'cu·ta'ne·ae' ab·dom'i·nis
—su'pra·re·na'les'
—su'pra·troch'le·ar'es'
—tem'po·ra'les' pro·fun'-dae'
—temporales su·per·fi'ci·a'-les'
—The·be'si·i'
—tho·ra'ci·cae' in·ter'nae'
—tho·ra·co·ep·i'gas'tri·cae'
—thy'mi·cae'
—thy're·oi'de·ae' in·fe'ri·o'-res'
—thyreoideae su·pe'ri·o'-res'
—thy'roi'de·ae' me'di·ae'
—tib'i·a'les' an·te'ri·o'res'
—tibiales pos·te'ri·o'res'
—tra'che·a'les'
—trans·ver'sae' col'li'
—tym'pan'i·cae'
—ul'nar'es'
—u·ter'i'nae'
—ves'i·ca'les
—ves·tib'u·lar'es'
—vor'ti·co'sae'
ve·na'tion
ve'nec·ta'si·a
ve'nec'to·my
ve·neer'
ven'e·na'tion
ven'e·nif'er·ous
ven'e·nous
ve·ne're·al
ve·ne're·ol'o·gist
ve·ne're·ol'o·gy
ve·ne're·ro·pho'bi·a
ven'er·y

ven'e·sec'tion *also* venisection
ven'e·su'ture *also* venisuture
ven'in
ven'i·punc'ture
ven'i·sec'tion *var. of* venesection
ven'i·su'ture *var. of* venesuture
ve·no·a'tri·al
ve·noc'ly·sis *pl.* -ses'
ve'no·fi·bro'sis
ve'no·gram'
ve'no·graph'ic
ve·nog'ra·phy
ven'om
ven·o·mo·sal'i·var'y
ve'no·mo'tor
ven'om·ous
ve·no-oc·clu'sive
ve'no·per'i·to·ne·os'to·my
ve'no·pres'sor
ve'no·scle·ro'sis *pl.* -ses'
ve'nose'
ve'no·si'nal
ve·nos'i·ty
ve·nos'ta·sis
ve'no·throm·bot'ic
ve·not'o·my
ve'nous
ve'no·ve·nos'to·my
vent
ven'ter
—anterior mus'cu·li' di·gas'tri·ci'
—fron·ta'lis mus'cu·li' oc·cip'i·to·fron·ta'lis
—inferior mus'cu·li' o'mo·hy·oi'de·i'
—mus'cu·li'
—oc·cip'i·ta'lis mus'cu·li' oc·cip'i·to·fron·ta'lis
—posterior mus'cu·li' di·gas'tri·ci'
—superior mus'cu·li' o'mo·hy·oi'de·i'
ven'ti·late', -lat'ed, -lat'ing
ven'ti·la'tion
ven'ti·la'tor
ven'ti·lom'e·ter
ven'trad'
ven'tral

ven·tra′lis
ven′tri·cle
—of A·ran′ti·us
—of Mor·ga′gni
ven′tri·cor′nu *pl.* -nu·a
ven′tri·cose′
ven·tric′u·lar
ven·tric′u·lar·is
ven·tric′u·li′tis
ven·tric′u·lo·a′tri·al
ven·tric′u·lo·a′tri·os·to·my
ven·tric′u·lo·cis′ter·nos′-
  to·my
ven·tric′u·lo·cor·dec′to·my
ven·tric′u·lo·gram′
ven·tric′u·log′ra·phy
ven·tric′u·lo·jug′u·lar
ven·tric′u·lo·mas′toid·os′-
  to·my
ven·tric′u·lom′e·try
ven·tric′u·lo·nec′tor
ven·tric′u·lo·per′i·to·ne′al
ven·tric′u·lo·pleu′ral
ven·tric′u·lo·punc′ture
ven·tric′u·lo·scope′
ven·tric′u·los′co·py
ven·tric′u·los′to·my
ven·tric′u·lo·sub′a·rach′-
  noid′
ven·tric′u·lo·ve′nous
ven·tric′u·lus *pl.* -li′
  —cer′e·bri′
  —cor′dis
  —dex′ter
  —la·ryn′gis
  —laryngis (Mor·ga′gni·i′)
  —lat′er·a′lis
  —me′di·us
  —op′ti·cus
  —quar′tus
  —si·nis′ter
  —ter′mi·na′lis
  —ter′ti·us
ven′tri·cum′bent
ven′tri·duct′
ven′tri·duc′tion
ven′tri·lat′er·al
ven′tri·me′sal
ven′trim·e′son
ven′tro·cys·tor′rha·phy
ven′tro·fix·a′tion
ven′tro·hys′ter·o·pex′y
ven′tro·lat′er·al

ven′tro·me′di·al
ven′tro·me′di·an
ven′tro·pos·te′ri·or
ven′trop·to′sis *pl.* -ses′
ven·tros′co·py
ven·trose′
ven·tros′i·ty
ven′tro·sus·pen′sion
ven·trot′o·my
ven′tro·ves′i·co·fix·a′tion
ven′tu·rim′e·ter
ven·u′la *pl.* -lae′
  —mac′u·lar′is inferior
  —mascularis superior
  —me′di·a′lis ret′i·nae′
  —na′sa′lis ret′i·nae′ inferior
  —nasalis retinae superior
  —tem′po·ra′lis ret′i·nae′
    inferior
  —temporalis retinae
    superior
ven·u′lae′
  —rec′tae′
  —stel·la′tae′
ven·u′lar
ven′ule′
ve′nus
ve·ra′pa·mil
ve·rat′ri·dine′
ver′a·trine′
ve·ra′trum vir′i·dae′
ver′bal
ver′bal·ly
ver·big′er·a′tion
ver′bo·ma′ni·a
ver′di·gris′
ver′do·glo′bin
ver′do·nych′i·a
ver′do·per·ox′i·dase′
Ver′ga ventricle
verge
ver′gence
ver′ge·ture
Ver′hoeff′ stain
ver′mi·cid′al
ver′mi·cide′
ver·mic′u·lar
ver·mic′u·late
ver·mic′u·la′tion
ver′mi·cule′
ver·mic′u·lose′
ver·mic′u·lous
ver·mic′u·lus *pl.* li′

ver′mi·form′
ver′mi·fu′gal
ver′mi·fuge′
ver′mi·lin′gual
ver·mil′ion
ver·mil′ion·ec′to·my
ver′min
ver′mi·na′tion
ver·min·o′sis *pl.* -ses′
ver′min·ous
ver′mis *pl.* -mes′
ver′nal
Ver′ner-Mor′ri·son
  syndrome
Ver·net′ syndrome
Ver·neuil′
  —bursitis
  —disease
  —neuroma
ver′ni·er
ver′nix ca·se·o′sa
Ver′o·cay′ bodies
ver·ru′ca *pl.* -cae′
  —a·cu′mi·na′ta
  —dig′i·ta′ta
  —fi′li·for′mis
  —nec′ro·gen′i·ca
  —pe·ru′a′na
  —pe·ru′vi·a′na
  —pla′na ju′ve·ni′lis
  —plan·tar′is
  —se·ni′lis
  —vul·gar′is
ver·ru′ci·form′
ver·ru′coid′
ver·ru′cose′
ver·ru·co′sis *pl.* -ses′
ver·ru′cous
ver·ru′ga pe·ru·a′na
ver′si·col′or
ver′sion
ver′te·bra *pl.* -brae′ *or* -bras
  —den·ta′ta
  —mag′na
  —pla′na
  —prom′i·nens
ver′te·brae′
  —cer′vi·ca′les′
  —coc·cyg′e·ae′
  —lum·ba′les′
  —sa·cra′les′
  —tho′ra·ca′les′
  —tho′ra·ci·cae′

ver'te·bral
ver'te·brar'i·um
ver'te·brar·te'ri·al
Ver'te·bra'ta
ver'te·brate
ver'te·brec'to·my
ver'te·bro·ar·te'ri·al
ver'te·bro·chon'dral
ver'te·bro·cos'tal
ver'te·bro·fem'o·ral
ver'te·bro·il'i·ac'
ver'te·bro·sa'cral
ver'te·bro·ster'nal
ver'tex' *pl.* -tex'es *or* -ti·ces'
　—cor'ne·ae'
　—ve·si'cae'
ver'ti·cal
ver'ti·ca'lis
ver'ti·cil
ver'ti·cil·late'
ver·tig'i·nous
ver'ti·go *pl.* -goes *or*
　vertig'i·nes'
　—par'a·ly'sant
　—te·neb'ri·co'sa
ver·tig'ra·phy
ver'u·mon'ta·ni'tis
ver'u·mon'ta'num
Ve·sa'li·us
　—foramen
　—ligament
ve·sa'ni·a
ve·sa'nic
ve·si'ca *pl.* -cae'
　—bi·par'ta
　—du'plex'
　—fel'le·a
　—um·bil'i·ca'lis
　—u'ri·nar'i·a
ves'i·cal (*pertaining to a bladder*)
　♦vesicle
ves'i·cant
ves'i·cate', -cat'ed, -cat'ing
ves'i·ca'tion
ves'i·ca·to'ry
ves'i·cle (*a small bladder; bulla*)
　♦vesical
ves'i·co·ab·dom'i·nal
ves'i·co·bul'lous
ves'i·co·cele'
ves'i·co·cer'vi·cal
ves'i·co·en·ter'ic
ves'i·co·fix·a'tion

ves'i·co·in·tes'ti·nal
ves'i·co·pros·tat'ic
ves'i·co·pu'bic
ves'i·co·pu·den'dal
ves'i·co·pus'tu·lar
ves'i·co·pus'tule'
ves'i·co·rec'tal
ves'i·co·rec'to·vag'i·nal
ves'i·co·re'nal
ves'i·co·sig'moid'
ves'i·co·sig'moid·os'to·my
ves'i·co·spi'nal
ves'i·cos'to·my
ves'i·cot'o·my
ves'i·co·um·bil'i·cal
ves'i·co·u·re'ter·al
ves'i·co·u·re'ter·o·gram'
ves'i·co·u·re'thral
ves'i·co·u·re'thro·vag'i·nal
ves'i·co·u'ter·ine
ves'i·co·u'ter·o·vag'i·nal
ves'i·co·vag'i·nal
ve·sic'u·la *pl.* -lae'
　—fel'le·a
　—oph·thal'mi·ca
　—op'ti·ca in·ver'sa
　—pros·tat'i·ca
　—sem'i·na'lis
ve·sic'u·lar
ve·sic'u·late'
ve·sic'u·la'tion
ve·sic'u·lec'to·my
ve·sic'u·li·form'
ve·sic'u·li'tis
ve·sic'u·lo·bron'chi·al
ve·sic'u·lo·bul'lous
ve·sic'u·lo·cav'ern·ous
ve·sic'u·lo·gram'
ve·sic'u·log'ra·phy
ve·sic'u·lo·pap'u·lar
ve·sic'u·lo·pus'tu·lar
ve·sic'u·lot'o·my
ve·sic'u·lo·tym·pan'ic
ves'sel
ves·tib'u·lar
ves'ti·bule'
ves·tib'u·li'tis
ves·tib'u·lo·cer'e·bel'lar
ves·tib'u·lo·coch'le·ar
ves·tib'u·lo·oc'u·lar
ves·tib'u·lo·plas'ty
ves·tib'u·lo·spi'nal
ves·tib'u·lot'o·my

ves·tib'u·lo·u·re'thral
ves·tib'u·lum *pl.* -la
　—au'ris in·ter'nae'
　—bur'sae' o'men·ta'lis
　—lab'y·rin'thi' os'se·i'
　—la·ryn'gis
　—na'si'
　—o'ris
　—va·gi'nae'
ves'tige
ves·tig'i·al
ves·tig'i·um *pl.* -i·a
　—pro·ces'sus vag'i·na'lis
ve'ta
vet'er·i·nar'i·an
vet'er·i·nar'y
ve'to
vi'a *pl.* vi'ae'
vi'a·bil'i·ty
vi'a·ble
vi'al
vi'be·sate'
vi'bex' *pl.* -bi·ces'
vi'brate', -brat'ed, -brat'ing
vi'bra·tile
vi'bra'tion
vi'bra'tor
vi'bra·to'ry
vib'ri·o'
Vib'ri·o'
　—chol'er·ae'
　—com'ma
　—fe'tus
vi·bri·on' sep·tique'
vib'ri·o'sis *pl.* -ses'
vi·bris'sa *pl.* -sae'
vi'bro·car'di·o·gram'
vi'bro·mas·sage'
vi'bro·ther'a·peu'tics
vi·car'i·ous
vice
vi'cious
Vicq d'A·zyr'
　—fasciculus
　—foramen
vi'da·ra·bine'
vid'e·o·an'gi·og'ra·phy
vid'e·o·fluo·rog'ra·phy
vid'e·o·fluo·ros'co·py
vid'e·og·no'sis
vid'e·o·ra'di·og'ra·phy
vid'i·an
Vieus·sens'

—annulus
—ansa
—ganglion
—isthmus
—loop
—ring
—valve
—ventricle
view
vig'il
vig·il·am'bu·lism
vig'i·lance
vig'or·ous
Vil·la·ret' syndrome
vil'li'
 —in·tes'ti·na'les'
 —pleu·ra'les'
 —sy·no'vi·a'les'
vil'i·ki'nin
vil·li'tis
vil·lo'ma pl. -mas or -ma·ta
vil'lose'
vil·lo·si'tis
vil·los'i·ty
vil'lous (pertaining to a villus)
 ♦villus
vil'lus (any minute projection
 arising from a mucous
 membrane), pl. -li'
 ♦villous
vil'lus·ec'to·my
vin·bar'bi·tal'
vin·blas'tine'
vin'ca·leu'ko·blas'tine'
Vin'ca ro'se·a
Vin'cent
 —angina
 —disease
 —gingivitis
 —infection
 —stomatitis
vin·cris'tine'
vin'cu·la
 —lin'gu·lae' cer'e·bel'li'
 —ten'di·num dig'i·to'rum
  ma'nus
 —tendinum digitorum
  pe'dis
vin'cu·lum pl. -la
 —brev'e'
 —lon'gum
 —ten'di·num
vin'de·sine'

Vine'berg' procedure
vin'e·gar
vin·gly'ci·nate'
vi'nic
vin·leu'ro·sine'
vi'nous
Vin'son syndrome
vi'nyl
vi'nyl·ben'zene'
vi'nyl·ene'
vi·nyl'i·dene'
vi'o·la'ceous
vi'o·la·quer'ci·trin
vi'o·la'tion
vi'o·my'cin
vi·os'ter·ol'
vi'per
Vi·per'i·dae'
vi·po'ma pl. -mas or -ma·ta
vi'ral
Vir'chow'
 —angle
 —cell
 —crystals
 —line
 —node
 —psammoma
Vir'chow-Rob'in spaces
vi·re'mi·a
vi·re'mic
vir'gin
vir'gin·al
vir·gin'i·ty
vir·gin'i·um
vir'i·dans'
vi·rid'in
vi·rid'o·ful'vin
vir'ile
vir'i·les'cence
vir'i·les'cent
vi·ril'i·a
vir'i·lism
vi·ril'i·ty
vir'i·li·za'tion
vir'i·lize', -ized', -liz'ing
vi'ri·on'
vi·rip'o·tent
vi'ro·cyte'
vi·rol'o·gist
vi·rol'o·gy
vi'ro·pex'is
vir'tu·al
vi'ru·cid'al

vi'ru·cide'
vir'u·lence
vir'u·lent
vi'ru·lif'er·ous
vi·ru'ri·a
vi'rus
vi'ru·stat'ic
vis pl. vi'res'
 —a fron'te'
 —a ter'go
 —con'ser'va'trix
 —for'ma'ti'va
 —in·er'ti·ae'
 —in si'tu'
 —med'i·ca'trix na·tu'rae'
 —vi'tae'
vis·am'min
vis'cer·ad'
vis'cer·al
vis'cer·a lar'va mi'grans'
vis'cer·al'gi·a
vis'cer·o·car'di·ac'
vis'cer·o·cep'tor
vis'cer·o·in·hib'i·to'ry
vis'cer·o·meg'a·ly
vis'cer·o·mo'tor
vis'cer·o·pa·ri'e·tal
vis'cer·o·per'i·to·ne'al
vis'cer·o·pleu'ral
vis'cer·op·to'sis pl. -ses'
vis'cer·o·sen'so·ry
vis'cer·o·skel'e·tal
vis'cer·o·so·mat'ic
vis'cer·o·tome'
vis'cer·ot'o·my
vis'cer·o·to'ni·a
vis'cer·o·ton'ic
vis'cer·o·troph'ic
vis'cer·o·trop'ic
vis'cid
vis·cid'i·ty
vis'co·e·las·tic'i·ty
vis·com'e·ter
vis·com'e·try
vis·co·sim'e·ter
vis·co·sim'e·try
vis·cos'i·ty
vis'cous (glutinous)
 ♦viscus
vis'cus (any of the organs
 enclosed in the cranium, thorax,
 abdomen, or pelvis), pl. -cer·a
 ♦viscous

vis'i·bil'i·ty
vis'i·ble
vis'i·bly
vi'sion
vis'u·al
vis'u·al·i·za'tion
vis'u·al·ize', -ized', -iz'ing
vis'u·o·au'di·to'ry
vis'u·og·no'sis
vis'u·o·mo'tor
vis'u·o·psy'chic
vis'u·o·sen'so·ry
vis'u·o·spa'tial
vi'sus
  —ac'ris
  —brev'i·or'
  —col'o·ra'tus
  —de·bil'i·tas
  —de·col'o·ra'tus
  —dim'i·di·a'tus
  —di·ur'nus
  —du'pli·ca'tus
  —heb'e·tu'do'
  —ju've·num
  —lu'ci·dus
  —mus·car'um
  —se·ni'lis
  —vi'tae'
vi'tal
vi'tal·ism
vi·tal'i·ty
vi'tal·ize', -ized', -iz'ing
vi'ta·lom'e·ter
vi'tals
vi'ta·mer
vi'ta·min
vit'el·lar'y
vi·tel'li·cle
vi·tel'li·form'
vi·tel'lin (a protein found in egg
  yolk)
  ♦vitelline
vi·tel'line' (pertaining to the
  vitellus)
  ♦vitellin
vi·tel'lo·gen'e·sis pl. -ses'
vi·tel'lo·lu'te·in
vi·tel'lo·mes'en·ter'ic
vi·tel'lo·ru'bin
vi·tel'lus pl. -li'
  —o'vi'
vi'ti·a'tion
vit'i·lig'i·nes'

vit'i·lig'i·nous
vit'i·li'go'
  —cap'i·tis
  —i'ri·dis
vi·trec'to·my
vi·trec'tor
vit're·o·den'tin
vit're·ous
vit're·um
vit'ric
vit'ri·fi·ca'tion
vi·tri'na
  —au'di·to'ri·a
  —au'ris
  —oc'u·lar'is
vit'ri·ol'
vit'ri·ol'ic
vit'ro·pres'sion
vit'rum
viv'i·di·al'y·sis
viv'i·dif·fu'sion
viv'i·fi·ca'tion
viv'i·par'i·ty
vi·vip'a·rous
viv'i·sect'
viv'i·sec'tion
viv'i·sec'tion·ist
viv'i·sec'tor
Vla'di·mir'off-Mik'u·licz
  amputation
vo'cal
vo·ca'lis
Vo'ges-Pros'kau'er
  —reaction
  —test
Vogt
  —disease
  —point
  —syndrome
voice, voiced, voic'ing
void
Voille·mier' point
vo'la
  —ma'nus
vo'lar
vo·la'ris
vol'a·tile
vol'a·til·i·za'tion
vol'a·til·ize', -ized', -iz'ing
vol·az'o·cine'
vo·le'mic
Vol'hard' test
vo·li'tion

vo·li'tion·al
Volk'mann
  —canals
  —contracture
vol'ley
Voll'mer patch test
volt
volt'age
vol·ta'ic
vol'ta·ism
volt'am'me'ter
volt'-am'pere'
volt'me'ter
Vol'to·li'ni disease
vol'ume
vol'u·me·nom'e·ter
vol'u·met'ric
vol'u·mom'e·ter
vol'un·tar'y
vo·lute'
vol'vu·lo'sis
vol'vu·lus
vo'mer
vo'mer·ine'
vo'mer·o·bas'i·lar
vom'er·o·na'sal
vom'i·cose'
vom'it
vom'i·tive
vóm'i·to' ne'gro'
vom'i·to'ry
vom'i·tu·ri'tion
vom'i·tus
  —cru·en'tes'
  —ma·ri'nus
  —mat'u·ti'nus
  —ni'ger
von Ec'o·no'mo disease
von Gier'ke disease
von Grae'fe sign
von Hip'pel-Lin'dau'
  disease
von Jaksch anemia
von Kós'sa stain
von Pir·quet' test
von Reck'ling·hau'sen
  —disease
  —hemofuscin
von Ro'ki·tan'sky disease
von Wil'le·brand' disease
Voor'hees bag
Voor'hoeve disease
vo·ra'cious

Vo'ro·noff' operation
vor'tex' *pl.* -ti·ces'
—coc·cyg'e·us
—cor'dis
—len'tis
vor'ti·ces' pi·lo'rum
vor'ti·cose'
Vos'si·us ring
vox
vo·yeur'
vo·yeur'ism
Vro'lik disease
vu'e·rom'e·ter
vul'can·ize', -ized', -iz'ing
vul·ga'ris
vul'ner·a·bil'i·ty
vul'ner·a·ble
vul'nus *pl.* -ner·a
Vul'pi·an
—atrophy
—effect
—reaction
Vul'pi·us-Com'pere
operation
vul·sel'lum *pl.* -la
vul'va
—con·ni'vens
—hi'ans'
vul'vae' a·cu'tum ul'cus
vul'val
vul'var
vul·vec'to·my
vul·vis'mus
vul·vi'tis
vul'vo·rec'tal
vul'vo·u'ter·ine
vul'vo·vag'i·nal
vul'vo·vag'i·ni'tis

W

Waar'den·burg syndrome
Wa'chen·stein-Zak'
method
Wa'da
—technique
—test
wad'ding
wad'dle
wa'fer
Wag'ner
—corpuscles
—operation

Wag'ner-Jau'regg'
treatment
Wag'staffe' fracture
Wahl sign
waist
waist'line'
wake'ful·ness
Wal'cher position
Wal'den·ström'
—disease
—macroglobulinemia
—syndrome
Wal'dey'er
—fossae
—glands
—ring
walk
walk'er
wall
Wal'lace-Di'a·mond
method
Wal'len·berg' syndrome
Wal·le'ri·an
—degeneration
—law
wall'eye'
Wal'thard' inclusions
Wal'ther
—ganglion
—ligament
Wal'ton operation
wan'der·ing
Wan'gen·steen'
—apparatus
—tube
Wang test
War'burg' apparatus
ward
War'dill
—method
—operation
War'drop
—disease
—method
Ward triangle
war'fa·rin
warm'-blood'ed
warmth
War'ner hand
War'ren
—incision
—operation
wart

War'ten·berg'
—disease
—sign
War'thin
—sign
—tumor
War'thin-Fin'kel·dey' cell
wart'y
wash'er
wash'ing
wash'out'
Was'ser·mann
—antibody
—test
Was'ser·mann-fast'
waste, wast'ed, wast'ing
wa'ter
wa'ter·fall'
Wa'ter·house-
Fri'der·ich·sen syndrome
wa'ters
Wa'ters
—projection
—view
wa'ter·shed'
wa'ter·y
Wat'son-Crick' model
Wat'son method
Wat'son-Schwartz' test
watt
watt'age
watt'me'ter
watt'-sec'ond
wave
wave'form'
wave'length'
wax
weak'ness
wean
web, webbed, web'bing
Web'er
—disease
—glands
—law
—organ
—paralysis
—syndrome
—test
Web'er-Chris'tian disease
Web'er-Di·mi'tri-
Ka'li·scher syndrome
Web'ster
—operation

—test
Wechs'ler Adult
  Intelligence Scale
Wechs'ler-Belle'vue'
  Intelligence Scale
We·den'sky
  —facilitation
  —inhibition
wedge
weep'ing
We'ge·ner granulomatosis
Weg'ner disease
Weich'sel·baum' coccus
Wei'del reaction
Wei'gert
  —law
  —method
  —stain
weight
weight'bear'ing
Weil
  —disease
  —stain
  —test
Weil'-Fe'lix
  —reaction
  —test
Wein'back' method
Wein'grow' reflex
Weir operation
Weis'bach' angle
Weis'mann theory
Weiss sign
Weit'brecht ligament
Welch bacillus
Wells facies
Wells'-Sten'ger test
wen
Wenck'e·bach'
  —block
  —period
  —phenomenon
Werd'nig-Hoff'mann
  atrophy
Werl'hof' disease
Wer'ne·kinck'
  commissure
Wer'ner
  —disease
  —syndrome
Wer'ner-His' disease
Wer'nick·e

—aphasia
—area
—disease
—encephalopathy
—syndrome
Wer'nick·e-Kor·sa'koff
  syndrome
Wer'nick·e-Mann'
  paralysis
Wert'heim' operation
Wert'heim-Schau'ta
  operation
Werth tumor
Wes'sels·bron' fever
Wes'ter·gren
  —method
  —sedimentation rate
West'phal'
  —disease
  —maneuver
  —nucleus
  —sign
West'phal-Pilcz' reflex
West'phal-Strüm'pell
  pseudosclerosis
West syndrome
Wet'zel grid
We'ver-Bray' phenomenon
Weyl test
Whar'ton
  —duct
  —jelly
  —tumor
wheal
wheel'chair'
Wheel'house' operation
wheeze, wheezed, wheez'ing
whey
whip'lash'
Whip'ple
  —disease
  —operation
  —triad
whip'worm'
whirl'pool'
whis'per
White
  —method
  —operation
white'head'
White'head'
  —deformity

—operation
white'pox'
Whit'field' ointment
whit'low'
Whit'man operation
Whit'more' bacillus
whole
whoop'ing cough
whorl
Whytt
  —disease
Wi'berg
  —classification
  —reflex
Wick'ham striae
wick'ing
Wi·dal'
  —syndrome
  —test
wide'spread'
Wig'and maneuver
Wil·cox'on test
Wild'bolz' reaction
Wil'der·muth ear
Wil'der test
Wilks
  —disease
  —syndrome
Wil'liam·son sign
Wil'liams syndrome
Wil'lis
  —circle
  —nerve
  —paracusis
Wilms tumor
Wil'son
  —disease
  —sign
Wil'son-Mik'i·ty syndrome
wince
Winck'el disease
wind'age
wind'burn'
wind'chill'
wind'kes'sel
win'dow
wind'pipe'
Win'i·war'ter-Buer'ger
  disease
Win'i·war'ter operation
Wins'low
  —foramen

—pancreas
—stars
Win'ter·bot'tom sign
Win'ter·nitz sound
Win'trich sign
Win'trobe'-Lands'berg' method
Win'trobe' method
wire
Wir'sung
—canal
—duct
wir'y
wish'-ful·fill'ment
Wis'kott-Al'drich syndrome
with·draw'al
with·drawn'
Wit'zel operation
wit'zel·sucht'
Wohl·fahr'ti·a
—mag·nif'i·ca
—o'pa·ca
—vig'il
Wohl'ge·muth' test
Wolff
—law
—method
Wolff'-Eis'ner test
wolff'i·an
Wolff'-Par'kin·son-White' syndrome
Wöl'fler operation
wolf'ram
Wol'fring glands
Wol·hyn'i·an fever
Wol'las·ton doublet
Wol'man disease
womb
Wong method
Wood
—light
—muscle
Wool'ner tip
wool'sort'ers disease
work'load'
work'up'
worm
wound
wo'ven
W'-plas'ty
wrap

wreath
Wre'den
—operation
—sign
Wre'den-Stone' operation
wrench
Wright
—stain
—syndrome
wrin'kle
Wris'berg'
—cartilage
—ganglion
—ligament
—nerve
wrist
wrist'drop'
wry'neck'
Wu'cher atrophy
Wu'cher·e'ri·a
—ban'crof'ti'
—ma·lay'i'
wu'cher·e·ri'a·sis pl. -ses'
Wun'der·lich curve
Wundt tetanus
Wy'lie operation

X

xan'thate'
xan'the·las'ma pl. -mas or -ma·ta
xan'the·las'ma·to'sis
xan·the'ma·tin
xan·the'mi·a
xan'thene' (non-nitrogenous compound)
♦ xanthine
xan'thic
xan'thine' (nitrogenous compound)
♦ xanthene
xan'thi·nol' ni'a·cin'ate'
xan'thi·nu'ri·a
xan'thi·nu'ric
xan'thi·u'ri·a
xan'tho·chro·mat'ic
xan'tho·chro'mi·a
xan'tho·chro'mic
xan'thoch'ro·ous
xan'tho·cy'a·nop'si·a
xan'tho·cy·no'pi·a

xan'tho·cyte'
xan'tho·der'ma
xan'tho·don'tous
xan'tho·fi·bro'ma the'co· cel'lu·lar'e'
xan'tho·gran'u·lo'ma
pl. -mas or -ma·ta
xan'tho·gran'u·lo'ma·to'sis
xan'tho·gran'u·lom'a·tous
xan'tho·ky·an·o'py
xan·tho'ma pl. -mas or -ma·ta
—di'a·bet'i·co'rum
—dis·sem'i·na'tum
—pal'pe·brar'um
—tu'ber·o'sum
—tuberosum mul'ti·plex'
xan·tho'ma·to'sis pl. -ses'
xan·tho'ma·tous
xan'thone'
xan'tho·phane'
xan'tho·phore'
xan'tho·phose'
xan'tho·phyll
xan·tho'pi·a
xan'tho·pro·te'ic
xan'tho·pro'tein'
xan·thop'si·a
xan·thop'sin
xan·thop'ter·in
xan'tho·rham'nin
xan'thor·rhe'a
xan'tho·sar·co'ma pl. -mas or -ma·ta
xan'tho·sine'
xan·tho'sis pl. -ses'
—fun'di' di'a·bet'i·ca
xan'tho·tox'in
xan'thous
xan'thu·re'nic
xan·thu'ri·a
xan·thy'drol'
xan·thyl'ic
xan'to·ru'bin
xen'o·bi·ot'ic
xen'o·di·ag·no'sis pl. -ses'
xen'o·ge·ne'ic
xen'o·gen'e·sis
xen'o·gen'ic
xe·nog'e·nous
xen'o·graft'
xe·nol'o·gy

xen′o·me′ni·a
xe′non′
xen′o·par′a·site′
xen′o·pho′bi·a
xen′o·pho′ni·a
xen′oph·thal′mi·a
xen′o·plas′tic
xen′o·plas′ty
Xen′op·syl′la
—che·o′pis
xe·ran′sis
xe·ran′tic
xe·ra′si·a
xe′ro·chei′li·a
xe′ro·der′ma
—pig′men·to′sum
xe′ro·der′mos·te·o′sis
xe·rog′ra·phy
xe·ro′ma *pl.* -mas *or* -ma·ta
xe′ro·mam·mog′ra·phy
xe′ro·me·ni·a
xe′ro·myc·te′ri·a
xe′ro·pha′gi·a
xe·roph′a·gy
xe′roph·thal′mi·a
xe′ro·ra′di·og′ra·phy
xe·ro′sis *pl.* -ses′
—con′junc·ti′vae′
—in·fan′ti·lis
xe′ro·sto′mi·a
xe′ro·tes′
xe·rot′ic
xe′ro·to′ci·a
xe′ro·trip′sis
xiph′i·ster′nal
xiph′i·ster′num
xiph′o·cos′tal
xi·phod′y·mus
xiph′o·dyn′i·a
xiph′oid′
xiph′oid·i′tis
xi·phop′a·gus
xiph′o·um·bil′i·cal
x′-ray′ *or* X′-ray′
xy·lam′i·dine′
xy′lene′
xy′le·nol′
xy′li·dine′ pon·ceau′
xy′lol′
xy′lo·me·taz′o·line′
xy′lose′
xy′lo·su′ri·a
xy′lyl

xy′ro·spasm
xys′ma
xys′ter

Y

YAG laser
yaw′ey
yawn
yaws
yeast
Yer·sin′i·a
—en′ter·o·co·lit′i·ca
—pes′tis
—pseu′do·tu·ber′cu·lo′sis
yer·sin′i·o′sis
yo′gurt
yo·him′bine′
yolk
York′-Yendt′ syndrome
Yo·shi′da tumor
Young
—method
—operation
y′per·ite′
yp·sil′i·form′
yt·ter′bi·um
yt′tri·um
Yu′ge syndrome
Y·von′ test

Z

Zang space
ze·a·tin
ze′a·xan′thin
Zee′man effect
Zeis glands
Zei·tels′ procedure
Zel′ler test
Zell′weg·er syndrome
Zen′ker
—degeneration
—diverticulum
—fixative
—pouch
ze′o·lite′
ze′ro
zeug′ma·tog′ra·phy
zi·do′vu·dine′
Zie′hen-Op′pen·heim′
  disease
Ziehl′-Neel′sen

—method
—stain
Ziems′sen point
Zieve syndrome
Zi′ka fever
Zim′mer·lin type
Zim′mer·mann
—corpuscle
—reaction
zinc
zinc·if′er·ous
zinc′oid′
zin′gi·ber
Zinn
—annulus
—artery
—ligament
zir·co′ni·um
zo′a·can·tho′sis *pl.* -ses′
zo·an′thro·py
zo·la·mine′
zo′ler·tine′
Zol′lin·ger-El′li·son
  syndrome
Zöll′ner lines
zo′me·pir′ac
zo′na *pl.* -nae′
—ar′cu·a′ta
—car′ti·la·gin′e·a
—cil′i·ar′is
—co′lum·nar′is rec′ti′
—cu·ta′ne·a rec′ti′
—den·tic′u·la′ta
—fas·cic′u·la′ta
—glo·mer′u·lo′sa
—hem′or·rhoi·da′lis
—in·cer′ta
—in′ter·me′di·a rec′ti′
—oph·thal′mi·ca
—or·bic′u·lar′is
—pec′ti·na′ta
—pel·lu′ci·da
—per′fo·ra′ta
—re·tic′u·lar′is
—spon′gi·o′sa
—tec′ta
zo′nal
zo′na·ry
zo′nate′
zone
zo′nes·the′si·a
zo·nif′u·gal
zon′ing

zo·nip'e·tal
zo·nog'ra·phy
zo'nu·la *pl.* -lae'
—ad·hae'rens
—cil'i·ar'is
—ciliaris (Zin'ni·i')
—oc·clu'dens
zo'nu·lar
zo'nule'
—of Zinn
zo'nu·li'tis
zo'nu·lol'y·sis
zo'nu·lot'o·my
zo'nu·ly'sis
zo'o·chem'is·try
zo'o·der'mic
zo'o·e·ras'ti·a
zo'o·gen'ic
zo·og'e·nous
zo·og'e·ny
zo'o·ge·og'ra·phy
zo'o·gle'a *pl.* -as *or* -ae'
zo·og'o·ny
zo'o·graft'
zo'o·graft'ing
zo'o·lag'ni·a
zo·ol'o·gist
zo·ol'o·gy
Zo'o·mas'ti·gi'na
zo'o·no'sis *pl.* -ses'
zo'o·not'ic
zo'o·par'a·site'
zo'o·par'a·sit'ic
zo'o·pa·thol'o·gy
zo·oph'a·gous
zo'o·phile'
zo'o·phil'ic
zo·oph'i·lism

zo'o·pho'bi·a
zo'o·plas'tic
zo'o·plas'ty
zo·op'si·a
zo'o·sperm'
zo'o·sper'mi·a
zo'o·spore'
zo·os'ter·ol'
zo'o·tech'nics
zo'o·tox'in
zo'o·troph'ic
zos'ter
—au·ric'u·lar'is
—bra'chi·a'lis
—fa·ci·a'lis
—fem'o·ra'lis
—oph·thal'mi·cus
zos·ter'i·form'
zos'ter·oid'
Z'-plas'ty
zuck'er·guss'
Zuck'er·kandl
—bodies
—convolution
zy'gal
zyg'a·poph'y·se'al
zyg'a·poph'y·sis *pl.* -ses'
zyg'i·on' *pl.* -i·a *or* -i·ons'
zy'go·dac'ty·ly
zy·go'ma *pl.* -ma·ta *or* -mas
zy'go·mat'ic
zy'go·mat'i·co·au·ric'u·lar'is *pl.* -es'
zy'go·mat'i·co·fa'cial
zy'go·mat'i·co·fron'tal
zy'go·mat'i·co·max'il·lar'y
zy'go·mat'i·co·or'bit·al
zy'go·mat'i·co·tem'po·ral

zy'go·mat'i·cus
zy'go·max'il·lar'y
zy'go·my'cete'
zy'go·my·ce'tous
zy'go·my·co'sis *pl.* -ses'
zy'gon
zy'go·ne'ma
zy·gos'i·ty
zy'go·sperm'
zy'go·spore'
zy'go·style'
zy'gote'
zy'go·tene'
zy·got'ic
zy'mase'
zyme
zy'mic
zy'mo·gen
zy'mo·gen'ic
zy·mog'e·nous
zy'mo·gram'
zy'mo·hex'ase'
zy'mo·hy·drol'y·sis *pl.* -ses'
zy'moid'
zy'mo·log'ic
zy·mol'o·gy
zy·mol'y·sis
zy'mo·lyte'
zy'mo·lyt'ic
zy'mom'e·ter
zy'mo·phore'
zy'mo·phor'ic
zy'mo·plas'tic
zy'mo·pro'tein'
zy·mo'sis *pl.* -ses'
zy·mos'ter·ol'
zy·xot'ic

Trade Names of Drugs

This list contains the names of many commonly used drugs.

Abbokinase	Akineton	Amino-Cerv	Antrocol
Abbo-Pac	Akrinol	Aminolete	Anturane
Accupril	Albalon	Amino Min D	Anusol-HC
Accurbron	Albamycin	Aminomine	Apatate
Accutane	Albuminar	Aminoplex	Aphrodyne
Aches-N-Pain	Albumotope	Aminostasis	Aplisol
Achromycin	Albutein	Aminosyn II	Aplitest
Achromycin V	Alcaine	Aminotate	Appecon
Aci-Jel	Aldactazide	Aminovirox	Apresazide
Aclovate	Aldactone	Aminoxin	Apresoline
Acnederm	Aldoclor	Amino Zn	AquaMephyton
Acnomel	Aldomet	Amipaque	Aquanil
Actahist	Aldoril	Amitril	Aquaphor
Acthar	Alfenta	Amnestrogen	Aquaphyllin
Actibine	Alferon N	Amoxil	AquaTar
Acticort	Alimentum	Amphicol	Aquatensen
Actidil	Alka-Mints	Amphojel	Aralen
Actidose	Alka-Seltzer	Anacin	Aramine
Actidose-Aqua	Alkeran	Anacin-3	Arco-Lase
Actifed	Allbee C	Anadrol-50	Arduan
Actigall	Allent	Anafranil	Arfonad
Actin-N	Allerest	Ana-Kit	Aristocort
Activase	Allerfed	Analpram-HC	Aristospan
Acutrim	Alphacaine	Anaprox	Arlidin
Acylanid	Alphacaine HCL	Anaspaz	Artane
Adagen	Alphaderm	Anatuss	Asbron G
Adalat	Alphadrol	Anavar	Ascriptin A/D
Adapin	Alpha Keri	Anbesol	Asendin
Adenocard	Alpha Plus	Ancef	Astramorph
Adipex-P	Alphatrex	Ancobon	Atabrine
Adipost	Alramucil	Androdiol	Atarax
Adrenalin	Altace	Android	Athrombin-K
Adriamycin PFS	Alterna	Anectine	Ativan
Adriamycin RDF	ALternaGEL	Anestacon	ATnativ Antithrom-
Advil	Alu-Cap	Anexsia	bin III
Aerobid	Aludrox	Angio-Conray	Atrac-Tain
AeroChamber	Alupent	Anhydron	Atrohist L.A.
Aerolate	Alurate	Ansaid	Atromid-S
Aerolate III	Alu-Tab	Anspor	Atrovent
Aerolate JR	Ambenyl	Antabuse	Attenuvax
Aerolate SR	Ambenyl-D	Antepar	Augmentin
Aerolone	Ambodryl	Anthra-Derm	Auralgan
Aeroseb-Dex	Amen	Anthramine	Aureomycin
Aeroseb-HC	Americaine	Antilirium	Autoplex T
Aerosporin	Amicar	Antiminth	Axid
Afrin	Amidate	Antivenin	Axsain
Afrinol	Amikin	Antivert	Aygestin
Aftate	Aminess	Antrenyl	Azactam

Azdone
Azlin
Azmacort
Azo Gantanol
Azo Gantrisin
Azulfidine

Baciguent
Bactine
Bactocill
Bactrim
Bactroban
Balmex
Balneol
Balnetar
Bancap HC
Banthine
Basaljel
Beano
Beclovent
Beconase
Beelith
Bellergal-S
Bell-O-Gesic
Benadryl
Benemid
Ben-Gay
Benoquin
Bentyl
Benylin
Benzac
Benzagel
Benzamycin
Benzedrex
Berocca
Berubigen
Beta-2
Betadine
Betapen-VK
Betatrex
Betoptic
Biavax
Bicillin
Bicitra
BiCNU
Bilezyme
Bilivist
Bilopaque
Bioscrub
Biltricide
Biocef
Biomox
Biotin Forte

Biphetamine
BlemErase
Blenoxane
Bleph-10
Bleph-30
Blinx
Blocadren
Bluboro
Bonine
Bontril
Breezee
Brethaire
Brethancer
Brethine
Bretylium
Bretylol
Brevibloc
Brevicon
Brevital
Brexin L.A.
Bricanyl
Bristamycin
Bromarest DX
Bromase
Bromfed
Bromfed-DM
Bromfed-PD
Broncholate
Bronkephrine
Bronkodyl
Bronkolixir
Bronkometer
Bronkosol/Bronko-
  meter
Bronkotabs
Bucladin-S
Bufferin
Bumex
Buminate
Buprenex
BuSpar
Buta-Barb
Butazolidin
Butesin
Butisol

Cafergot
Calan SR
Cal-Bid
Calcet
Calcibind
Calci-Chew
Calcidrine

Calcimar
Calci-Mix
Calciparine
CaldeCORT
Calderol
Caldesene
Calel-D
Calphosan
Cal-Plus
Caltrate
Cama
Camalox
Camoquin
Cantharone
Cantil
Capastat
Capitrol
Capoten
Capozide
Carafate
Carbocaine
Cardene
Cardilate
Cardiografin
Cardiolite
Cardioquin
Cardiotec
Cardizem
Cardizem SR
Cardura
Carmol
Carnitor
Carotene-E
Carpuject
Cartrol
Castellani Paint
Catapres
Catemine
Ceclor
Cedilanid-D
CeeNU
Cefadyl
Cefizox
Cefobid
Cefol
Cefotan
Ceftin
Cefzil
Celestone
Celontin
Centrax
Centrum
Ceo-Two
Cēpacol

CEPASTAT
Cephulac
Cerose-DM
Cerubidine
Cerumenex
Cetacaine
Cetaphil
Cetylcide
Cevi-Bid
Cevi-Fer
Chemstrip
Cheracol
Chlor-3
Chlorafed
Chloraseptic
Chloresium
Chloromycetin
Chloroptic
Chlor-Trimeton
Cholac
Cholebrine
Choledyl
Cholografin
Choloxin
Cholybar
Chromagen
Chronulac
Cibalith-S
Cinobac
Cipro
Citanest
Citrical
Citrolith
Claforan
Clear Eyes
Clearasil
Cleocin
Clinoril
Clistin
Clofibrate
Clomid
Clorpactin
Cloxapen
Clozaril
CoAdvil
Codiclear DH
Codimal DH
Codimal DM
Codimal-L.A.
Codimal PH
Cogentin
Co-Gesic
Colace
ColBENEMID

Colestid
Collyrium Fresh
ColoCare
ColoScreen
Coly-Mycin M
Coly-Mycin S
Colyte
Combipres
Comhist LA
Compazine
Complete
Complex-Cho
Comtrex
Conceptrol
Congespirin
Congestac
Conray
Constant-T
Constilac
Contac
Coppertone
Cordarone
Cordran
Cordran-N
Cordran SP
Corgard
Coricidin
Correctol
Cortaid
Cort-Dome
Cortef
Cortenema
Cortifoam
Cortisporin
Cortone
Cortril
Cortrosyn
Corzide
Cosmegen
Cotazym
Cotazym-S
Cotrim
Coumadin
Creon
Cruex
Crystodigin
Cuprimine
Curretab
Cyclapen-W
Cyclocort
Cyclogyl
Cyclopar
Cylert
Cycrin

Cyklockapron
Cylert
Cysto-Conray
Cystospaz
Cystospaz M
Cytadren
Cytomel
Cytosar-U
Cytotec
Cytovene
Cytoxan

Dalalone D.P.
Dalgan
Dallergy
Dalmane
Damason-P
Danex
Danocrine
Dantrium
Daranide
Daraprim
Darbid
Daricon
Darvocet-N
Darvon
Darvon-N
Datril
Dayalets
Deapril-ST
Debrisan
Debrox
Decaderm
Decadron
Deca-Durabolin
Decapryn
Decaspray
Decholin
Declomycin
Deconamine SR
Deconsal
Delalutin
Delatestryl
Delestrogen
Delfen
Delta-Cortef
Deltalin
Deltasone
Demazin
Demerol
Demi-Regroton
Demser
Demulen

Denorex
Depakene
Depakote
Depen
Depo-Estradiol
Depo-Medrol
Deponit NTG
Depo-Provera
Depo-Testosterone
Deprol
Derifil
Dermaide
Dermolate
Dermoplast
Desenex
Desferal
Desitin
DesOwen
Desoxyn
Despec
Desquam-E
Desquam-X
Desyrel
Dexedrine
DiaBeta
Diabinese
Dialose
Diamox
Diapid
Dibenzyline
Dical-D
Dicumarol
Dicurin
Didrex
Didronel
Diflucan
Di-Gel
Digestol
Digibind
Dilantin-30
Dilantin Infatabs
Dilantin Kapseals
Dilantin-SR
Dilaudid
Dilaudid H-P
Dilor
Dimacol
Dimetane
Dimetane-DC
Dimetane-DX
Dimetapp
Dimetapp-DM
Dionosil
Diprivan

Diprolene
Diprosone
Diquinol
Disalcid
Disipal
Disonate
Disophrol
Ditropan
Diucardin
Diulo
Diupres
Diuril
Diutensen-R
Doan's Pills
Dobutrex
Doca
Dolacet
Dolene
Dolobid
Dolophine
Domeboro
Donatussin
Donnagel
Donnagel-PG
Donnatal
Donnazyme
Dopar
Dopram
Doral
Dorcol
Doriden
Doryx
Doxidan
Doxychel
Dramamine
Drisdol
Dristan
Drithocreme
Dritho-Scalp
Drixoral
Drize
Drolban
Drysol
Dulcolax
DuoCet
DuoDERM
Duofilm
Duo-Medihaler
Duoplant
Duphalac
Durabolin
Duracillin
Dura-Gest
Duramorph

Duranest
Duraquin
Dura-Tap
Dura-Vent/A
Dura-Vent/DA
Duricef
Duvoid
Dyazide
Dycill
Dyclone
Dymelor
DynaCirc
Dynapen
Dyrenium
Dytuss

Easprin
Ecotrin
Edecrin
Efudex
Elase
Elavil
Eldecort
Eldepryl
Eldercaps
Eldertonic
Eldopaque
Eldoquin Forte
Elemite
Elixophyllin
Elocon
Elspar
Emcyt
Emete-con
Emetrol
Eminase
Emko
Empirin
Emulsoil
Endal-HD
Endep
Endorphan
Endorphenyl
Enduron
Enduronyl
Enduronyl Forte
Energix-B
Enkaid
Enlon
Enovid
Enrich
Ensure
Entex

Entex LA
Entolase-HP
Entozyme
Entuss
Entuss-D
Epifoam
EpiPen
Epitrate
Epogen
Eppy/N
Equagesic
Equani
Ergamisol
Ergomar
Ergostat
Ergotrate Maleate
ERYC
Erycette
EryDerm
Erygel
Erymax
EryPed
Ery-Tab
Erythrocin
Esgic-Plus
Esidrix
Esimil
Eskalith
Eskalith CR
Esotérica
Estar Gel
Estinyl
Estrace
Estraderm
Estradurin
Estratab
Estratest
Estrovis
Ethamide
Ethamolin
Ethiodol
Ethmozine
Ethrane
Ethril
Etrafon-A
Etrafon Forte
Eucerin
Eulexin
Eurax
Euthroid
Eutonyl
Eutron
Evac-Q-Kit
Evac-Q-Kwik

Excedrin
Exelderm
Exna
Exorbin
Exsel
Extendryl

Factrel
Fansidar
Fastin
Fedahist
Feen-A-Mint
Feldene
Femogen
Femstat
Fenesin
Fenoprofen
Fentanyl
Feosol
Feostat
Ferancee
Ferancee-HP
Fero-Folic-500
Fero-Grad-500
Fero-Gradumet
Ferralet
Ferro-Sequels
Festal II
Fetrin
Feverall
Fiberall
FiberCon
Fibermed
Fibrad
Filibon
Fioricet
Fiorinal
Flagyl
Flatulex
Flaxedil
Fleet
Flexeril
Flintstones
Florinef
Florone
Floropryl
Florvite
Flu-Imune
Fluogen
Fluonid
Fluori-Methane
Flouritab
Flurorplex

Fluorouracil
Fluothane
Fluress
Fluro-Ethyl
Folex
Folex PFS
Follutein
Folvite
Forane
Fortaz
Fosfree
Fototar
FreAmine
Ful-Glo
Fulvicin P/G
Fulvicin-U/F
Fungi-Nail
Fungizone
Fungoid HC
Furacin
Furadantin
Furoxone

Gammar
Gammar-IV
Gamophen
Gamulin Rh
Gantanol
Gantrisin
Garamycin
Gastrocrom
Gastrosed
Gas-X
Gaviscon
Gelpirin
Gelpirin-CCF
Gemonil
Gen-XENE
Geocillin
Geopen
Gerimed
Geriplex-FS
Geritonic
Gevrabon
Gevral T
Glucern
Glucotrol
Glutofac
Glutose
Gly-Oxide
GoLYTELY
Granulex
Grifulvin V

Grisactin
Gris-PEG
Guaifed
Guaitab
Gustase
Gyne-Lotrimin
Gynol II

Halcion
Haldol
Haldrone
Halog
Halog-E
Halotestin
Halotex
Haltran
Harmonyl
Head & Shoulders
Hedulin
Hemaspan
Hemocyte
Hemocyte-F
Hemofil M
Hemopad
Hep-B-Gammagee
Hep-Forte
Hep-Lock
Hep-Lock U/P
Heptavax-B
Heptuna Plus
Herpecin-L
Herplex
Hespan
Hexa-Betalin
Hexabrix
Hexadrol
Hibiclens
Hibistat
HibTITER
Hippuran
Hipputope
Hiprex
Hismanal
Hispril
Histalog
Histor-D
Histussin HC
Humate P
Humatin
Humatrope
Humibid
Humorsol
Humulin

Hurricaine
Hy-C
Hycodan
Hycomine
Hyco-Pap
Hycotuss
Hydeltrasol
Hydeltra-T.B.A.
Hydergine
Hydra-Zide
Hydrea
Hydrisalic
Hydrisinol
Hydrocet
Hydrocil
Hydrocortone
HydroDIURIL
Hydromox
Hydropres
Hydroserpine Plus
Hygroton
Hylorel
Hypaque
Hyperstat
Hy-Phen
Hyskon
Hytone
Hytrin

Iberet
Iberet-500
Iberet-Folic-500
Icy Hot
Identi-Code
Identi-Dose
IFEX
Iletin
Ilosone
Ilotycin
Imferon
Imodium
Imogam
Imovax
Impregon
Imuran
Inapsine
Incremin
Inderal
Inderide
Indocin
Indocin SR
Infatabs
Inflamase

Inhal-Aid
Innovar
Inocor
InspirEase
Instat
Insulatard NPH
Intal
Interceed
Intralipid
Introlite
Intron A
Intropin
Inversine
Iodotope
Ionamin
Ionil
Ionosol
IoTuss
Ipsatol
Ircon
Ircon-FA
Iromin-G
Irospan
Ismelin
Iso-B
Iso-Bid
Isoclor
Isocom
Isomil
Isomil SF
Isopaque
Isoptin
Isopto Cetamide
Isordil
Isovex
Isoxsuprine
Isuprel
Itch-X
Ivadantin

Janimine
Jevity

Kabikinase
Kafocin
Kantrex
Kaolin-Pectin
Kaon-CL
Kaopectate
Kappadione
Kasof
Kato

Kay Ciel
Kayexalate
K-Dur
Keflex
Keflin
Keftab
Kefurox
Kefzol
Kemadrin
Kenacort
Kenalog
Kenwood
Keralyt
Keri
Kerlone
Ketalar
Ketamine
Kinesed
K-Lease
Klonopin
K-Lor
Klor-Con
Klorvess
Klotrix
K-Lyte
Kolyum
Komed
Komex
Konakion
Koromex
Kronofed-A
K-Tab
Kutrase
Ku-Zyme
Kwelcof
Kwell

Lac-Hydrin
Lacril
Lacri-Lube
Lacrisert
Lactaid
LactiCare-HC
Lactinex
Lactisol
Lactocal-F
Lactrase
Lamprene
Laniazid
Lanoxicaps
Lanoxin
Largon
Lariam

Larobec
Larodopa
Larotid
Larylseptic
Lasix
Lazer
LazerFormalyde
LazerSporin-C
Ledercillin VK
Lederplex
Lente
Leritine
Leukeran
Levatol
Levlen
Levo-Dromoran
Levophed
Levoprome
Levothroid
Levoxine
Levsin
Levsinex
Levsin/SL
Librax
Libritabs
Librium
Lidex
Limbitrol
Lincocin
Lioresal
Lipo Gantrisin
Liposyn
Liquaemin
Liquamar
Liqui-Cal
Liqui-Cher
Liquid Pred
Liquifilm Forte
Lithane
Lithobid
Lithonate
Lithostat
Loestrin
Lomotil
Loniten
Lo/Ovral
Lopid
Lopressor
Loprox
Lopurin
Lorabid
Lorcet-HD
Lorcet Plus
Lorelco

Lorfan
Lortab
Lotrimin
Lotrisone
Lotusate
Lowila Cake
Loxitane
Lozol
Lubraseptic
Lubrin
Ludiomil
Lufyllin
Lufyllin-GG
Lupron
Luride
Lurine PMS
Luroscrub
Lutrepulse
Lynoral
Lysodren

Maalox
Macrodantin
Macrodex
Mag-L
Magnacort
Magnatril
Magonate
Mag-Ox 400
Magsal
Mag-Tab SR
Maltsupex
Mandelamine
Mandol
Maolate
Marax
Marblen
Marcaine
Marezine
Marinol
Marlyn
Marplan
Massé
Massengill
Materna
Matulane
Maxair
MaxEPA
Maxibolin
Maxidex
Maxiflor
Maxitrol
Maxivate

Maxovite
Maxzide
May-Vita
Mazanor
Mazicon
MD-60
MD-76
MD-Gastroview
Mebaral
Meclan
Meclomen
Mediatric
Medicone
Medigesic
Medihaler-Epi
Medihaler-Iso
Medilax
Medipren
Medrol
Mefoxin
Mega-B
Megace
Megadose
Mega-Max EPA
Megestrol
Melfiat
Mellaril
Mellaril-S
Menrium
Mepergan
Mepergan Fortis
Mephyton
Mepiridine
Meprospan
Meruvax
Mesantoin
Mesnex
Mestinon
Metahydrin
Metamucil
Metandren
Metaprel
Metatensin
Methalgen
Methergine
Meticortelone
Meticorten
Metopirone
Metreton
Metric 21
Metrodin
Metrogel
Metubine Iodide
Mevacor

Mevanin-C
Mexate
Mexate-AQ
Mexitil
Mezlin
Micro-Guard
Micro-K
Micronase
Micronor
Microsulfon
Midamor
Midol
Midrin
Miles Nervine
Milk of Magnesia
Milontin
Miltown
Mini-Gamulin
Minipress
Minitran
Minizide
Minocin
Minoxidil
Mintezol
Miochol
Mio-Rel
Miostat
Miradon
Mission
Mithracin
Mitrolan
Mixtard
Moban
Mobigesic
Mobisyl
Modane
Moderil
Modicon
Moduretic
Moisturel
Mol-Iron
Monistat
Monistat-Derm
Monocid
Monoclate-P
Monodox
Mono-Gesic
Mono-Vacc
Motofen
Motrin
Mucomyst
Mudrane-2
Mudrane GG
Multitest CMI

Mulvidren-F
Mumpsvax
Murine
Mustargen
Mutamycin
Myambutol
Mycelex
Mycelex-G
Mycifradin
Myciguent
Mycitracin
Mycolog II
Mycostatin
Mydriacyl
Mykrox
Mylanta
Mylaxen
Myleran
Mylicon
Myochrysine
Myotonachol
Mysoline
Mytelase
Mytrex

Nafcil
Naftin
Nail Scrub
Naldecon
Nalfon
Naloxone
Naphcon-A
Naprosyn
Naqua
Naquival
Narcan
Nardil
Nasalcrom
Nasalide
Natabec
Natacyn
Natalins
Naturetin
Navane
Nebcin
NebuPent
NegGram
Nelova
Nembutal
Neo-Calglucon
Neo-Cortef
NeoDecadron
Neo-Delta-Cortef

Neo-Hydeltrasol
Neoloid
Neo-Medrol
Neosar
Neosporin
Neo-Synalar
Neo-Synephrine
Neotrizine
Nephro-Calci
Nephrocaps
Nephro-Derm
Nephro-Fer
Nephro-Vite
Nephrox
Neptazane
Nesacaine
Nesacaine-MPF
Nestabs FA
Netromycin
Neutra-Phos
Neutra-Phos-K
Nia-Bid
Niacels
Niacor
Niaplus
Niclocide
Nicobid
Nicolar
Nicorette
Nicotinex
Niferex
Niferex-PN Forte
Night Cast
Nilstat
Nimotop
Nipride
Nitro-Bid
Nitrodisc
Nitro-Dur
Nitrogard
Nitrol
Nitrolingual
Nitrong
Nitrostat
Nix
Nizoral
N'Odor
No Doz
Nolahist
Nolamine
Nolex LA
Noludar
Nordette
Norethin

Norflex
Norgesic
Norgesic Forte
Norinyl
Norisodrine
Norlestrin
Norlutate
Norlutin
Normodyne
Normozide
Noroxin
Norpace
Norpace CR
Norplant
Norpramin
Nor-QD
Norzine
Novafed
Novahistine
Novamine
Novantrone
Novocain
Novolin
NovolinPen
NovoPen
Nubain
Nucofed
Nu-Iron
Numorphan
Nupercainal
Nuprin
Nursoy
Nutracort
Nutraderm
Nutrox
Nydrazid
Nylidrin
Nystex

Occlusal
Occlusal-HP
Occucoat
Octamide PFS
OcuClear
Ogen
Omnipaque
Omnipen
Omnipen-N
Oncovin
One-A-Day
Ophthaine
Ophthetic
Opticrom

Optilets-500
Optilets-M-500
Optimine
Optiray
Orabase HCA
Oragrafin
Orap
Orazinc
Oretic
Oreticyl
Oreton
Orexin
Organidin
Orimune
Orinase
Ornade
Ornex
Ornidyl
Orphengesic
Ortho
Ortho Dienestrol
Orthoclone
Ortho-Creme
Ortho-Gynol
Ortho-Novum
Orudis
Os-Cal
Osmolite
Osti-Derm
Otic Domeboro
Otic Tridesilon
Otobiotic
Otocort
Otrivin
Ovcon
Ovral
Ovrette
Ovulen
Oxistat
Oxsoralen
Oxsoralen-Ultra
Oxy Clean
Oxy Night Watch

Pacaps
PALS
Pamelor
Pamine
Panafil
Panafil-White
Panalgesic Gold
Pancrease
Pancrease MT

Panhematin	Pentrax	Plasma-Plex	Pre-Pen
Panmycin	Pen•Vee K	Plasmatein	Pre-Sate
PanOxyl	Pepcid	Platinol	PreSun
Pantopaque	Peptavlon	Platinol-AQ	PreviDent
Pantopon	Pepto-Bismol	Plegine	Prilosec
Panwarfin	Percocet	Pneumovax 23	Primatene
Paradione	Percodan	Pnu-Imune 23	Primaxin
Paraflex	Percodan-Demi	Pod-Ben-25	Principen
Parafon Forte	Percogesic	Point-Two	Prinivil
ParaGard	Percorten	Polaramine	Prinzide
Paraplatin	Perdium	Polocaine	Priscoline
Parasal	Pergonal	Polycillin	Privine
Parathar	Periactin	Polycillin-N	Pro-Banthine
Par-Decon	Peri-Colace	Polycillin-PRB	Probec-T
Parepectolin	Peridex	Polycitra	Procan SR
Par-Glycerol	Peridin-C	Polycitra-K	Procardia
Par-Glycerol C	Peritinic	Polycitra-LC	Procardia XL
Par-Glycerol DM	Peritrate	Polycose	Pro-Ception
Parlodel	Peritrate SA	Poly-Histine CS	Proctocort
Parnate	Permapen	Poly-Histine-D	ProctoCream-HC
Parsidol	Permax	Poly-Histine DM	ProctoFoam
Paskalium	Permitil	Polymox	ProctoFoam-HC
Pathocil	Persa-Gel	Polysporin	Profasi
Pavabid	Persantine	Poly-Vi-Flor	Profilate OSD
Pavabid HP	Pertofrane	Ponaris	Profilnine
Pavulon	Pfizerpen	Pondimin	Proglycem
Paxipam	Pfizerpen-AS	Ponstel	Pro-Hepatone
Pazo	PharmaCreme	Pontocaine	ProHIBit
Pedameth	Phazyme	Posture	Proketazine
PediaCare	PhenaCal	Posture-D	Prolixin
Pediacof	Phenaphen	Potaba	Proloid
Pediaflor	Phenergan	Povan	Proloprim
Pedialyte	Phenergan-D	PrameGel	Promaquid
Pediamycin	Phenergan VC	Pramet FA	ProMod
Pediapred	Phenurone	Pramilet FA	Pronestyl
PediaProfen	Phenytoin	Pramosone	Pronestyl-SR
PediaSure	pHisoDerm	Prantal	Propacet
Pediazole	pHisoHex	Pravachol	Propagest
Pedi-Boro	PhosChol	Prax	Prophyllin
Pedi-Dri	Phos-Ex	Prazosin	Propine
PediOtic	Phos-Flur	Prazosin HCL	Proplex T
Pedi-Pro	pHos-pHaid	Predcef	Prostaphlin
PedvaxHIB	Phospholine Iodide	Pred Forte	Prostigmin
Peganone	Photoplex	Pred Mild	Prostin VR
Penapar-VK	Phrenilin	Prednicen-M	Protid
Penbritin-S	Phrenilin Forte	Prefrin	Protopam
Penecort	Phyllocontin	Pregnyl	Protostat
Penetrex	Pilopine HS	Prelone	Prototropin
Pen•Kera	Pima	Prelu-2	Proventil
Pentam 300	Pipracil	Preludin	Provera
Pentaspan	Pitocin	Premarin	Provocholine
Penthrane	Pitressin	Prenatal/Zinc	Prozac
Pentids	Placidyl	Prenate 90	Prulet
Pentothal	Plaquenil Sulfate	Preparation H	Psorcon

Psorion
Pulmocare
Pure-E
Purge
Puri-Clens
Purinethol
Purpose
Pyopen
Pyridium
Pyridoxal-5-Phos-
   phate
Pyrroxate

Quadrinal
Quarzan
Quelicin
Quelidrine
Questran
Quibron
Quibron-T
Quibron-T/SR
Quide
Quinaglute
Quinalan
Quinamm
Quinidex
Quinora

Ramipril
Raudixin
Rau-Sed
Rautensin
Rauwiloid
Rauzide
Recombivax HB
Redisol
Redutemp
Refresh
Regitine
Reglan
Regonol
Regroton
Regutol
Rela
Relafen
Relefact TRH
Remular-S
Renacidin
Renese
Renese-R
Renografin
Reno-M

Renoquid
Renovist
Repan
Replena
Replens
Respaire-SR
Respbid
Restoril
Retin-A
Retrovir
Reversol
Rheaban
Rheomacrodex
Rheumatrex
Rhindecon
Rhinolar
Rhinolar-EX
RhoGAM
Ribo-2
Ridaura
Rifadin
Rifamate
Rimactane
Rimso-50
Riopan
Ritalin
Ritalin-SR
Robaxin
Robaxisal
Robimycin
Robinul
Robitussin
Robitussin A-C
Robitussin-CF
Robitussin-DAC
Robitussin-DM
Robitussin-PE
Rocaltrol
Rocephin
Roferon-A
Rogaine
Rondec
Rondec-DM
Rondec-TR
Ross
Ross SLD
Rowasa
Roxanol
Roxanol SR
Roxanol UD
Roxicet
Roxicodone
Roxiprin
Rubex

Rubramin
Rufen
Rum-K
Ru-Tuss II
Ru-Tuss DE
Rxosine
Ryna
Ryna-C
Ryna-CX
Rynatan
Rynatan S
Rynatuss
Rythmol

Saave
SalAc
Sal-Acid
Salactic Film
Salflex
Salinex
Sal-Plant
Salsalate
Salsitab
Saluron
Salutensin
Sam-E.P.A.
Sandimmune
Sandoglobulin
Sandostatin
Sandril
Sanorex
Sansert
Sarapin
Scleromate
Sebulex
Sebutone
Seconal
Secretin-Ferring 75
   CU
Sectral
Sedapap
Seldane
Selsun Blue
Semicid
Semilente
Seniors
Senokot
Senokot-S
SenokotXTRA
Sensorcaine
Septra
Ser-Ap-Es

Serax
Serentil
Seromycin
Serophene
Serpasil
Serpasil-Apresoline
Serpasil-Esidrix
Sethotope
Shade
Sigtab
Silvadene
Similac
Sinarest
Sine-Aid
Sinemet
Sine-Off
Sinequan
Singlet
Sinografin
Sinufed
Sinulin
Sinumist-SR
Skelaxin
Slo-bid Gyrocaps
Slo-Niacin
Slo-phyllin
Slow Fe
Slow-K
Solaquin Forte
Solarcaine
Solatene
Solbar PF
Solbar Plus
Solfoton
Solganal
Solu-Cortef
Solu-Medrol
Soma
Somophyllin
Somophyllin-CRT
Somophyllin-DF
Somophyllin-T
Sorbitrate
Sotradecol
Sparine
Spectazole
Spectrobid
Stadol
Staphage Lysate
Staphcillin
Statobex
Star-Otic
Stelazine
Sterane

Sterapred
Stilphostrol
Stoxil
Streptase
Stresscaps
Stresstabs
Strovite Plus
Stuartinic
Stuartnatal
Sublimaze
Sucostrin
Sudafed
Sufenta
Sulfacet-R
Sulfamylon
Sulfose
Sulfoxyl
Sulla
Sultrin
Summer's Eve
Sumycin
Sunkist
Supac
SuperEPA
Superkids
Suprax
Surbex
Surbex-T
Surfak
Surital
Surmontil
Sus-Phrine
Sustaire
Sween
Sween-A-Peel
Sween Prep
Syllact
Symmetrel
Synacort
Synalar
Synalar-HP
Synalgos-DC
Synarel
Synemol
Synkayvite
Synophylate
Synthroid
Syntocinon
Syprine
Sytobex

Tacaryl
TACE

Tagamet
Talacen
Talwin
Talwin Nx
Tambocor
Tandearil
Tao
Tapazole
Taractan
Tavist
Tavist-D
Tazicef
Tazidime
Tears Naturale II
Tears Plus
Tedral SA
Tegison
Tegopen
Tegretol
Teldrin
Tel-E-Dose
Telepaque
Temaril
Temovate
Tencet
Tencon
Tenex
Ten-K
Tenoretic
Tenormin
Tensilon
Tenuate
Tepanil
Terazol
Terra-Cortril
Terramycin
Teslac
Tessalon
Tes-Tape
Testred
Tetrex
Thalitone
Tham
Tham-E
Theelin
Theo-24
Theochron
Theoclear
Theo-Dur
Theolair
Theolair-SR
Theolixir
Theo-Organidin
Theophyl

Theostat 80
Therabid
TheraCys BCG
TheraFlu
Thera-Flur
Thera-Flur-N
Thera-Gesic
Theragran
Theragran-M
Therevac
Thiacide
Thiamilate
Thioguanine
Thiola
Thiosulfil
Thiotepa
Thorazine
Threostat
Thrombinar
Thrombostat
Thyrar
Thyrolar
Thytropar
Ticar
Tigan
Timentin
Timolide
Timolol
Timoptic
Tinactin
Tindal
Tinver
Tobrex
Tofranil
Tofranil-PM
Tolectin
Tolerex
Tolfrinic
Tolinase
Tolmetin
Tonocard
Topicort
ToppTrims
Toradol IM
Torecan
Tornalate
Totacillin-N
Tracrium
Tral
Trancopal
Trandate HCT
Transderm
Transderm-Nitro
Transderm-Scop

Trans-Plantar
Trans-Ver-Sal
Tranxene-SD
Tranxene T-TAB
Travase
Travert
Trecator-SC
Trental
Trest
Trexan
Triaminic
Triaminicin
Triaminicol
Triavil
Triclos
Tridesilon
Tridil
Tridione
Tri-Immunol
Trilafon
Tri-Levien
Trilisate
Trimox
Trimpex
Trinalin
Tri-Norinyl
Trinsicon
Triphasil
Triplevite/Fluoride
Trisoralen
Trisulfam
Tri-Vi-Flor
Trobicin
Tronolane
Tropamine
Troph-Iron
Trophite
Trymex
Tryptoplex
Trypto-Som
Trysul
Tubasal
Tubex
Tubizid
Tums
Tussafed
Tussar
Tussar DM
Tussar SF
Tussionex
Tussi-Organidin
Tuss-Ornade
TwoCal HN
Tylenol

Tylox
Tyzine

Ultracef
Ultracholine
Ultralente
Unasyn
Unicap
Unifiber
Unilax
Unipen
Uniphyl
Unipres
Unisom
Ureacin
Urecholine
Urex
Urised
Urispas
Urobiotic-250
Urocit-K
Uro-KP-Neutral
Urolene Blue
Uro-Mag
Uro-Phosphate
Uroquid-Acid
Uticillin VK
Uticort

Vagisec
Vagisec Plus
Vagistat
Vagitrol
Valisone
Valium
Valmid
Valpin 50

Valrelease
Vancenase
Vanceril
Vancocin HCL
Vancoled
Vancor
Vanobid
Vanoxide-HC
Vanseb
Vanseb-T
Vari-Flavors
Vascor
Vascoray
Vaseretic
Vasocidin
Vasocon
Vasotec
Vasoxyl
V-Cillin
V-Cillin K
Veetids
Velban
Velosef
Velosulin
Ventolin
VePesid
Verelan
Vermox
Verr-Canth
Verrex
Verrusol
Versapen
Versapen-K
Versed
Vesprin
Vibramycin
Vibra-Tabs
Vicks
Vicodin

Vicodin ES
Vicon Forte
Vi-Daylin
Vi-Daylin/F
Vioform
Viokase
Vira-A
Viranol
Virazole
Virilon
Viroptic
Visine
Visken
Vistaril
Vitafol
Vita-Kid
Vita-Min
Vivacil
Vivonex
Voltaren
Vontrol
VoSoL
Vytone

Wart-Off
Water Babies
Wehless-105
Wellbutrin
Westcort
Wigraine
Winstrol
Wyamine
Wyamycin E
Wyamycin S
Wyanoids
Wycillin
Wydase
Wygesic

Wymox
Wytensin

Xanax
Xerac
Xylocaine

Yocon
Yodoxin
Yohimex
Yutopar

Zanosar
Zantac
Zarontin
Zaroxolyn
Zefazone
Zenate
Zephiran
Zephrex
Zestoretic
Zestril
Zetar
Zinacef
Zincon
Zocor
Zoladex
Zolicef
Zolyse
Zone-A
Zorprin
Zostrix
Zovirax
Zydone
Zyloprim
Zymase

Sound-Spelling Correspondences

The following table is designed to aid the user in locating in the list words whose pronunciation is known but whose spelling presents difficulties. Such difficulties are caused by the fact that so many speech sounds can be spelled in more than one way, since the standard alphabet has twenty-six characters to represent the forty or more sounds used in the English language. If you are unable to find a word when you look it up, check this table and try another combination of letters that represent the same sound.

Sound	Spelling	In these sample words
a (as in pat)	ai	plaid
	al	half-life
	au	laugh
a (as in mane)	ai	pain
	ao	gaol
	au	gauge
	ay	pay
	e	suede
	ea	break
	ei	vein
	eig	feign
	eigh	eight, neighbor
	ey	prey
a (as in father)	ah	ah
	al	balm
	e	sergeant
	ea	heart
b (as in bib)	bb	blubber
	bh	bhang
	pb	cupboard, raspberry
ch (as in church)	c	cello
	Cz	Czech
	tch	patch, stitch
	ti	question
	tu	denture
d (as in deed)	bd	bdellium
	dd	ladder
	ed	mailed
	dh	dhobie
e (as in pet)	a	any
	ae	aesthetic
	ai	said
	ay	says
	ea	thread

Sound	Spelling	In these sample words
e (as in p**e**t)	ei	h**ei**fer
	eo	l**eo**pard
	ie	fr**ie**ndly
	oe	r**oe**ntgen
	u	b**u**rial
e (as in b**e**)	ae	C**ae**sar
	ay	qu**ay**
	ea	**ea**ch, b**ea**ch
	ee	b**ee**t
	ei	conc**ei**t
	eo	p**eo**ple
	ey	k**ey**
	i	p**i**ano, card**i**ac
	ie	s**ie**ge
	oe	ph**oe**nix, am**oe**ba
	y	icht**y**osis, tracheot-om**y**
f (as in **fif**e)	ff	sti**ff**
	gh	enou**gh**
	lf	ha**lf**
	ph	**ph**os**ph**ate, gra**ph**
g (as in **g**a**g**)	gg	bra**gg**ed
	gh	**gh**ost
	gu	**gu**est
	gue	epilo**gue**
h (as in **h**at)	wh	**wh**ole
	g	**G**ila monster
	j	**J**erez
i (as in p**i**t)	a	vill**a**ge, clim**a**te
	e	**e**nough
	ee	b**ee**n
	ia	carr**ia**ge
	ie	s**ie**ve
	o	w**o**men
	u	b**u**sy
	ui	b**ui**lt
	y	c**y**st, phar**y**nx
i (as in **i**dle)	ai	gu**ai**ac
	ay	b**ay**ou
	ei	h**ei**ght, m**ei**osis
	ie	l**ie**
	igh	s**igh**, r**igh**t
	is	**is**land, **is**let
	uy	b**uy**
	y	sk**y**, m**y**ograph, ach**y**lia

Sound	Spelling	In these sample words
i (as in idle)	ye	rye
j (as in jar)	d	gradual
	dg	lodging
	di	soldier
	dj	adjective
	g	register, geriatric, argyria
	ge	vengeance
	gg	exaggerate
k (as in kite)	c	call, ecstasy
	cc	account, saccular
	cch	acchymosis, saccharin
	ch	cochlea, chyle, schizophrenia
	ck	crack
	cqu	lacquer
	cu	biscuit
	lk	talk
	q	Aqaba
	qu	quay
	que	plaque
l (as in lid)	ll	tall, llama
	lh	Lhasa
m (as in mum)	chm	drachm
	gm	paradigm, phlegm
	lm	balm
	mb	plumb
	mm	hammer
	mn	solemn
n (as in no)	cn	cnemis, gastrocnemium
	gn	gnat, gnathic, gnosis
	kn	knife
	mn	mnemasthenia
	nn	canny, inn
	pn	pneumonia, pnigma
ng (as in thing)	n	congress, ink
	ngue	tongue
o (as in pot)	a	waffle, watch
	ho	honest
	ou	trough
o (as in no)	au	hautboy, mauve
	eau	beau, bureau

Sound	Spelling	In these sample words
o (as in no)	eo	yeoman
	ew	sew
	oa	foal, foam
	oe	Joe
	oh	ohm
	oo	brooch
	ou	shoulder
	ough	borough, dough
	ow	low, row
	owe	owe, Marlowe
o (as in for)	a	all, warm
	al	talk
	ah	Utah
	as	Arkansas
	au	caught, gaunt
	aw	awful
	oa	broad
	ough	bought
oi (as in noise)	oy	boy
ou (as in out)	au	sauerkraut
	hou	hour
	ough	bough
	ow	scowl, sow
oo (as in took)	o	woman, wolf
	ou	should
	u	cushion, full
oo (as in boot)	eu	leukemia, maneuver
	ew	shrew
	ieu	lieutenant
	o	do, move, two
	oe	canoe
	ou	group, soup
	ough	through
	u	rude
	ue	blue, flue
	ui	bruise, fruit
p (as in pop)	pp	happy
r (as in roar)	rh	rhythm
	rr	cherry
	rrh	cirrhosis, hemorrhoid
	wr	write
s (as in say)	c	cellar, cyst, lecithin
	ce	sauce

Sound	Spelling	In these sample words
s (as in say)	ps	pseudocyst, ili-opsoas
	sc	sciatic, abscess
	sch	schism
	ss	pass, byssinosis
	sth	isthmus
sh (as in ship)	ce	oceanic
	ch	chandelier, chancre
	ci	special, deficient
	psh	pshaw
	s	sugar
	sc	conscience
	sch	schist, schistosis
	se	nauseous
	si	pension
	ss	tissue, mission
	ti	election, nation
t (as in tie)	ct	ctenoids
	ed	stopped
	ght	caught
	phth	phthisis
	pt	ptosis, ptyalism
	th	Thomas
	tt	letter
	tw	two
th (as in think)	chth	chthonophagy
	phth	phthalic, phthiocol
u (as in cut)	o	son, income
	oe	does
	oo	blood
	ou	couple, trouble
u (as in use)	eau	beautiful
	eu	feud, eugenic
	eue	queue
	ew	pew
	ieu	adieu
	iew	view
	u	ulotomy, unipennate
	ue	cue
	you	youth
	yu	yule
v (as in valve)	f	of
	ph	Stephen
w (as in with)	o	one
	ou	ouabain

Sound	Spelling	In these sample words
w (as in **with**)	u	g**u**anese, q**u**ick
y (as in **yes**)	i	on**i**on
	j	**J**ung, halleluj**ah**
z (as in **zebra**)	cz	**cz**ar
	s	ri**s**e, her**s**
	ss	de**ss**ert
	x	**x**iphoid, ilio**x**iphop-agus
	zz	fu**zz**

Note: the letter *x* spells six sounds in English: ks, as in box, exit; gz, as in exact, exist; sh, as in anxious; gzh, as in luxurious, luxury; ksh (a variant of gzh), also as in luxurious, luxury; and z, as in anxiety, Xerox.

Abbreviations

In accordance with the style preferred by the American Medical Association, no periods are used in the following list of abbreviations.

A absolute; acetum; area of heart shadow; mass number
A absorbance
A₂ aortic second sound
Å angstrom unit
a accommodation; anterior; aqua; arteria
a absorptivity
AA achievement; age; Alcoholics Anonymous
abd abdomen
abort abortion
AC air conduction; alternating current; anodic closure; axiocervical
Ac acetyl
ac, a-c alternating current
ACE adrenocortical extract
ACG apex cardiogram
acG accelerator globulin (factor V)
AcPase acid phosphatase
ACTH adrenocorticotropic hormone
AD right ear (*auris dextra*)
Ad anisotropic disk
ADC anodic duration contraction; axiodistocervical
ADH antidiuretic hormone
A disk anisotropic disk
ADP adenosine diphosphate
ADPase adenosine diphosphatase
AGA accelerated growth area
A/G ratio albumin-globulin ratio
ah hypermetropic astigmatism
AHF antihemophilic factor (factor VIII)

AHG antihemophilic globulin (factor VIII)
AI aortic insufficiency
AJ ankle jerk
AK above knee
alb albumin
AM amperemeter
am ametropia; meter-angle; myopic astigmatism
AMA against medical advice
AMI acute myocardial infarction
AML acute myoblastic leukemia
AMP adenosine monophosphate
amp amperage; ampere; ampule
AMpase adenosine monophosphatase
An anisometropia; anodal; anode
anat anatomic; anatomical; anatomy
ANS anterior nasal spine; autonomic nervous system
A-P anteroposterior
A+P auscultation and percussion
APC aspirin, phenacetin, and caffeine
APC virus adenovirus
A-P&Lat anteroposterior and lateral
APF animal protein factor (vitamin B₁₂)
AQ achievement quotient
AQRS mean manifest electrical axis of the QRS complex
AR alarm reaction
ARD acute respiratory disease

AS left ear (*auris sinister*)
ASCVD arteriosclerotic cardiovascular disease
ASLO antistreptolysin-O
Ast astigmatism
AT mean manifest magnitude of repolarization of the myocardium
ATCC American Type Culture Collection
atm atmosphere
ATN acute tubular necrosis
ATP adenosine triphosphate
ATPase adenosine triphosphatase
ATS equine antitetanus serum
at vol atomic volume
at wt atomic weight
AV arteriovenous; atrioventricular; auriculoventricular
Av avoirdupois weight
aV augmented unipolar limb lead
ax axis
Az azote
AZT Aschheim-Zondek test

B bacillus; boils at; buccal
BBB bundle branch block
BBT basal body temperature
BE barium enema
bev billion electron volts
BFP biologic false positive reaction
BM bowel movement
BMR basal metabolic rate
BNA Basle Nomina Anatomica

BP blood pressure; British Pharmacopoeia
bp boiling point
BR British or Birmingham Revision
BS blood sugar; breath sounds
BSA body surface area
BSR blood sedimentation rate
BTU British thermal unit
BUN blood urea nitrogen

C canine of second dentition; cathode; Celsius; centigrade; chest; closure; contraction; cylinder
c centum; deciduous canine
CA chronological age
Ca cancer
Cal large calorie
cal small calorie
CAR conditioned avoidance response
CBC complete blood count
CBG corticosteroid-binding globulin
CBS chronic brain syndrome
CC chief complaint
cc cubic centimeter
Ccr creatinine clearance
CCU coronary care unit
cd candela
CDC Center for Disease Control
CER conditioned escape response
CFT complement-fixation test
cg centigram
CHD congenital heart disease; coronary heart disease
CHINA chronic infectious neuropathic agent
CI color index
Ci curie
CID cytomegalic inclusion disease

cl centiliter
CLSH corpus luteum stimulating hormone
cm centimeter
cmm cubic millimeter
CMR cerebral metabolic rate
CNS central nevous system
CoA coenzyme A
COPD chronic obstructive pulmonary disease
CP chemically pure
CPD cephalopelvic disproportion
cpm cycles per minute
cps cycles per second
CR conditioned reflex; conditioned response
CRM cross-reacting material
CRS Chinese restaurant syndrom
CS conditioned stimulus
CSF cerbrospinal fluid
CSM cerebrospinal meningitis
CSR corrected sedimentation rate
CST convulsive shock therapy
CTR cardiothoracic ratio
cu ft cubic foot
cu in cubic inch
cu m cubic meter
CV cardiovascular
CVA cardiovascular accident; costovertebral angle
CVD cardiovascular disease
cwt hundredweight
Cx cervix
Cyl cylinder; cylindrical lens

D, d dead; deciduous; density; dexter; died; diopter; distal; dorsal; dose; duration; give (*da*); let it be given (*detur*)
ᴅ de

d dextrorotatory
DA developmental age
D&C dilatation and curettage
dB decibel
dc, d-c direct current
dg decigram
DIP distal interphalangeal
DJD degenerative joint disease
dl deciliter
dm decimeter
DOA dead on arrival
DOE dyspnea on exertion
DQ developmental quotient
dr dram
DT delirium tremens
DTR deep tendon reflex
dx diagnosis

E einstein; elecromotive force
e electron
EA educational age
ECG electrocardiogram
ECS electroconvulsive shock
ECT electroconvulsive therapy
ED effective dose; erythema dose
ED$_{50}$ median effective dose
EDR effective direct radiation; electrodermal response
EEG electroencephalogram; electroencephalograph; electroencephalography
EHBF estimated hepatic blood flow
EKG electrocardiogram
EKY electrokymogram
EMC encephalomyocarditis
EMF electromotive force; erythrocyte maturation factor
EMG electromyogram
ENT ear, nose, and throat
EOM extraocular movement

ERBF effective renal blood flow
ERG electroretinogram
ERPF effective renal plasma flow
ERV expiratory reserve volume
EQ educational quotient
ESP extrasensory perception
ESR erythrocyte sedimentation rate
EST electroshock therapy
eV electron volt

F Fahrenheit; fellow; fluorine; formula
FB foreign body
fb finger-breadth
FBS fasting blood sugar
FD focal distance
FFA free fatty acids
FFT flicker fusion threshold
FH family history
fl fluid
fl dr fluid dram
fl oz fluid ounce
fp foot-pound
FRC functional residual capacity
FRF follicle-stimulating hormone releasing factor
FSF fibrin stabilizing factor
FSH follicle-stimulating hormone
ft foot
FUO fever of undetermined origin
fx fracture

G gonidial (colony)
g gram
G, g gauge; gravitational constant
G, Ĝ, g, ĝ ventricular gradient
gal gallon
GBS gallbladder series
GI gastrointestinal

gl gland; glands (*glandula; glandulae*)
GOT glutamicoxaloacetic transaminase
GP general paresis; general practitioner
GPT glutamic-pyruvic transaminase
GTH gonadatropic hormone
GU genitourinary
GYN gynecology

H henry; horizontal; hour
H+ hydrogen ion
h height; hundred; Planck constant
HAA hepatitis-associated antigen
hb hemoglobin
HCG human chorionic gonadotropin
HCT hematocrit
HEENT head, eye, ear, nose, and throat
HF Hageman factor (factor XII)
hg hyperglycemic factor (hectogram)
hgb hemoglobin
HGF hyperglycemic factor (hyperglycemic-glycogenolytic factor)
hl hectoliter
hm hectometer
HOP high-pressure oxygen
Hp haptoglobin
hpf high-power field
HSV herpes simplex virus
HVD hypertensive vascular disease
Hz hertz

IB inclusion body
IC inspiratory capacity
ICT insulin coma therapy
ICU intensive care unit
I&D incision and drainage
ID intradermal
Ig immunoglobulin

IH infectious hepatitis
IHSS idiopathic hypertrophic subaortic stenosis
IM intramuscular
in inch
IOP intraocular pressure
IP interphalangeal
IPPB intermittent positive pressure breathing
IQ intelligence quotient
IS intercostal space
IST insulin shock therapy
IU immunizing unit; international unit
IUD intrauterine contraceptive device
IV, iv intravenous
IVCD intraventricular conduction delay
IVP intravenous pyelogram

J joule
JNA Jena Nomina Anatomica

kc kilocycle
kcal kilocalorie
kCi kilocurie
kcps kilocycle per second
keV kiloelectron volt
kg kilogram
Kg-cal kilogram-calorie
kHz kilohertz
km kilometer
kMc kilomegacycle
kMcps kilomegacycles per second
KUB kidney, ureter, and bladder
kV kilovolt
kW kilowatt
kW-hr kilowatt hour

L Latin
l left; lethal
L&A light and accommodation
lab laboratory

LATS long-acting thyroid stimulator
LD lethal dose
LE lupus erythematosus
LLL lower left lobe
LLQ left lowerquadrant
LMP last menstrual period
LNMP last normal menstrual period
LP lumbar puncture
lpf low-power field
LPN licensed practical nurse
LS lumbosacral
LUL left upper lobe
LUQ left upper quadrant
LVH left ventricular hypertrophy
lymphs lymphocytes

M Micrococcus; muscle
m meter
MA mental age
mA milliampere
MBC maximum breathing capacity
Mc megacycle
mcg microgram
MCH mean corpuscular hemoglobin
mch millicurie hour
MCHC mean corpuscular hemoglobin concentration
MCi megacurie
mCi millicurie
MCV mean corpuscular volumn
MD Doctor of Medicine (*Medicinae Doctor*)
MED minimal effective dose; minimum erythema dose
mEq milliequivalent
mg milligram
mHg millimeters of mercury
MHz megahertz
ml milliliter
MLD minimum lethal dose
MM mucous membranes
mm millimeter
mono monocyte

MP metacarpophalangeal (wrist); metatarsophalangeal (ankle)
mp melting point
MRD minimum reacting dose
mrd millirutherford
MS mitral stenosis; multiple sclerosis
msec millisecond
MSL midsternal line
myelo myelocyte

N normal
NA Nomina Anatomica
NAD no appreciable disease
nc nanocurie
NG nasogastric
ng nanogram
nl nanoliter
nm nanometer
NPO nothing by mouth
NSR normal sinus rhythm
NTP normal temperature and pressure

O occiput; oculus (eye); oxygen
O$_2$cap oxygen capacity
O$_2$sat oxygen saturation
OB obstetrics
OD right eye (*oculus dexter*)
OFC occipitofrontal circumference
OPD outpatient department
OR operating room
OS left eye (*oculus sinister*)

P position; premolar; pulse; pupil
P radiant flux
P$_2$ pulmonic second heart sound
PA posteroanterior projection
P&A percussion and auscultation
PBI protein-bound iodine

PCG phonocardiogram
pCi picocurie
PD doctor of pharmacy; interpupillary distance
pd prism diopter; pupillary distance
PE physical examination
PEG pneumoencephalogram; pneumoencephalography
pg picogram
PH past history; Pharmacopeia
pH hydrogen ion concentration
ph phenyl
PI present illness; protamine insulin
PIP proximal interphalangeal
PKU phenylketonuria
PMB polymorphonuclear basophil leukocytes
PME ploymorphonuclear eosinophil leukocytes
PMI point of maximal impulse
PMN polymorphonuclear neutrophil leukocytes
PP near point (*punctum proximum*)
PPD purified protein derivative
ppg picopicogram
Pr presbyopia; prism
psi pounds per square inch
PT physical therapy
PTT partial thromboplastin time
PVC premature ventricular contraction
PZI protamine zinc insulin

Q electric quantity
qt quart

R electrical resistance; regression coefficient; respiration; right
r roentgen

RBC, rbc red blood cell; red blood count
rd rutherford
Rh Rhesus blood factor
RHD relative hepatitic dullness
RLL right lower lobe
RM repiratory movement
RN registered nurse
R/O rule out
RPF renal plasma flow
rpm revolutions per minute
RQ respiratory quotient
RUL right upper lobe
RV residual volume
RVH right ventricular hypertrophy

S spherical; spherical lens
s left (*sinister*); half (*semis*)
SA sinoatrial
sat saturated
sc subcutaneously
SCAT sheep cell aglutination test
SD skin dose; standard deviation
SE standard error
SED skin eurythema dose
sed rate erythrocyte sedimentation rate
SFW slow-filling wave
SGOT serum glutamic oxaloacetic transaminase
SGPT serum glutamic pyruvic transaminase
SH serum hepatitis; social history

SI soluble insulin
SIADH syndrome of inappropriate antidiuretic hormone
sp gr specific gravity
SQ subcutaneous
SR review of systems; sedimentation rate
Staph Staphylococcus
STD skin test dose
STREP Streptococcus
STS serologic test for syphillus
sym symmetrical

T temperature; thoracic
t temporal
tab tablet
T&A tonsillectomy and adenoidectomy
TAT Thematic Appercption Test; toxin-antitoxin
TB tuberculosis
tbsp tablespoon
TGA thyroglobin antibodies
TLC tender loving care; total lung capacity
TPR temperature, pulse, and respiration
tr tincture
TS test solution
TSH thyroid-stimulating hormone
tsp teaspoon
TU toxic unit
tus a cough (*tussis*)

U unit
UGI upper gastrointestinal
UP uteropelvic
USP United States Pharmacopeia
URI upper respiratory infection
UV uterovesical

V vision; visual acuity; volt
VC vital capacity
VCG vectorcardiogram
VD venereal disease
VDH valvular disease of the heart
VDRL Venereal Disease Research Laboratories
VF vocal fremitus
vf field of vision
VPB ventricular premature beat
VR vocal resonance

W watt
WBC, wbc white blood cell; white blood count
WD well developed
WN well nourished
wt weight

X Kienböck unit of x-ray dosage
yd yard
Z contraction (*Zuckung*)
z atomic number

Medical Signs and Symbols

$\bar{a}\bar{a}$, $\overline{AA}$	of each
A, Å	angstrom unit
C′	complement
E_0	electroaffinity
F_1	first filial generation
F_2	second filial generation
L_+	limes death
L_0	limes zero
Q_{O_2}	oxygen consumption
m-	meta-
o-	ortho-
p-	para
℞	(*L. recipe*). Take
S.	(*L. signa*). Write
c̄, c	(*L. cum*). With
ss, ss	(*L. semis*). One half
m, M	(*L. misce*). Mix
O.	(*L. octarius*). Pint
C.	(*L. congius*). Gallon
C	Centigrade (Celsius)
F	Farenheit
°	degree
℞, ℞	minim
Э	scruple
Э i	one scruple
Э ss′	half a scruple
ʒ	dram (apothecaries′)
ʒ i	one dram
fʒ	fluid dram
℥	ounce (troy)
℥i	one ounce
℥ss	half an ounce
℥iss	an ounce and a half
℥ij	two ounces
f℥	fluid ounce
′	foot, minute, univalent
″	inch, second, bivalent

‴	line (1/12 inch), trivalent
μ	micron
$\mu\mu$	micromicron
$m\mu$	millimicron, micromillimeter
σ	1/1000 of a second
π	3.1416—ratio of circumference of a circle to its diameter
®	registered trademark status
mg %	milligrams per cent
vol. %	volume per cent
μg	microgram
gr.	grain
□, ♀	male
○, ♂	female
*	birth
†	death
∞	infinity
:	ratio
::	equality between ratios
−	negative, levorotatory
+	positive, dextrorotatory
±	either positive or negative, not definite, racemic
÷	divided by
×	multiplied by
=	equal to
>	greater than
<	less than
$\sqrt{}$	root, square root
$\sqrt[2]{}$	square root
$\sqrt[3]{}$	cube root
⇌	denotes a reversible reaction
#	number
∧	value considered as a vector in electrocardiography
w/v	weight in volume

Common Latin and Greek Terms
Used In Prescription Writing

Latin or Greek word or phrase	Abbreviation	English meaning
ad	ad	to, up to
ad libitum	ad lib.	freely
alternis horis	alternis horis	every other hour
ana	āā, AA	of each
ante	ante	before
ante cibum	a.c.	before meals
aqua	aq.	water
aqua destillata	aq. dest.	distilled water
bis	bis	twice
bis in die	b.i.d.	twice a day
capsula	caps.	capsule
charta	chart.	paper
collyrium	collyr.	eyewash
cum	c̄, c	with
dentur tales doses	d.t.d.	give of such doses
divide	divid.	divide (thou)
elixir	elix.	elixir
enema	enem.	enema
et	et	and
fac, fiat, fiant	ft.	make
fiant chartulae vi	ft. chart. vi	let 6 powders be made
fiat pulvis	ft. pulv.	make a powder
fluidextractum	fldxt.	fluid extract
gutta, guttae	gtt.	drop, drops
hora	h., H.	an hour
hora somni	H.S., hor. som.	just before sleep
in die	in d.	in a day
infusum	inf.	an infusion
injectio	inj.	an injection
inter	inter	between
linimentum	lin.	liniment
liquor	liquor, liq.	a solution
lotio	lot.	lotion
minimum	m., min.	a minim
misce	M.	mix (thou)
mistura	mist.	mixture
nocte, noctis	noct., noctis	at night
non	non	not
non repetatur	non rep.	do not repeat
numero, numerus	no.	number
oculo dextro	O.D.	in the right eye
oculo laevus	O.L.	in the left eye
omni hora	omn. hor.	every hour
omni nocte	omn. noct.	every night
pilula (e)	pil.	pill(s)
post cibum, cibos	p.c.	after meals
pro re nata	p.r.n.	as occasion arises
pulvis, pulveres, pulveratus	pulv.	powder, powders, powdered
quantum sufficiat	q.s.	a sufficient quantity
quaque hora	qq. hor., q.h.	every hour
quaque secunda hora	qq. 2 hor., q. 2h	every two hours

Latin or Greek word or phrase	Abbreviation	English meaning
quater in die	q.i.d.	four times a day
secundum artem	s.a., S.A.	according to art
semi, semis	sem., s̄s̄, ss	a half
signa	sig., s.	write, label
sine	sine	without
solutio	sol.	a solution
spiritus	sp.	spirit
suppositorium	suppos.	a suppository
syrupus	syr.	syrup
tabella	tabel.	a lozenge
talis, tales	talis, tales	such, like this
ter die	t.d.	three times a day
ter in die	t.i.d.	three times a day
tinctura	tinct., tr.	a tincture
unguentum	ung.	an ointment
ut dictum	ut dict.	as directed

Table of the Elements

Name	Symbol	Atomic Weight*	Atomic Number	Name	Symbol	Atomic Weight*	Atomic Number
Actinium	Ac	(227)	89	Mendelevium	Md	(258)	101
Aluminum	Al	26.9815	13	Mercury	Hg	200.59	80
Americium	Am	(243)	95	Molybdenum	Mo	95.94	42
Antimony	Sb	121.75	51	Neodymium	Nd	144.24	60
Argon	Ar	39.948	18	Neon	Ne	20.183	10
Arsenic	As	74.9216	33	Neptunium	Np	(237)	93
Astatine	At	(210)	85	Nickel	Ni	58.71	28
Barium	Ba	137.34	56	Niobium	Nb	92.906	41
Berkelium	Bk	(247)	97	Nitrogen	N	14.0067	7
Beryllium	Be	9.0122	4	Nobelium	No	(255)	102
Bismuth	Bi	208.980	83	Osmium	Os	190.2	76
Boron	B	10.811	5	Oxygen	O	15.9994	8
Bromine	Br	79.909	35	Palladium	Pd	106.4	46
Cadmium	Cd	112.40	48	Phosphorus	P	30.9738	15
Calcium	Ca	40.08	20	Platinum	Pt	195.09	78
Californium	Cf	(251)	98	Plutonium	Pu	(244)	94
Carbon	C	12.01115	6	Polonium	Po	(209)	84
Cerium	Ce	140.12	58	Potassium	K	39.102	19
Cesium	Cs	132.905	55	Praseodymium	Pr	140.907	59
Chlorine	Cl	35.453	17	Promethium	Pm	(145)	61
Chromium	Cr	51.996	24	Protactinium	Pa	(231)	91
Cobalt	Co	58.9332	27	Radium	Ra	(226)	88
Copper	Cu	63.546	29	Radon	Rn	(222)	86
Curium	Cm	(247)	96	Rhenium	Re	186.2	75
Dysprosium	Dy	162.50	66	Rhodium	Rh	102.905	45
Einsteinium	Es	(254)	99	Rubidium	Rb	85.47	37
Element 104			104	Ruthenium	Ru	101.07	44
Erbium	Er	167.26	68	Samarium	Sm	150.35	62
Europium	Eu	151.96	63	Scandium	Sc	44.956	21
Fermium	Fm	(257)	100	Selenium	Se	78.96	34
Fluorine	F	18.9984	9	Silicon	Si	28.086	14
Francium	Fr	(223)	87	Silver	Ag	107.870	47
Gadolinium	Gd	157.25	64	Sodium	Na	22.9898	11
Gallium	Ga	69.72	31	Strontium	Sr	87.62	38
Germanium	Ge	72.59	32	Sulfur	S	32.064	16
Gold	Au	196.967	79	Tantalum	Ta	180.948	73
Hafnium	Hf	178.49	72	Technetium	Tc	(97)	43
Helium	He	4.0026	2	Tellurium	Te	127.60	52
Holmium	Ho	164.930	67	Terbium	Tb	158.924	65
Hydrogen	H	1.00797	1	Thallium	Tl	204.37	81
Indium	In	114.82	49	Thorium	Th	(232)	90
Iodine	I	126.9044	53	Thulium	Tm	168.934	69
Iridium	Ir	192.2	77	Tin	Sn	118.69	50
Iron	Fe	55.847	26	Titanium	Ti	47.90	22
Krypton	Kr	83.80	36	Tungsten	W	183.85	74
Lanthanum	La	138.91	57	Uranium	U	(238)	92
Lawrencium	Lr	(256)	103	Vanadium	V	50.942	23
Lead	Pb	207.19	82	Xenon	Xe	131.30	54
Lithium	Li	6.939	3	Ytterbium	Yb	173.04	70
Lutetium	Lu	174.97	71	Yttrium	Y	88.905	39
Magnesium	Mg	24.312	12	Zinc	Zn	65.37	30
Manganese	Mn	54.9380	25	Zirconium	Zr	91.22	40

*A number in parentheses indicates the mass number of the most stable isotope.

Weights and Measures

Metric Weights

		Grams*		Grains		Av. Ounces
Milligram	=	0.001	=	0.01543		
Centigram	=	0.01	=	0.15432		
Decigram	=	0.1	=	1.54324		
Gram	=	1	=	15.43236	=	0.03527
Decagram	=	10	=		=	0.3527
Hectogram	=	100	=		=	3.52739
Kilogram	=	1000	=		=	35.2739

* 1 gram = 1 cubic centimeter of distilled water at 4° C

Metric Linear Measure

		Meter		U.S. Inches		Feet		Yards		Miles
Millimeter	=	0.001	=	0.03937	=	0.00328				
Centimeter	=	0.01	=	0.3937	=	0.03280				
Decimeter	=	0.1	=	3.937	=	0.32808	=	0.10936		
Meter	=	1	=	39.37	=	3.2808	=	1.0936		
Decameter	=	10	=			32.808	=	10.936		
Hectometer	=	100	=			328.08	=	109.36	=	0.062137
Kilometer	=	1000	=			3280.8	=	1093.6	=	0.62137

Troy Weights

Pound*		Ounces		Penny-weights		Grains
1	=	12	=	240	=	5760
		1	=	20	=	480
				1	=	24

* 1 pound = 22.816 cubic inches of distilled water at 62° F

Apothecaries' Weights

Pound*		Ounces		Drams		Scruples		Grains
1	=	12	=	96	=	288	=	5760
		1	=	8	=	24	=	480
				1	=	3	=	60
						1	=	20

* 1 pound = 1 pound troy

Avoirdupois Weights

Pound*		Ounces		Drams		Grains
1	=	16	=	256	=	7000
		1	=	16	=	437.5
				1	=	27.34375

* 1 pound = 1.2153 pounds troy

U.S. Apothecaries' Measures

Gallon		Quarts		Pints		Fluid Ounces		Fluid drams		Minims
1	=	4	=	8	=	128	=	1024	=	61,440
		1	=	2	=	32	=	256	=	15,360
				1	=	16	=	128	=	7680
						1	=	8	=	480
								1	=	60

Imperial Apothecaries' Measures

Gallon		Quarts		Pints		Fluid Ounces		Fluid drams		Minims
1	=	4	=	8	=	160	=	1280	=	76,800
		1	=	2	=	40	=	320	=	19,200
				1	=	20	=	160	=	9,600
						1	=	8	=	480
								1	=	60

The minim, fluid dram, and fluid ounce of the U.S. apothecaries' measures are slightly larger than the corresponding denominations of the Imperial (British) measures; the pint, quart, and gallon, on the other hand, are smaller.

	U.S.		Imp.	Imp.		U.S.
Minim, fluid dram, fluid ounce	1	=	1.0406	1	=	0.9609
Pint, quart, gallon	1	=	0.8325	1	=	1.2011

Conversion Tables

Metric Equivalents of Apothecaries' Weights

Grains	Grams	Grains	Grams	Grains	Grams	Grains	Grams
1/50	0.00130	18	1.166	50	3.240	82	5.314
1/32	0.00202	19	1.231	51	3.305	83	5.378
1/20	0.00324	20	1.296	52	3.370	84	5.443
1/18	0.00360	21	1.361	53	3.434	85	5.508
1/16	0.00405	22	1.426	54	3.499	86	5.573
1/15	0.00432	23	1.490	55	3.564	87	5.638
1/12	0.00540	24	1.555	56	3.629	88	5.702
1/10	0.00648	25	1.620	57	3.694	89	5.767
1/8	0.00810	26	1.685	58	3.758	90	5.832
1/6	0.01080	27	1.749	59	3.823	91	5.897
1/5	0.01296	28	1.814	60	3.888	92	5.962
1/4	0.01620	29	1.879	61	3.953	93	6.026
1/3	0.02160	30	1.944	62	4.018	94	6.091
1/2	0.03240	31	2.009	63	4.082	95	6.156
3/4	0.04860	32	2.074	64	4.147	96	6.221
1	0.0648	33	2.138	65	4.212	97	6.286
2	0.1296	34	2.203	66	4.277	98	6.350
3	0.1944	35	2.268	67	4.342	99	6.415
4	0.2592	36	2.333	68	4.406	100	6.480
5	0.3240	37	2.398	69	4.471	120	7.776
6	0.3888	38	2.462	70	4.536	180	11.664
7	0.4536	39	2.527	71	4.601	200	12.960
8	0.5184	40	2.592	72	4.666	240	15.552
9	0.5832	41	2.657	73	4.730	300	19.440
10	0.6480	42	2.722	74	4.795	360	23.328
11	0.7128	43	2.786	75	4.860	400	25.920
12	0.7776	44	2.851	76	4.925	500	32.399
13	0.8424	45	2.916	77	4.990	600	38.879
14	0.9072	46	2.981	78	5.054	700	45.359
15	0.9720	47	3.046	79	5.119	800	51.839
16	1.037	48	3.110	80	5.184	900	58.319
17	1.102	49	3.175	81	5.249	1000	64.799

Equivalents of Metric in Apothecaries' Weights

Grams	Grains	Grams	Grains	Grams	Grains	Grams	Grains
0.01	0.1543	0.7	10.803	13	200.621	28	432.106
0.02	0.3086	0.8	12.346	14	216.054	29	447.538
0.03	0.4630	0.9	13.889	15	231.486	30	462.971
0.04	0.6173	1	15.432	16	246.918	35	540.133
0.05	0.7716	2	30.865	17	262.350	40	617.294
0.06	0.9259	3	46.297	18	277.782	45	694.456
0.07	1.0803	4	61.730	19	293.215	50	771.618
0.08	1.2346	5	77.162	20	308.647	55	848.780
0.09	1.3889	6	92.594	21	324.080	60	925.941
0.1	1.543	7	108.027	22	339.512	70	1080.265
0.2	3.086	8	123.459	23	354.944	80	1234.589
0.3	4.630	9	138.892	24	370.377	90	1388.912
0.4	6.173	10	154.324	25	385.809	100	1534.236
0.5	7.716	11	169.756	26	401.241		
0.6	9.259	12	185.189	27	416.674		

Equivalents of Metric in U.S. Apothecaries' Measures

Cubic centimeters	Minims	Cubic centimeters	Fluid drams
0.01	0.16	5	1.35
0.02	0.32	6	1.62
0.03	0.49	7	1.89
0.04	0.65	8	2.17
0.05	0.81	9	2.43
0.06	0.97	10	2.71
0.07	1.14	25	6.76
0.08	1.30		Fluid
0.09	1.46		ounces
0.1	1.62	30	1.01
0.2	3.25	50	1.69
0.3	4.87	75	2.54
0.4	6.49	100	3.38
0.5	8.12	200	6.76
0.6	9.74	300	10.15
0.7	11.36	400	13.53
0.8	12.99	500	16.91
0.9	14.61	600	20.29
1	16.23	700	23.67
2	32.47	800	27.05
3	48.70	900	30.43
4	64.94	1000	33.82

Metric Equivalents of Avoirdupois Weights

Av. Ounces	Grams	Av. Pounds	Grams
1/16	1.772	1	453.59
1/8	3.544	2	907.18
1/4	7.088	2.2	1000
1/2	14.175	3	1360.78
1	28.350	4	1814.37
2	56.699	5	2267.96
3	85.049	6	2721.55
4	113.398	7	3175.15
5	141.748	8	3628.74
6	170.097	9	4082.33
7	198.447	10	4535.92
8	226.796		
9	255.146		
10	283.495		
11	311.845		
12	340.194		
13	368.544		
14	396.893		
15	425.243		

Metric Equivalents of U.S. Apothecaries' Measures

Minims	Cubic centimeters	Minims	Cubic centimeters	Fluid ounces	Cubic centimeters	Fluid Ounces	Cubic centimeters
1	0.06	25	1.54	1	29.57	21	621.03
2	0.12	30	1.85	2	59.15	22	650.60
3	0.19	35	2.16	3	88.72	23	680.18
4	0.25	40	2.46	4	118.29	24	709.75
5	0.31	45	2.77	5	147.87	25	739.32
6	0.37	50	3.08	6	177.44	26	768.90
7	0.43	55	3.39	7	207.01	27	798.47
8	0.49			8	236.58	28	828.04
9	0.55			9	266.16	29	857.61
10	0.62	Fluid		10	295.73	30	887.19
11	0.68	drams		11	325.30	31	916.76
12	0.74	1	3.70	12	354.88	32	946.33
13	0.80	2	7.39	13	384.45	48	1419.49
14	0.86	3	11.09	14	414.02	56	1656.08
15	0.92	4	14.79	15	443.59	64	1892.66
16	0.99	5	18.48	16	473.17	72	2129.25
17	1.05	6	22.18	17	502.74	80	2365.83
18	1.11	7	25.88	18	532.31	96	2839.00
19	1.17			19	561.89	112	3312.16
20	1.23			20	591.46	128	3785.32

Temperature Conversion Table

This table permits one to convert from Celsius degrees to Farenheit degrees or from Farenheit degrees to Celsius degrees. The conversion is accomplished by first locating in a column printed in boldface type the number that is to be converted. If the number to be converted is in Farenheit degrees, one may find its equivalent in Celsius degrees by reading to the left. If the number to be converted is in Celsius degrees, one may find its equivalent in Farenheit degrees by reading to the right. Celsius degrees are identical to Centigrade degrees.

The approved international symbolic abbreviation for Celsius degrees is °C, whereas for Farenheit degrees it is °F. The relation between Farenheit degrees and Celsius degrees may be expressed by

$$°C = 5/9 \ °F - 32$$
or
$$°F = 9/5 \ °C + 32$$

To °C	To convert ↕°F or °C↕	To °F	To °C	To convert ↕°F or °C↕	To °F	To °C	To convert ↕°F or °C↕	To °F
−28.89	−20	−4	−6.67	20	68	15.56	60	140
−28.33	−19	−2.2	−6.11	21	69.8	16.11	61	141.8
−27.78	−18	−0.4	−5.56	22	71.6	16.67	62	143.6
−27.22	−17	1.4	−5	23	73.4	17.22	63	145.4
−26.67	−16	3.2	−4.44	24	75.2	17.78	64	147.2
−26.11	−15	5	−3.89	25	77	18.33	65	149
−25.56	−14	6.8	−3.33	26	78.8	18.89	66	150.8
−25	−13	8.6	−2.78	27	80.6	19.44	67	152.6
−24.44	−12	10.4	−2.22	28	82.4	20	68	154.4
−23.89	−11	12.2	−1.67	29	84.2	20.56	69	156.2
−23.33	−10	14	−1.11	30	86	21.11	70	158
−22.78	−9	15.8	−0.56	31	87.8	21.67	71	159.8
−22.22	−8	17.6	.0	32	89.6	22.22	72	161.6
−21.67	−7	19.4	.56	33	91.4	22.78	73	163.4
−21.11	−6	21.2	1.11	34	93.2	23.33	74	165.2
−20.56	−5	23	1.67	35	95	23.89	75	167
−20	−4	24.8	2.22	36	96.8	24.44	76	168.8
−19.44	−3	26.6	2.78	37	98.6	25	77	170.6
−18.89	−2	28.4	3.33	38	100.4	25.56	78	172.4
−18.33	−1	30.2	3.89	39	102.2	26.11	79	174.2
−17.78	0	32	4.44	40	104	26.67	80	176
−17.22	1	33.8	5	41	105.8	27.22	81	177.8
−16.67	2	35.6	5.56	42	107.6	27.78	82	179.6
−16.11	3	37.4	6.11	43	109.4	28.33	83	181.4
−15.56	4	39.2	6.67	44	111.2	28.89	84	183.2
−15	5	41	7.22	45	113	29.44	85	185
−14.44	6	42.8	7.78	46	114.8	30	86	186.8
−13.89	7	44.6	8.33	47	116.6	30.56	87	188.6
−13.33	8	46.4	8.89	48	118.4	31.11	88	190.4
−12.78	9	48.2	9.44	49	120.2	31.67	89	192.2
−12.22	10	50	10	50	122	32.22	90	194
−11.67	11	51.8	10.56	51	123.8	32.78	91	195.8
−11.11	12	53.6	11.11	52	125.6	33.33	92	197.6
−10.56	13	55.4	11.67	53	127.4	33.89	93	199.4
−10	14	57.2	12.22	54	129.2	34.44	94	201.2
−9.44	15	59	12.78	55	131	35	95	203
−8.89	16	60.8	13.33	56	132.8	35.56	96	204.8
−8.33	17	62.6	13.89	57	134.6	36.11	97	206.6
−7.78	18	64.4	14.44	58	136.4	36.67	98	208.4
−7.22	19	66.2	15	59	138.2	37.22	99	210.2

To °C	To convert ◆°F or °C◆	To °F	To °C	To convert ◆°F or °C◆	To °F	To °C	To convert ◆°F or °C◆	To °F
37.78	100	212	70.56	159	318.2	103.33	218	424.4
38.33	101	213.8	71.11	160	320	103.89	219	426.2
38.89	102	215.6	71.67	161	321.8	104.44	220	428
39.44	103	217.4	72.22	162	323.6	105	221	429.8
40	104	219.2	72.78	163	325.4	105.56	222	431.6
40.56	105	221	73.33	164	327.2	106.11	223	433.4
41.11	106	222.8	73.89	165	329	106.67	224	435.2
41.67	107	224.6	74.44	166	330.8	107.22	225	437
42.22	108	226.4	75	167	332.6	107.78	226	438.8
42.78	109	228.2	75.56	168	334.4	108.33	227	440.6
43.33	110	230	76.11	169	336.2	108.89	228	442.4
43.89	111	231.8	76.67	170	338	109.44	229	444.2
44.44	112	233.6	77.22	171	339.8	110	230	446
45	113	235.4	77.78	172	341.6	110.56	231	447.8
45.56	114	237.2	78.33	173	343.4	111.11	232	449.6
46.11	115	239	78.89	174	345.2	111.67	233	451.4
46.67	116	240.8	79.44	175	347	112.22	234	453.2
47.22	117	242.6	80	176	348.8	112.78	235	455
47.78	118	244.4	80.56	177	350.6	113.33	236	456.8
48.33	119	246.2	81.11	178	352.4	113.89	237	458.6
48.89	120	248	81.67	179	354.2	114.44	238	460.4
49.44	121	249.8	82.22	180	356	115	239	462.2
50	122	251.6	82.78	181	357.8	115.56	240	464
50.56	123	253.4	83.33	182	359.6	116.11	241	465.8
51.11	124	255.2	83.89	183	361.4	116.67	242	467.6
51.67	125	257	84.44	184	363.2	117.22	243	469.4
52.22	126	258.8	85	185	365	117.78	244	471.2
52.78	127	260.6	85.56	186	366.8	118.33	245	473
53.33	128	262.4	86.11	187	368.6	118.89	246	474.8
53.89	129	264.2	86.67	188	370.4	119.44	247	476.6
54.44	130	266	87.22	189	372.2	120	248	478.4
55	131	267.8	87.78	190	374	120.56	249	480.2
55.56	132	269.6	88.33	191	375.8	121.11	250	482
56.11	133	271.4	88.89	192	377.6	121.67	251	483.8
56.67	134	273.2	89.44	193	379.4	122.22	252	485.6
57.22	135	275	90	194	381.2	122.78	253	487.4
57.78	136	276.8	90.56	195	383	123.33	254	489.2
58.33	137	278.6	91.11	196	384.8	123.89	255	491
58.89	138	280.4	91.67	197	386.6	124.44	256	492.8
59.44	139	282.2	92.22	198	388.4	125	257	494.6
60	140	284	92.78	199	390.2	125.56	258	496.4
60.56	141	285.8	93.33	200	392	126.11	259	498.2
61.11	142	287.6	93.89	201	393.8	126.67	260	500
61.67	143	289.4	94.44	202	395.6	127.22	261	501.8
62.22	144	291.2	95	203	397.4	127.78	262	503.6
62.78	145	293	95.56	204	399.2	128.33	263	505.4
63.33	146	294.8	96.11	205	401	128.89	264	507.2
63.89	147	296.6	96.67	206	402.8	129.44	265	509
64.44	148	298.4	97.22	207	404.6	130	266	510.8
65	149	300.2	97.78	208	406.4	130.56	267	512.6
65.56	150	302	98.33	209	408.2	131.11	268	514.4
66.11	151	303.8	98.89	210	410	131.67	269	516.2
66.67	152	305.6	99.44	211	411.8	132.22	270	518
67.22	153	307.4	100	212	413.6	132.78	271	519.8
67.78	154	309.2	100.56	213	415.4	133.33	272	521.6
68.33	155	311	101.11	214	417.2	133.89	273	523.4
68.89	156	312.8	101.67	215	419	134.44	274	525.2
69.44	157	314.6	102.22	216	420.8	135	275	527
70	158	316.4	102.78	217	422.6	135.56	276	528.8

To °C	To convert ◀ °F or °C ▶	To °F	To °C	To convert ◀ °F or °C ▶	To °F	To °C	To convert ◀ °F or °C ▶	To °F
136.11	277	530.6	151.67	305	581	167.22	333	631.4
136.67	278	532.4	152.22	306	582.8	167.78	334	633.2
137.22	279	534.2	152.78	307	584.6	168.33	335	635
137.78	280	536	153.33	308	586.4	168.89	336	636.8
138.33	281	537.8	153.89	309	588.2	169.44	337	638.6
138.89	282	539.6	154.44	310	590	170	338	640.4
139.44	283	541.4	155	311	591.8	170.56	339	642.2
140	284	543.2	155.56	312	593.6	171.11	340	644
140.56	285	545	156.11	313	595.4	171.67	341	645.8
141.11	286	546.8	156.67	314	597.2	172.22	342	647.6
141.67	287	548.6	157.22	315	599	172.78	343	649.4
142.22	288	550.4	157.78	316	600.8	173.33	344	651.2
142.78	289	552.2	158.33	317	602.6	173.89	345	653
143.33	290	554	158.89	318	604.4	174.44	346	654.8
143.89	291	555.8	159.44	319	606.2	175	347	656.6
144.44	292	557.6	160	320	608	175.56	348	658.4
145	293	559.4	160.56	321	609.8	176.11	349	660.2
145.56	294	561.2	161.11	322	611.6	176.67	350	662
146.11	295	563	161.67	323	613.4	177.22	351	663.8
146.67	296	564.8	162.22	324	615.2	177.78	352	665.6
147.22	297	566.6	162.78	325	617	178.33	353	667.4
147.78	298	568.4	163.33	326	618.8	178.89	354	669.2
148.33	299	570.2	163.89	327	620.6	179.44	355	671
148.89	300	572	164.44	328	622.4	180	356	672.8
149.44	301	573.8	165	329	624.2	180.56	357	674.6
150	302	575.6	165.56	330	626	181.11	358	676.4
150.56	303	577.4	166.11	331	627.8	181.67	359	678.2
151.11	304	579.2	166.67	332	629.6	182.22	360	680